Handbook of NEURAL NETWORK SIGNAL PROCESSING

THE ELECTRICAL ENGINEERING AND APPLIED SIGNAL PROCESSING SERIES

Edited by Alexander Poularikas

The Advanced Signal Processing Handbook: Theory and Implementation for Radar, Sonar, and Medical Imaging Real-Time Systems
Stergios Stergiopoulos

The Transform and Data Compression Handbook
K.R. Rao and P.C. Yip

Handbook of Multisensor Data Fusion
David Hall and James Llinas

Handbook of Neural Network Signal Processing
Yu Hen Hu and Jenq-Neng Hwang

Handbook of Antennas in Wireless Communications
Lal Chand Godara

Forthcoming Titles

Propagation Data Handbook for Wireless Communications
Robert Crane

The Digital Color Imaging Handbook
Guarav Sharma

Applications in Time Frequency Signal Processing
Antonia Papandreou-Suppappola

Noise Reduction in Speech Applications
Gillian Davis

Signal Processing in Noise
Vyacheslav Tuzlukov

Electromagnetic Radiation and the Human Body: Effects, Diagnosis, and Therapeutic Technologies
Nikolaos Uzunoglu and Konstantina S. Nikita

Digital Signal Processing with Examples in MATLAB®
Samuel Stearns

Smart Antennas
Lal Chand Godara

Pattern Recognition in Speech and Language Processing
Wu Chou and Bing Huang Juang

Handbook of NEURAL NETWORK SIGNAL PROCESSING

Edited by
YU HEN HU
JENQ-NENG HWANG

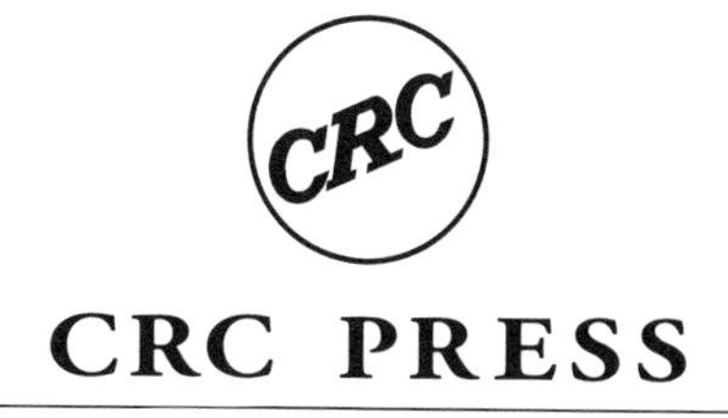

CRC PRESS
Boca Raton London New York Washington, D.C.

Library of Congress Cataloging-in-Publication Data

Handbook of neural network signal processing / editors, Yu Hen Hu, Jenq-Neng Hwang.
p. cm.— (Electrical engineering and applied signal processing (Series))
Includes bibliographical references and index.
ISBN 0-8493-2359-2
1. Neural networks (Computer science)—Handbooks, manuals, etc. 2. Signal processing—Handbooks, manuals, etc. I. Hu, Yu Hen. II. Hwang, Jenq-Neng. III. Electrical engineering and signal processing series.

QA76.87 H345 2001
006.3′2—dc21 2001035674

Direct all inquiries to CRC Press LLC, 2000 N.W. Corporate Blvd., Boca Raton, Florida 33431.

Visit the CRC Press Web site at www.crcpress.com

International Standard Book Number 0-8493-2359-2
Library of Congress Card Number 2001035674
Printed in the United States of America 1 2 3 4 5 6 7 8 9 0
Printed on acid-free paper

Preface

The field of artificial neural networks has made tremendous progress in the past 20 years in terms of theory, algorithms, and applications. Notably, the majority of real world neural network applications have involved the solution of difficult statistical signal processing problems. Compared to conventional signal processing algorithms that are mainly based on linear models, artificial neural networks offer an attractive alternative by providing nonlinear parametric models with universal approximation power, as well as adaptive training algorithms. The availability of such powerful modeling tools motivated numerous research efforts to explore new signal processing applications of artificial neural networks. During the course of the research, many neural network paradigms were proposed. Some of them are merely reincarnations of existing algorithms formulated in a neural network-like setting, while the others provide new perspectives toward solving nonlinear adaptive signal processing. More importantly, there are a number of emergent neural network paradigms that have found successful real world applications.

The purpose of this handbook is to survey recent progress in artificial neural network theory, algorithms (paradigms) with a special emphasis on signal processing applications. We invited a panel of internationally well known researchers who have worked on both theory and applications of neural networks for signal processing to write each chapter. There are a total of 12 chapters plus one introductory chapter in this handbook. The chapters are categorized into three groups. The first group contains in-depth surveys of recent progress in neural network computing paradigms. It contains five chapters, including the introduction, that deal with multilayer perceptrons, radial basis functions, kernel-based learning, and committee machines. The second part of this handbook surveys the neural network implementations of important signal processing problems. This part contains four chapters, dealing with a dynamic neural network for optimal signal processing, blind signal separation and blind deconvolution, a neural network for principal component analysis, and applications of neural networks to time series predictions. The third part of this handbook examines signal processing applications and systems that use neural network methods. This part contains chapters dealing with applications of artificial neural networks (ANNs) to speech processing, learning and adaptive characterization of visual content in image retrieval systems, applications of neural networks to biomedical image processing, and a hierarchical fuzzy neural network for pattern classification.

The theory and design of artificial neural networks have advanced significantly during the past 20 years. Much of that progress has a direct bearing on signal processing. In particular, the nonlinear nature of neural networks, the ability of neural networks to learn from their environments in supervised and/or unsupervised ways, as well as the universal approximation property of neural networks make them highly suited for solving difficult signal processing problems.

From a signal processing perspective, it is imperative to develop a proper understanding of basic neural network structures and how they impact signal processing algorithms and applications. A challenge in surveying the field of neural network paradigms is to distinguish those neural network structures that have been successfully applied to solve real world problems from those that are still under development or have difficulty scaling up to solve realistic problems. When dealing with signal processing applications, it is critical to understand the nature of the problem formulation so that the most appropriate neural network paradigm can be applied. In addition, it is also important to assess the impact of neural networks on the performance, robustness, and cost-effectiveness of signal processing systems and develop methodologies for integrating neural networks with other signal processing algorithms.

We would like to express our sincere thanks to all the authors who contributed to this handbook: Michael T. Manry, Hema Chandrasekaran, and Cheng-Hsiung Hsieh (Chapter 2); Andrew D. Back (Chapter 3); Klaus-Robert Müller, Sebastian Mika, Gunnar Rätsch, Koji Tsuda, and Bernhard Scholköpf (Chapter 4); Volker Tresp (Chapter 5); Jose C. Principe (Chapter 6); Scott C. Douglas (Chapter 7); Konstantinos I. Diamantaras (Chapter 8); Yuansong Liao, John Moody, and Lizhong Wu (Chapter 9); Shigeru Katagirig (Chapter 10); Paisarn Muneesawang, Hau-San Wong, Jose Lay, and Ling Guan (Chapter 11); Tülay Adali, Yue Wang, and Huai Li (Chapter 12); and Jinshiuh Taur, Sun-Yuan Kung, and Shang-Hung Lin (Chapter 13). Many reviewers have carefully read the manuscript and provided many constructive suggestions. We are most grateful for their efforts. They are Andrew D. Back, David G. Brown, Laiwan Chan, Konstantinos I. Diamantaras, Adriana Dumitras, Mark Girolami, Ling Guan, Kuldip Paliwal, Amanda Sharkey, and Jinshiuh Taur.

We would like to thank the editor-in-chief of this series of handbooks, Dr. Alexander D. Poularikas, for his encouragement. Our most sincere appreciation to Nora Konopka at CRC Press for her infinite patience and understanding throughout this project.

Editors

Yu Hen Hu received a B.S.E.E. degree from National Taiwan University, Taipei, Taiwan, in 1976. He received M.S.E.E. and Ph.D. degrees in electrical engineering from the University of Southern California in Los Angeles, in 1980 and 1982, respectively. From 1983 to 1987, he was an assistant professor in the electrical engineering department of Southern Methodist University in Dallas, Texas. He joined the department of electrical and computer engineering at the University of Wisconsin in Madison, as an assistant professor in 1987, and he is currently an associate professor. His research interests include multimedia signal processing, artificial neural networks, fast algorithms and design methodology for application specific micro-architectures, as well as computer aided design tools for VLSI using artificial intelligence. He has published more than 170 technical papers in these areas. His recent research interests have focused on image and video processing and human computer interface.

Dr. Hu is a former associate editor for *IEEE Transactions of Acoustic, Speech, and Signal Processing* in the areas of system identification and fast algorithms. He is currently associate editor of the *Journal of VLSI Signal Processing.* He is a founding member of the Neural Network Signal Processing Technical Committee of the IEEE Signal Processing Society and served as committee chair from 1993 to 1996. He is a former member of the VLSI Signal Processing Technical Committee of the Signal Processing Society. Recently, he served as the secretary of the IEEE Signal Processing Society (1996–1998).

Dr. Hu is a fellow of the IEEE.

Jenq-Neng Hwang holds B.S. and M.S. degrees in electrical engineering from the National Taiwan University, Taipei, Taiwan. After completing two years of obligatory military services after college, he enrolled as a research assistant at the Signal and Image Processing Institute of the department of electrical engineering at the University of Southern California, where he received his Ph.D. degree in December 1988. He was also a visiting student at Princeton University from 1987 to 1989.

In the summer of 1989, Dr. Hwang joined the Department of Electrical Engineering of the University of Washington in Seattle, where he is currently a professor. He has published more than 150 journal and conference papers and book chapters in the areas of image/video signal processing, computational neural networks, and multimedia system integration and networking. He received the 1995 IEEE Signal Processing Society's Annual Best Paper Award (with Shyh-Rong Lay and Alan Lippman) in the area of neural networks for signal processing.

Dr. Hwang is a fellow of the IEEE. He served as the secretary of the Neural Systems and Applications Committee of the IEEE Circuits and Systems Society from 1989 to 1991, and he was a member of the Design and Implementation of Signal Processing Systems Technical Committee of the IEEE Signal Processing Society. He is also a founding member of the Multimedia Signal Processing Technical Committee of the IEEE Signal Processing Society. He served as the chairman of the Neural Networks Signal Processing Technical Committee of the IEEE Signal Processing Society from 1996 to 1998, and he is currently the Society's representative to the IEEE Neural Network Council. He served as an associate editor for *IEEE Transactions on Signal Processing* from 1992 to 1994 and currently is the associate editor for *IEEE Transactions on Neural Networks* and *IEEE Transactions on Circuits and Systems for Video Technology.* He is also on the editorial board of the *Journal of VLSI Signal Processing Systems for Signal, Image, and Video Technology.* Dr. Hwang was the conference program chair of the 1994 IEEE Workshop on Neural Networks for Signal Processing held in Ermioni, Greece in September 1994. He was the general co-chair of the International Symposium on

Artificial Neural Networks held in Hsinchu, Taiwan in December 1995. He also chaired the tutorial committee for the IEEE International Conference on Neural Networks held in Washington, D.C. in June 1996. He was the program co-chair of the International Conference on Acoustics, Speech, and Signal Processing in Seattle, Washington in 1998.

Contributors

Tülay Adali
University of Maryland
Baltimore, Maryland

Andrew D. Back
Windale Technologies
Brisbane, Australia

Hema Chandrasekaran
U.S. Wireless Corporation
San Ramon, California

Konstantinos I. Diamantaras
Technological Education Institute of Thessaloniki
Sindos, Greece

Scott C. Douglas
Southern Methodist University
Dallas, Texas

Ling Guan
University of Sydney
Sydney, Australia

Cheng-Hsiung Hsieh
Chien Kou Institute of Technology
Changwa
Taiwan, China

Yu Hen Hu
University of Wisconsin
Madison, Wisconsin

Jenq-Neug Hwang
University of Washington
Seattle, Washington

Shigeru Katagiri
Intelligent Communication Science Laboratories
Kyoto, Japan

Sun-Yuan Kung
Princeton University
Princeton, New Jersey

Jose Lay
University of Sydney
Sydney, Australia

Huai Li
University of Maryland
Baltimore, Maryland

Yuansong Liao
Oregon Graduate Institute of Science and Technology
Beaverton, Oregon

Shang-Hung Lin
EPSON Palo Alto Laboratories ERD
Palo Alto, California

Michael T. Manry
University of Texas
Arlington, Texas

Sebastian Mika
GMD FIRST
Berlin, Germany

John Moody
Oregon Graduate Institute of Science and Technology
Beaverton, Oregon

Klaus-Robert Müler
GMD FIRST and University of Potsdam
Berlin, Germany

Paisarn Muneesawang
University of Sydney
Sydney, Australia

Jose C. Principe
University of Florida
Gainesville, Florida

Gunnar Rätsch
GMD FIRST and University of Potsdam
Berlin, Germany

Bernhard Schölkopf
Max-Planck-Institut für Biologische Kybernetik
Tübingen, Germany

Junshiuh Taur
National Chung-Hsing University
Taichung
Taiwan, China

Volker Tresp
Siemens AG
Corporate Technology
Munich, Germany

Koji Tsuda
AIST Computational Biology Research Center
Tokyo, Japan

Yue Wang
The Catholic Universtiy of America
Washington, DC

Hau-San Wong
University of Sydney
Sydney, Australia

Lizhong Wu
HNC Software, Inc.
San Diego, California

Contents

1

Introduction to Neural Networks for Signal Processing

Yu Hen Hu
University of Wisconsin

Jenq-Neng Hwang
University of Washington

1.1 Introduction

The theory and design of artificial neural networks have advanced significantly during the past 20 years. Much of that progress has a direct bearing on signal processing. In particular, the non-linear nature of neural networks, the ability of neural networks to learn from their environments in supervised as well as unsupervised ways, as well as the universal approximation property of neural networks make them highly suited for solving difficult signal processing problems.

From a signal processing perspective, it is imperative to develop a proper understanding of basic neural network structures and how they impact signal processing algorithms and applications. A challenge in surveying the field of neural network paradigms is to identify those neural network structures that have been successfully applied to solve real world problems from those that are still under development or have difficulty scaling up to solve realistic problems. When dealing with signal processing applications, it is critical to understand the nature of the problem formulation so that the most appropriate neural network paradigm can be applied. In addition, it is also important to assess the impact of neural networks on the performance, robustness, and cost-effectiveness of signal processing systems and develop methodologies for integrating neural networks with other signal processing algorithms. Another important issue is how to evaluate neural network paradigms, learning algorithms, and neural network structures and identify those that do and do not work reliably for solving signal processing problems.

This chapter provides an overview of the topic of this handbook — neural networks for signal processing. The chapter first discusses the definition of a neural network for signal processing and why it is important. It then surveys several modern neural network models that have found successful signal processing applications. Examples are cited relating to how to apply these nonlinear

0-8493-2359-2/01/$0.00+$1.50

computation paradigms to solve signal processing problems. Finally, this chapter highlights the remaining contents of this book.

1.2 Artificial Neural Network (ANN) Models — An Overview

1.2.1 Basic Neural Network Components

A neural network is a general mathematical computing paradigm that models the operations of biological neural systems. In 1943, McCulloch, a neurobiologist, and Pitts, a statistician, published a seminal paper titled "A logical calculus of ideas imminent in nervous activity" in *Bulletin of Mathematical Biophysics* [1]. This paper inspired the development of the modern digital computer, or the electronic brain, as John von Neumann called it. At approximately the same time, Frank Rosenblatt was also motivated by this paper to investigate the computation of the eye, which eventually led to the first generation of neural networks, known as the perceptron [2]. This section provides a brief overview of ANN models. Many of these topics will be treated in greater detail in later chapters. The purpose of this chapter, therefore, is to highlight the basic concept of these neural network models to prepare the readers for later chapters.

1.2.1.1 McCulloch and Pitts' Neuron Model

Among numerous neural network models that have been proposed over the years, all share a common building block known as a neuron and a networked interconnection structure. The most widely used neuron model is based on McCulloch and Pitts' work and is illustrated in Figure 1.1.

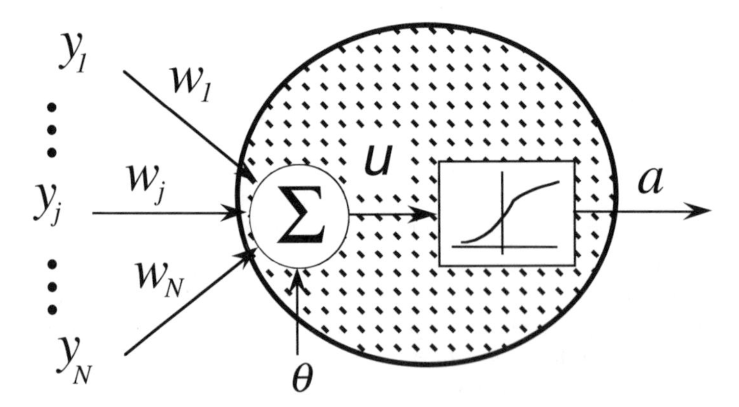

1.1 McCulloch and Pitts' neuron model.

In Figure 1.1, each neuron consists of two parts: the net function and the activation function. The net function determines how the network inputs $\{y_j; 1 \leq j \leq N\}$ are combined inside the neuron. In this figure, a weighted linear combination is adopted:

$$u = \sum_{j=1}^{N} w_j y_j + \theta \tag{1.1}$$

$\{w_j; 1 \leq j \leq N\}$ are parameters known as synaptic weights. The quantity θ is called the bias (or threshold) and is used to model the threshold. In the literature, other types of network input combination methods have been proposed as well. They are summarized in Table 1.1.

TABLE 1.1 Summary of Net Functions

Net Functions	Formula	Comments
Linear	$u = \sum_{j=1}^{N} w_j y_j + \theta$	Most commonly used
Higher order (2nd order formula exhibited)	$u = \sum_{j=1}^{N} \sum_{k=1}^{N} w_{jk} y_j y_k + \theta$	u_i is a weighted linear combination of higher order polynomial terms of input variable. The number of input terms equals N^d, where d is the order of the polynomial
Delta ($\sum - \prod$)	$u = \prod_{j=1}^{N} w_j y_j$	Seldom used

The output of the neuron, denoted by a_i in this figure, is related to the network input u_i via a linear or nonlinear transformation called the activation function:

$$a = f(u) . \tag{1.2}$$

In various neural network models, different activation functions have been proposed. The most commonly used activation functions are summarized in Table 1.2.

TABLE 1.2 Neuron Activation Functions

Activation Function	Formula $a = f(u)$	Derivatives $\frac{df(u)}{du}$	Comments
Sigmoid	$f(u) = \frac{1}{1+e^{-u/T}}$	$f(u)[1 - f(u)]/T$	Commonly used; derivative can be computed from $f(u)$ directly.
Hyperbolic tangent	$f(u) \tanh\left(\frac{u}{T}\right)$	$\left(1 - [f(u)]^2\right)/T$	T = temperature parameter
Inverse tangent	$f(u) = \frac{2}{\pi} \tan^{-1}\left(\frac{u}{T}\right)$	$\frac{2}{\pi T} \cdot \frac{1}{1+(u/T)^2}$	Less frequently used
Threshold	$f(u) = \begin{cases} 1 & u > 0; \\ -1 & u < 0. \end{cases}$	Derivatives do not exist at $u = 0$	
Gaussian radial basis	$f(u) = \exp\left[-\lVert u - m \rVert^2/\sigma^2\right]$	$-2(u - m) \cdot f(u)/\sigma^2$	Used for radial basis neural network; m and σ^2 are parameters to be specified
Linear	$f(u) = au + b$	a	

Table 1.2 lists both the activation functions as well as their derivatives (provided they exist). In both sigmoid and hyperbolic tangent activation functions, derivatives can be computed directly from the knowledge of $f(u)$.

1.2.1.2 Neural Network Topology

In a neural network, multiple neurons are interconnected to form a network to facilitate distributed computing. The configuration of the interconnections can be described efficiently with a directed graph. A directed graph consists of nodes (in the case of a neural network, neurons, as well as external inputs) and directed arcs (in the case of a neural network, synaptic links).

The topology of the graph can be categorized as either acyclic or cyclic. Refer to Figure 1.2a; a neural network with acyclic topology consists of no feedback loops. Such an acyclic neural network is often used to approximate a nonlinear mapping between its inputs and outputs. As shown in Figure 1.2b, a neural network with cyclic topology contains at least one cycle formed by directed arcs. Such a neural network is also known as a recurrent network. Due to the feedback loop, a recurrent network leads to a nonlinear dynamic system model that contains internal memory. Recurrent neural networks often exhibit complex behaviors and remain an active research topic in the field of artificial neural networks.

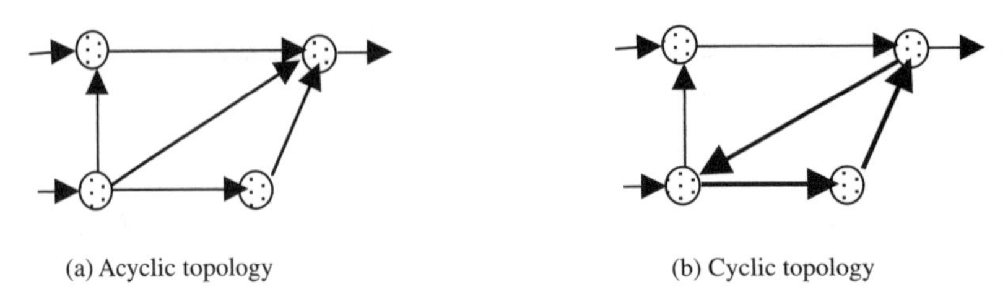

(a) Acyclic topology (b) Cyclic topology

1.2 Illustration of (a) an acyclic graph and (b) a cyclic graph. The cycle in (b) is emphasized with thick lines.

1.2.2 Multilayer Perceptron (MLP) Model

The multilayer perceptron [3] is by far the most well known and most popular neural network among all the existing neural network paradigms. To introduce the MLP, let us first discuss the perceptron model.

1.2.2.1 Perceptron Model

An MLP is a variant of the original perceptron model proposed by Rosenblatt in the 1950s [2]. In the perceptron model, a single neuron with a linear weighted net function and a threshold activation function is employed. The input to this neuron $\underline{x} = (x_1, x_2, \ldots, x_n)$ is a feature vector in an n-dimensional feature space. The net function $u(\underline{x})$ is the weighted sum of the inputs:

$$u(\underline{x}) = w_0 + \sum_{i=1}^{n} w_i x_i \tag{1.3}$$

and the output $y(\underline{x})$ is obtained from $u(\underline{x})$ via a threshold activation function:

$$y(\underline{x}) = \begin{cases} 1 & u(\underline{x}) \geq 0 \\ 0 & u(\underline{x}) < 0 \,. \end{cases} \tag{1.4}$$

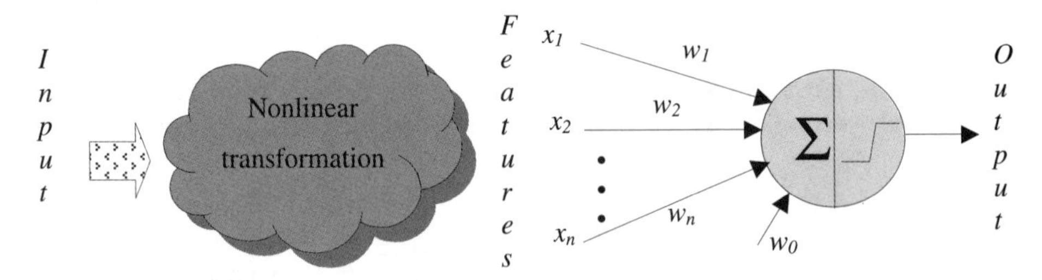

1.3 A perceptron neural network model.

The perceptron neuron model can be used for detection and classification. For example, the weight vector $\underline{w} = (w_1, w_2, \ldots, w_n)$ may represent the template of a certain target. If the input feature vector $\underline{x}$ closely matches $\underline{w}$ such that their inner product exceeds a threshold $-w_0$, then the output will become $+1$, indicating the detection of a target.

The weight vector $\underline{w}$ needs to be determined in order to apply the perceptron model. Often, a set of training samples $\{(\underline{x}(i), d(i)); i \in I_r\}$ and testing samples $\{(\underline{x}(i), d(i)); i \in I_t\}$ are given. Here, $d(i) (\in \{0, 1\})$ is the desired output value of $y(\underline{x}(i))$ if the weight vector $\underline{w}$ is chosen correctly, and I_r and I_t are disjoined index sets. A sequential online perceptron learning algorithm can be applied to iteratively estimate the correct value of $\underline{w}$ by presenting the training samples to the perceptron neuron in a random, sequential order. The learning algorithm has the following formulation:

$$\underline{w}(k+1) = \underline{w}(k) + \eta(d(k) - y(k))\underline{x}(k) \tag{1.5}$$

where $y(k)$ is computed using Equations (1.3) and (1.4). In Equation (1.5), the learning rate $\eta (0 < \eta < 1/|\underline{x}(k)|_{\max})$ is a parameter chosen by the user, where $|\underline{x}(k)|_{\max}$ is the maximum magnitude of the training samples $\{\underline{x}(k)\}$. The index k is used to indicate that the training samples are applied sequentially to the perceptron in a random order. Each time a training sample is applied, the corresponding output of the perceptron $y(k)$ is to be compared with the desired output $d(k)$. If they are the same, meaning the weight vector $\underline{w}$ is correct for this training sample, the weights will remain unchanged. On the other hand, if $y(k) \neq d(k)$, then $\underline{w}$ will be updated with a small step along the direction of the input vector $\underline{x}(k)$. It has been proven that if the training samples are linearly separable, the perceptron learning algorithm will converge to a feasible solution of the weight vector within a finite number of iterations. On the other hand, if the training samples are not linearly separable, the algorithm will not converge with a fixed, nonzero value of η.

<u>*MATLAB Demonstration*</u> Using MATLAB m-files `perceptron.m`, `datasepf.m`, and `sline.m`, we conducted a simulation of a perceptron neuron model to distinguish two separable data samples in a two-dimensional unit square. Sample results are shown in Figure 1.4.

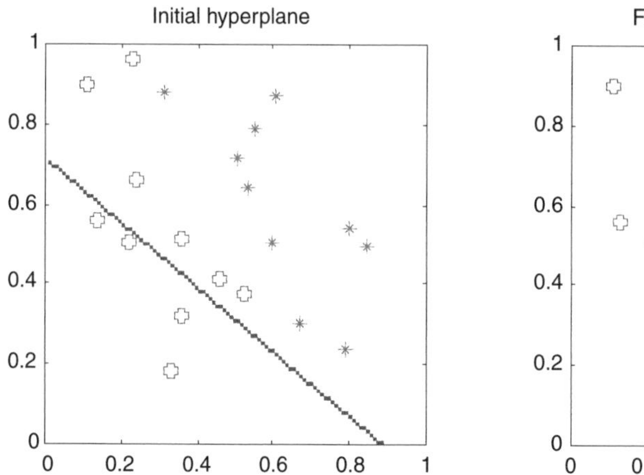

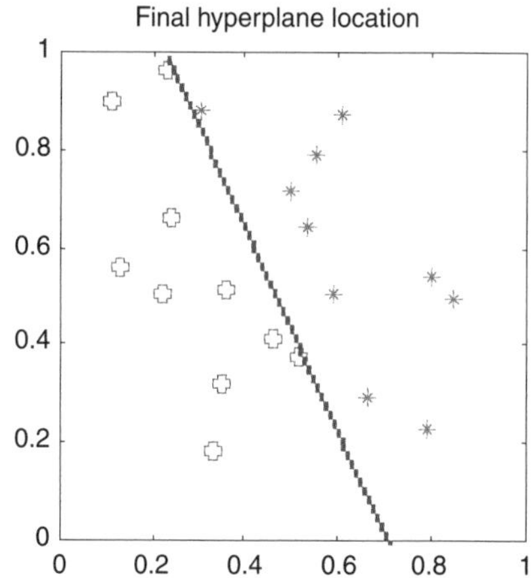

1.4 Perceptron simulation results. The figure on the left-hand side depicts the data samples and the initial position of the separating hyperplane, whose normal vector contains the weights to the perceptron. The right-hand side illustrates that the learning is successful as the final hyperplane separates the two classes of data samples.

1.2.2.1.1 Applications of the Perceptron Neuron Model

There are several major difficulties in applying the perceptron neuron model to solve real world pattern classification and signal detection problems:

1. The nonlinear transformation that extracts the appropriate feature vector x is not specified.
2. The perceptron learning algorithm will not converge for a fixed value of learning rate η if the training feature patterns are not linearly separable.
3. Even though the feature patterns are linearly separable, it is not known how long it takes for the algorithm to converge to a weight vector that corresponds to a hyperplane that separates the feature patterns.

1.2.2.2 Multilayer Perceptron

A multilayer perceptron (MLP) neural network model consists of a feed-forward, layered network of McCulloch and Pitts' neurons. Each neuron in an MLP has a nonlinear activation function that is often continuously differentiable. Some of the most frequently used activation functions for MLP include the sigmoid function and the hyperbolic tangent function.

A typical MLP configuration is depicted in Figure 1.5. Each circle represents an individual neuron. These neurons are organized in layers, labeled as the hidden layer #1, hidden layer #2, and the output layer in this figure. While the inputs at the bottom are also labeled as the input layer, there is usually no neuron model implemented in that layer. The name *hidden layer* refers to the fact that the output of these neurons will be fed into upper layer neurons and, therefore, is hidden from the user who only observes the output of neurons at the output layer. Figure 1.5 illustrates a popular configuration of MLP where interconnections are provided only between neurons of successive layers in the network. In practice, any acyclic interconnections between neurons are allowed.

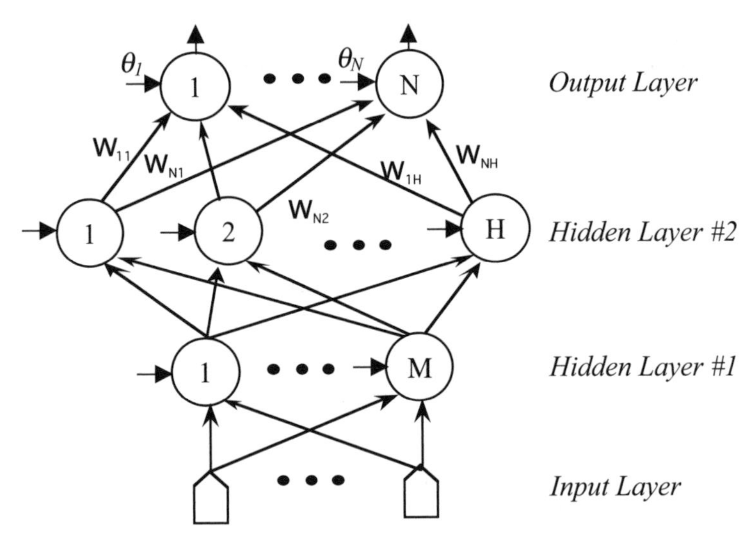

1.5 A three-layer multilayer perceptron configuration.

An MLP provides a nonlinear mapping between its input and output. For example, consider the following MLP structure (Figure 1.6) where the input samples are two-dimensional grid points, and the output is the z-axis value. Three hidden nodes are used, and the sigmoid function has a parameter $T = 0.5$. The mapping is plotted on the right side of Figure 1.6. The nonlinear nature of this mapping is quite clear from the figure. The MATLAB m-files used in this demonstration are `mlpdemo1.m` and `mlp2.m`.

It has been proven that with a sufficient number of hidden neurons, an MLP with as few as two hidden layer neurons is capable of approximating an arbitrarily complex mapping within a finite support [4].

1.2.2.3 Error Back-Propagation Training of MLP

A key step in applying an MLP model is to choose the weight matrices. Assuming a layered MLP structure, the weights feeding into each layer of neurons form a weight matrix of that layer (the input layer does not have a weight matrix as it contains no neurons). The values of these weights are found using the error back-propagation training method.

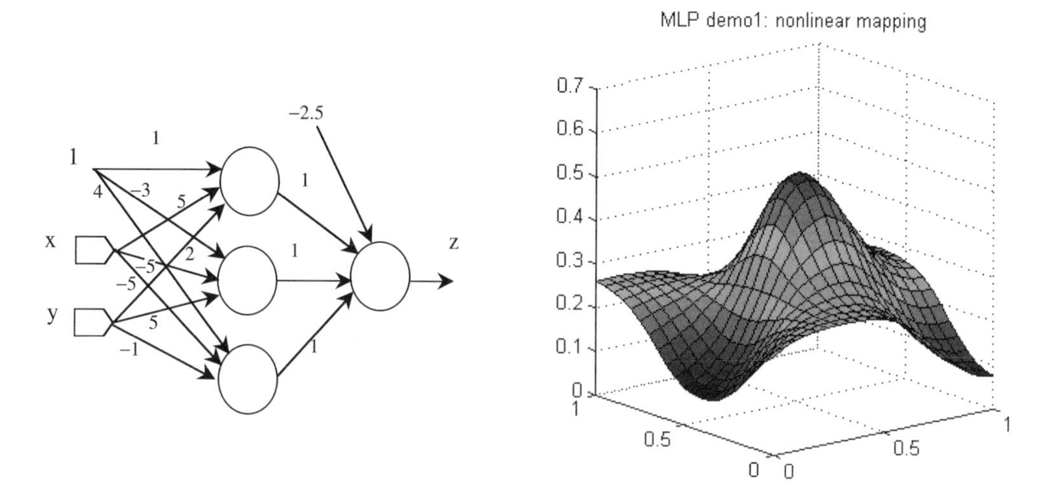

1.6 Demonstration of nonlinear mapping property of MLP.

1.2.2.3.1 *Finding the Weights of a Single Neuron MLP*

For convenience, let us first consider a simple example consisting of a single neuron to illustrate this procedure. For clarity of explanation, Figure 1.7 represents the neuron in two separate parts: a summation unit to compute the net functions u, and a nonlinear activation function $z = f(u)$. The

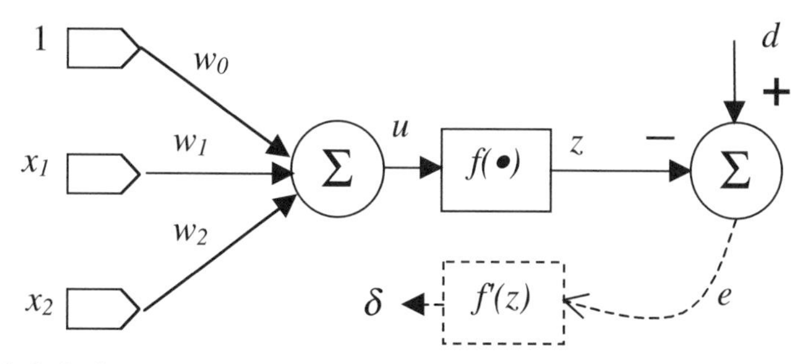

1.7 MLP example for back-propagation training — single neuron case.

output z is to be compared with a desired target value d, and their difference, the error $e = d - z$, will be computed. There are two inputs $[x_1 \quad x_2]$ with corresponding weights w_1 and w_2. The input labeled with a constant 1 represents the bias term θ shown in Figures 1.1 and 1.5 above. Here, the bias term is labeled w_0. The net function is computed as:

$$u = \sum_{i=0}^{2} w_i x_i = \mathbf{W}\mathbf{x} \tag{1.6}$$

where $x_0 = 1$, $\mathbf{W} = [w_0\, w_1\, w_2]$ is the weight matrix, and $\mathbf{x} = [1\, x_1\, x_2]^T$ is the input vector.

Given a set of training samples $\{(\mathbf{x}(k), d(k)); 1 \le k \le K\}$, the error back-propagation training begins by feeding all K inputs through the MLP network and computing the corresponding output $\{z(k); 1 \le k \le K\}$. Here we use an initial guess for the weight matrix $\mathbf{W}$. Then a sum of square error will be computed as:

$$E = \sum_{k=1}^{K} [e(k)]^2 = \sum_{k=1}^{K} [d(k) - z(k)]^2 = \sum_{k=1}^{K} [d(k) - f(\mathbf{Wx}(k))]^2 . \tag{1.7}$$

The objective is to adjust the weight matrix $\mathbf{W}$ to minimize the error E. This leads to a nonlinear least square optimization problem. There are numerous nonlinear optimization algorithms available to solve this problem. Basically, these algorithms adopt a similar iterative formulation:

$$\mathbf{W}(t+1) = \mathbf{W}(t) + \Delta\mathbf{W}(t) \tag{1.8}$$

where $\Delta\mathbf{W}(t)$ is the correction made to the current weights $\mathbf{W}(t)$. Different algorithms differ in the form of $\Delta\mathbf{W}(t)$. Some of the important algorithms are listed in Table 1.3.

TABLE 1.3 Iterative Nonlinear Optimization Algorithms to Solve for MLP Weights

Algorithm	$\Delta\mathbf{W}(t)$	Comments
Steepest descend gradient method	$= -\eta \mathbf{g}(t) = -\eta \; dE/d\mathbf{W}$	$\mathbf{g}$ is known as the gradient vector. η is the step size or learning rate. This is also known as error back-propagation learning.
Newton's method	$= -\boldsymbol{H}^{-1}\mathbf{g}(t)$	$\mathbf{H}$ is known as the Hessian matrix. There are several different ways to estimate it.
	$= -\left[d^2E/d\mathbf{W}^2\right]^{-1} (dE/d\mathbf{W})$	
Conjugate-Gradient method	$= \eta\mathbf{p}(t)$ where $\mathbf{p}(t+1) = -\mathbf{g}(t+1) + \beta \; \mathbf{p}(t)$	

This section focuses on the steepest descend gradient method that is also the basis of the error back-propagation learning algorithm. The derivative of the scalar quantity E with respect to individual weights can be computed as follows:

$$\frac{\partial E}{\partial w_i} = \sum_{k=1}^{K} \frac{\partial [e(k)]^2}{\partial w_i} = \sum_{k=1}^{K} 2[d(k) - z(k)] \left(-\frac{\partial z(k)}{\partial w_i} \right) \quad \text{for } i = 0, 1, 2 \tag{1.9}$$

where

$$\frac{\partial z(k)}{\partial w_i} = \frac{\partial f(u)}{\partial u} \frac{\partial u}{\partial w_i} = f'(u) \frac{\partial}{\partial w_i} \left(\sum_{j=0}^{2} w_j x_j \right) = f'(u) x_i \tag{1.10}$$

Hence,

$$\frac{\partial E}{\partial w_i} = -2 \sum_{k=1}^{K} [d(k) - z(k)] f'(u(k)) x_i(k) . \tag{1.11}$$

With $\delta(k) = [d(k) - z(k)] f'(u(k))$, the above equation can be expressed as:

$$\frac{\partial E}{\partial w_i} = -2 \sum_{k=1}^{K} \delta(k) x_i(k) \tag{1.12}$$

$\delta(k)$ is the error signal $e(k) = d(k) - z(k)$ modulated by the derivative of the activation function $f'(u(k))$ and hence represents the amount of correction needed to be applied to the weight w_i for the given input $x_i(k)$. The overall change Δw_i is thus the sum of such contribution over all K training samples. Therefore, the weight update formula has the format of:

$$w_i(t+1) = w_i(t) + \eta \sum_{k=1}^{K} \delta(k) x_i(k) \; . \tag{1.13}$$

If a sigmoid activation function as defined in Table 1.1 is used, then $\delta(k)$ can be computed as:

$$\delta(k) = \frac{\partial E}{\partial u} = [d(k) - z(k)] \cdot z(k) \cdot [1 - z(k)] \; . \tag{1.14}$$

Note that the derivative $f'(u)$ can be evaluated exactly without any approximation. Each time the weights are updated is called an epoch. In this example, K training samples are applied to update the weights once. Thus, we say the epoch size is K. In practice, the epoch size may vary between one and the total number of samples.

1.2.2.3.2 *Error Back-Propagation in a Multiple Layer Perceptron*

So far, this chapter has discussed how to adjust the weights (training) of an MLP with a single layer of neurons. This section discusses how to perform training for a multiple layer MLP. First, some new notations are adopted to distinguish neurons at different layers. In Figure 1.8, the net-function and output corresponding to the kth training sample of the jth neuron of the $(L-1)$th are denoted by $u_j^{L-1}(k)$ and $z_j^{L-1}(k)$, respectively. The input layer is the *zero*th layer. In particular, $z_j^0(k) = x_j(k)$. The output is fed into the ith neuron of the Lth layer via a synaptic weight denoted by $w_{ij}^L(t)$ or, for simplicity, w_{ij}^L, since we are concerned with the weight update formulation within a single training epoch.

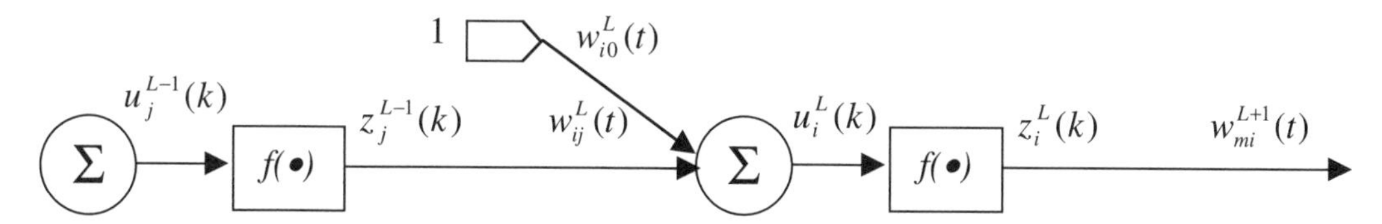

1.8 Notations used in a multiple-layer MLP neural network model.

To derive the weight adaptation equation, $\partial E/\partial w_{ij}^L$ must be computed:

$$\begin{aligned}\frac{\partial E}{\partial w_{ij}^L} &= -2\sum_{k=1}^{K} \frac{\partial E}{\partial u_i^L(k)} \cdot \frac{\partial u_i^L(k)}{\partial w_{ij}^L} = -2\sum_{k=1}^{K}\left[\delta_i^L(k) \cdot \frac{\partial}{\partial w_{ij}^L}\sum_m w_{im}^L z_m^{L-1}(k)\right] \\ &= -2\sum_{k=1}^{K} \delta_i^L(k) \cdot z_j^{L-1}(k) \; . \end{aligned} \tag{1.15}$$

In Equation (1.15), the output $z_j^{L-1}(k)$ can be evaluated by applying the kth training sample $\mathbf{x(k)}$ to the MLP with weights fixed to w_{ij}^L. However, the delta error term $\delta_i^L(k)$ is not readily available and has to be computed.

Recall that the delta error is defined as $\delta_i^L(k) = \partial E/\partial u_i^L(k)$. Figure 1.9 is now used to illustrate how to iteratively compute $\delta_i^L(k)$ from $\delta_m^{L+1}(k)$ and weights of the $(L+1)$th layer.

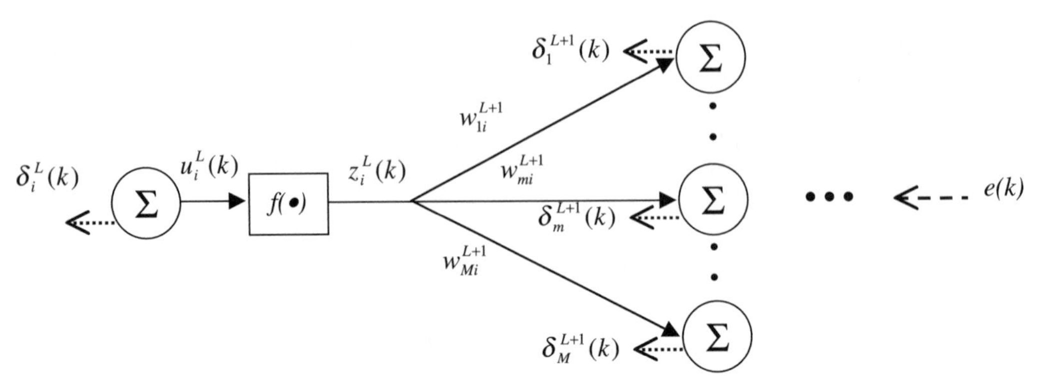

1.9 Illustration of how the error back-propagation is computed.

Note that $z_i^L(k)$ is fed into all M neurons in the $(L+1)$th layer. Hence:

$$\begin{aligned}\delta_i^L(k) &= \frac{\partial E}{\partial u_i^L(k)} = \sum_{m=1}^{M} \frac{\partial E}{\partial u_m^{L+1}(k)} \cdot \frac{\partial u_m^{L+1}(k)}{\partial u_i^L(k)} = \sum_{m=1}^{M}\left[\delta_m^{L+1}(k) \cdot \frac{\partial}{\partial u_i^L(k)} \sum_{j=1}^{J} w_{mj}^L f\left(u_j^L(k)\right)\right] \\ &= f'\left(u_i^L(k)\right) \cdot \sum_{m=1}^{M} \delta_m^{L+1}(k) \cdot w_{mi}^L \,. \end{aligned} \tag{1.16}$$

Equation (1.16) is the error back-propagation formula that computes the delta error from the output layer back toward the input layer, in a layer-by-layer manner.

1.2.2.3.3 Weight Update Formulation with Momentum and Noise

Given the delta error, the weights will be updated according to a modified formulation of Equation (1.13):

$$w_{ij}^L(t+1) = w_{ij}^L(t) + \eta \cdot \sum_{k=1}^{K} \delta_i^L(k) z_j^{L-1}(k) + \mu\left[w_{ij}^L(t) - w_{ij}^L(t-1)\right] + \varepsilon_{ij}^L(t) \,. \tag{1.17}$$

On the right hand side of Equation (1.17), the second term is the gradient of the mean square error with respect to w_{ij}^L. The third term is known as a momentum term. It provides a mechanism to adaptively adjust the step size. When the gradient vectors in successive epochs point to the same direction, the effective step size will increase (gaining momentum). When successive gradient vectors form a zigzag search pattern, the effective gradient direction will be regulated by this momentum term so that it helps minimize the mean-square error.

There are two parameters that must be chosen: the learning rate, or step size η, and the momentum constant μ. Both of these parameters should be chosen from the interval of [0 1]. In practice, η often assumes a smaller value, e.g., $0 < \eta < 0.3$, and μ usually assumes a larger value, e.g., $0.6 < \mu < 0.9$.

The last term in Equation (1.17) is a small random noise term that will have little effect when the second or the third terms have larger magnitudes. When the search reaches a local minimum or a plateau, the magnitude of the corresponding gradient vector or the momentum term is likely to diminish. In such a situation, the noise term can help the learning algorithm leap out of the local minimum and continue to search for the globally optimal solution.

1.2.2.3.4 Implementation of the Back-Propagation Learning Algorithm

With the new notations and the error back-propagation formula, the back-propagation training algorithm for MLP can be summarized below in the MATLAB m-file format:

Algorithm Listing: Back-Propagation Training Algorithm for MLP

```
% configure the MLP network and learning parameters.
bpconfig;     % call mfile bpconfig.m

% BP iterations begins
while not_converged==1,
 % start a new epoch
 % Randomly select K training samples from the training set.
 [train,ptr,train0]=rsample(train0,K,Kr,ptr); % train is K by M+N
 z{1}=(train(:,1:M))'; % input sample matrix  M by K, layer# = 1
 d=train(:,M+1:MN)';    % corresponding target value  N by K

 % Feed-forward phase, compute sum of square errors
 for l=2:L,                 % the l-th layer
    u{l}=w{l}*[ones(1,K);z{l-1}]; % u{l} is n(l) by K
    z{l}=actfun(u{l},atype(l));
 end
 error=d-z{L};              % error is N by K
 E(t)=sum(sum(error.*error));

 % Error back-propagation phase, compute delta error
 delta{L}=actfunp(u{L},atype(L)).*error;  % N (=n(L)) by K
 if L>2,
    for l=L-1:-1:2,
      delta{l}=(w{l+1}(:,2:n(l)+1))'*delta{l+1}...
               .*actfunp(u{l},atype(l));
    end
 end

 % update the weight matrix using gradient,
 % momentum and random perturbation
 for l=2:L,
    dw{l}=alpha*delta{l}*[ones(1,K);z{l-1}]'+...
          mom*dw{l}+randn(size(w{l}))*0.005;
    w{l}=w{l}+dw{l};
 end

 % display the training error
 bpdisplay;    % call mfile bpdisplay.m

 % Test convergence to see if the convergence
 % condition is satisfied,
 cvgtest;      % call mfile cvgtest.m
 t = t + 1;    % increment epoch count
end % while loop
```

This m-file, called `bp.m`, together with related m-files `bpconfig.m`, `cvgtest.m`, `bpdisplay.m`, and supporting functions, can be downloaded from the CRC website for the convenience of readers.

There are numerous commercial software packages that implement the multilayer perceptron neural network structure. Notably, the MATLAB neural network toolbox^{TM} from Mathwork is a sophisticated software package. Software packages in C++ programming language that are available free for non-commercial use include PDP++ (http://www.cnbc.cmu.edu/PDP++/PDP++.html) and MLC++ (http://www.sgi.com/tech/mlc/).

1.2.3 Radial Basis Networks

A radial basis network is a feed-forward neural network using the radial basis activation function. A radial basis function has the general form of $f(||\mathbf{x} - \mathbf{m_0}||) = f(\mathbf{r})$. Such a function is symmetric with respect to a center point $\mathbf{x}_0$. Some examples of radial basis functions in one-dimensional space are depicted in Figure 1.10.

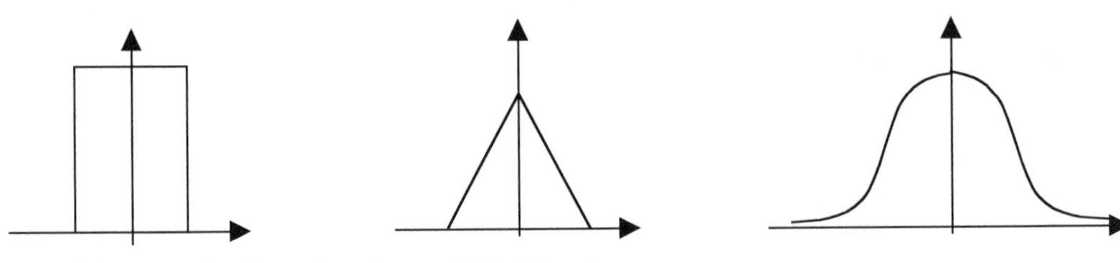

1.10 Three examples of one-dimensional radial basis functions.

Radial basis functions can be used to approximate a given function. For example, as illustrated in Figure 1.11, a rectangular-shaped radial basis function can be used to construct a staircase approximation of a function, and a triangular-shaped radial basis function can be used to construct a trapezoidal approximation of a function.

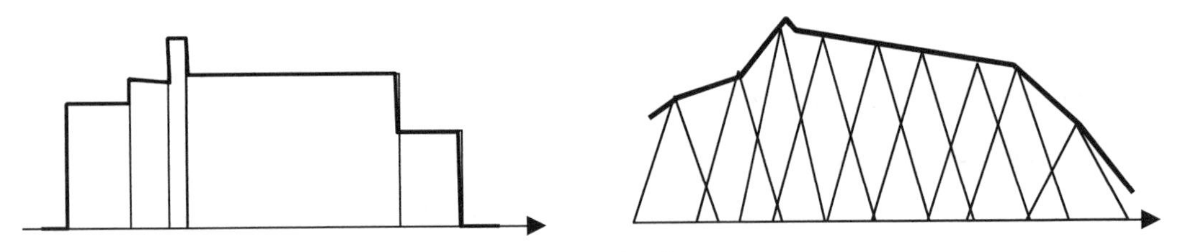

1.11 Two examples illustrating radial basis function approximation.

In each of the examples in Figure 1.11, the approximated function can be represented as a weighted linear combination of a family of radial basis functions with different scaling and translations:

$$\hat{F}(x) = \sum_{i=1}^{C} w_i \varphi\left(\|x - m_i\| / \sigma_i\right) . \tag{1.18}$$

This function can be realized with a radial basis network, as shown in Figure 1.12.

There are two types of radial basis networks based on how the radial basis functions are placed and shaped. To introduce these radial basis networks, let us present the function approximation problem formulation:

Radial Basis Function Approximation Problem Given a set of points $\{\mathbf{x}(k); 1 \le k \le K\}$ and the values of an unknown function $F(\mathbf{x})$ evaluated on these K points $\{d(k) = F(\mathbf{x}(k)); 1 \le k \le K\}$, find an approximation of $F(\mathbf{x})$ in the form of Equation (1.18) such that the sum of square approximation

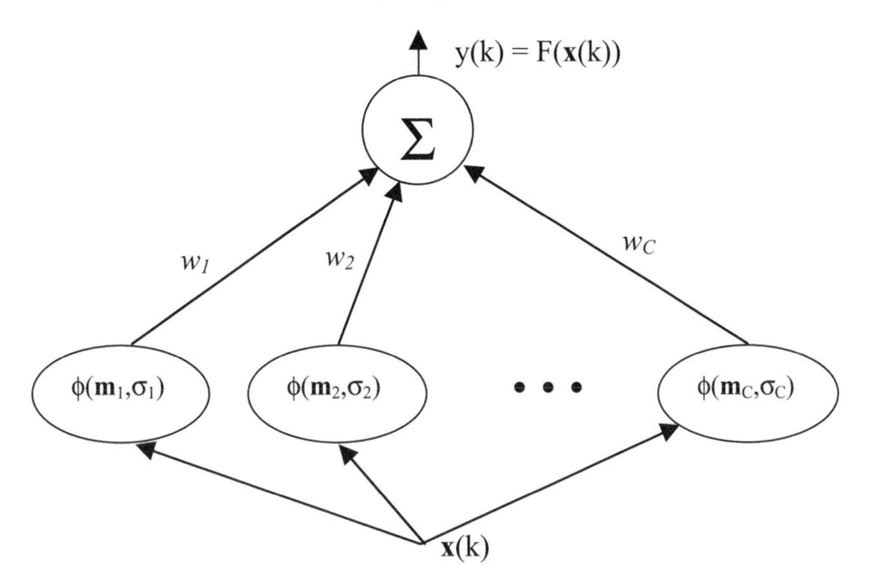

1.12 A radial basis network.

error at these sets of training samples,

$$\sum_{k=1}^{K}\left[d(k) - \hat{F}(x(k))\right]^2$$

is minimized.

1.2.3.1 Type I Radial Basis Network

The first type of radial basis network chooses every training sample as the location of a radial basis function [5]. In other words, it sets $C = K$ and $\mathbf{m}_i = \mathbf{x}(i)$, where $1 \le i \le K$. Furthermore, a fixed constant scaling parameter σ is chosen for every radial basis function. For convenience, $\sigma = 1$ in the derivation below. That is, $\sigma_i = \sigma$ for $1 \le k \le K$. Now rewrite Equation (1.18) in a vector inner product formulation:

$$[\phi\left(\|x(k) - m_1\|\right) \quad \phi\left(\|x(k) - m_2\|\right) \quad \cdots \quad \phi\left(\|x(k) - m_C\|\right)]\begin{bmatrix} w_1 \\ w_2 \\ \vdots \\ w_C \end{bmatrix} = d(k)\,. \tag{1.19}$$

Substituting $k = 1, 2, \ldots, K$, Equation (1.19) becomes a matrix equation $\mathbf{\Phi w} = \mathbf{d}$:

$$\underbrace{\begin{bmatrix} \phi\left(\|x(1) - m_1\|\right) & \phi\left(\|x(1) - m_2\|\right) & \cdots & \phi\left(\|x(1) - m_C\|\right) \\ \phi\left(\|x(2) - m_1\|\right) & \phi\left(\|x(2) - m_2\|\right) & \cdots & \phi\left(\|x(2) - m_C\|\right) \\ \vdots & \vdots & \ddots & \vdots \\ \phi\left(\|x(K) - m_1\|\right) & \phi\left(\|x(K) - m_2\|\right) & \cdots & \phi\left(\|x(K) - m_C\|\right) \end{bmatrix}}_{\mathbf{\Phi}} \underbrace{\begin{bmatrix} w_1 \\ w_2 \\ \vdots \\ w_C \end{bmatrix}}_{\mathbf{w}} = \underbrace{\begin{bmatrix} d(1) \\ d(2) \\ \vdots \\ d(K) \end{bmatrix}}_{\mathbf{d}} \tag{1.20}$$

$\mathbf{\Phi}$ is a $K \times C$ square matrix (note that $C = K$), and is generally positive for commonly used radial basis functions. Thus, the weight vector $\mathbf{w}$ can be found as:

$$\mathbf{w} = \mathbf{\Phi}^{-1}\mathbf{d} . \tag{1.21a}$$

However, in practical applications, the $\mathbf{\Phi}$ matrix may be nearly singular, leading to a numerically unstable solution of $\mathbf{w}$. This can happen when two or more samples $\mathbf{x}(k)$s are too close to each other. Several different approaches can be applied to alleviate this problem.

1.2.3.1.1 *Method 1: Regularization*

For a small positive number λ, a small diagonal matrix is added to the radial basis coefficient matrix $\mathbf{\Phi}$ such that

$$\mathbf{w} = (\mathbf{\Phi} + \lambda\mathbf{I})^{-1}\mathbf{d} . \tag{1.21b}$$

1.2.3.1.2 *Method 2: Least Square Using Pseudo-Inverse*

The goal is to find a least square solution $\mathbf{w}_{\mathrm{LS}}$ such that $||\mathbf{\Phi w} - \mathbf{d}||^2$ is minimized. Hence,

$$\mathbf{w} = \mathbf{\Phi}^{+}\mathbf{d} \tag{1.22}$$

where $\mathbf{\Phi}^{+}$ is the pseudo-inverse matrix of $\mathbf{\Phi}$ and can be found using singular value decomposition.

1.2.3.2 Type II Radial Basis Network

The type II radial basis network is rooted in the regularization theory [6]. The radial basis function of choice is the Gaussian radial basis function:

$$\phi(\|x - m\|) = \exp\left[-\frac{\|x - m\|^2}{2\sigma^2}\right] .$$

The locations of these Gaussian radial basis function are obtained by clustering the input samples $\{\mathbf{x}(k); 1 \leq k \leq K\}$. Known clustering algorithms such as the k-means clustering algorithm can be applied to serve this purpose. However, there is no objective method to determine the number of clusters. Some experimentation will be needed to find an adequate number of clusters $C(< K)$. Once the cluster is completed, the mean and variance of each cluster can be used as the center location and the spread of the radial basis function. A type II radial basis network gives the solution to the following regularization problem:

Type II Radial Basis Network Approximation Problem Find $\mathbf{w}$ such that $\|\mathbf{Gw}-\mathbf{d}\|^2$ is minimized subject to the constraint $\mathbf{w}^{\mathrm{T}}\mathbf{G}_0\mathbf{w} = \mathbf{a}$ constant.

In the above, $\mathbf{G}$ is a $K \times C$ matrix similar to the $\mathbf{\Phi}$ matrix in Equation (1.20) and is defined as:

$$\mathbf{G} = \begin{bmatrix} \exp\left[-\frac{(x(1)-m_1)^2}{2\sigma_1^2}\right] & \exp\left[-\frac{(x(1)-m_2)^2}{2\sigma_2^2}\right] & \cdots & \exp\left[-\frac{(x(1)-m_C)^2}{2\sigma_C^2}\right] \\ \exp\left[-\frac{(x(2)-m_1)^2}{2\sigma_1^2}\right] & \exp\left[-\frac{(x(2)-m_2)^2}{2\sigma_2^2}\right] & \cdots & \exp\left[-\frac{(x(2)-m_C)^2}{2\sigma_C^2}\right] \\ \vdots & \vdots & \ddots & \vdots \\ \exp\left[-\frac{(x(K)-m_1)^2}{2\sigma_1^2}\right] & \exp\left[-\frac{(x(K)-m_2)^2}{2\sigma_2^2}\right] & \cdots & \exp\left[-\frac{(x(K)-m_C)^2}{2\sigma_C^2}\right] \end{bmatrix}$$

and $\mathbf{G_0}$ is a $C \times C$ symmetric square matrix defined as:

$$\mathbf{G_0} = \begin{bmatrix} \exp\left[-\frac{(m_1-m_1)^2}{2\sigma_1^2}\right] & \exp\left[-\frac{(m_1-m_2)^2}{2\sigma_2^2}\right] & \cdots & \exp\left[-\frac{(m_1-m_C)^2}{2\sigma_C^2}\right] \\ \exp\left[-\frac{(m_2-m_1)^2}{2\sigma_1^2}\right] & \exp\left[-\frac{(m_2-m_2)^2}{2\sigma_2^2}\right] & \cdots & \exp\left[-\frac{(m_2-m_C)^2}{2\sigma_C^2}\right] \\ \vdots & \vdots & \ddots & \vdots \\ \exp\left[-\frac{(m_C-m_1)^2}{2\sigma_1^2}\right] & \exp\left[-\frac{(m_C-m_2)^2}{2\sigma_2^2}\right] & \cdots & \exp\left[-\frac{(m_C-m_C)^2}{2\sigma_C^2}\right] \end{bmatrix}$$

The solution to the constrained optimization problem can be found as:

$$\mathbf{w} = \left(\mathbf{G}^T\mathbf{G} + \lambda\mathbf{G_0}\right)^{-1} \mathbf{G}^T\mathbf{d} \tag{1.23}$$

where λ is a regularization parameter and is usually selected as a very small non-negative number. As $\lambda \to 0$, Equation (1.23) becomes the least square solution.

MATLAB Implementation The type I and type II radial basis networks have been implemented in a MATLAB m-file called `rbn.m`. Using this function, we developed a demonstration program called `rbndemo.m` that can illustrate the properties of these two types of radial basis networks. Twenty training samples are regularly spaced in $[-0.5\ 0.5]$, and the function to be approximated is a piecewise linear function. For the type I RBN network, 20 Gaussian basis functions located at each training sample are used. The standard deviation of each Gaussian basis function is the same and equals the average distance between two basis functions. For the type II RBN network, ten Gaussian basis functions are generated using k-means clustering algorithm. The variance of each Gaussian basis function is the variance of samples within the corresponding cluster.

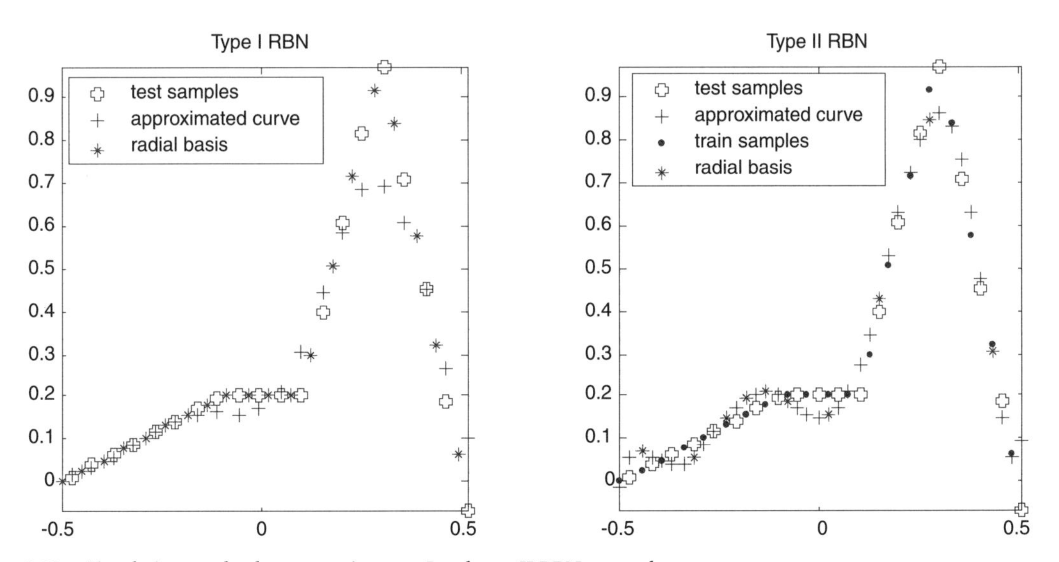

1.13 Simulation results demonstrating type I and type II RBN networks.

1.2.4 Competitive Learning Networks

Both the multilayer perceptron and the radial basis network are based on the popular learning paradigm of error-correction learning. The synaptic weights of these networks are adjusted to reduce the difference (error) between the desired target value and corresponding output. For competitive learning networks, a competitive learning paradigm is incorporated.

With the competitive learning paradigm, a single-layer of neurons compete among themselves to represent the current input vector. The winning neuron will adjust its own weight to be closer to the input pattern. As such, competitive learning can be regarded as a sequential clustering algorithm.

1.2.4.1 Orthogonal Linear Networks

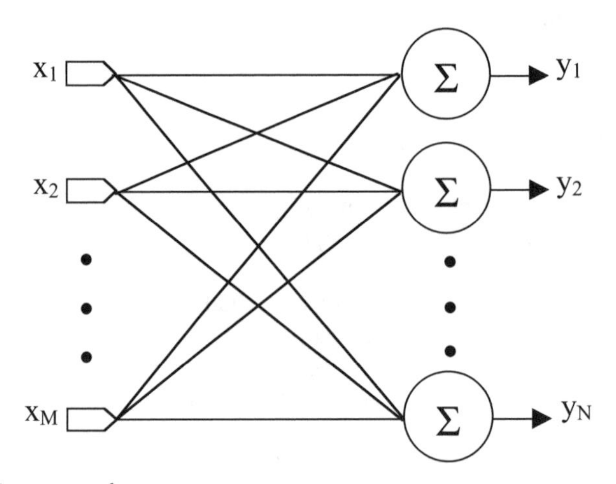

1.14 An orthogonal linear network.

In a single-layer, linear network, the output $y_n(t) = \Sigma_{m=1}^{M} w_{nm}(t)x_m(t)$. The synaptic weights are updated according to a generalized Hebbian learning rule [7]:

$$\Delta w_{nm}(t) = w_{nm}(t+1) - w_{nm}(t) = \eta y_n(t) \left[x_m(t) - \sum_{k=1}^{n} w_{km}(t) y_k(t) \right] .$$

As such, the weight vector $\mathbf{w}_n = [w_{n1}\, w_{n2} \ldots w_{nM}]^T$ will converge to the eigenvector of the nth largest eigenvalue of the sample covariance matrix formed by the input vectors

$$\mathbf{C} = \sum_t \mathbf{x}(t)\mathbf{x}^T(t)$$

where

$$\mathbf{x}^T(t) = [x_1(t)\, x_2(t)\, \ldots x_M(t)] .$$

Therefore, upon convergence, such a generalized Hebbian learning network will produce the principal components (eigenvectors) of the sample covariance matrix of the input samples. Principal component analysis (PCA) has found numerous applications in data compression and data analysis tasks. For the signal processing applications, PCA based on an orthogonal linear network has been applied to image compression [7].

A MATLAB implementation of the generalized Hebbian learning algorithm and its demonstration can be found in `ghademo.m` and `ghafun.m`.

1.2.4.2 Self-Organizing Maps

A self-organizing map [8] is a single-layer, competitive neural network that imposes a preassigned ordering among the neurons. For example, in Figure 1.15, the shaded circles represent a 6×5 array of neurons, each labeled with a preassigned index (i, j), $1 \leq i \leq 6, 1 \leq j \leq 5$. In1

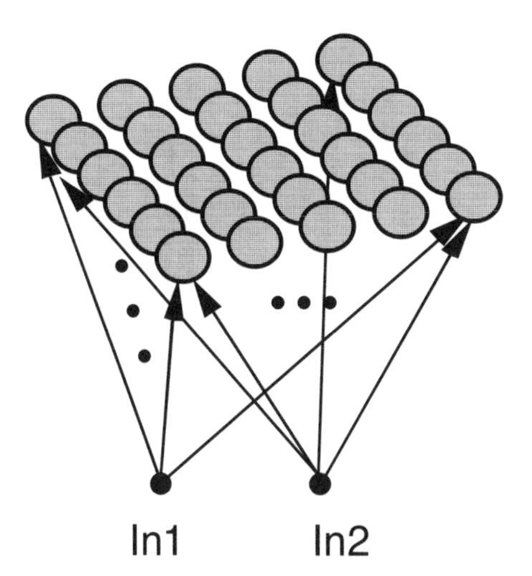

1.15 A two-dimensional self-organizing map neural network structure.

and In2 are two-dimensional inputs. Given a specific neuron, e.g., (3,2), one may identify its four nearest neighbors as (3,1), (2,2), (4,2), and (3,3). Each neuron has two synaptic connections to the two inputs. The weights of these two connections give a two-dimensional coordinate to represent the location of the neuron in the input feature space. If the input (In1, In2) is very close to the two weights of a neuron, that neuron will give an output 1, signifying it is the winner to represent the current input feature vector. The remaining losing neurons will have their output remain at 0. Therefore, the self-organizing map is a neural network whose behavior is governed by competitive learning. In the ideal situation, each neuron will represent a cluster of input feature vectors (points) that may share some common semantic meaning. Consequently, the 6×5 array of neurons can be regarded as a mapping from points in the input feature space to a coarsely partitioned label space through the process of clustering. The initial labeling of individual neurons allows features of similar semantic meaning to be grouped into closer clusters. In this sense, the self-organizing map provides an efficient method to visualize high-dimensional data samples in low-dimensional display.

1.2.4.2.1 Basic Formulation of Self-Organizing Maps (SOMs)

Initialization: Choose weight vectors $\{w_m(0); 1 \leq m \leq M\}$ randomly. Set iteration count $t = 0$.
While Not_Converged
  Choose the next x and compute $d(x, w_m(t))$; $1 \leq m \leq M$.
  Select $m^* = \text{mim}_m d(x, w_m(t))$

$$w_m(t+1) = \begin{cases} w_m(t) + \eta(x - w_m(t)) & m \in N(m^*, t); \\ w_m(t) & m \notin N(m^*, t) \end{cases}$$

  % Update node m^* and its neighborhood nodes:
  If Not_converged, then $t = t + 1$
End % while loop

This algorithm is demonstrated in a MATLAB program `somdemo.m`. A plot is given in Figure 1.16. In the public domain, SOMPAK is the official implementation of SOM (http://www.cis.hut.fi/research/som-research/nnrc-programs.shtml). A MATLAB toolbox is also available at http://www.cis.hut.fi/projects/somtoolbox/.

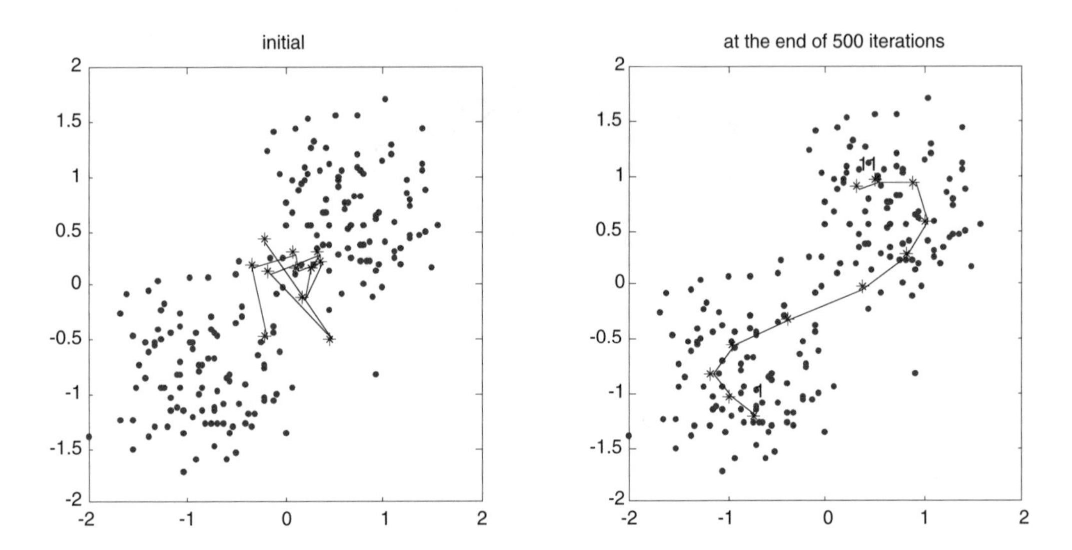

1.16 The neurons are initially placed randomly in the feature space as shown to the left of the figure. After 500 iterations, they are distributed evenly to represent the underlying feature vector distribution.

1.2.5 Committee Machines

A committee machine consists of multiple modules of neural networks. The same inputs will be applied to each module. The outputs of individual modules will be combined to form the final output. Thus, the modules in a committee machine work like the members in a committee to make collective decisions. Based on how the committee combines its members' outputs, there are two basic types of committee machines: (1) ensemble network and (2) mixture of experts.

1.2.5.1 Ensemble Network

In an ensemble network [9]–[12], individual modular neural networks will be developed separately, independent of other modules. Then, an ensemble of these trained neural network modules will be combined using various methods including majority vote and other weighted voting or combination schemes. However, regardless of which combination method is used, the rule of combination will be independent of the specific data inputs.

An ensemble network is a very flexible architecture. Each modular classifier can be independently developed and the combination rule itself can create a pattern classifier that takes the output of modular classifiers as its input to make the final decisions. In fact, additional layers may be added to build a hierarchical structure. In this sense, a multilayer perceptron can be regarded as a special case of an ensemble network.

1.2.5.2 Mixture of Expert (MoE) Network

In a mixture of expert (MoE) network [13], each individual neural network module will specialize over a subregion within the feature space. Hence each module becomes an expert of features

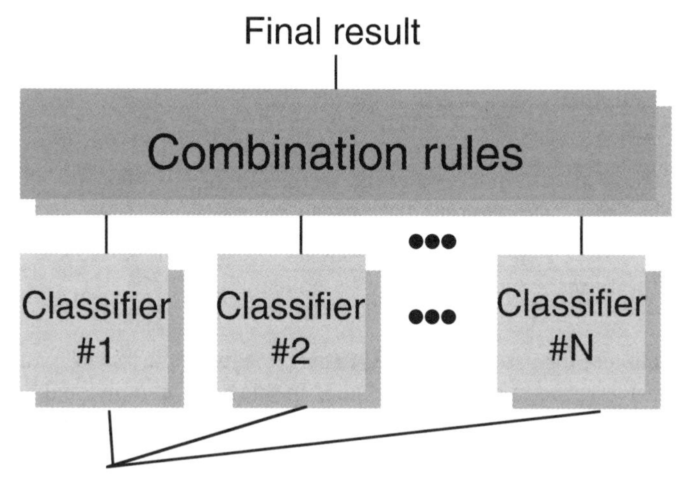

1.17 Ensemble network structure.

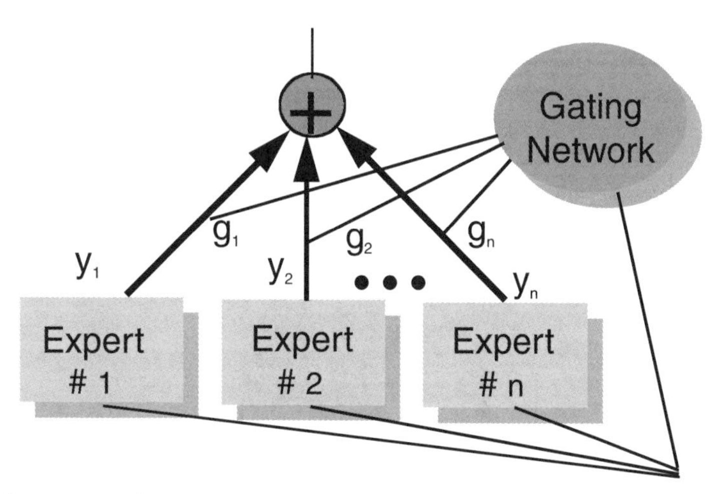

1.18 Mixture of expert network structure.

in the subregion. A gating network will examine the input vector and then assign it to a particular expert neural network module. In other words, the combination rule of an MoE is dependent on the input feature vectors. This is the key difference between an MoE and an ensemble network.

Let $z(\mathbf{x})$ be the output of the MoE network, then

$$z(\mathbf{x}) = \sum_{i=1}^{n} g_i(\mathbf{x}) y_i(\mathbf{x}) \qquad \text{subject to:} \qquad \sum_{i=1}^{n} g_i(\mathbf{x}) = 1$$

where $y_i(\mathbf{x})$ is the output of the ith expert module network, and the corresponding weight $g_i(\mathbf{x})$ is the output of a gating network that also observes the input feature vector $\mathbf{x}$. Jacobs et al. [13] proposed an expectation–maximization (EM) algorithm-based training method to determine the structure of both $g_i(\mathbf{x})$ and $y_i(\mathbf{x})$. Here, a more general formulation for the development of an MoE network is presented:

Repeat until training is completed.
For each training sample $\mathbf{x}$,
Assign $\mathbf{x}$ to expert i if $g_i(\mathbf{x}) > g_k(\mathbf{x})$ for $k \neq i$.

Assume that $g_i(\mathbf{x}) = 1$ (hence $g_k(\mathbf{x}) = 0, k \neq i$), update the expert i based on output error. Update gating network so that $g_i(\mathbf{x})$ is even closer to unity.

Alternatively, a batch training method can be adopted:

1. Apply a clustering algorithm to cluster the set of training samples into n clusters. Use the membership information to train the gating network.
2. Assign each cluster to an expert module and train the corresponding expert module.
3. Fine-tune the performance using gradient-based learning.

Note that the function of the gating network is to partition the feature space into largely disjointed regions and assign each region to an expert module. In this way, an individual expert module only needs to learn a subregion in the feature space and is likely to yield better performance.

Combining n expert modules under the gating network, the overall performance is expected to improve. Figure 1.19 shows an example using the batch training method presented above. The dots are the training and testing samples. The circles are the cluster centers that represent individual experts. These cluster centers are found by applying the k-means clustering algorithm on the training samples. The gating network output is proportional to the inverse of the square distance from each sample to all three cluster centers. The output value is normalized so that the sum equals unity. Each expert module implements a simple linear model (a straight line in this example). We did not implement the third step, so the results are obtained without fine-tuning. The corresponding MATLAB m-files are `moedemo.m` and `moegate.m`.

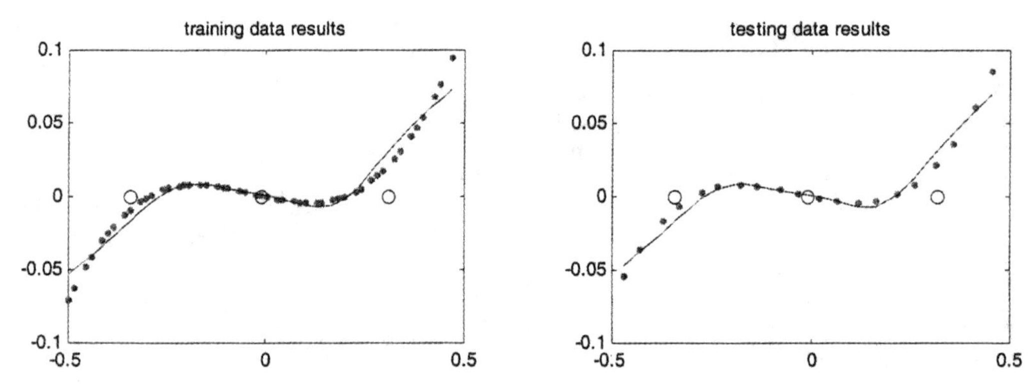

1.19 Illustration of mixture of expert network using batched training method.

1.2.6 Support Vector Machines (SVMs)

A support vector machine [14] has a basic format, as depicted in Figure 1.20, where $\varphi_k(\mathbf{x})$ is a nonlinear transformation of the input feature vector $\mathbf{x}$ into a high-dimensional space new feature vector $\boldsymbol{\varphi}(\mathbf{x}) = [\varphi_1(\mathbf{x})\, \varphi_2(\mathbf{x}) \ldots \varphi_p(\mathbf{x})]$. The output y is computed as:

$$y(\mathbf{x}) = \sum_{k=1}^{p} w_k \varphi_k(\mathbf{x}) + b = \varphi(\mathbf{x})\mathbf{w}^{\mathrm{T}} + b$$

where $\mathbf{w} = [w_1\, w_2 \ldots w_p]$ is the $1 \times p$ weight vector, and b is the bias term. The dimension of $\boldsymbol{\varphi}(\mathbf{x})(= p)$ is usually much larger than that of the original feature vector $(= m)$. It has been argued that mapping a low-dimensional feature into a higher-dimensional feature space will likely make the resulting feature vectors linearly separable. In other words, using $\boldsymbol{\varphi}$ as a feature vector is likely to result in better pattern classification results.

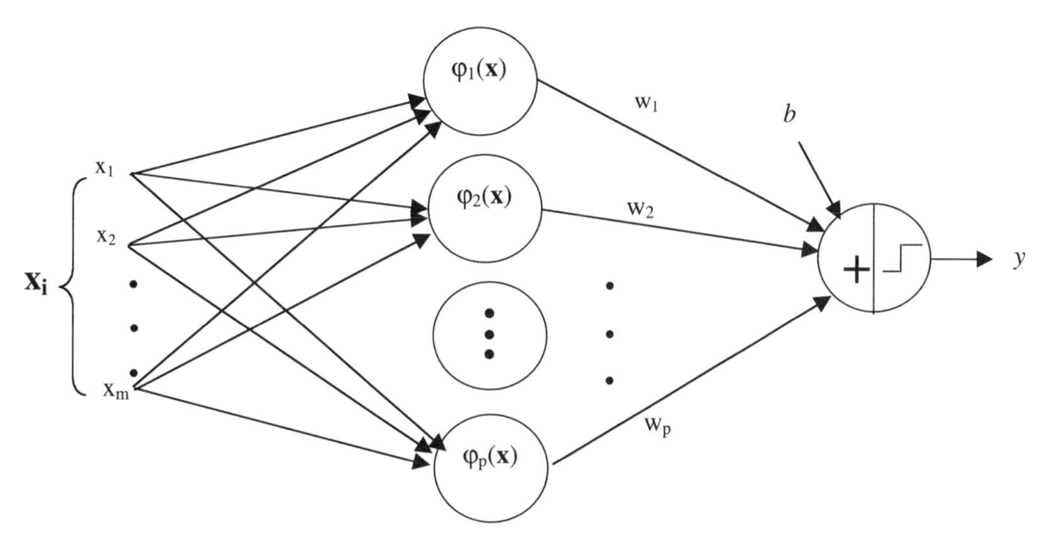

1.20 An SVM neural network structure.

Given a set of training vectors $\{\mathbf{x}(i);\ 1 \le i \le N\}$, one can solve the weight vector $\mathbf{w}$ as:

$$\mathbf{w} = \sum_{i=1}^{N} \gamma_i \varphi(\mathbf{x}(i)) = \gamma \Phi$$

where $\Phi = [\varphi(\mathbf{x}(1))\ \varphi(\mathbf{x}(2))\ \ldots \varphi(\mathbf{x}(N))]^{\mathrm{T}}$ is an $N \times p$ matrix, and γ is a $1 \times N$ vector. Substituting $\mathbf{w}$ into $y(\mathbf{x})$ yields:

$$y(\mathbf{x}) = \varphi(\mathbf{x})\mathbf{w}^{\mathrm{T}} + b = \sum_{i=1}^{N} \gamma_i \varphi(\mathbf{x})\varphi^{\mathrm{T}}(\mathbf{x}(i)) + b = \sum_{i=1}^{N} \gamma_i K(\mathbf{x}, \mathbf{x}(i)) + b$$

where the kernel $K(\mathbf{x}, \mathbf{x}(i))$ is a scalar-valued function of the testing sample $\mathbf{x}$ and a training sample $\mathbf{x(i)}$. For $N << p$, one may choose to use γ and $K(\mathbf{x}, \mathbf{x}(i))$ to evaluate $y(\mathbf{x})$ instead of using $\mathbf{w}$ and $\varphi(\mathbf{x})$ explicitly. For this purpose, one must estimate γ and b and identify a set of support vectors $\{\mathbf{x}(i);\ 1 \le i \le N\}$ that may be a subset of the entire training set of data samples.

Commonly used kernel functions are summarized in Table 1.4.

TABLE 1.4 List of Commonly Used Kernel Functions for Support Vector Machines (SVMs)

Type of SVM	$K(x, y)$	Comments
Polynomial learning machine	$\left(\mathbf{x}^{\mathrm{T}}\mathbf{y} + 1\right)^{p}$	p: selected *a priori*
Radial basis function	$\exp\left(-\frac{1}{2\sigma^2}\|\mathbf{x} - \mathbf{y}\|^2\right)$	σ^2: selected *a priori*
Two-layer perceptron	$\tanh\left(\beta_o \mathbf{x}^{\mathrm{T}}\mathbf{y} + \beta_1\right)$	Only some β_o and β_1 values are feasible

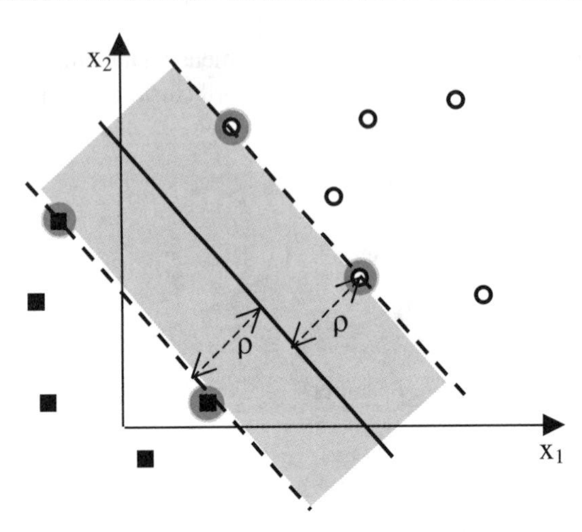

1.21 A linearly separable pattern classification example. ρ is the distance between each class to the decision boundary.

To identify the support vectors from a set of training data samples, consider the linearly separable pattern classification example shown in Figure 1.21. According to Cortes and Vapnik [15], the empirical risk is minimized in a linearly separable two-class pattern classification problem, as shown in Figure 1.21, if the decision boundary is located such that the minimum distance from each training sample of each class to the decision boundary is maximized. In other words, the parameter ρ in Figure 1.21 should be maximized subject to the constraints that all "o" class samples should be on one side of the decision boundary, and all "x" class samples should be on the other side of the decision boundary. This can be formulated as a nonlinear constrained quadratic optimization problem. Using a Karush–Kühn–Tucker condition, it can be shown that not all training samples will contribute to the determination of the decision boundary. In fact, as shown in Figure 1.21, only those training samples that are closest to the decision boundary (marked with color in the figure) will contribute to the solution of $\mathbf{w}$ and b. These training samples will then be identified as the support vectors.

There are many public domain implementations of SVM. They include a support vector machine MATLAB toolbox (S.R.Gunn@ecs.soton.ac.uk), a C implementation SVM_light (http://ais.gmd.de/~thorsten/svm_light/), and a recent release of BSVM (http://www.csie.ntu.edu.tw/~cjlin/). Figure 1.22 shows an example using an SVM toolbox to solve a linearly separable problem with a radial basis kernel. The three support vectors are labeled with white dots and the decision boundary and the gap are also illustrated.

1.3 Neural Network Solutions to Signal Processing Problems

1.3.1 Digital Signal Processing

In the most general sense a signal is a physical quantity that is a function of one or more independent variables such as time or spatial coordinates. A signal can be naturally occurring or artificially synthesized. It can be the temperature variations in a building, a stock price quote, the faint radiation from a distant galaxy, or the brain waves from a human body.

How do we use the signals obtained from various measurements? Simply put, a signal carries information. Based on building temperature readings, we may turn the building's heater on or off. Based on a stock price quote, we may buy or sell stocks. The faint radiation from a distant galaxy may reveal the secret of the universe. Brain waves from a human body may be used to communicate and control external devices. In short, the purpose of signal processing is to exploit inherent information

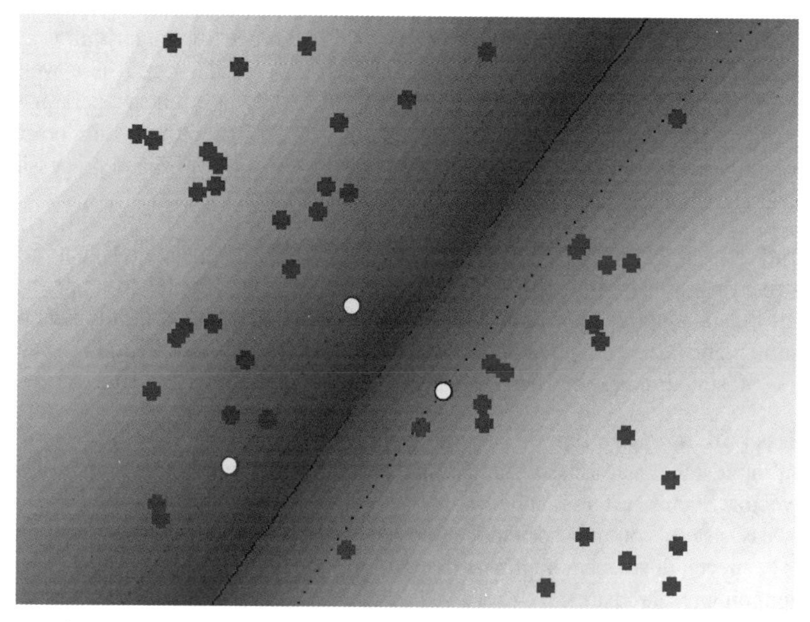

1.22 Illustration of support vector machine classification result.

carried by the signal. More specifically, by processing a signal, we can manipulate the information by injecting new information into the signal or by extracting inherent information from the signal. There are many ways to process signals. One may filter, transform, transmit, estimate, detect, recognize, synthesize, record, or reproduce a signal.

Perhaps the most comprehensive definition of signal processing is the Field of Interests statement of the IEEE (Institute of Electrical and Electronics Engineering) Signal Processing Society, which states that signal processing concerns

> *... theory and application of filtering, coding, transmitting, estimating, detecting, analyzing, recognizing, synthesizing, recording, and reproducing signals by digital or analog devices or techniques. The term "signal" includes audio, video, speech, image, communications, geophysical, sonar, radar, medical, musical, and other signals.*

If a signal is a function of time only, it is a one-dimensional signal. If the time variable is continuous, the corresponding signal is a continuous time signal. Most real world signals are continuous time signals. A continuous time signal can be sampled at regular time intervals to yield a discrete time signal. A discrete time signal can be described using a sequence of numbers. To process a discrete time signal using digital computers, the value of each discrete time sample may also be quantized to finite precision to fit into the internal word length of the computer.

1.3.1.1 A Taxonomy of Digital Signal Processing (DSP) Algorithms

A DSP algorithm describes how to process a given signal. Depending on their assumptions of the underlying signal, the mathematical formulations, DSP algorithms can be characterized in a number of different dimensions:

Deterministic vs. statistical signal processing — In a statistical DSP algorithm, it is assumed that the underlying signal is generated from a probabilistic model. No such model is assumed in a deterministic DSP algorithm. Almost all the neural network application examples we encountered concerned statistical signal processing applications.

Linear vs. nonlinear signal processing — A linear signal processing algorithm is a linear system (linear operator) operating on the incoming signal. If a particular signal is a weighted sum of two different signals, then the output of this signal after applying a linear operator will also be a weighted sum of the outputs of those two different signals. This superimposition property is unique to linear signal processing algorithms. Neural network applications to signal processing are mostly for nonlinear signal processing algorithms.

Data-adaptive vs. data-independent formulation — A data-independent signal processing algorithm has fixed parameters that do not depend on specific data samples to be processed. On the other hand, a data-adaptive algorithm will adjust its parameters based on the signal presented to the algorithm. Thus, data-adaptive algorithms need a training phase to acquire specific values of parameters. Most neural network based signal processing algorithms are data adaptive.

Memoryless vs. dynamic system — The output of a signal processing algorithm may depend on both the present input signal as well as a signal in the past. Usually, the signal in the past is summarized as a state vector. Such a system is called a dynamic system that has memory (remembering the past). A memoryless system's output is dependent only on the present input. While linear dynamic system theory has been well developed, nonlinear dynamic system theory that incorporates neural networks is still an ongoing research area.

1.3.1.2 Nonlinear Filtering

There are many reports on using artificial neural networks to perform nonlinear filtering of a signal for the purposes of noise reduction and signal enhancement. However, due to the nonlinear nature, most applications must be developed for specific training corpus and are data dependent. Therefore, to apply ANN for nonlinear filtering, one must be able to collect an extensive set of training samples to cover all possible situations and develop a neural network to adapt to the given training set.

For example [16], an MLP-based neural filter is developed to remove quantum noise from X-ray images, while at the same time trying to enhance the edge of the images. The purpose is to replace current high dosage X-ray film with low dosage X-ray while improving the quality of the image. In this application, high dosage X-ray film with high-pass filtered edge enhancement is used as the target. A simulated low-dosage X-ray image, derived from the original high-dosage X-ray image, is used as the input to the MLP. The resulting SNR improvement of a testing data set is used to gauge the effectiveness of this approach.

1.3.1.3 Linear Transformations

A linear transformation transforms a block (vector) of signal into a different vector space where special properties may be exploited. For example, a discrete Fourier transform transforms a time domain signal into frequencies in the frequency domain. A discrete wavelet transform transforms to and back from scale space representation of the signal. A very important application of linear transformation is the transform-based signal compression. The original signal is first transformed using a linear transformation such as the fast Fourier transform, the discrete cosine transform, or the discrete wavelet transform into the frequency domain. The purpose is to compact the energy in the original signal into a few large frequency coefficients. By encoding these very few large frequency coefficients, the original signal can be compressed with a high compression ratio.

Another popular data-dependent linear transform is called principal component analysis (PCA) or, sometimes, Karhunen–Loeve expansion (KL expansion). The main difference between PCA and other types of linear transforms is that the transformation depends on the inherent structure of the data. Hence, PCA can achieve optimal performance in terms of energy compaction. The generalized

Hebbian learning neural network structure can be regarded as an online approximation of PCA, and hence can be applied to tasks that would require PCA.

1.3.1.4 Pattern Classification

Pattern classification is perhaps the most important application of artificial neural networks. In fact, a majority of neural network applications can be categorized as solving complex pattern classification problems. In the area of signal processing, pattern classification has been employed in speech recognition, optical (handwritten) character recognition, bar code recognition, human face recognition, fingerprint recognition, radar/sonar target identification, biomedical signal diagnosis, and numerous other areas.

Given a set of feature vectors $\{\mathbf{x}; \mathbf{x} \in \Re^n\}$ of an object of interest, we assume that the (probabilistic) state of nature of each object can be designated with a label $\omega \in \Omega$, where Ω is the set of all possible labels. We denote the prior probability $p(\omega)$ to be the probability that a feature vector is assigned by nature of the object to the label ω_c. We may also define a posterior probability $p(\omega|\mathbf{x})$ to be the probability that a feature vector $\mathbf{x}$ has label ω_c given the observation of the feature vector $\mathbf{x}$.

A minimum error statistical pattern classifier is one that maps each feature vector $\mathbf{x}$ to an element in Ω such that the probability that the mapped label is different from the label assigned by the nature of the object (the probability of misclassification) is minimized. To achieve this minimum error rate, for a given feature vector $\mathbf{x}$, one must

$$\text{Decide } \mathbf{x} \text{ has label } \omega_i \text{ if } \quad p(\omega_i|\mathbf{x}) > p(\omega_j|\mathbf{x}) \quad \text{for } j \neq i, \omega_i, \omega_j \in \Omega\,.$$

In practice, it is very difficult to evaluate the posterior probability in close form. Instead, one may use an appropriate discriminant function $g_i(\mathbf{x})$ that satisfies

$$g_i(\mathbf{x}) > g_j(\mathbf{x}) \text{ if } \quad p(\omega_i|\mathbf{x}) > p(\omega_j|\mathbf{x}) \quad \text{for } j \neq i, \omega_i, \omega_j \in \Omega\,.$$

Then, the minimum error pattern classification can be achieved by

$$\text{Decide } \mathbf{x} \text{ has label } \omega_i \text{ if } \quad g_i(\mathbf{x}) > g_j(\mathbf{x}) \quad \text{for } j \neq i, \omega_i, \in \Omega\,.$$

The minimum probability of misclassification is also known as the Bayes error, and a minimum error classifier is also known as a maximum *a posteriori* probability (MAP) classifier.

In applying the MAP classifier to real world applications, one must find an estimate of the posterior probability $p(\omega|\mathbf{x})$ or, equivalently, a discriminant function $g(\mathbf{x})$ based on a set of training data. Thus, a neural network such as the multilayer perceptron can be a good candidate for such a purpose. A support vector machine is another neural network structure that directly estimates a discriminant function.

One may apply the Bayes rule to express the posterior probability as:

$$p(\omega|\mathbf{x}) = p(\mathbf{x}|\omega)p(\omega)/p(\mathbf{x})$$

where $p(\mathbf{x}|\omega)$ is called the likelihood function, $p(\omega)$ is the prior probability distribution of class label ω, and $p(\mathbf{x})$ is the marginal probability distribution of the feature vector $\mathbf{x}$. Since $p(\mathbf{x})$ is independent of ω_i, the MAP decision rule can be expressed as:

$$\text{Decide } \mathbf{x} \text{ has label } \omega_i \text{ if } \quad p(\mathbf{x}|\omega_i)p(\omega_i) > p(\mathbf{x}|\omega_j)p(\omega_j) \quad \text{for } j \neq i, \omega_i, \omega_j \in \Omega\,.$$

$p(\omega_i)$ can be estimated from the training data samples as the percentage of training samples that are labeled ω_i. Thus, only the likelihood function needs to be estimated. One popular model for such a purpose is a mixture of the Gaussian model:

$$p(\mathbf{x}|\omega_i) = \sum_{k=1}^{K_i} \nu_{ki} \exp\left[-(\mathbf{x} - \mathbf{m}_{ki})^2 / \left(2\sigma_{ki}^2\right)\right].$$

To deduce the model parameters, $\{(\nu_{ki}, \mathbf{m}_{ki}, \sigma_{ki}^2); 1 \le k \le K_i, 1 \le i \le C\}$ $(C = |\Omega|)$. Obviously, a radial basis neural network structure will be handy here to model the mixture of Gaussian likelihood function.

Since the weighted sum of the mixture of Gaussian density functions is still a mixture of a Gaussian density function, one may choose instead to model the marginal distribution $p(\mathbf{x})$ with a mixture of a Gaussian model. Each individual Gaussian density function in the mixture model will be assigned to a particular class label based on a majority voting of training samples assigned to that particular Gaussian density function. Additional fine-tuning can be applied to enhance the probability of classification. This is the approach implemented in the learning vector quantization (LVQ) neural network. The above discussion is summarized in Table 1.5.

TABLE 1.5 Pattern Classification Methods and Corresponding Neural Network Implementations

Pattern Classification Methods	Neural Network Implementations
MAP: maximize posterior probability $p(\omega\|\mathbf{x})$	Multilayer perceptron
MAP: maximize discriminant function $g(\mathbf{x})$	Support vector machine
ML: maximize product of likelihood function and prior distribution $p(\mathbf{x}\|\omega)p(\omega)$	Radial basis network, LVQ

1.3.1.5 Detection

Detection can be regarded as a special case of pattern classification where only two class labels are used: detect or no-detect. The purpose of signal detection is to detect the presence of a known signal in the presence of additive noise. It is assumed that the received signal (often a vector) $\mathbf{x}$ may consist of the true signal vector $\mathbf{s}$ and an additive statistical noise vector $\mathbf{n}$:

$$\mathbf{x} = \mathbf{s} + \mathbf{n}$$

or simply the noise vector:

$$\mathbf{x} = \mathbf{n} \, .$$

Assuming that the probability density function of the noise vector $\mathbf{n}$ is known, one may apply statistical hypothesis testing procedure to determine whether $\mathbf{x}$ contains the known signal $\mathbf{s}$. For example, we may calculate the log-likelihood function and compare it to a predefined threshold in order to maximize the probability of detection subject to an upper bound of a prespecified false alarm rate.

One popular assumption is that the noise vector $\mathbf{n}$ has a multivariate Gaussian distribution with zero mean and known covariance matrix. In this case, the inner product $\mathbf{s}^T\mathbf{x}$ is a sufficient statistic, known as a matched filter signal detector.

A single neuron perceptron can be used to implement the matched filter computation. The signal template $\mathbf{s}$ will be the weight vector, and the observation $\mathbf{x}$ is applied as its input. The bias term is threshold, and the output $= 1$ if the presence of the signal is detected. A multilayer perceptron can also be used to implement a nonlinear matched filter if the output activation function is a threshold function. By the same token, a support vector machine is also a plausible neural network structure to realize a nonlinear matched filter.

1.3.1.6 Time Series Modeling

A time series is a sequence of readings as a function of time. It arises in numerous practical applications, including stock prices, weather readings (e.g., temperature), utility demand, etc. A central issue in time series modeling is to predict the future time series outcomes. There are three different ways of predicting a time series $\{y(t)\}$:

1. Predicting $y(t)$ based on past observations $\{y(t-1), y(t-2), \dots\}$. That is,

$$\hat{y}(t) = E\{y(t)|y(t-1), y(t-2), \dots\}\,.$$

2. Predicting $y(t)$ based on observation of other relevant time series $\{x(t); x(t), x(t-1), \dots\}$:

$$\hat{y}(t) = E\{y(t)|x(t), x(t-1), x(t-2), \dots\}\,.$$

3. Predicting $y(t+1)$ based on both $\{y(t-k); k = 1, 2, \dots\}$ and $\{x(t-m); m = 0, 1, 2, \dots\}$:

$$\hat{y}(t) = E\{y(t)|x(t), x(t-1), x(t-2), \dots, y(t-1), y(t-2), \dots\}\,.$$

Both $\{x(t)\}$ and $\{y(t)\}$ can be vector valued time series. If the conditional expectation is a linear function, then these formulae lead to three popular linear time series models:

Auto-regressive (AR)	$y(t) = \sum_{k=1}^{N} a(k)y(t-k) + e(t)$
Moving average (MA)	$y(t) = \sum_{m=0}^{M} b(m)x(t-m)$
Auto-regressive moving average (ARMA)	$y(t) = \sum_{m=0}^{M} b(m)x(t-m) + \sum_{k=1}^{N} a(k)y(t-k) + e(t)$

In the AR and ARMA models, $e(t)$ is a zero-mean, uncorrelated innovation process representing a random persistent excitation of the system. Neural network models can be incorporated into these time series models to facilitate nonlinear time series prediction. Specifically, one may use the generalized state vector s as an input to a neural network and obtain the output $y(t)$ from the output of the neural network.

One such example is the time-delayed neural network (TDNN) that can be described as:

$$y(n) = \varphi(x(n), x(n-1), \dots, x(n-M))$$

$\varphi(\bullet)$ is a nonlinear transformation of its arguments, and it is implemented with a multilayer perceptron in TDNN.

1.3.1.7 System Identification

System identification is a modeling problem. Given a black box system, the goal of system identification is to develop a mathematical model to describe the relation between the input and output of the unknown system.

If the system under consideration is memoryless, the implication is that the output of this system is a function of present input only and bears no relation to past input. In this situation, the system identification problem becomes a function approximation problem.

1.3.1.7.1 Function Approximation

Assume a set of training samples $\{(\mathbf{u}(i), \mathbf{y}(i))\}$, where $\mathbf{u}(i)$ is the input vector and $\mathbf{y}(i)$ is the output vector. The purpose of function approximation is to identify a mapping from $\mathbf{x}$ to $\mathbf{y}$, that is,

$$\mathbf{y} = \varphi(\mathbf{u})$$

such that the expected sum of square approximation error $E\{|\mathbf{y} - \varphi(\mathbf{u})|^2\}$ is minimized.

Neural network structures such as the multilayer perceptron and radial basis network are both good candidate algorithms to realize the $\varphi(\mathbf{u})$ function.

1.3.1.7.2 Dynamic System Identification

If the system to be identified is a dynamic system, then the present input $\mathbf{u}(t)$ alone is not sufficient to determine the output $\mathbf{y}(t)$. Instead, $\mathbf{y}(t)$ will be a function of both $\mathbf{u}(t)$ and a present state vector $\mathbf{x}(t)$. The state vector can be regarded as a summary of all the input in the past. Unfortunately, for many systems, only input and outputs are observable. In this situation, previous outputs within a time window may be used as a generalized state vector.

To derive the mapping from $\mathbf{u}(t)$ and $\mathbf{x}(t)$ to $\mathbf{y}(t)$, one may gather a sufficient amount of training data and then develop a mapping $\mathbf{y}(t) = \varphi(\mathbf{u}(t), \mathbf{x}(t))$ using, for example, a linear model or a nonlinear model such as an artificial neural network structure. In practice, however, such training process is conducted using online learning. This is illustrated in Figure 1.23.

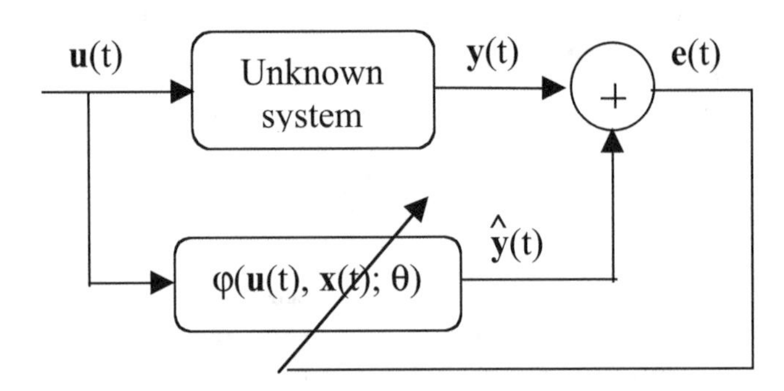

1.23 Illustration of online dynamic system identification. The error $\mathbf{e}(t)$ is fed back to the model to update model parameters θ.

With online learning, the mathematical dynamic model receives the same inputs as the real, unknown system, and produces an output $\hat{y}(t)$ to approximate the true output $\mathbf{y}(t)$. The difference between these two quantities will then be fed back to update the mathematical model.

1.4 Overview of the Handbook

This handbook is organized into three complementary parts: neural network fundamentals, neural network solutions to statistical signal processing problems, and signal processing applications using neural networks. In the first part, in-depth surveys of recent progress of neural network computing paradigms are presented. Part One consists of five chapters:

- **Chapter 1: Introduction to Neural Networks for Signal Processing.** This chapter has provided an overview of topics discussed in this handbook so that the reader is better prepared for the in-depth discussion in later chapters.
- **Chapter 2: Signal Processing Using the Multilayer Perceptron.** In this chapter, Manry, Chandrasekaran, and Hsieh discuss the training strategies of the multilayer perceptron and methods to estimate testing error from the training error. A potential application of MLP to flight load synthesis is also presented.
- **Chapter 3: Radial Basis Functions.** In this chapter, Back presents a complete review of the theory, algorithm, and five real world applications of radial basis network: time series modeling, option pricing in the financial market, phoneme classification, channel equalization, and symbolic signal processing.
- **Chapter 4: An Introduction to Kernel-Based Learning Algorithms.** In this chapter, Müller, Mika, Rätsch, Tsuda, and Schölkopf introduce three important kernel-based

learning algorithms: support vector machine, kernel Fisher discriminant analysis, and kernel PCA. In addition to clear theoretical derivations, two impressive signal processing applications, optical character recognition and DNA sequencing analysis, are presented.

- **Chapter 5: Committee Machines.** Tresp gives three convincing arguments in this chapter as to why a committee machine is important: (a) performance enhancement using averaging, bagging, and boosting; (b) modularity with a mixture of expert networks; and (c) computation complexity reduction as illustrated with the introduction of a Bayesian committee machine.

The second part of this handbook surveys the neural network implementations of important signal processing problems. These include the following chapters:

- **Chapter 6: Dynamic Neural Networks and Optimal Signal Processing.** In this chapter, Principe casts the problem of optimal signal processing in terms of a more general mathematical problem of function approximation. Then, a general family of nonlinear filter structures, called a dynamic neural network, that consists of a bank of linear filters followed by static nonlinear operators, is presented. Finally, a discussion of generalized delay operators is given.
- **Chapter 7: Blind Signal Separation and Blind Deconvolution.** In this chapter, Douglas discusses the recent progress of blind signal separation and blind deconvolution. Given two or more mixture signals, the purpose of blind separation and deconvolution is to identify the independent components in a statistical mixture of the signal.
- **Chapter 8: Neural Networks and Principal Component Analysis.** In this chapter, Diamantaras presents a detailed survey on using neural network Hebbian learning to realize principal component analysis (PCA). Also discussed in this chapter is nonlinear principal component analysis as an extension of the conventional PCA.
- **Chapter 9: Applications of Artificial Neural Networks to Time Series Prediction.** In this chapter, Liao, Moody, and Wu provide a technical overview of neural network approaches to time series prediction problems. Three techniques — sensitivity-based input selection and pruning, constructing a committee prediction model using input feature grouping, and smoothing regularization for recurrent neural networks — are reviewed, and applications to financial time series prediction are discussed.

The last part of this handbook examines signal processing applications and systems that use neural network methods. The chapters in this part include:

- **Chapter 10: Applications of ANNs to Speech Processing.** Katagiri surveys the recent work in applying neural network techniques to aid speech processing tasks. Four topics are discussed: (a) the generalized gradient descent learning method, (b) recurrent neural networks, (c) support vector machines, and (c) signal separation techniques. Instead of just introducing these techniques, the focus is on how to apply them to enhance the performance of current speech processing systems.
- **Chapter 11: Learning and Adaptive Characterization of Visual Content in Image Retrieval Systems.** In this chapter, Muneesawang, Wong, Lay, and Guan discuss the application of a radial basis network to adaptively characterize the similarity of image content to support content-based image retrieval in modern multimedia signal processing systems.
- **Chapter 12: Applications of Neural Networks to Biomedical Image Processing.** In this chapter, Adali, Wang, and Li summarize recent progress in applying neural networks to biomedical image processing. Two specific areas, image analysis and computer assisted diagnosis, are discussed in great detail.

- **Chapter 13: Hierarchical Fuzzy Neural Networks for Pattern Classification.** In this chapter, Taur, Kung, and Lin introduce the decision-based neural network, a modular network, and its applications to a number of pattern classification applications, including texture classification, video browsing, and face and currency recognition. The authors also introduce the incorporation of fuzzy logic inference into the neural network for rule-based inference and classification.

References

[1] W. McCulloch and W. Pitts, A logical calculus of ideas imminent in nervous activity, *Bulletin of Mathematical Biophysics,* vol. 5, pp. 115–133, 1943.

[2] F. Rosenblatt, The perceptron: a probabilistic model for information storage and organization in the brain, *Psychological Review,* vol. 65, pp. 386–408, 1958.

[3] D.E. Rumelhart and J.L. MacClelland, *Parallel Distributed Processing: Explorations in the Microstructure of Cognition,* vol. I, MIT Press, Cambridge, MA, 1986.

[4] G. Cybenko, Approximation by superpositions of a sigmoidal function, University of Illinois, Department of Electrical and Computer Engineering, Technical Report 856, 1988.

[5] M.J.D. Powell, Radial basis functions for multivariable interpolation, presented at the IMA Conference on Algorithms for the Approximation of Functions and Data, Shrivenham, UK, pp. 143–167, 1985.

[6] T. Poggio and F. Girosi, Networks for approximation and learning, *Proceedings of the IEEE,* vol. 78, pp. 1481–1497, 1990.

[7] T.D. Sanger, Optimal unsupervised learning in a single layer linear feed-forward neural network, *Neural Networks,* vol. 12, pp. 459–473, 1989.

[8] T. Kohonen, The self-organizing map, *Proceedings of the IEEE,* vol. 78, pp. 1464–1480, 1990.

[9] M.P. Perrone and L.N. Cooper, When networks disagree: ensemble method for neural networks, in *Neural Networks for Speeach and Image Processing,* R.J. Mammone, Ed., Chapman & Hall, Boca Raton, FL, 1993.

[10] A. Krogh and J. Vedelsby, Neural networks ensembles, cross validation and active learning, in *Advances in Neural Information Processing Systems 7,* MIT Press, Cambridge, MA, 1995.

[11] L.K. Hansen and P. Salamon, Neural network ensembles, *IEEE Trans.,* PAMI, vol. 12, pp. 993–1001, 1990.

[12] K. Tumer and J. Ghosh, Error correlation and error reduction in ensemble classifiers, *Connection Science* [special issue on combining neural networks, to appear].

[13] R.A. Jacobs, M.I. Jordan, S. Nowlan, and G.E. Hinton, Adaptive mixtures of local experts, *Neural Computation,* vol. 3, pp. 79–87, 1991.

[14] V.N. Vapnik, *The Nature of Statistical Learning Theory,* Springer-Verlag, New York, 1995.

[15] C. Cortes and V. Vapnik, Support vector networks, *Machine Learning,* vol. 20, pp. 273–297, 1995.

[16] K. Suzuki, I. Horiba, and N. Sugie, Efficient approximation of a neural filter for quantum noise removal in X-ray images, presented at the *IEEE Workshop on Neural Networks for Signal Processing,* Madison, WI, pp. 370–379, 1999.

2

Signal Processing Using the Multilayer Perceptron

Michael T. Manry
University of Texas

Hema Chandrasekaran
U.S. Wireless Corporation

Cheng-Hsiung Hsieh
Chien Kou Institute of Technology

2.1 Introduction

Multilayer perceptron (MLP) neural networks with sufficiently many nonlinear units in a single hidden layer have been established as universal function approximators [1, 2]. MLPs have several significant advantages over conventional approximations. First, MLP basis functions (hidden unit outputs) change adaptively during training, making it unnecessary for the user to choose them beforehand. Second, the number of free parameters in the MLP can be unambiguously increased in small increments by simply increasing the number of hidden units. Third, MLP basis functions are bounded, making round-off and overflow errors unlikely.

Disadvantages of the MLP relative to conventional approximations include its long training time and its sensitivity to initial weight values. In addition, MLPs have the following problems:

1. MLP training algorithms are excessively time-consuming and do not always converge.
2. MLP training error vs. network topology is unknown. Selecting the topology for a single hidden layer MLP is reduced to choosing the correct number of hidden units N_h. If the MLP does not have enough hidden units, it is not sufficiently complex to solve the function approximation problem and it underfits the data, producing excessive error at the outputs. If the MLP has too many hidden units, then it may fit the noise and outliers,

0-8493-2359-2/01/$0.00+$1.50

leading to overfitting [3, 4]. Such an MLP performs well on the training set but poorly on new input vectors or a testing set. Current approaches for choosing N_h include growing methods [5, 6], pruning methods [7, 8], and approaches based upon Akaike's information criterion [9, 10]. Unfortunately, these methods are very time consuming.

3. MLP training performance relative to conventional nonlinear networks is unknown. As a result, users are more likely to use Volterra filters [11, 12] and piecewise linear approximations [13, 14] than they are to use neural networks.
4. MLP testing error is difficult to predict from training data. The leave-one-out cross validation technique can be used, but it is very time consuming.
5. Determining the optimal amount of training for an MLP is difficult. A common solution to this problem involves stopping the training when the validation error starts to increase [15]. However, this approach does not guarantee that optimal performance on a test set has been reached.

This chapter attacks all five of the problems listed above. Section 2.2 attacks the first problem by presenting a fast, convergent algorithm for training the MLP. Section 2.3 develops and demonstrates an algorithm that sizes the MLP by relating it to a piecewise linear network (PLN) with the same pattern storage. The performance of the MLP and PLN on random data is also summarized. Thus, problems 2 and 3 above are attacked. Section 2.4 describes a method for obtaining Cramer–Rao maximum *a posteriori* lower bounds [16] on the estimation error variance. The bounds also allow determination of how close to optimal the MLP's performance is [17]–[19], and they allow us to attack problems 4 and 5 above. Section 2.5 applies the techniques of Sections 2.2, 2.3, and 2.4 to an application: flight load synthesis in helicopters.

2.2 Training of the Multilayer Perceptron

Several global neural network architectures have been developed over the last few decades, including the MLP [20], the cascade correlation network [21], and the radial basis function (RBF) network [22]. Since the MLP has emerged as the most successful network, we limit our attention to MLP alone.

2.2.1 Structure and Operation of the MLP

Multilayer feed-forward networks consist of units arranged in layers with only forward connections to units in subsequent layers. The connections have weights associated with them. Each signal traveling along the link is multiplied by the connection weight. The first layer is the input layer, and the input units distribute the inputs to units in subsequent layers. In the following layers, each unit sums its inputs and adds a bias or threshold term to the sum and nonlinearly transforms the sum to produce an output. This nonlinear transformation is called the activation function of the unit. The output layer units often have linear activations. In the remainder of this chapter, linear output layer activations are assumed. The layers sandwiched between the input layer and output layer are called hidden layers, and units in hidden layers are called hidden units. Such a network is shown in Figure 2.1. The training data set consists of N_v training patterns $\{(\boldsymbol{x}_p, \boldsymbol{t}_p)\}$, where p is the pattern number. The input vector $\boldsymbol{x}_p$ and desired output vector $\boldsymbol{t}_p$ have dimensions N and M, respectively. $\boldsymbol{y}_p$ is the network output vector for the pth pattern. The thresholds are handled by augmenting the input vector with an element $\boldsymbol{x}_p(N+1)$ and setting it equal to one. For the jth hidden unit, the net

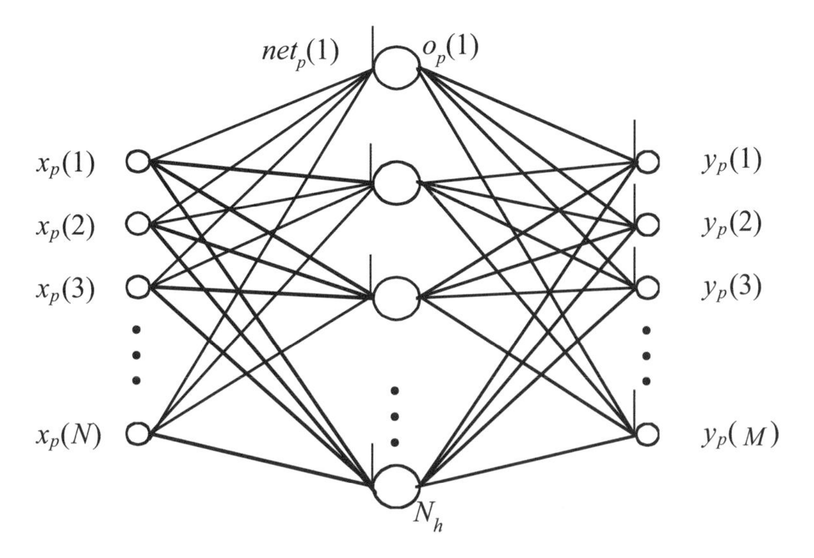

2.1 Feed-forward network with one hidden layer. (With permission from C-H Hsieh, M.T. Manry, and H. Chandrasekaran, Near optimal flight load synthesis using neural networks, NNSP '99, *IEEE*, 1999.)

input $\text{net}_p(j)$ and the output activation $O_p(j)$ for the pth training pattern are

$$\begin{aligned} \text{net}_p(j) &= \sum_{i=1}^{N+1} w(j,i) \cdot x_p(i), \quad 1 \le j \le N_h \\ O_p(j) &= f\left(\text{net}_p(j)\right) \end{aligned} \tag{2.1}$$

where $w(j,i)$ denotes the weight connecting the ith input unit to the jth hidden unit. For MLP networks, a typical activation function f is the sigmoid

$$f\left(\text{net}_p(j)\right) = \frac{1}{1+e^{-\text{net}_p(j)}} . \tag{2.2}$$

For trigonometric networks [23], the activations are sines and cosines. The kth output for the pth training pattern is y_{pk} and is given by

$$y_{pk} = \sum_{i=1}^{N+1} w_{io}(k,i) \cdot x_p(i) + \sum_{j=1}^{Nh} w_{ho}(k,j) \cdot O_p(j), \quad 1 \le k \le M \tag{2.3}$$

where $w_{io}(k,i)$ denotes the output weight connecting the ith input unit to the kth output unit and $w_{ho}(k,j)$ denotes the output weight connecting the jth hidden unit to the kth output unit. The mapping error for the pth pattern is

$$E_p = \sum_{k=1}^{M} \left[t_{pk} - y_{pk}\right]^2 \tag{2.4}$$

where t_{pk} denotes the kth element of the pth desired output vector. In order to train a neural network in batch mode, the mapping error for the kth output unit is defined as

$$E(k) = \frac{1}{N_v} \sum_{p=1}^{N_v} \left[t_{pk} - y_{pk}\right]^2 . \tag{2.5}$$

The overall performance of an MLP neural network, measured as mean square error (MSE), can be written as

$$E = \sum_{k=1}^{M} E(k) = \frac{1}{N_v} \sum_{p=1}^{N_v} E_p \,. \tag{2.6}$$

2.2.2 Training the MLP Using OWO-HWO

Several investigators have devised fast training techniques that require the solution of sets of linear equations [24]–[29]. In output weight optimization-back propagation [27] (OWO-BP), linear equations are solved to find output weights and back propagation [20] is used to find hidden weights (those which feed into the hidden units). Unfortunately, back propagation is not a very effective method for updating hidden weights [30, 31]. Some researchers [32]–[35] have used the Levenberg–Marquardt (LM) method to train the MLP. While this method has better convergence properties [36] than the conventional back propagation method, it requires storage on the order of $O(N^2)$ and calculations on the order of $O(N^2)$, where N is the total number of weights in an MLP [37]. Hence, training an MLP using the LM method is impractical for all but small networks.

Scalero and Tepedelenlioglu [38] have developed a non-batching approach for finding all MLP weights by minimizing separate error functions for each hidden unit. Although their technique is more effective than back propagation, it does not use OWO to optimally find the output weights, and it does not use full batching. Therefore, its convergence is unproven. Our approach has adapted their idea of minimizing a separate error function for each hidden unit to find the hidden weights; this technique has been termed hidden weight optimization (HWO).

In this section, MLPs with a single hidden layer are trained with hidden weight optimization-output weight optimization (OWO-HWO) [29]. In each training iteration, output weight optimization (OWO) solves linear equations to find the output weights, which are those connecting to linear output units. The HWO step uses separate error functions for each hidden unit and solves multiple sets of linear equations to find the optimal weights connecting to the hidden units. By minimizing many simple error functions instead of one large one, it is hoped that the training speed and convergence can be improved. However, this requires desired hidden net functions, which are not normally available. The desired net function can be constructed as

$$\text{net}_{pd}(j) \cong \text{net}_p(j) + Z \cdot \delta_p(j) \tag{2.7}$$

where $\text{net}_{pd}(j)$ is the desired net function and $\text{net}_p(j)$ is the actual net function for jth unit and the pth pattern. Z is the learning factor and $\delta_p(j)$ is the delta function [20] defined as

$$\delta_p(j) = \frac{-\partial E_p}{\partial \text{net}_p(j)} \,. \tag{2.8}$$

The calculations of the delta functions for output units and hidden units are, respectively [20],

$$\begin{aligned} \delta_{po}(j) &= f'\left(\text{net}_j\right) \cdot \left(t_{pj} - O_p(j)\right) \\ \delta_p(j) &= f'\left(\text{net}_j\right) \sum_n \delta_{po}(n) w_{ho}(n, j) \end{aligned} \tag{2.9}$$

where n is the index of units in the following layers which are connected to the jth unit. Elements $e(j, i)$ of the hidden weight change matrix are found by minimizing

$$E_\delta(j) = \sum_{p=1}^{N_v} \left[\delta_p(j) - \sum_i e(j, i) x_p(i) \right]^2 \tag{2.10}$$

with respect to the desired weight changes $e(j, i)$. We then update the hidden weights $w(j, i)$ by adding

$$\Delta w(j, i) = Z \cdot e(j, i) \tag{2.11}$$

to the weights $w(j, i)$. In a given iteration, the total change in the error function E, due to changes in all hidden weights, becomes approximately

$$\Delta E \cong -Z \frac{1}{N_v} \sum_{j=1}^{Nh} \sum_{p=1}^{N_v} \delta_p^2(j) \,. \tag{2.12}$$

First consider the case where the learning factor Z is positive and small enough to make the above approximation (Equation (2.12)) valid. Let E_k denote the training error in the kth iteration. Since the ΔE sequence is nonpositive, the E_k sequence is nonincreasing. Since nonincreasing sequences of nonnegative real numbers converge, E_k converges.

When the error surface is highly curved, the approximation of Equation (2.12) may be invalid in some iterations, resulting in increases in E_k. In such a case, the algorithm reduces Z and restores the previous optimum network. This sequence of events need only be repeated a finite number of times before E_k is again decreasing, since the error surface is continuous. After removing parts of the E_k sequence which are increasing, we again have convergence. It should be pointed out that this training algorithm also works for radial basis function (RBF) networks [22] and trigonometric networks [23].

2.3 A Sizing Algorithm for the Multilayer Perceptron

It has been observed that different kinds of nonlinear networks with the same theoretical pattern storage (or pattern memorization) produce very similar values of the training error E [39, 40]. In order to verify the observation with networks having many free parameters, however, very efficient training methods are required. This section analyzes and relates the performances of the MLP and the piecewise linear network (PLN). The PLN is a piecewise linear approximation to the training data. Using the relationship, we develop a sizing algorithm for the MLP, thus solving problems 1 and 2 from Section 2.1. In Section 2.3.1, we develop bounds on MLP training error in terms of pattern storage for the case of random training patterns. In Section 2.3.2, we obtain an expression for the PLN training error as a function of pattern storage for the case of random training patterns. In Section 2.3.3, we relate the pattern storages of PLN and MLP networks and describe the resulting sizing algorithm. In Section 2.3.4, we present numerical results that demonstrate the effectiveness of the sizing algorithm using several well known benchmark data sets.

2.3.1 Bounding MLP Performance

Our goal in this subsection is to bound MLP training error performance as a function of pattern storage when the training pattern elements x_k and t_n, $1 \le k \le N$, $1 \le n \le M$, and the training patterns $(\boldsymbol{x}_p, \boldsymbol{t}_p)$ and $(\boldsymbol{x}_q, \boldsymbol{t}_q)$, $p \ne q$ are statistically independent. A brute force approach to this problem would involve: (1) completely training tens of MLP networks of each size with different initial weights and (2) selecting the best network of each size from the trained networks. This approach is computationally very expensive and, therefore, impractical. A simpler but analyzable approach that we have taken involves the following steps: (1) train a large MLP network to zero error, (2) employ the modified Gram–Schmidt (GS) vector orthogonalization procedure [41, 42] on the hidden unit basis functions, (3) order the hidden unit basis functions by repeatedly applying the

GS procedure, and (4) predict the performance of MLPs of each size by plotting MLP training error as a function of hidden unit orthogonal basis functions weights.

We want to emphasize the fact that building an ordered orthonormal basis using the Gram–Schmidt procedure is suboptimal. In general, there is no reason why a subset of N_h hidden units' basis functions should contain the best subset of $(N_h - 1)$ hidden unit basis functions [41]–[43]. Yet, unlike the brute force method of selecting the optimal MLP of each size, the GS procedure is mathematically tractable and provides an upper bound on the training MSE reached by MLP networks of each size.

2.3.1.1 MLP Pattern Storage

The pattern storage of a network is the number of randomly chosen input–output pairs the network can be trained to memorize without error. Consider a fully connected MLP, which includes bypass weights, thresholds in the hidden layer, and thresholds in the output layer. The MLP can memorize a minimum number of patterns equal to the number of output weights connecting to one output unit. Therefore, its pattern storage, S_{MLP}, has a lower bound of $(N + N_h + 1)$ [25, 30]. The upper bound on the MLP's pattern storage is P_{MLP}/M, where P_{MLP} is the total number of free parameters in the network. This is the same formula used for polynomial network pattern storage. It has been shown [30] that this bound is fairly tight. Therefore, assume that

$$S_{\mathrm{MLP}}(N_h) = \left(\frac{(N+1+M)}{M}\right) \cdot N_h + (N+1)\,. \tag{2.13}$$

We notice that the MLP's pattern storage is a constant plus a linear function of the number of hidden units N_h.

2.3.1.2 Discussion of the Shape of the MSE vs. N_h Curve

Consider a single hidden-layer fully connected MLP with N inputs, N_h hidden units, and M outputs, as before. Each output receives connections from N inputs, N_h hidden units, and a threshold, so there are a total of $N_u = N + 1 + N_h$ basis functions in the MLP. Let the initial raw basis functions be $\sigma_1, \sigma_2, \sigma_3, \sigma_4, \ldots, \sigma_{Nu}$, where $\sigma_1 = 1$ for thresholds, $\sigma_2 = x_1, \sigma_3 = x_2, \ldots, \sigma_{N+1} = x_N$ for input units, and $\sigma_{N+2} = O_p(1), \sigma_{N+3} = O_p(2), \ldots, \sigma_{Nu} = O_p(N_h)$ for hidden units.

Construct an orthonormal basis by applying the modified Gram–Schmidt procedure on the basis functions. Order the orthonormal basis functions by choosing the normalized threshold, $1/N_v$, as the first basis function, followed by the normalized inputs. Let the first $(N+1)$ ordered orthonormal basis functions be $\phi_1, \phi_2, \phi_3, \ldots, \phi_{N+1}$.

Next, proceed with ordering the hidden units' orthonormal basis functions. Consider two consecutive hidden units i and $i+1$, $i \geq (N+2)$. Removing the effect of first $i-1$ basis functions from the remaining basis functions i through N_u, we have

$$\nu_{pm} = \sigma_{pm} - D_{1m}\phi_{p1} - D_{2m}\phi_{p2} - \cdots - D_{(i-1)m}\phi_{p(i-1)} \tag{2.14}$$

where $i \leq m \leq N_u$, p is the pattern number, and $1 \leq p \leq N_\nu$. The D_{1m} coefficients are inner products [44], defined as:

$$D_{1m} = \langle \phi_1, \sigma_m \rangle = \frac{1}{N_\nu}\sum_{p=1}^{N_\nu} \phi_{1p} \cdot \sigma_{mp}, \quad \cdots \quad D_{i-1m} = \langle \phi_{i-1}, \sigma_m \rangle = \frac{1}{N_\nu}\sum_{p=1}^{N_\nu} \phi_{(i-1)p} \cdot \sigma_{mp}\,. \tag{2.15}$$

Similarly, removing the effect of first $i-1$ basis functions from the desired output t_{pk},

$$t'_{pk} = t_{pk} - \sum_{n=1}^{i-1} \phi_{pn} C_n \tag{2.16}$$

where the C_n are weights for orthonormal basis functions, found as $C_n = \langle \phi_n, t' \rangle$.

Consider the basis functions ν_i and ν_{i+1}. Without loss of generality, they will be referred to as basis functions 1 and 2 from now on. Also, we now consider only one output. Define

$$P_{11} = \langle \nu_1, \nu_1 \rangle, P_{12} = \langle \nu_1, \nu_2 \rangle, Q_1 = \langle \nu_1, t' \rangle, Q_2 = \langle \nu_2, t' \rangle . \tag{2.17}$$

Next, orthonormalize hidden unit basis functions ν_1, ν_2 as:

$$\nu_1^I = \frac{\nu_1}{\sqrt{P_{11}}}, \qquad \nu_1^I = \phi_i \tag{2.18}$$

$$\nu_2^{II} = \frac{\nu_2 - \langle \nu_1^I, \nu_2 \rangle \nu_1^I}{\left\| \nu_2 - \frac{P_{12}}{P_{11}} \cdot \nu_1 \right\|} = \frac{\nu_2 - \frac{P_{12}}{P_{11}} \nu_1}{\sqrt{P_{22} - \frac{P_{12}^2}{P_{11}}}} = \frac{P_{11} \cdot \nu_2 - P_{12} \cdot \nu_1}{\sqrt{P_{11}} \sqrt{P_{11} \cdot P_{22} - P_{12}^2}}, \tag{2.19}$$

$$\nu_2^{II} = \phi_{i+1} .$$

Here, the superscripts I and II on ν_1^I and υ_2^{II} indicate that ν_1 is chosen as the first basis function and ν_2 is the second basis function in the ordered basis. Let C_1 and C_2 be the orthonormal weights connecting ν_1^I and υ_2^{II} to one output t. Then C_1 and C_2 are found as:

$$\begin{aligned} C_1 &= \langle \nu_1^I, t' \rangle = \frac{Q_1}{\sqrt{P_{11}}} \\ C_2 &= \langle \nu_2^{II}, t' \rangle = \frac{\langle P_{11} \cdot \nu_2 - P_{12} \cdot \nu_1, t' \rangle}{\sqrt{P_{11}} \sqrt{P_{11} \cdot P_{22} - P_{12}^2}} = \frac{P_{11} \cdot Q_2 - P_{12} \cdot Q_1}{\sqrt{P_{11}} \sqrt{P_{11} \cdot P_{22} - P_{12}^2}} . \end{aligned} \tag{2.20}$$

Then

$$C_1^2 - C_2^2 = \frac{\left(P_{11} P_{22} Q_1^2 - P_{11}^2 Q_2^2\right) + 2\left(P_{11} P_{12} Q_1 Q_2 - P_{12}^2 Q_1^2\right)}{P_{11}\left(P_{11} P_{22} - P_{12}^2\right)} . \tag{2.21}$$

If we force ν_2 to be the first basis function and ν_1 the second, then the corresponding orthonormal weights would be

$$\begin{aligned} C_1' &= \langle \nu_2^I, t' \rangle = \frac{Q_2}{\sqrt{P_{22}}} \\ C_2' &= \langle \nu_1^{II}, t' \rangle = \frac{\langle P_{22} \cdot \nu_1 - P_{12} \cdot \nu_2, t' \rangle}{\sqrt{P_{22}} \sqrt{P_{11} \cdot P_{22} - P_{12}^2}} = \frac{P_{22} \cdot Q_1 - P_{12} \cdot Q_2}{\sqrt{P_{22}} \sqrt{P_{11} \cdot P_{22} - P_{12}^2}} . \end{aligned} \tag{2.22}$$

Then

$$C_1'^2 - C_2'^2 = \frac{\left(P_{11} P_{22} Q_2^2 - P_{22}^2 Q_1^2\right) + 2\left(P_{22} P_{12} Q_1 Q_2 - P_{12}^2 Q_2^2\right)}{P_{22}\left(P_{11} P_{22} - P_{12}^2\right)} . \tag{2.23}$$

While building an ordered orthonormal basis, if $C_1^2 \geq C_1'^2$, we retain ν_1 as the first basis function and we consider $C_1^2 - C_2^2$ for subsequent discussions. If, on the other hand, $C_1^2 < C_1'^2$, we retain ν_2 as the first basis function and we consider $C_1'^2 - C_2'^2$ for subsequent discussions. Without loss of generality, we assume that $C_1^2 \geq C_1'^2$.

We know the following facts from Schmidt procedure ordering:

Since $C_1^2 \geq C_1'^2$, we consider Equation (2.21) and

$$\frac{Q_1^2}{P_{11}} > \frac{Q_2^2}{P_{22}} \qquad \text{or} \qquad P_{11} P_{22} Q_1^2 > P_{11}^2 Q_2^2 .$$

The term $(P_{11}P_{22}Q_1^2 - P_{11}^2 Q_2^2)$ is always positive.

$P_{11}P_{22} > P_{12}^2$ (since $\frac{P_{11}P_{22}-P_{12}^2}{P_{11}} = \left\| v_2 - \langle v_1^I, v_2 \rangle v_1^I \right\|$ and P_{11} is positive).

We cannot say whether the second term $(P_{11}P_{12}Q_1Q_2 - P_{12}^2 Q_1^2)$ in Equation (2.21) is positive or negative for a particular realization of the network. Consider an MLP with N_h hidden units, which has been trained to memorize all the patterns and whose hidden unit basis functions have been ordered using a modified Gram–Schmidt procedure. Then

- $C_i^2 \neq 0,\ 1 \leq i \leq N_h$, where C_i is the orthonormal weight from ith orthonormal hidden unit basis function to the output (all the basis functions are linearly independent; if not, we can always eliminate those dependent hidden units).
- The mean squared error E is given by

$$E = E\left[t'^2\right] - \left(C_{N+2}^2 + C_{N+3}^2 + \cdots + C_{N+1+N_h}^2\right) \tag{2.24}$$

  where t' is the output from which linear mapping between inputs and target has been removed, as in Equation (2.16), and $E[\cdot]$ denotes the expected value.

E in Equation (2.24) is plotted vs. N_h in Figure 2.2, where the weight energies are (1) in strictly decreasing order, (2) in strictly increasing order, and (3) all equal.

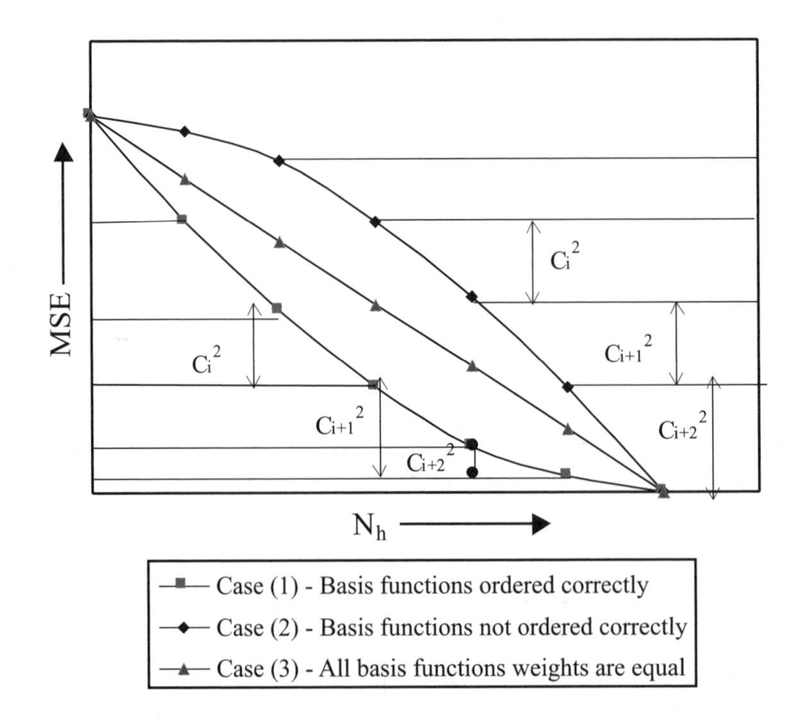

2.2 MLP hidden unit basis functions ordered using GS procedure. (With permission from C-H Hsieh, M.T. Manry, and H. Chandrasekaran, Near optimal flight load synthesis using neural networks, NNSP '99, *IEEE*, 1999.)

2.3.1.3 Convexity of the MSE vs. N_h Curve

A convex function is a function whose value at the midpoint of every interval in its domain does not exceed the average of its values at the ends of the interval [45]. In other words, a function

$f(x)$ is convex on an interval $[a, b]$ if, for any two points x_1 and x_2 in $[a, b]$, $f[\frac{1}{2}(x_1 + x_2)] \leq \frac{1}{2}[f(x_1) + f(x_2)]$. If $f(x)$ has a second derivative in $[a, b]$, then a necessary and sufficient condition for it to be convex on that interval is that the second derivative $f''(x) > 0$ for all x in $[a, b]$.

LEMMA 2.1 The MSE vs. N_h curve is convex if hidden unit basis functions are ordered such that

$$C_1^2 > C_{i+1}^2, \qquad 1 \leq i \leq (N_h - 1) \ .$$

This is easily proven using the definition of convexity and Equation (2.24). Therefore, the average MSE vs. N_h curve is convex if the hidden unit basis functions are ordered such that their weight magnitudes are in strictly descending order.

2.3.1.4 Finding the Shape of the Average MSE vs. N_h Curve

In Section 2.3.1.3, we proved that the average MSE vs. N_h curve is convex if we can order the hidden units' basis functions such that the C_i^2 sequence is strictly decreasing. In Section 2.3.1.2, we obtained an expression for $C_1^2 - C_2^2$, where C_1 and C_2 are the weights from two consecutive hidden units' orthonormal basis functions to the output.

Consider the ensemble average of $(P_{11}P_{12}Q_1Q_2 - P_{12}^2Q_1^2)$, which can be written as

$$\begin{aligned} E\left[P_{11}P_{12}Q_1Q_2 - P_{12}^2Q_1^2\right] &= \sum_{k=1}^{Nv}\sum_{j=1}^{Nv}\sum_{m=1}^{Nv}\sum_{n=1}^{Nv} E\left[v_{1k}^2 v_{1m} v_{2m} v_{1n} t_n' v_{2j} t_j'\right] \\ &\quad - \sum_{k=1}^{Nv}\sum_{j=1}^{Nv}\sum_{m=1}^{Nv}\sum_{n=1}^{Nv} E\left[v_{1k} v_{2k} v_{1j} v_{2j} v_{1m} t_m' v_{1n} t_n'\right] \ . \qquad (2.25) \end{aligned}$$

Here j, k, m, and n are pattern numbers within the same data set. The following assumption is made about the training data: training patterns $(\boldsymbol{x}_p, \boldsymbol{t}_p)$ and $(\boldsymbol{x}_q, \boldsymbol{t}_q)$ are also statistically independent for $p \neq q$.

Since the sigmoid activation function is an odd function after subtracting the constant basis function, it is possible to derive [40]

$$\begin{aligned} E\left[P_{11}P_{12}Q_1Q_2 - P_{12}^2Q_1^2\right] &= \sum_{k=1}^{Nv}\sum_{m=1}^{Nv} E\left[v_{1k}^2\right] E\left[v_{1m}^2 v_{2m}^2 t_m'^2\right] \\ &\quad - \sum_{k=1}^{Nv}\sum_{m=1}^{Nv} E\left[v_{1k}^2 v_{2k}^2\right] E\left[v_{1m}^2 t_m'^2\right] \ . \qquad (2.26) \end{aligned}$$

Using Schwarz's inequality, it is easily shown that

LEMMA 2.2

$$\sum_{k=1}^{Nv}\sum_{m=1}^{Nv} E\left[v_{1k}^2\right] \cdot E\left[v_{1m}^2 v_{2m}^2 t_m'^2\right] \geq \sum_{k=1}^{Nv}\sum_{m=1}^{Nv} E\left[v_{1k}^2 v_{2k}^2\right] \cdot E\left[v_{1m}^2 t_m'^2\right] \ .$$

Thus, $E\left[P_{11}P_{12}Q_1Q_2 - P_{12}^2Q_1^2\right]$ is net positive. Therefore $C_1^2 - C_2^2$ is positive in an ensemble average sense, and the average MSE vs. N_h curve is convex. This result is true even if there are multiple outputs, since $\Sigma_{k=1}^{M} E\left[C_{1k}^2 - C_{2k}^2\right] > 0$.

The average MSE vs. N_h curve is convex, even for nonrandom training data, provided the training patterns $(\boldsymbol{x}_p, \boldsymbol{t}_p)$ and $(\boldsymbol{x}_q, \boldsymbol{t}_q)$ are statistically independent for $p \neq q$.

THEOREM 2.1 *The average mean square training error E of an MLP as a function of pattern storage S_{MLP}, is bounded above by a straight line $E(S_{MLP}) \leq A - B \cdot S_{MLP}$ under the following conditions:*

1. *The training patterns $(\boldsymbol{x}_p, \boldsymbol{t}_p)$ and $(\boldsymbol{x}_q, \boldsymbol{t}_q)$ are statistically independent for $p \neq q$.*
2. *The activation function of the MLP hidden units is odd symmetric or odd symmetric + a constant.*

In Sections 2.3.1.2 and 2.3.1.3, we proved that the MLP training error vs. N_h curve is convex if the hidden unit orthonormal basis functions are ordered such that the basis function weights are in descending order of magnitude. The MLP pattern storage S_{MLP} is a constant plus a linear function of N_h. Therefore, the MSE vs. S_{MLP} curve also is convex under the same conditions, as illustrated in Figure 2.3.

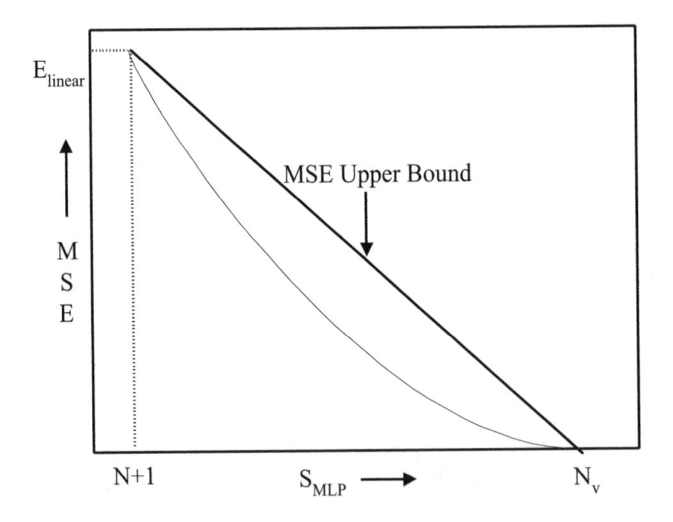

2.3 MLP training MSE vs. pattern storage S_{MLP}. (With permission from C-H Hsieh, M.T. Manry, and H. Chandrasekaran, Near optimal flight load synthesis using neural networks, NNSP '99, *IEEE*, 1999.)

2.3.2 Estimating PLN Performance

Our goal in this subsection is to introduce a specific PLN, describe its training, analyze its performance, and find its pattern storage. Our PLN for N inputs and M outputs contains N_c modules, each of which has an N-dimensional center vector $\boldsymbol{m}_n$ and a matrix $\boldsymbol{W}_{pwl}(\boldsymbol{n})$ of dimension $M \times (N+1)$. Such a network is shown in Figure 2.4. The network employs a weighted sum of square distance measure $d(\cdot)$. If the input vector x belongs to the nth cluster such that $d(\boldsymbol{x}, \boldsymbol{m}_n) = \min_k d(\boldsymbol{x}, \boldsymbol{m}_k)$, then the output vector is $\boldsymbol{y} = \boldsymbol{W}_{pwl}(\boldsymbol{n}) \cdot (\boldsymbol{x}^T : 1)^T$. This PLN provides a conventional way to

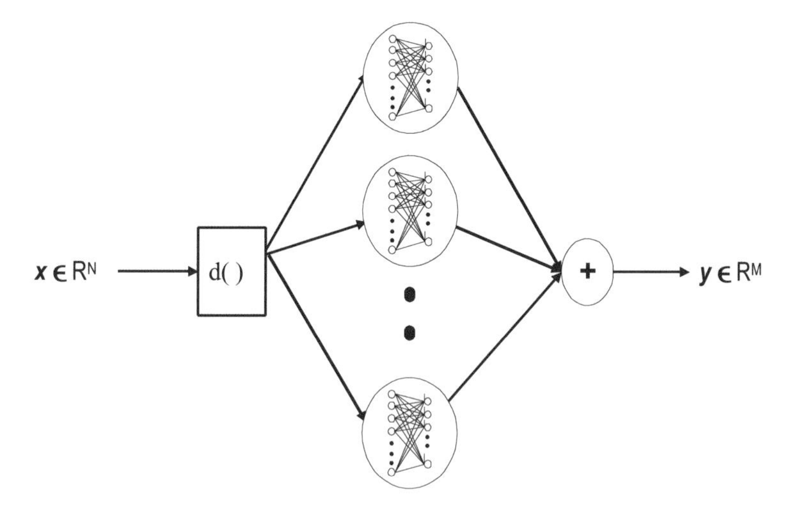

2.4 Piecewise linear network architecture. (With permission from C-H Hsieh, M.T. Manry, and H. Chandrasekaran, Near optimal flight load synthesis using neural networks, NNSP '99, *IEEE*, 1999.)

approximate nonlinear functions. The PLN trains much more quickly than the MLP, but it produces discontinuous approximations and generalizes less dependably.

2.3.2.1 Convergent PLN Training Algorithm

A convergent training algorithm for the piecewise linear network [40, 46] is described in the following section.

1. Weights of the distance measure which de-emphasize less useful inputs are found, following the approach of Subbarayan et al. [47].
2. We initialize the network with one cluster centered at the mean vector of input vectors. Two new cluster centers are found by perturbing this mean and reassigning patterns. A linear mapping is designed for each module or cluster through regression. In each iteration, a new cluster is added by splitting one of the existing clusters. This method of clustering falls under the category of hierarchical clustering [48, 49] utilizing a divisive method. Each cluster is then fitted with a linear mapping.
3. Four (or existing) clusters with the most mapping errors are identified as candidates for splitting.
4. The candidate cluster is optimally split into two. Now we have one more cluster than in the previous iteration. Each cluster is fitted with a linear mapping and the total mapping error E is calculated.
5. If the mapping error decreases, we save the new configuration and update the bound on the mapping error as $E_{\min} = E$. We now backtrack the network to the configuration that existed in step 3.
6. Finally, the configuration that leads to the lowest actual bound on the mapping error is retained. This method of finding the optimal placement of a new hyperplane can be termed a limited branch and bound method [50, 51], which is a special variation of the backtracking algorithm.
7. If the new module results in a decrease in E, the next iteration proceeds by repeating steps 3 through 6. Otherwise, the algorithm terminates.

2.3.2.2 PLN Pattern Storage

The pattern storage of a network is the number of randomly chosen input–output pairs the network can be trained to memorize without error. The pattern storage of the piecewise linear network is N_c multiplied by the storage per module,

$$S_{PLN} = N_c \cdot (N + 1) . \tag{2.27}$$

This pattern storage is attainable only if the training algorithm efficiently assigns patterns to the modules.

2.3.2.3 Calculating PLN Training Error

Here, we develop bounds on the PLN training error performance as a function of the number of modules in the network when the training pattern elements x_k and t_n, $1 \leq k \leq N, 1 \leq n \leq M$, and the training patterns $(\boldsymbol{x}_p, \boldsymbol{t}_p)$ and $(\boldsymbol{x}_q, \boldsymbol{t}_q)$, $p \neq q$ are statistically independent.

THEOREM 2.2 *The average mean square error expression for a piecewise linear network with N_c modules trained using random numbers for inputs and outputs is given by*

$$E = \frac{\sum_{p=1}^{Nv} \sum_{k=1}^{M} t_{pk}^2}{N_v} \left(1 - \frac{N_c(N+1)}{N_v}\right) \tag{2.28}$$

where N_v is the total number of training patterns, N is the number of inputs, and M is the number of outputs. This is easily proven [40] by finding and manipulating the singular value decomposition (SVD) [52, 53] of the matrix $\boldsymbol{D}$ of size $(N + 1) \times N_v$, each of whose columns consists of an N-dimensional input vector augmented with a one.

From Equation (2.28), we observe that the average MSE vs. the number of modules in a PLN curve is a straight line. Since the pattern storage S_{PLN} of a PLN with N_c modules is $N_c \cdot (N + 1)$, the average MSE vs. S_{PLN} curve is also linear and it coincides with the upper bound on the MSE vs. S_{MLP} curve in Figure 2.3. Thus, PLN and MLP networks have similar training errors when the training patterns are completely random.

2.3.3 Sizing Algorithm

We have seen that networks with similar pattern storage have similar training error when the training patterns have statistically independent elements. Here, we develop a sizing algorithm for the MLP based on the heuristic assumption that our result is valid when the patterns are not statistically independent.

Consider the PLN trained for N_{it} iterations. Let $E_t(i)$ be the training error and $N_c(i)$ be the number of modules in the ith iteration. Following Equation (2.27), the pattern storage $S_{PLN}(i)$ in the ith iteration is given by

$$S_{PLN}(i) = N_c(i) \cdot (N + 1) . \tag{2.29}$$

Equating the pattern memorization of the MLP in Equation (2.13) to that of the PLN in Equation (2.29), we have

$$N_h(i) \equiv N_h\left(S_{PLN}(i)\right) = \frac{M \cdot (N+1) \cdot (N_c(i) - 1)}{N + M + 1} . \tag{2.30}$$

This formula helps us estimate the number of hidden units in an equivalent MLP for various $E_t(i)$, $i = 1, 2, \ldots N_{it}$.

Case $M = 1$*:* When the number of outputs $M = 1$, Equation (2.30) approximately reduces to $N_h = (N_c - 1)$.

Case $M > 1$*:* In this case, overly large MLP networks result when the desired outputs are correlated and many free parameters are redundant. Then, an SVD technique is employed to detect whether outputs can be compressed without significantly degrading the MSE performance. Compressing the outputs allows the sizing algorithm to predict a smaller, less complex MLP. The resulting mean square error E_t', after we compress the M outputs down to M', is given by

$$E_t' = E_t + \sum_{i=M'+1}^{M} \lambda_i$$

where λ_is are the ith singular values of the desired outputs' covariance matrix. For each value of i, the sizing algorithm generates all possible MLP configurations and their predicted training MSE using M' values between 1 and M. The algorithm sifts through these potential configurations and saves those that have the lowest training MSE for a given number of hidden units. The final output of our algorithm is the sequence of ordered pairs, $\left\{E_t'(i), N_h(i)\right\}$.

Recall that the MLP's training error has that of the PLN as an upper bound for statistically independent patterns. It is therefore reasonable to expect that the MLP can perform better than predicted by the sizing algorithm.

2.3.4 Numerical Results

This section presents simulation results based on our approach to the MLP sizing problem. The PLN network is obtained through forward training without any pruning.

The data set `Single2.tra` has 16 inputs and 3 outputs and represents the training set for inversion of surface permittivity ε, the normalized surface rms roughness $k\sigma$, and the surface correlation length kL found in backscattering models from randomly rough dielectric surfaces [56]. The training set contains 5992 patterns. The three outputs can be compressed down to one with less than 1% increase in training MSE of an equivalent MLP. The results, illustrated in Figure 2.5, show good performance by the sizing algorithm.

The file `build3.tra` is part of the `Proben1` [57] benchmarking data sets. The data set represents the problem of predicting the hourly consumption of electrical energy, hot water, and cold water based on the date, time of day, outside temperature, outside air humidity, solar radiation, and wind speed. There are 8 inputs, 3 outputs, and 2104 training patterns in this data set. All three outputs are relevant, and no compression of the outputs is possible. The predicted and actual E vs. N_h curves, illustrated in Figure 2.6, are not very disparate.

The data set `oh7.tra` contains VV and HH polarization at L 30°, 40°, C 10°, 30°, 40°, 50°, 60°, and X 30°, 40°, 50° along with the corresponding unknowns rms surface height, surface correlation length, and volumetric soil moisture content in g/cubic cm [58]. There are 10,453 training patterns, 20 inputs, and 3 outputs in the `oh7.tra` data set. The predicted and actual E vs. N_h curves are illustrated in Figure 2.7. For the first time, the predicted MSE values are 60% higher than the actual MSE values for $2 \leq N_h \leq 12$.

The data set `matrix.tra` provides the data for inversion of random two-by-two matrices. Each pattern consists of four input features and four output features. The input features, which are uniformly distributed between 0 and 1, represent a matrix, and the four output features are elements of the corresponding inverse matrix. The determinants of the input matrices are constrained to be

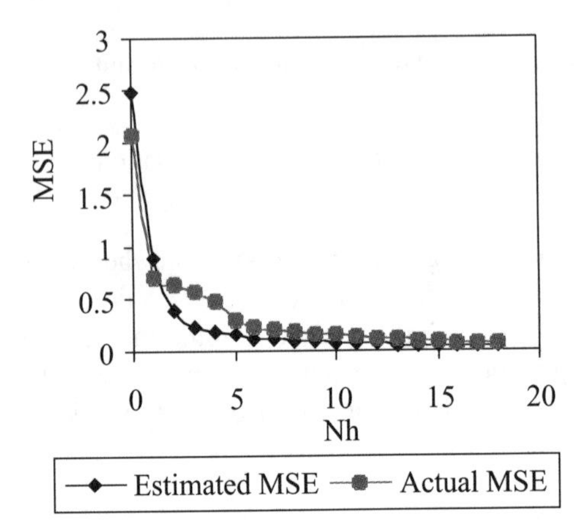

2.5 MLP sizing performance on `single2.tra`. (With permission from C-H Hsieh, M.T. Manry, and H. Chandrasekaran, Near optimal flight load synthesis using neural networks, NNSP '99, *IEEE*, 1999.)

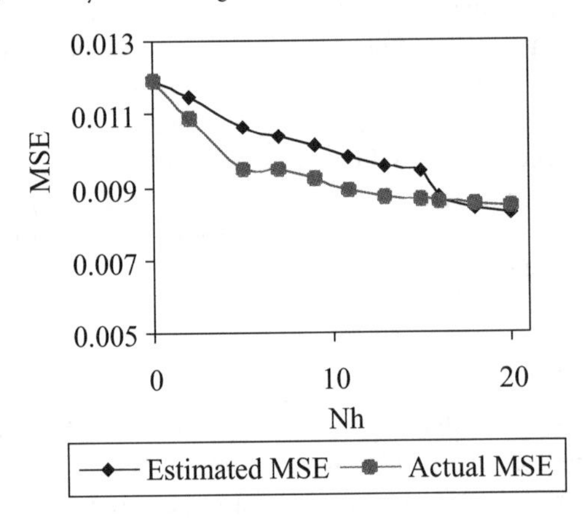

2.6 MLP sizing performance on `build3.tra`. (With permission from C-H Hsieh, M.T. Manry, and H. Chandrasekaran, Near optimal flight load synthesis using neural networks, NNSP '99, *IEEE*, 1999.)

between 0.3 and 2. There are 2000 training patterns in the data set. The predicted and actual E vs. N_h curves are illustrated in Figure 2.8. The predicted MSE curve seems to reflect the trend in the actual MSE vs. N_h curve, but with an offset.

The data set `Twod.tra` contains simulated data used in the task of inverting the surface scattering parameters from an inhomogeneous layer above a homogeneous half space, where both interfaces are randomly rough [56]. The data set has 8 inputs, 7 outputs, and 1768 training patterns. The predicted and actual E vs. N_h curves are illustrated in Figure 2.9. The predicted MSE curve seems to reflect the trend in the actual MSE vs. N_h curve, but with an offset.

The synthetic data set `parabolic.tra` contains 8 inputs, 3 outputs, and 2000 training patterns. The target outputs are defined as

$$\begin{aligned}
t_1 &= 10x_1^2 + 11x_2^2 + (x_3 - 0.5) - 3.5x_4 + 20\,(x_5 - 0.5) + 10x_6 + 5x_7 + n \\
t_2 &= 1.35x_1x_2 + 15x_3 + 2.79x_4x_5 + 7x_6 - 6.5x_8 + n \\
t_3 &= x_3^2 + 2.33x_2x_4 - 17.11x_5 + x_6 + 23x_7 + n
\end{aligned}$$

where n is zero mean Gaussian noise with 0.1 variance. The inputs $x_1 \ldots x_8$ are sampled independently from a uniform distribution over the interval [0, 1]. The predicted and actual E vs. N_h curves, illustrated in Figure 2.10, again show that the sizing algorithm is very useful.

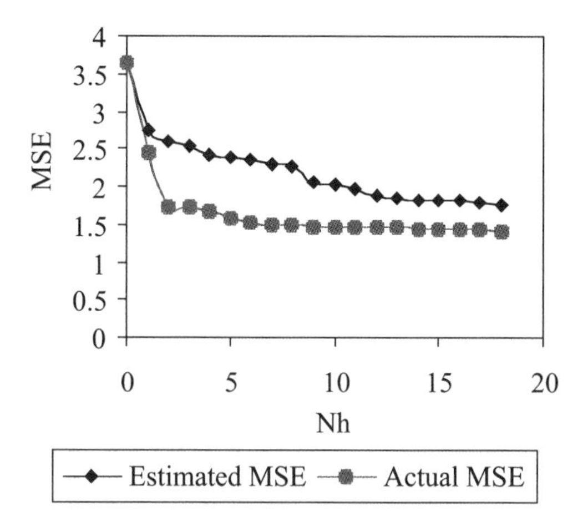

2.7 MLP sizing performance on `oh7.tra`. (With permission from C-H Hsieh, M.T. Manry, and H. Chandrasekaran, Near optimal flight load synthesis using neural networks, NNSP '99, *IEEE*, 1999.)

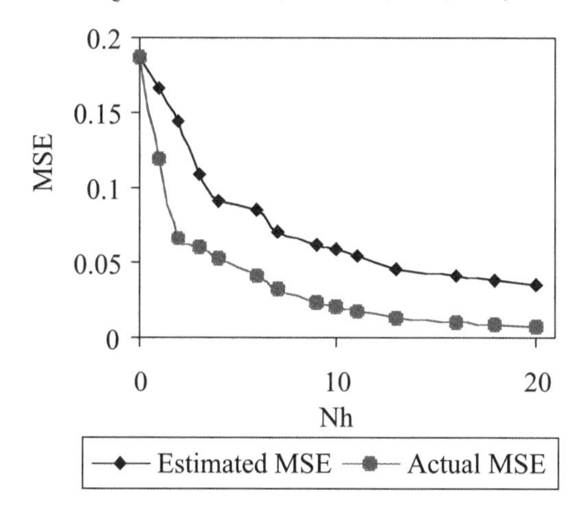

2.8 MLP sizing performance on `matrix.tra`. (With permission from C-H Hsieh, M.T. Manry, and H. Chandrasekaran, Near optimal flight load synthesis using neural networks, NNSP '99, *IEEE*, 1999.)

Using several standard benchmark data sets, we have experimentally verified that the sizing algorithm works and is an order of magnitude faster than the brute force design of multiple MLPs. Although the sizing algorithm often accurately forecasts the training error E as a function of N_h, it remains for us to pick a specific value of N_h from the curve. One method is to find where the E vs. N_h curve flattens out. A second method is suggested in the following subsection.

2.4 Bounding MLP Testing Errors from Training Data

In designing nonlinear estimators from training data, it is very useful to have known lower bounds on the testing error. By stopping training when the training error approaches the bounds, we can avoid overtraining of the network. Also, superimposing the bound on the forecast training error vs. N_h curve of the previous subsection, we can pick the N_h value seen at the intersection of the two curves. This section describes a method for obtaining Cramer–Rao maximum *a posteriori* (CRMAP) bounds [16] on the MLP testing error.

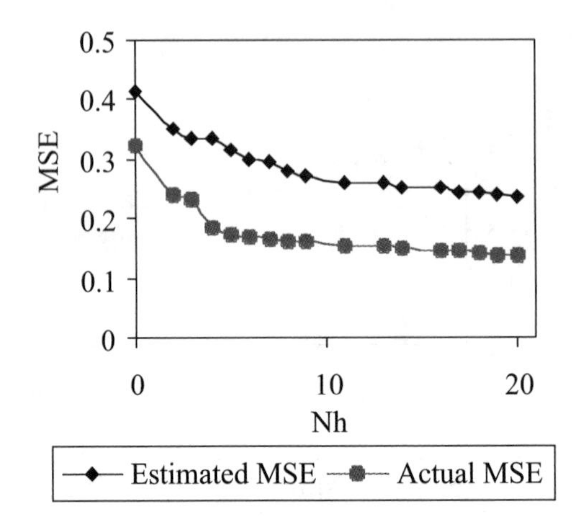

2.9 MLP sizing performance on `twod.tra`. (With permission from C-H Hsieh, M.T. Manry, and H. Chandrasekaran, Near optimal flight load synthesis using neural networks, NNSP '99, *IEEE*, 1999.)

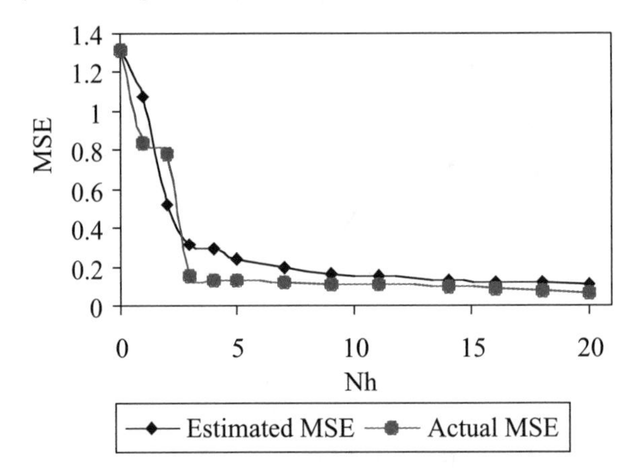

2.10 MLP sizing performance on `parabolic.tra`. (With permission from C-H Hsieh, M.T. Manry, and H. Chandrasekaran, Near optimal flight load synthesis using neural networks, NNSP '99, *IEEE*, 1999.)

2.4.1 Bounds on Estimation Error

CRMAP bounds [16] have been shown to provide lower bounds on neural network testing error [17, 18]. Specifically, let the neural network error E be defined as

$$E \equiv \sum_{i=1}^{M} E(i) \tag{2.31}$$

where $E(i)$ denotes the error for the ith output parameter and M denotes the number of outputs, as in Section 2.2. E and $E(i)$ denote training error or testing error, depending upon the situation. The CRMAP bound on $var(\theta_i' - \theta_i)$, the variance of the error between the ith output θ_i and the ith output's estimate θ_i', is denoted by B_i. Therefore,

$$\begin{aligned} E(i) &\geq B_i \\ E &\geq \sum_{i=1}^{M} B_i \,. \end{aligned} \tag{2.32}$$

When we have equality in Equation (2.32), the estimates are usually optimal. This section shows the details of how CRMAP bounds are calculated from training data.

2.4.2 Obtaining the Bounds

This subsection describes how to calculate the $M \times M$ MAP Fisher information matrix (FIM) [16], given statistics on the training data. Let $\{\boldsymbol{x}_p, \boldsymbol{\theta}_p\}$ for $1 \leq p \leq N_v$ represent the training set for a neural network. Here, $\boldsymbol{x}_p$ represents the pth example of the N-dimensional random input vector $\boldsymbol{x}$, and $\boldsymbol{\theta}_p$ represents the pth example of the M-dimensional random parameter vector $\boldsymbol{\theta}$.

Elements of the $M \times M$ MAP FIM, $\boldsymbol{J}^{MAP}$ are defined as

$$\begin{aligned} J_{ij}^{MAP} &= E_\theta\left[J_{ij}^{MLE}\right] + E_\theta\left[\frac{\partial \Lambda^{AP}}{\partial \theta_i}\frac{\partial \Lambda^{AP}}{\partial \theta_j}\right] \\ J_{ij}^{MLE} &= E_n\left[\frac{\partial \Lambda^{MLE}}{\partial \theta_i}\frac{\partial \Lambda^{MLE}}{\partial \theta_j}\right] \end{aligned} \tag{2.33}$$

where $E_\theta[\cdot]$ denotes expected value over the parameter vector $\boldsymbol{\theta}$ and $E_n[\cdot]$ denotes expected value over the noise, where $\Lambda^{MAP} = \ell n(p_{\theta|x}(\boldsymbol{\theta}|\boldsymbol{x}))$, $\Lambda^{MLE} = \ell n(p_{x|\theta}(\boldsymbol{x}|\boldsymbol{\theta})$, and $\Lambda^{AP} = \ell n(p_\theta(\boldsymbol{\theta}))$. Assume that the elements $x(k)$ of $\boldsymbol{x}$ are modeled as

$$x(k) = s(k) + n(k) \tag{2.34}$$

where the elements $s(n)$ and $n(n)$ are, respectively, elements of the signal and noise vectors $\boldsymbol{s}$ and $\boldsymbol{n}$, respectively. $\boldsymbol{s}$ is a deterministic function of the parameter vector $\boldsymbol{\theta}$. The $N \times N$ covariance matrix of $\boldsymbol{x}$ or $\boldsymbol{n}$ is denoted by $\boldsymbol{C}_{nn}$. The elements of $\boldsymbol{J}^{MAP}$ in Equation (2.33) can now be evaluated as:

$$\begin{aligned} E_\theta\left[J_{ij}^{MLE}\right] &= E_\theta\left[\left(\frac{\partial \boldsymbol{s}}{\partial \theta_i}\right)^T C_{nn}^{-1}\left(\frac{\partial \boldsymbol{s}}{\partial \theta_j}\right)\right] \\ E_\theta\left[\frac{\partial \Lambda^{AP}}{\partial \theta_i}\frac{\partial \Lambda^{AP}}{\partial \theta_j}\right] &= d_\theta(i,j) \end{aligned} \tag{2.35}$$

where $\boldsymbol{C}_\theta$ denotes the $M \times M$ covariance matrix of the M-dimensional parameter vector $\boldsymbol{\theta}$ and $d_\theta(i,j)$ denotes an element of $\boldsymbol{C}_\theta^{-1}$. Let $\left(J^{MAP}\right)^{ij}$ denote an element of $\left(\boldsymbol{J}^{MAP}\right)^{-1}$. Then [59],

$$var\left(\theta_i' - \theta_i\right) \geq \left(\boldsymbol{J}^{MAP}\right)^{ii} \tag{2.36}$$

where θ_i' can be any estimate of θ_i. The B_i in Equation (2.32) are the $\left(\boldsymbol{J}^{MAP}\right)^{ii}$ of Equation (2.36). In order to calculate the log-likelihood functions and the CRMAP lower bounds on the variance of the parameter estimates, a statistical model of the input vector $\boldsymbol{x}$ is required. This model consists of a deterministic expression for the signal vector $\boldsymbol{s}$ in terms of the parameter vector $\boldsymbol{\theta}$, the joint probability density of the additive noise vector $\boldsymbol{n}$. In most applications however, the signal model is unknown and bound calculation is not possible. One approach to this problem is to create an approximate signal model from the given training data.

2.4.2.1 Signal Modeling

Given the training patterns for our estimator, we want to find the signal component model and noise probability density function (pdf). We make the following assumptions, which make this problem solvable.

A1. The unknown, exact signal model of Equation (2.34) can be written in vector form as

$$\boldsymbol{x}_p = \boldsymbol{s}_p + \boldsymbol{n}_p \tag{2.37}$$

where $\boldsymbol{x}_p$ and $\boldsymbol{\theta}_p$ are defined as before, $\boldsymbol{s}_p$ denotes the pth example of $\boldsymbol{s}$, and $\boldsymbol{n}_p$ denotes the noise component of $\boldsymbol{x}_p$.

A2. The elements $\theta(k)$ of θ are statistically independent of $\boldsymbol{n}$.

A3. The noise vector $\boldsymbol{n}$ has independent elements with a jointly Gaussian pdf.

A4. The mapping $\boldsymbol{s}(\boldsymbol{\theta})$ is one-to-one.

2.4.2.2 Basic Approach

From Equation (2.35) and the above assumptions, we need to find a differentiable deterministic input signal model $\boldsymbol{s}(\boldsymbol{\theta})$ and the statistics of $\boldsymbol{n}$ and $\boldsymbol{\theta}$. Our first step is to rewrite the signal model of Equation (2.37) as:

$$\boldsymbol{x}_p = \boldsymbol{s'}_p + \boldsymbol{n'}_p \tag{2.38}$$

where $\boldsymbol{s'}_p$ and $\boldsymbol{n'}_p$ denote approximations to $\boldsymbol{s}_p$ and $\boldsymbol{n}_p$, respectively. Noting that $\boldsymbol{s}$ is a function of the desired output $\boldsymbol{\theta}$, we propose to approximate the nth element of $\boldsymbol{s}_p$ with an inverse neural net,

$$s'_p(n, \mathbf{w}) = \sum_{k=1}^{N_u} w_O(n, k) f_p(k, \mathbf{w}_i) \tag{2.39}$$

for $1 \le n \le N$, where $w_o(n, k)$ denotes the coefficient of $f_p(k, \boldsymbol{w}_i)$ in the approximation to $s_p(n)$, $f_p(k, \boldsymbol{w}_i)$ is the kth input or hidden unit in the network, $\boldsymbol{w}_i$ is a vector of weights connecting the input layer to a single hidden layer, and N_u is the number of units feeding the output layer. This is an inverse network in the sense that desired outputs are mapped back to inputs. The vector $\boldsymbol{w}$ is the concatenation of the input weight vector $\boldsymbol{w}_i$ with the output weight vector whose elements are $w_o(n, k)$. Note that $f_p(k, \boldsymbol{w}_i)$ can represent a multinomial function of parameter vector $\boldsymbol{\theta}$ in a functional link network [60], or a hidden unit output in an MLP or radial basis function network [22]. Because of the capabilities of the MLP [2, 61] and PLN for approximating derivatives, either of these networks would be a good choice for generating $\boldsymbol{s'}$.

Before we can find the neural net weight vector $\boldsymbol{w}$ in Equation (2.39), we must have an error function to minimize during training, which includes desired output vectors. Since we want $\boldsymbol{s'}_p$ to approximate $\boldsymbol{s}_p$, the natural choice for the desired output is $\boldsymbol{s}_p$. Because $\boldsymbol{s}_p$ is unavailable, we can try using $\boldsymbol{x}_p$ as the desired output vector, which yields the error function for the nth output node,

$$E_x(n) = \frac{1}{N_v} \sum_{p=1}^{N_v} \left[x_p(n) - s'_p(n, \boldsymbol{w}) \right]^2 . \tag{2.40}$$

The hope is that by minimizing $E_x(n)$ with respect to $\boldsymbol{w}$, we are simultaneously approximately minimizing

$$E_s(n) = \frac{1}{N_v} \sum_{p=1}^{N_v} \left[s_p(n) - s'_p(n, \boldsymbol{w}) \right]^2 . \tag{2.41}$$

The signal model is determined from the noisy data by using a gradient approach, such as back propagation (BP) or output weight optimization (OWO) [27, 29], to minimize $E_x(n)$ with respect to

w, whose elements are denoted by $w(m)$. The gradient of $E_n(n)$ is

$$\frac{\partial E_x(n)}{\partial w(m)} = \frac{-2}{N_\nu} \sum_{p=1}^{N_\nu} \left[x_p(n) - s'_p(n, \boldsymbol{w}) \right]^2 \frac{\partial s'_p(n, \boldsymbol{w})}{\partial w(m)} . \tag{2.42}$$

An MLP network for obtaining the signal model is shown in Figure 2.11.

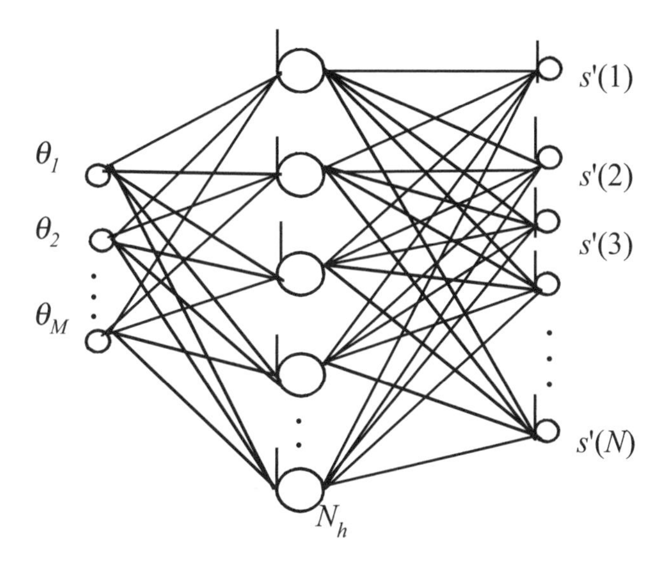

2.11 Inverse network for signal modeling. (With permission from C-H Hsieh, M.T. Manry, and H. Chandrasekaran, Near optimal flight load synthesis using neural networks, NNSP '99, *IEEE*, 1999.)

Given a model $\boldsymbol{s'}_p$ for the deterministic signal component, and given the noisy input vectors $\boldsymbol{x}_p$, we get $\boldsymbol{n'}_p$ from Equation (2.38) as:

$$\boldsymbol{n'}_p = \boldsymbol{x}_p - \boldsymbol{s'}_p .$$

The mean vector and covariance matrix of the noise component are then estimated as

$$\begin{aligned} \boldsymbol{m'}_n &= \frac{1}{N_\nu} \sum_{p=1}^{N_\nu} \boldsymbol{n'}_p \\ \boldsymbol{C'}_{nn} &= \frac{1}{N_\nu} \sum_{p=1}^{N_\nu} \left(\boldsymbol{n'}_p - \boldsymbol{m'}_p\right) \left(\boldsymbol{n'}_p - \boldsymbol{m'}_p\right)^T . \end{aligned} \tag{2.43}$$

In addition to the statistics of $\boldsymbol{n}$, calculation of the CRMAP bounds in Equation (2.33) requires knowledge of the statistics of $\boldsymbol{\theta}$, which are

$$\begin{aligned} \boldsymbol{m'}_\theta &= \frac{1}{N_\nu} \sum_{p=1}^{N_\nu} \boldsymbol{\theta}_p \\ \boldsymbol{C'}_\theta &= \frac{1}{N_\nu} \sum_{p=1}^{N_\nu} \left(\boldsymbol{\theta}_p - \boldsymbol{m'}_\theta\right) \left(\boldsymbol{\theta}_p - \boldsymbol{m'}_\theta\right)^T . \end{aligned} \tag{2.44}$$

When $\boldsymbol{\theta}$ is non-Gaussian, it is still possible to calculate good bounds using our approach. Theoretical justification of this can be found in the literature [62, 63].

2.4.3 Convergence of the Method

Since we are minimizing $E_x(n)$ rather than $E_s(n)$ in the previous subsection, it is not clear that $\mathbf{s'}_p$ is a good model for $\mathbf{s}_p$. This subsection analyzes the convergence of the gradient of $E_x(n)$ to the gradient of $E_s(n)$ with the following theorem.

THEOREM 2.3 *Assume that the training of the input weight vector $\mathbf{w}_i$ is stopped after iteration number N_{it}, which is fixed and bounded, and that training of the output weights $w_o(n,k)$ is allowed to proceed. Then, in the limit as N_v approaches infinity, $\partial E_x(n)/\partial w(m) = \partial E_s(n)/\partial w(m)$.*

PROOF 2.1 The proof is divided into three parts.

Part 1: Energy of the Gradient Noise
Continuing Equation (2.42), we get

$$\begin{aligned} \frac{\partial E_x(n)}{\partial w(m)} &= \frac{-2}{N_v}\sum_{p=1}^{N_v}\left[s_p(n) - s'_p(n,w)\right]\frac{\partial s'_p(n,w)}{\partial w(m)} + e_{nm} \\ &= \frac{\partial E_s(n)}{\partial w(m)} + e_{nm} \qquad (2.45) \\ e_{nm} &= -\frac{2}{N_v}\sum_{p=1}^{N_v} n_p(n)\frac{\partial s'_p(n,w)}{\partial w(m)} . \end{aligned}$$

Using the fact that

$$E\left[n_p(n)n_q(n)\right] = \sigma_n^2 \cdot \delta(p-q)$$

the mean square of the noise term e_{nm} is evaluated as

$$\begin{aligned} E\left[e_{nm}^2\right] &= \frac{4}{N_v^2}\sum_{p=1}^{N_v}\sum_{q=1}^{N_v} E\left[n_p(n)n_q(n)\right]\frac{\partial s'_p(n,\mathbf{w})}{\partial w(m)}\frac{\partial s'_q(n,\mathbf{w})}{\partial w(m)} \\ &= \frac{4\sigma_n^2}{N_v^2}\sum_{p=1}^{N_v}\left(\frac{\partial s'_p(n,\mathbf{w})}{\partial w(m)}\right)^2 \qquad (2.46) \\ &= \frac{4\sigma_n^2 \cdot E_m}{N_v} \end{aligned}$$

where E_m is the average energy of the partial derivative of $s'_p(n,w)$ with respect to $\mathbf{w}(m)$ and σ_n^2 is the variance of $n(n)$. It remains for us to show that E_m is bounded.

Part 2: E_m for the Output Weight Case
First, assume that $w(m)$ corresponds to an output weight $w_o(n,j)$. Then, from Equation (2.39),

$$\begin{aligned} \frac{\partial s'_p(n,\mathbf{w})}{\partial w(m)} &= f_p\left(j,\mathbf{w}_i\right) \\ E_m &= \frac{1}{N_v}\sum_{p=1}^{N_v} f_p^2\left(j,\mathbf{w}_i\right) . \qquad (2.47) \end{aligned}$$

Here, the terms in E_m are input or hidden unit activations or multinomial combinations of inputs for the functional link case. These terms in E_m are bounded if the inverse network inputs (θ_i) are bounded and if the activation functions are bounded. If Equation (2.39) represents a functional link net, bounding of the inputs produces bounding of the multinomials $f_p(j, \boldsymbol{w}_i)$ and E_m.

Part 3: E_m for the Input Weight Case
Assume that $w(m)$ corresponds to a weight $w_i(u)$ which feeds unit number j (a hidden unit). Then

$$\begin{aligned}\frac{\partial s'_p(n, \boldsymbol{w})}{\partial w(m)} &= w_o(n, j)\frac{\partial f_p\,(j, \boldsymbol{w}_i)}{\partial w_i(u)} \\ E_m &= \frac{w_o^2(n, j)}{N_v} \cdot \sum_{p=1}^{N_v} \left(\frac{\partial f_p\,(j, \boldsymbol{w}_i)}{\partial w_i(u)}\right)^2 . \qquad (2.48)\end{aligned}$$

Functional link nets have no input weight vector and have $E_m = 0$ for the input weight case. For MLP and RBF networks, consider the two factors in E_m separately. In the second factor, partials of $f_p(j, \boldsymbol{w}_i)$ are bounded for bounded activations. Unfortunately, the $w_o^2(n, j)$ term in the first factor in Equation (2.48) is not bounded in general. Its value depends upon the initial weight values, the training method chosen, and the learning parameters. This can be solved by stopping the training of the input weight vector $\boldsymbol{w}_i$ after a bounded number of iterations, N_{it}. After this iteration, the vector $\boldsymbol{w}$ consists only of elements $w_o(n, k)$, and we are left with only the output weight case.

In the limit, $E_x(n)$ and $E_s(n)$ have equal derivatives and the same local and global minima. In the next section, we develop CRMAP lower bounds on output error variance given a data file, using the approach described in this section.

2.5 Designing Networks for Flight Load Synthesis

This section describes the use of MLPs for near-optimal helicopter flight load synthesis (FLS), which is the process of estimating mechanical loads during helicopter flight using cockpit measurements. The sizing, bounding, and training methods described earlier are applied here.

2.5.1 Description of Data Files

The FLS data were obtained from the M430 flight load level survey conducted in Mirabel, Canada, in 1995 by Bell Helicopter Textron. The input features, which are measurements available in the cockpit, include: (1) CG F/A load factor, (2) CG lateral load factor, (3) CG normal load factor, (4) pitch attitude, (5) pitch rate, (6) roll attitude, (7) roll rate, (8) yaw rate, (9) corrected airspeed, (10) rate of climb, (11) longitudinal cyclic stick position, (12) pedal position, (13) collective stick position, (14) lateral cyclic stick position, (15) main rotor mast torque, (16) main rotor mast rpm, (17) density ratio, (18) F/A acceleration, transmission, (19) lateral acceleration, transmission, (20) vertical acceleration, transmission, (21) left-hand forward pylon link, (22) right-hand forward pylon link, (23) left-hand aft pylon link, and (24) right-hand aft pylon link.

The desired outputs are the helicopter loads which are the strains on mechanical parts. These are not available in a typical helicopter, but need to be estimated throughout the flight so that mechanics know when to replace critical parts. During test flights, the loads are measured by strain gauges which are temporarily attached to the critical parts. The desired output loads are as follows: (1) fore/aft cyclic boost tube oscillatory axial load (OAL), (2) lateral cyclic boost tube OAL, (3) collective boost tube OAL, (4) main rotor (MR) pitch link OAL, (5) MR mast oscillatory perpendicular bending smoothed time average (STA), (6) MR yoke oscillatory beam bending STA, (7) MR blade oscillatory beam bending STA, (8) MR yoke oscillatory chord bending STA, and (9) resultant mast bending STA position.

Three training data files were produced. File `F17.dat` used features 1 through 17 and all 9 output loads. File `F20.dat` used features 1 through 20 and all nine output loads. File `F24.dat` used features 1 through 24 and all 9 output loads.

2.5.2 CRMAP Bounds and Sizing of FLS Neural Nets

After training signal models for the three data files, as in Section 2.4, we estimated CRMAP bounds on E, as in Equation (2.32). The bound values for 17, 20, and 24 inputs were 0.30×10^8, 0.29×10^8, and 0.22×10^8, respectively. In obtaining the bounds, the 17- and 20-input signal models were produced by training PLNs. The discontinuous nature of the PLN's mapping causes no difficulties when calculating derivatives for the CRMAP bounds. For the 24-input data in file `F24.dat`, the signal modeling was done with an MLP.

After finding the bounds on the training error E, we ran the sizing algorithm of Section 2.3 on each of the three data files. Figures 2.12, 2.13, and 2.14 show the forecast training errors vs. the

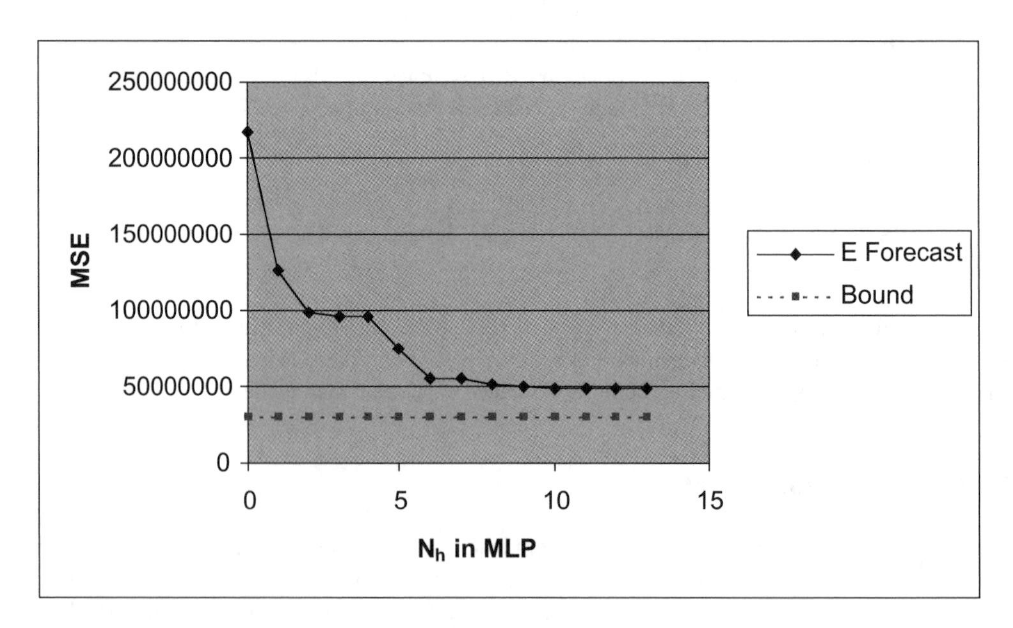

2.12 Forecast training error and bound vs. N_h for `F17.dat`. (With permission from C-H Hsieh, M.T. Manry, and H. Chandrasekaran, Near optimal flight load synthesis using neural networks, NNSP '99, *IEEE*, 1999.)

numbers of hidden units for each data file. Also shown are the CRMAP bounds on E. Ideally, we want to see the forecast E curve cross the bound curve. We can then use a number of hidden units equal to the value of N_h at the intersection, as mentioned earlier. As seen in Figure 2.12, however,

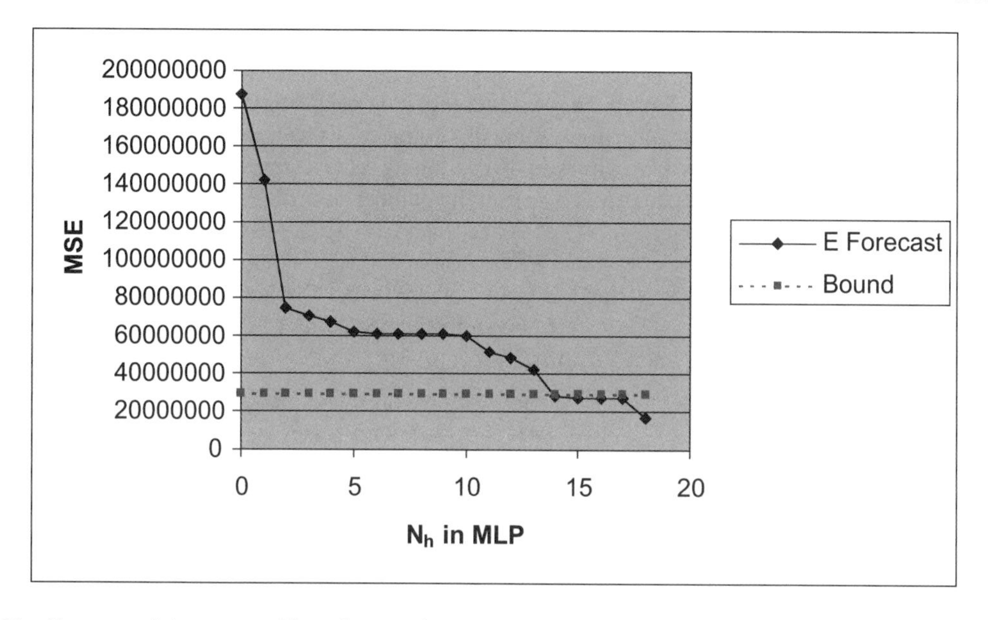

2.13 Forecast training error and bound vs. N_h for F20.dat. (With permission from C-H Hsieh, M.T. Manry, and H. Chandrasekaran, Near optimal flight load synthesis using neural networks, NNSP '99, *IEEE*, 1999.)

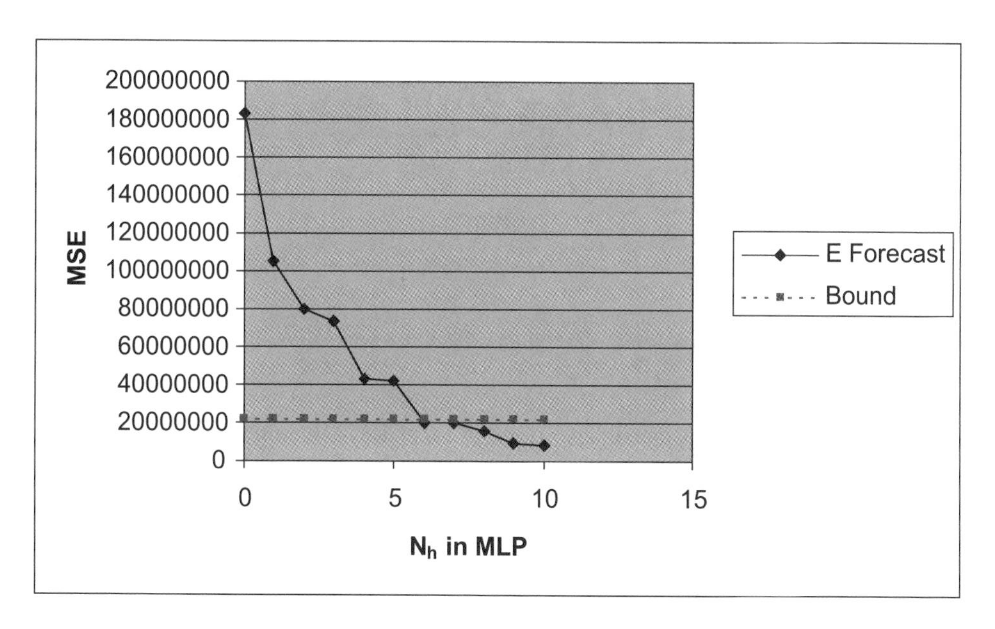

2.14 Forecast training error and bound vs. N_h for F24.dat. (With permission from C-H Hsieh, M.T. Manry, and H. Chandrasekaran, Near optimal flight load synthesis using neural networks, NNSP '99, *IEEE*, 1999.)

the curves do not intersect, so we arbitrarily chose N_h to be 13 for file `F17.dat`. From Figures 2.13 and 2.14, we easily chose N_h to be 13 and 6, respectively, for files `F20.dat` and `F24.dat`.

The methodology used here often works when valid CRMAP bounds can be calculated. When the bounds or the forecast E curve are in error, as when the forecast E is much greater than or much less than the bound, one can look for a place on the forecast E curve where the curve flattens out.

2.5.3 MLP Training and Testing Results

Lacking testing data for the FLS problem, we randomly split each original FLS data set into two subsets: one for training and the other for testing. By doing so, we can evaluate the generalization ability of the designed FLS networks. The ratio of the training set to testing set sizes is approximately 1 to 4. The number of training patterns is 896, and the number of testing patterns is 3849. For the new training data sets, the structures 17-13-9, 20-13-9, and 24-6-9 are used for 17-input, 20-input, and 24-input files, respectively, as suggested by the results in the previous subsection. All networks were trained for 50 iterations. The testing MSEs are obtained every five iterations during the training process. The training and testing results are shown in Figures 2.15–2.17, which are, respectively, for files `F17.dat`, `F20.dat`, and `F24.dat`.

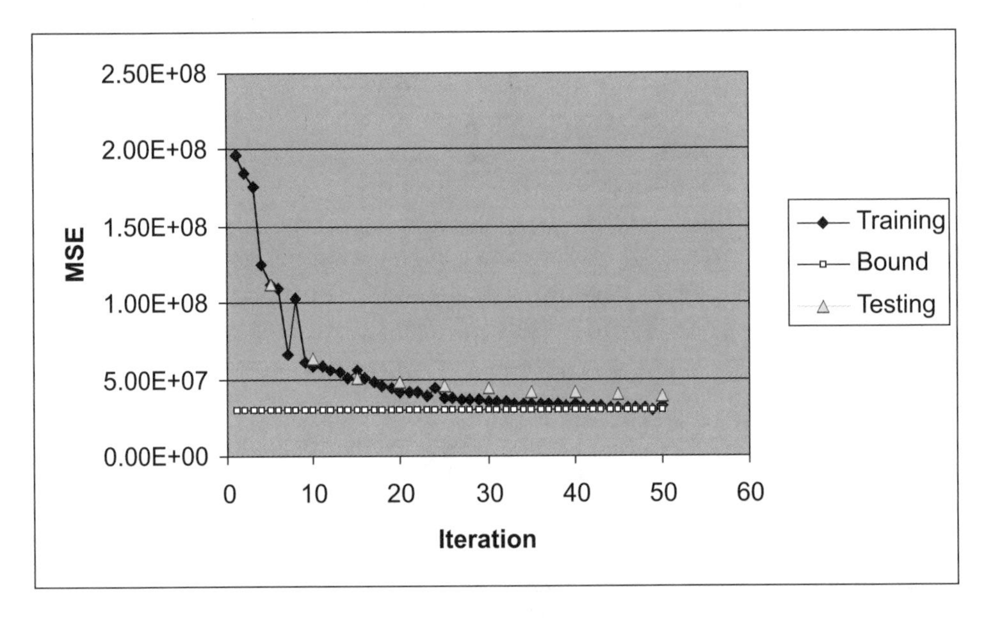

2.15 MLP training and testing errors and bound vs. iteration number for `F17.dat`. (With permission from C-H Hsieh, M.T. Manry, and H. Chandrasekaran, Near optimal flight load synthesis using neural networks, NNSP '99, *IEEE*, 1999.)

Figures 2.12–2.17 show that the sizing algorithm and CRMAP bounds have provided us with fairly good estimates of the required network sizes. Also, the OWO-HWO training algorithm has provided near optimal MLP networks for the FLS application.

2.6 Conclusions

This chapter has presented three algorithms which help researchers apply the MLP to signal processing problems. First, the chapter described a fast, convergent training method for the MLP. Next, a theory that relates MLP and PLN training errors through their pattern storages was described, and a sizing algorithm for the MLP was developed. We provided numerical results that demonstrate the effectiveness of the sizing algorithm. Lastly, this chapter described a method for calculating CRMAP bounds on neural network testing error.

We successfully applied the three algorithms to MLPs used for flight load synthesis in helicopters and showed that MLPs could be trained to attain near-optimal performance, as indicated by CRMAP bounds.

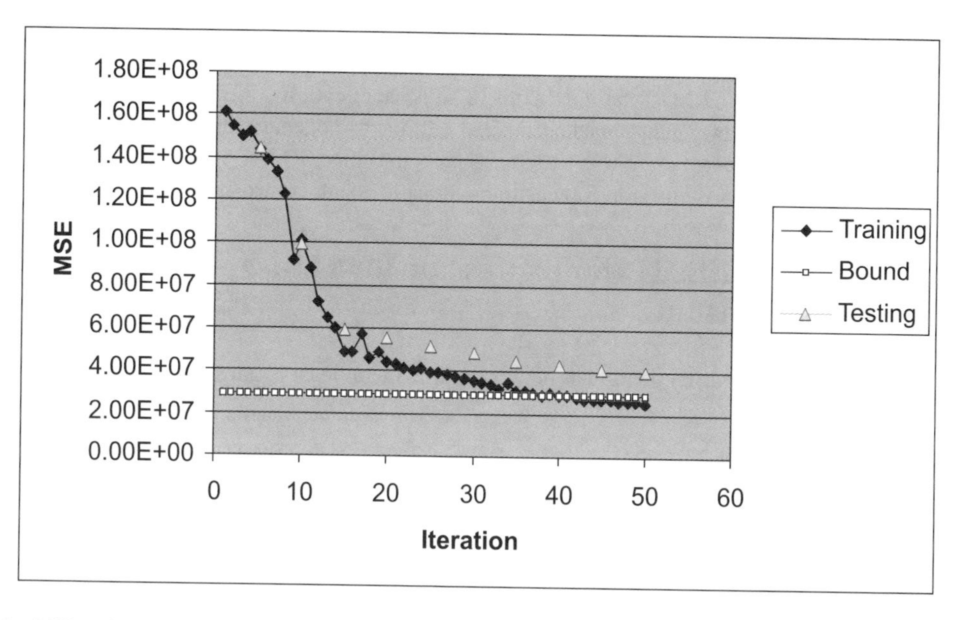

2.16 MLP training and testing errors and bound vs. iteration number for `F20.dat`. (With permission from C-H Hsieh, M.T. Manry, and H. Chandrasekaran, Near optimal flight load synthesis using neural networks, NNSP '99, *IEEE*, 1999.)

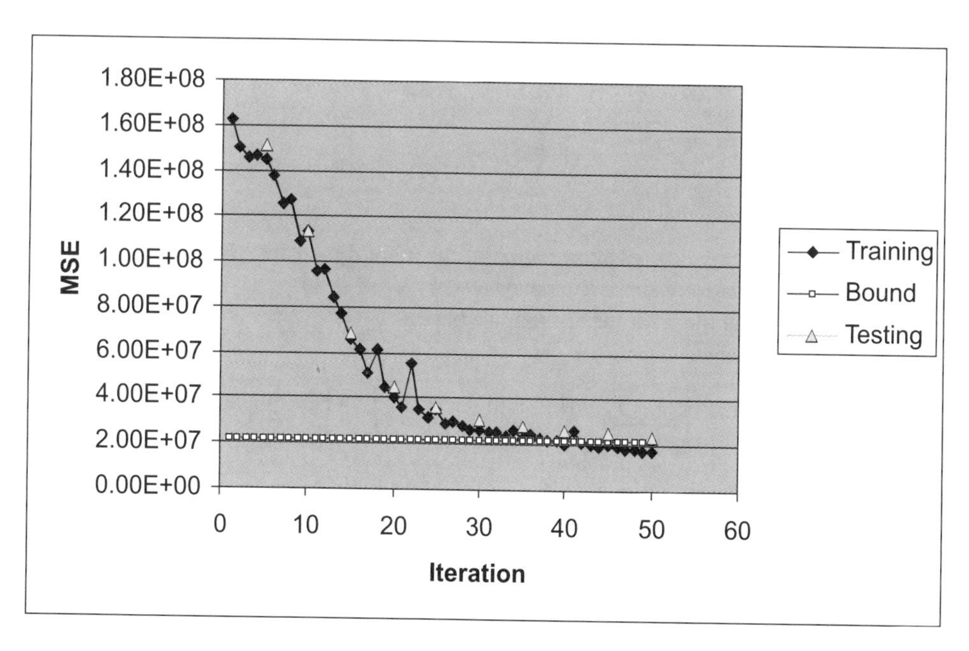

2.17 MLP training and testing errors and bound vs. iteration number for `F24.dat`. (With permission from C-H Hsieh, M.T. Manry, and H. Chandrasekaran, Near optimal flight load synthesis using neural networks, NNSP '99, *IEEE*, 1999.)

Much work remains to be done. Training algorithms for the MLP need to be improved further. For example, currently available training algorithms cannot reliably train an MLP to memorize, even when the network is large enough to do so. If we can design optimal PLNs, the Akaike procedure [9] could be applied to the PLN's E vs. N_h curve to forecast the testing error performance of MLPs. Although the estimated CRMAP bounds work in some applications, they can be calculated only when the signal model, mapping noiseless desired outputs to noiseless inputs, is one-to-one. The bounds should be extended to non one-to-one cases so that the CRMAP bounds can be applied to more data sets, such as those used in forecasting applications and control.

Appendix: Simplified Error Expression for a Linear Network Trained with LMS Algorithm

The mean square error (MSE) of a linear network trained with least mean squares (LMS) algorithm is given by

$$E = \frac{1}{N_v} \sum_{p=1}^{N_v} \left[t_p - \left(\sum_{j=1}^{N+1} w(j) \cdot x_p(j) \right) \right]^2 . \tag{A.1}$$

Taking the partial derivative of E with respect to $w(j)$, we obtain

$$\frac{\partial E}{\partial w(j)} = \frac{1}{N_v} \sum_{p=1}^{N_v} -2 \cdot \left[t_p - \sum_k w(k) \cdot x_p(k) \right] \cdot x_p(j) . \tag{A.2}$$

Setting this partial derivative equal to zero, we get

$$\sum_p t_p \cdot x_p(j) = \sum_k w(k) \left(\sum_p x_p(k) \cdot x_p(j) \right)$$

$$c(j) = \sum_{k=1}^{N+1} w(k) \cdot r(k, j) . \tag{A.3}$$

Here, $c(j)$ is an element of the cross-correlation vector $\boldsymbol{C}$ of dimension $(N+1)$, and $r(k, j)$ is an element of the autocorrelation matrix $\boldsymbol{R}$ of size $(N+1) \times (N+1)$.

Expanding the terms of the error expression, we have

$$E = \frac{1}{N_v} \left[\left(\sum_{p=1}^{N_v} t_p^2 \right) + \left(\sum_k \sum_j w(k) \cdot w(j) \cdot r(j, k) \right) - \left(2 \cdot \sum_j w(j) \cdot c(j) \right) \right] . \tag{A.4}$$

Substituting Equation (A.3) into Equation (A.4) we get a simplified expression for E:

$$E = \frac{1}{N_v} \left[\left(\sum_{p=1}^{N_v} t_p^2 \right) - \left(\sum_j w(j) \cdot c(j) \right) \right] \tag{A.5}$$

or, in vector, notation

$$E = \frac{1}{N_v} \left[\left(\sum_{p=1}^{N_v} t_p^2 \right) - \boldsymbol{C}^T \cdot \boldsymbol{W} \right] . \tag{A.6}$$

From Equation (A.3), we can write in matrix form

$$\boldsymbol{R} \cdot \boldsymbol{W} = \boldsymbol{C} \tag{A.7}$$

where $\boldsymbol{W}$ is the weight vector of dimension $(N+1)$ and whose elements are $w(j)$.

The solution vector $\boldsymbol{W}$ is obtained as

$$\boldsymbol{W} = \boldsymbol{R}^{-1} \cdot \boldsymbol{C}\,. \tag{A.8}$$

Acknowledgments

This work was supported by the state of Texas through the Advanced Technology Program under grant number 003656-063. Sections 2.4 and 2.5 are reprinted, with permission, from *Proceedings of NNSP'99,* August 23–25, 1999, Madison, Wisconsin, pp. 535–544.

References

[1] K. Hornik, M. Stinchcombe, and H. White, Multilayer feedforward networks are universal approximators, *Neural Networks,* vol. 2, no. 5, pp. 359–366, 1989.
[2] K. Hornik, M. Stinchcombe, and H. White, Universal approximation of an unknown mapping and its derivatives using multilayer feedforward networks, *Neural Networks,* vol. 3, no. 5, pp. 551–560, 1990.
[3] S. Geman, E. Bienenstock, and R. Doursat, Neural networks and the bias/variance dilemma, *Neural Computation,* vol. 4, no. 1, pp. 1–58, 1992.
[4] T. Masters, *Practical Neural Network Recipes in C++,* Academic Press, New York, 1993.
[5] B. Fritzke, Growing cell structures—a self-organizing network for unsupervised and supervised learning, *Neural Networks,* vol. 7, no. 9, pp. 1441–1460, 1994.
[6] J.N. Hwang, S.S. You, S.R. Lay, and I.C. Jou, Cascade correlation learning: a projection pursuit learning perspective, *IEEE Transactions on Neural Networks,* vol. 7, no. 2, pp. 278–289, 1996.
[7] B. Hassibi, D.G. Stork, and G.J. Wolff, Optimal brain surgeon and general network pruning, *1993 IEEE International Conference on Neural Networks,* pp. 293–299, March 1993.
[8] Z.J. Yang, Hidden-layer size reducing for multilayer neural networks using the orthogonal least-squares method, *Proceedings of the 1997 36th IEEE Society of Instrument and Control Engineers (SICE) Annual Conference,* pp. 1089–1092, July 1997.
[9] H. Akaike, A new look at the statistical model identification, *IEEE Transactions on Automatic Control,* vol. AC-19, no. 6, pp. 716–723, 1974.
[10] D.B. Fogel, An information criterion for optimal neural network selection, *IEEE Transactions on Neural Networks,* vol. 2, no. 5, pp. 490–497, 1991.
[11] V. Volterra, Sopra le funzioni che dipendono da altre funzioni, *Rend. Regia Academia dei Lince,* 20 Sem., pp. 97–105, 141–146, 153–158, 1887.
[12] K.I. Kim and E.J. Powers, A digital method of modeling quadratically nonlinear systems with a general random input, *IEEE Transactions on Acoustics, Speech, and Signal Processing,* vol. 36, no. 11, pp. 1758–1769, 1988.
[13] S.M. Kang and L.O. Chua, A global representation of multi-dimensional piecewise-linear functions, *IEEE Transactions on Circuits and Systems,* vol. 25, pp. 938–940, 1978.
[14] C. Kahlert and L.O. Chua, A generalized canonical piecewise-linear representation, *IEEE Transactions on Circuits and Systems,* vol. 37, no. 4, pp. 373–383, 1990.
[15] W. Finnof, F. Hergert, and H.G. Zimmermann, Improving model selection by nonconvergent methods, *Neural Networks,* vol. 6, pp. 771–783, 1993.
[16] H.L. Van Trees, *Detection, Estimation, and Modulation Theory*—Part I, John Wiley & Sons, New York, 1968.

[17] S.J. Apollo, M.T. Manry, L.S. Allen, and W.D. Lyle, Optimality of transforms for parameter estimation, *Conference Record of the 26th Annual Asilomar Conference on Signals, Systems, and Computers,* vol. 1, pp. 294–298, October 1992.

[18] M.T. Manry, S.J. Apollo, and Q. Yu, Minimum mean square estimation and neural networks, *Neurocomputing,* vol. 13, pp. 59–74, 1996.

[19] M.T. Manry, C.H. Hsieh, and H. Chandrasekaran, Near-optimal flight load synthesis using neural nets, *Neural Networks for Signal Processing IX, Proceedings of the 1999 IEEE Signal Processing Society Workshop,* pp. 535–544, August 1999.

[20] D.E. Rumelhart, G.E. Hinton, and R.J. Williams, Learning internal representations by error propagation, in *Parallel Distributed Processing,* Vol. 1, D.E. Rumelhart and J.L. McClelland, Eds., MIT Press, Cambridge, MA, 1986.

[21] S.E. Fahlman and C. Lebiere, The cascade correlation learning architecture, *Neural Information Processing Systems,* vol. 2, pp. 524–532, 1990.

[22] S. Chen, C.F.N. Cowan, and P.M. Grant, Orthogonal least squares learning algorithm for radial basis function networks, *IEEE Transactions on Neural Networks,* vol. 2, pp. 302–307, 1991.

[23] I.I. Sakhnini, M.T. Manry, and H. Chandrasekaran, Iterative improvement of trigonometric networks, *International Joint Conference on Neural Networks* (IJCNN'99), July 1999.

[24] S.A. Barton, A matrix method for optimizing a neural network, *Neural Computation,* vol. 3, no. 3, pp. 450–459, 1991.

[25] M.A. Sartori and P.J. Antsaklis, A simple method to derive bounds on the size and to train multilayer neural networks, *IEEE Transactions on Neural Networks,* vol. 2, no. 4, pp. 467–471, 1991.

[26] M.S. Chen and M.T. Manry, Back-propagation representation theorem using power series, *Proceedings of the International Joint Conference on Neural Networks,* San Diego, vol. 1, pp. 643–648, 1990.

[27] M.T. Manry et al., Fast training of neural networks for remote sensing, *Remote Sensing Reviews,* vol. 9, pp. 77–96, 1994.

[28] J.N. Hwang, S.R. Lay, M. Maechler, R.D. Martin, and J. Schimert, Regression modeling in back-propagation and projection pursuit learning, *IEEE Transactions on Neural Networks,* vol. 5, no. 3, pp. 342–353, 1994.

[29] H.H. Chen, M.T. Manry, and H. Chandrasekaran, A neural network training algorithm utilizing multiple sets of linear equations, *Neurocomputing,* vol. 25, no. 1–3, pp. 55–72, 1999.

[30] A. Gopalakrishnan, X. Jiang, M.S. Chen, and M.T. Manry, Constructive proof of efficient pattern storage in the multilayer perceptron, *Conference Record of the 27th Asilomar Conference on Signals, Systems, and Computers,* vol. 1, pp. 386–390, Nov. 1993.

[31] P. Werbos, Backpropagation: past and future, *Proceedings of the IEEE International Conference on Neural Networks,* pp. 343–353, 1988.

[32] M.H. Fun and M.T. Hagan, Levenberg–Marquardt training for modular networks, *Proceedings of the 1996 IEEE International Conference on Neural Networks,* vol. 1, pp. 468–473, 1996.

[33] M.T. Hagan and M.B. Menhaj, Training feedforward networks with the Marquardt algorithm, *IEEE Transactions on Neural Networks,* vol. 5, no. 6, pp. 989–993, 1994.

[34] S. Kollias and D. Anastassiou, An adaptive least squares algorithm for the efficient training of artificial neural networks, *IEEE Transactions on Circuits and Systems,* vol. 36, no. 8, pp. 1092–1101, 1989.

[35] S. McLoone, M.D. Brown, G. Irwin, and G. Lightbody, A hybrid linear/nonlinear training algorithm for feedforward neural networks, *IEEE Transactions on Neural Networks,* vol. 9, no. 9, pp. 669–683, 1998.

[36] R. Battiti, First- and second-order methods for learning: between steepest descent and Newton's method, *Neural Computation,* vol. 4, no. 2, pp. 141–166, 1992.

[37] T. Masters, *Neural, Novel and Hybrid Algorithms for Time Series Prediction,* John Wiley & Sons, New York, 1995.

[38] R.S. Scalero and N. Tepedelenlioglu, A fast new algorithm for training feedforward neural networks, *IEEE Transactions on Signal Processing,* vol. 40, no. 1, pp. 202–210, 1992.

[39] K.K. Kim and M.T. Manry, A complexity algorithm for estimating the size of the multilayer perceptron, *Conference Record of the 29th Annual Asilomar Conference on Signals, Systems, and Computers,* vol. 2, pp. 899–903, October 1995.

[40] H. Chandrasekaran, Analysis and convergent design of piecewise linear networks, Ph.D. dissertation, The University of Texas at Arlington, May 2000.

[41] A.J. Miller, *Subset Selection in Regression,* Chapman and Hall, New York, 1990.

[42] W.J. Kennedy, Jr. and J.E. Gentle, *Statistical Computing,* Marcel Dekker, New York, 1980.

[43] K. Fukunaga, *Introduction to Statistical Pattern Recognition,* Academic Press, New York, 1990.

[44] A. Papoulis, *Probability, Random Variables, and Stochastic Processes,* McGraw-Hill, New York, 1991.

[45] I.S. Gradshteyn and I.M. Ryzhik, *Tables of Integrals, Series, and Products,* A. Jeffrey, Ed., translated from Russian by Scripta Technica, 1994.

[46] H. Chandrasekaran and M.T. Manry, Convergent design of a piecewise linear neural network, *Proceedings of the International Joint Conference on Neural Networks,* July 1999.

[47] S. Subbarayan, K. Kim, M.T. Manry, V. Devarajan, and H. Chen, Modular neural network architecture using piecewise linear mapping, *Conference Record of the 30th Asilomar Conference on Signals, Systems, and Computers,* vol. 2, pp. 1171–1175, 1996.

[48] R. Gnanadesikan, *Methods for Statistical Data Analysis of Multivariate Observations,* John Wiley & Sons, New York, 1997.

[49] H. Späth, *Cluster Analysis Algorithms for Data Reduction and Classification of Objects,* Ellis Horwood Limited, Chichester, U.K., 1980.

[50] G.M. Furnival and R.W. Wilson, Regression by leaps and bounds, *Technometrics,* vol. 16, no. 4, pp. 499–511, 1974.

[51] W.L.G. Koontz, P.M. Narendra, and K. Fukunaga, Branch and bound clustering algorithm, *IEEE Transactions on Computers,* vol. C-24, no. 9, pp. 908–915, 1975.

[52] W.H. Press, S.A. Teukolsky, W.T. Vetterling, and B.P. Flannery, *Numerical Recipes in C: The Art of Scientific Computing,* Cambridge University Press, New York, 1992.

[53] S.R. Searle, *Matrix Algebra Useful for Statistics,* John Wiley & Sons, New York, 1982.

[54] A. Lapedes and R. Farber, Nonlinear signal processing using neural networks: prediction and system modeling, Technical Report LA-UR-87-2662, Los Alamos National Laboratory, Los Alamos, NM, 1987.

[55] Delve: Data for Evaluating Learning in Valid Experiments, URL: http://www.cs.utoronto.ca/~delve/data/datasets.html.

[56] A.K. Fung, Z. Li, and K.S. Chen, Backscattering from a randomly rough dielectric surface, *IEEE Transactions on Geoscience and Remote Sensing,* vol. 30, no. 2, pp. 356–369, 1992.

[57] Proben1, URL: ftp://ftp.ira.uka.de/pub/neuron/proben1.tar.gz.

[58] Y. Oh, K. Sarabandi, and F.T. Ulaby, An empirical model and an inversion technique for radar scattering from bare soil surfaces, *IEEE Transactions on Geoscience and Remote Sensing,* vol. 30, no. 2, pp. 370–381, 1992.

[59] S.J. Apollo, M.T. Manry, L.S. Allen, and W.D. Lyle, Optimality of transforms for parameter estimation, *Conference Record of the 26th Annual Asilomar Conference on Signals, Systems, and Computers,* vol. 1, pp. 294–298, October 1992.

[60] Y.H. Pao, *Adaptive Pattern Recognition and Neural Networks,* Addison-Wesley, New York, 1989.

[61] W. Liang, M.T. Manry, Q. Yu, S.J. Apollo, M.S. Dawson, and A.K. Fung, Bounding the performance of neural network estimators, given only a set of training data, *Conference Record of the 28th Annual Asilomar Conference on Signals, Systems, and Computers,* vol. 2, pp. 912–916, November 1994.

[62] M.T. Manry, C.H. Hsieh, M.S. Dawson, A.K. Fung, and S.J. Apollo, Cramer Rao maximum a posteriori bounds on neural network training error for non-Gaussian signals and parameters, *International Journal of Intelligent Control and Systems,* vol. 1, no. 3, pp. 381–391, 1996.

[63] C.H. Hsieh, M.T. Manry, and H.H. Chen, Cramer Rao maximum *a posteriori* bounds for a finite number of non-Gaussian parameters, *Conference Record of the 30th Asilomar Conference on Signals, Systems, and Computers,* vol. 2, pp. 1161–1165, November 1996.

3

Radial Basis Functions

Andrew D. Back
Windale Technologies

3.1 Introduction

In classical signal processing, we typically consider a single-input single-output (SISO) discrete-time, causal, infinite-dimensional, time-invariant dynamical system described by

$$y(t) = \sum_{k=p}^{\infty} h(k)x(t-k) + v(t) \tag{3.1}$$

where $\{h(k)\} \in \Re^1$ is a weighting sequence, $\{v(t)\}$ is a disturbance sequence of zero-mean, independent and identically distributed random variables, and $x(t)$ is the input to the model at time t.

A common task is to approximate $\{y(t)\}$ by a finite-dimensional signal model, producing an output $\{\hat{y}(t)\}$ and resulting in an output prediction error sequence $\{e(t)\}$.[1] The system output $y(t)$ can be represented as

$$y(t) = \hat{y}(t) + e(t) \; . \tag{3.2}$$

[1] $e(t)$ is different from $v(t)$ because we assume that the plant could be infinite-dimensional and the signal model is finite-dimensional.

0-8493-2359-2/01/$0.00+$1.50

In Equation (3.1), for $p = 0$, we arrive at the classical system identification problem. For $p = 1$ and $x(t) = y(t)$, the problem is the one-step-ahead time series prediction. Hence, in this framework, both system modeling (identification) and time series prediction can be accommodated.

In this framework, there is a basic assumption that a linear relationship exists between inputs and outputs and can be described by a linear transfer function. A linear discrete time time-invariant signal model is given by

$$\hat{y}(t) = G(z, \theta)x(t) \tag{3.3}$$

$$= \varphi'(t)\theta \tag{3.4}$$

where $G(z, \theta)$ is a linear transfer function, z is the usual shift operator defined as $z^{-1}x(t) \triangleq x(t-1)$, and θ is some parameter vector. $\varphi(t)$ is a vector dependent only on the system input $x(t)$ and its past values and past values of the system output $y(t)$. The prime operator $'$ represents the vector or matrix transpose.

A finite impulse response (FIR) signal model is defined as

$$G(z, \theta) = \sum_{i=0}^{M} b_i z^{-i} \tag{3.5}$$

where $\theta = [b_0, \ldots, b_M]'$, $\varphi(t) = [x(t), \ldots, x(t - M)]'$.

In some applications, where a linear relationship between the input variables and the outputs of the model does not exist, it is necessary to use a nonlinear model.

In contrast to conventional linear signal processing models, we consider the use of a class of nonlinear model, written as

$$\hat{y}(t) = F[x(t), x(t-1), \ldots, x(t - M)] \tag{3.6}$$

where F is a nonlinear functional, mapping the input sequence $\{x(t)\}$ to the output $\hat{y}(t)$. Throughout this book, a range of nonlinear models are considered, each with different properties and subsequent advantages and disadvantages.

This chapter considers radial basis function (RBF) networks. Radial basis function networks originated from multidimensional interpolation models and have been described in the literature since 1985 [5, 24, 32, 33].

A radial basis function network can be described as a parametrized model used to approximate an arbitrary function by means of a linear combination of basis functions. RBF networks belong to the class of kernel function networks where the inputs to the model are passed through kernel functions which limit the response of the network to a local region in the input space for each kernel or basis function. The output from each basis function is weighted and summed and possibly offset by some amount to provide the output of the network.

Since there is such a wide range of nonlinear models, it is valid to ask "What are the relative advantages of using a radial basis function network?" Why, indeed, should we consider using an RBF network from among the many other neural network types offered? To answer this question, it is helpful to consider the reason why simple linear models have been popularly used.

Linear time-invariant transfer functions have the advantage of properties such as:

- Understandability
- Ease of parametrization (or training) for FIR (finite impulse response) models
- Low computational complexity

- Low memory requirements[2]
- Stability
- Robustness

A significant factor in the widespread success of linear models is their advantage in each of the above areas. The recent introduction of multilayer sigmoidal neural networks and the back-propagation algorithm has led to widespread interest in nonlinear models. However, a significant amount of research over the last 10 years has been aimed at improving the performance of multilayer neural networks in the performance areas listed above.

While there has been much success in developing nonlinear neural network models, in particular multilayer networks trained by back-propagation, researchers, and practitioners have found that, in some cases, it can be difficult to train a multilayer network and obtain good performance without resorting to sophisticated algorithms.

The main reason it is difficult to train a multilayer network is that such networks are nonlinear in the parameters. This means that learning algorithms typically use gradient descent approaches as a means of solving the nonlinear optimization problem.

It is desirable, therefore, to obtain models which can overcome this problem of training. RBF networks do offer a means of avoiding exactly this problem. Later in the chapter, we describe learning algorithms for RBF networks and show how they can overcome the problem of training that normally occurs in multilayer networks.

This chapter explores the use of RBF networks in terms of basic theory, architectures, learning algorithms, and applications to signal processing. From this perspective, the user may wish to examine the literature in more depth where more advanced techniques are desired. As with most of the techniques presented in this book, there are a number of more advanced research topics which are beyond the scope of this work and, hence, are not discussed here. Hopefully, the material presented here will serve as an introduction to the use of RBF networks in signal processing applications.

3.2 Architecture

3.2.1 Overview

An RBF network generally consists of two weight layers — the hidden layer and the output layer. They can be described by the following equation:

$$y = w_0 + \sum_{i=1}^{n_h} w_i f\left(\|\mathbf{x} - \mathbf{c}_i\|\right) \tag{3.7}$$

where f are the radial basis functions, w_i are the output layer weights, w_0 is the output offset, $\mathbf{x}$ are the inputs to the network, $\mathbf{c}_i$ are the centers associated with the basis functions, n_h is the number of basis functions in the network, and $||\cdot||$ denotes the Euclidean norm.

Given the vector

$$\mathbf{x} = [x_1, \ldots, x_n]' \tag{3.8}$$

on $\Re^n$, the Euclidean norm on this space measures the size of the vector in a general sense and is

[2]This depends on the application. IIR (infinite impulse response) models may be considered when the memory complexity is a problem, although such models need stability checking to be included.

defined as

$$\begin{aligned} ||\mathbf{x}|| &= \left(\sum_{i=1}^{n} x_i^2\right)^{\frac{1}{2}} \\ &= \left(\mathbf{x}'\mathbf{x}\right)^{\frac{1}{2}} . \end{aligned} \tag{3.9}$$

The basic operation of an RBF network can be thought of as follows. Each input vector $\mathbf{x}$ passed to the network is shifted in $\Re^n$ space according to some stored parameters (the "centers") in the network. The Euclidean norm is computed for each of these shifted vectors $\mathbf{x} - \mathbf{c}_j$ for $j = 1, \ldots, n_h$. Each $\mathbf{c}_j$ is a vector with the same number of elements as the input vector $\mathbf{x}$. Note that there is one comparison or shifting operation for each $\mathbf{c}_j$ stored in the network, and one center is defined for each radial basis function in the network. Centers which are closest to the input data vector will have the smallest output, the limiting case being where a center exactly coincides with an input vector. In this case, the Euclidean distance is zero. Conversely, when the data are further away from a given center, the output will become larger. In that case, the Euclidean distance will also become large.

Now consider the action of the Gaussian basis function on the resulting outputs from the Euclidean distance measures. For data which are far away from the centers, the output from the corresponding basis functions will be small, approaching zero with increased distance. On the other hand, for data which are close to the centers, the output from the corresponding basis functions will be larger, approaching one with decreased distance.

Hence, radial basis function networks are able to model data in a local sense. For each input data vector, one or more basis functions provide an output. In the extreme case, one basis function is used for every input data vector, and the centers themselves are identical to the data vectors. Therefore, it is then a simple matter to map the output from the basis function to any required output value by means of the output layer weights.

3.2.2 Basis Functions

The nonlinear basis function f can be formed using a number of different functions. Some common examples include [35]:

- Gaussian function

$$f(x) = e^{\frac{-(x-c)^2}{r^2}} \tag{3.10}$$

  where $c \in \Re$ is the center of the basis function which has radius r. The Gaussian radial basis function monotonically decreases with distance from the center, as shown in Figure 3.1.

- Multiquadric (Figure 3.2)

$$f(x) = \left((x-c)^2 + r^2\right)^{1/2} \tag{3.11}$$

- Inverse multiquadric (Figure 3.3)

$$f(x) = \frac{\left((x-c)^2 + r^2\right)^{-1/2}}{r} \tag{3.12}$$

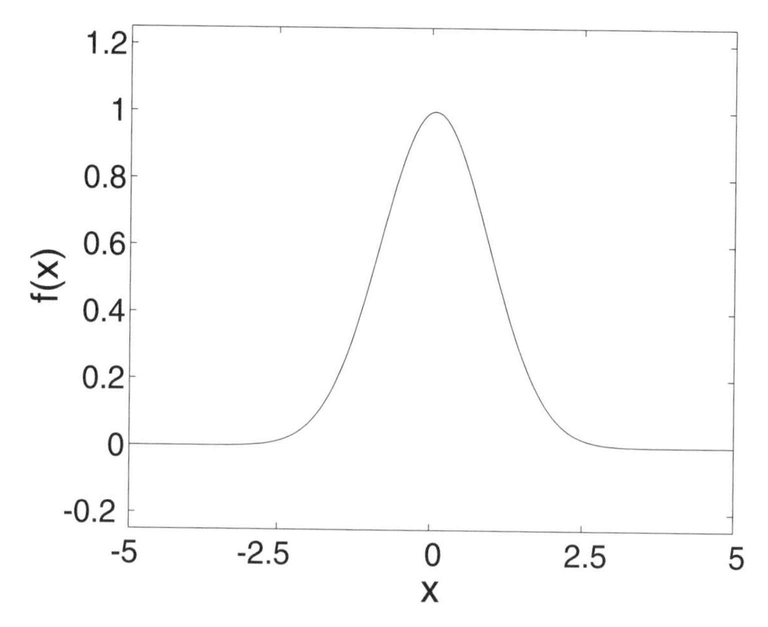

3.1 The Gaussian radial basis function with center $c = 0$ and radius $r = 1$.

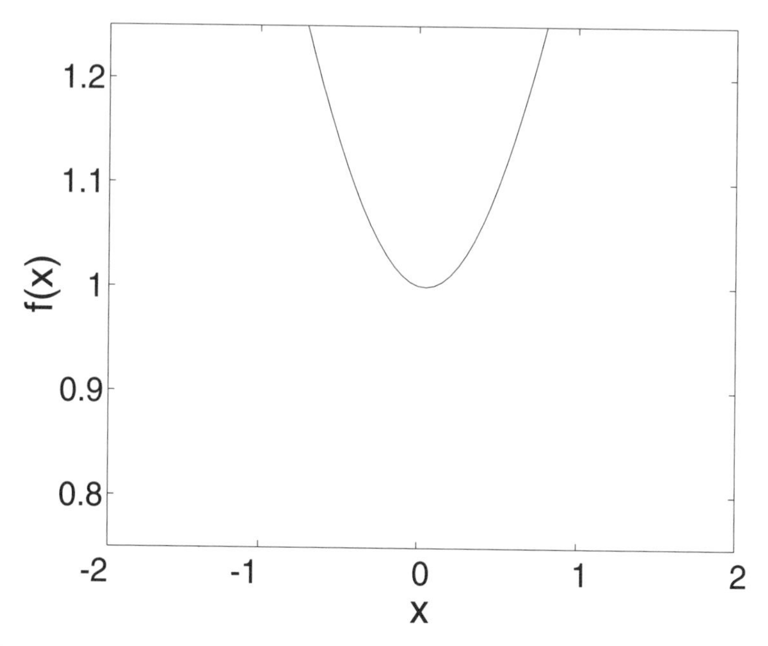

3.2 The multiquadric radial basis function with center $c = 0$ and radius $r = 1$.

- Cauchy function (Figure 3.4)

$$f(x) = \frac{\left((x-c)^2 + r^2\right)^{-1}}{r} \tag{3.13}$$

Clearly, it is possible to introduce other radial basis functions which will have similar properties to those described above. An interesting relationship that can be drawn between RBF networks and

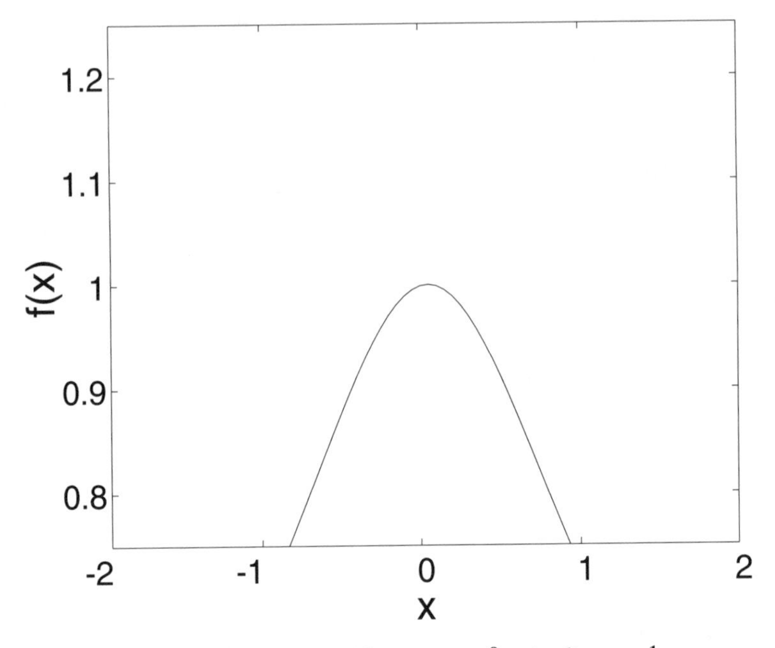

3.3 The inverse multiquadric radial basis function with center $c = 0$ and radius $r = 1$.

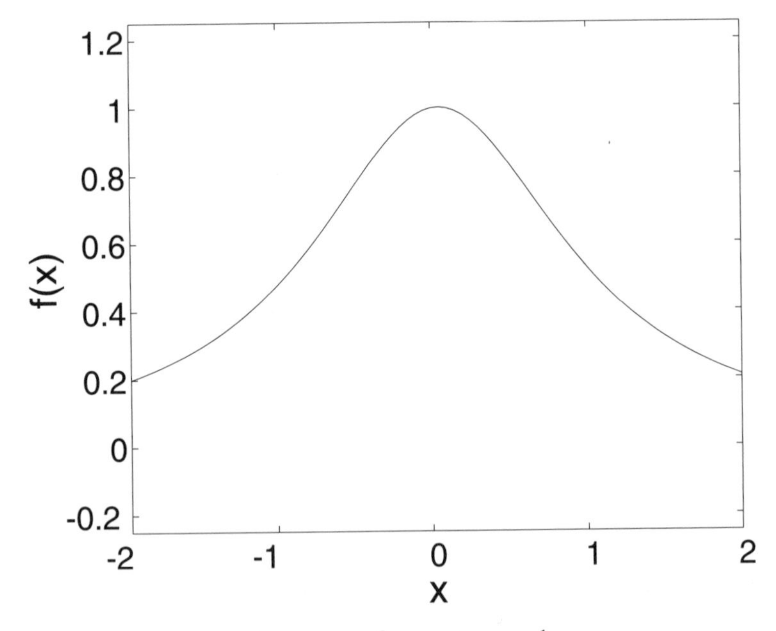

3.4 The Cauchy radial basis function with center $c = 0$ and radius $r = 1$.

probabilistic framework is that when a Gaussian basis function is used, the model can be viewed as a mixture of normal density functions. Such an approach is commonly used to approximate an unknown probability density function [35].

The choice of basis function may be dictated by particular implementation requirements or constraints, although from a theoretical perspective, the choice is arbitrary.[3] Possibly the most common choice for basis functions is the Gaussian which is used in this chapter.

3.2.3 Gaussian RBF Network

The Gaussian RBF network can be written using conventional time series notation as

$$y(t) = \mathbf{z}'(t)\mathbf{w} \tag{3.14}$$

where $\mathbf{w}$ is the output layer weight vector and $\mathbf{z}(t)$ is the basis function output vector at time t given, respectively, by

$$\begin{aligned}
\mathbf{w} &= \left[w_0, w_1, \ldots, w_{n_h}\right]' \\
\mathbf{z} &= \left[1, z_1(t), \ldots, z_{n_h}(t)\right]' \\
z_i(t) &= e^{\frac{-\|\mathbf{x}(t)-\mathbf{c}_i\|^2}{r_i^2}} \\
\mathbf{c}_i &= i\text{th basis function center vector} \\
r_i &= i\text{th basis function width.}
\end{aligned} \tag{3.15}$$

Note that z_i corresponds to the output from the ith basis function unit due to the input vector $\mathbf{x}(t)$ presented to the network at time t defined by

$$\mathbf{x}(t) = \left[x_1(t), \ldots, x_{n_h}(t)\right]' . \tag{3.16}$$

It is also possible to write the radial basis in vector notation for sequences of input and output data, as follows:

$$\mathbf{y} = \mathbf{Z}'\mathbf{w} \tag{3.17}$$

where

$$\begin{aligned}
\mathbf{y} &= [y_1, \ldots, y_m]' \\
\mathbf{Z} &= \left[\mathbf{z}_1', \ldots, \mathbf{z}_m'\right]' \\
\mathbf{z}_j &= \left[1, z_{j1}, \ldots, z_{jn_h}\right]' \qquad j = 1, \ldots, m \\
z_{ji} &= e^{\frac{-\|\mathbf{x}_j-\mathbf{c}_i\|^2}{r_i^2}} .
\end{aligned} \tag{3.18}$$

Here, z_{ji} corresponds to the output from the ith basis function unit due to the jth input vector $\mathbf{x}_j$, defined by

$$\mathbf{x}_j = \left[x_{j1}, \ldots, x_{jn_h}\right]' . \tag{3.19}$$

[3]The choice of basis function should, of course, be restricted to functions which have the characteristic "bump" shape in order to be used in this particular architecture. Functions which do not meet this requirement, e.g., polynomials, would dramatically change the properties of the network.

3.2.4 Example of How an RBF Network Works

As a simple example, consider the following two input RBF networks. Suppose there are four input data vectors, well separated in $\Re^4$:

$$\begin{aligned} \mathbf{x}_1 &= [0, 0]' \\ \mathbf{x}_2 &= [0, 10]' \\ \mathbf{x}_3 &= [10, 0]' \\ \mathbf{x}_4 &= [10, 10]' . \end{aligned} \tag{3.20}$$

The desired outputs for each of these inputs is:

$$\begin{aligned} \mathbf{d}_1 &= 3.5 \\ \mathbf{d}_2 &= 1.2 \\ \mathbf{d}_3 &= 4.7 \\ \mathbf{d}_4 &= 0.9 . \end{aligned} \tag{3.21}$$

We may choose the centers for each of the basis functions to be equal to the data vectors themselves. Hence we have

$$\begin{aligned} \mathbf{c}_1 &= [0, 0]' \\ \mathbf{c}_2 &= [0, 10]' \\ \mathbf{c}_3 &= [10, 0]' \\ \mathbf{c}_4 &= [10, 10]' . \end{aligned} \tag{3.22}$$

For convenience, we choose the radii of the basis functions to be unity, i.e., $r_i = 1, i = 1, \ldots, 4$. Consider the presentation of the first data vector to the network:

$$z_i = e^{\frac{-||\mathbf{x}_1 - \mathbf{c}_i||^2}{r_i^2}} \qquad i = 1, \ldots, 4 . \tag{3.23}$$

This results in the following basis function outputs

$$\begin{aligned} z_1 &= e^{-||\mathbf{x}_1 - \mathbf{c}_1||^2} \\ &= e^0 \\ &= 1 \end{aligned} \tag{3.24}$$

$$\begin{aligned} z_2 &= e^{-||\mathbf{x}_1 - \mathbf{c}_2||^2} \\ &= e^{-10} \\ &= 4.5 \times 10^{-5} \end{aligned} \tag{3.25}$$

$$z_3 = 4.5 \times 10^{-5} \tag{3.26}$$

$$z_4 = 4.5 \times 10^{-5} . \tag{3.27}$$

To obtain the desired outputs, in this case it is a simple matter to set the output layer weights equal to the desired values:

$$\begin{aligned} \mathbf{w}_1 &= 3.5 \\ \mathbf{w}_2 &= 1.2 \\ \mathbf{w}_3 &= 4.7 \\ \mathbf{w}_4 &= 0.9 . \end{aligned} \tag{3.28}$$

The most accurate means of setting the output layer weights comes from applying the least squares algorithm to the model. Hence we have

$$\mathbf{y} = \mathbf{Z}'\mathbf{w} \tag{3.29}$$

where

$$\mathbf{Z} = \left[1, \mathbf{z}_1', \ldots, \mathbf{z}_4'\right]' . \tag{3.30}$$

The least squares error between the desired outputs and the actual outputs is given by

$$\begin{aligned} \mathbf{J} &= \frac{1}{2}\mathbf{e}'\mathbf{e} \\ \mathbf{e} &= \mathbf{d} - \mathbf{y} \end{aligned} \tag{3.31}$$

where $\mathbf{e}$ is an $m \times 1$ error vector. The least squares solution to minimizing $\mathbf{J}$ is found as

$$\mathbf{w} = \left(\mathbf{Z}'\mathbf{Z}\right)^{-1}\mathbf{Z}'\mathbf{d} . \tag{3.32}$$

Using this approach, the weight vectors for the network can be found as

$$\begin{aligned} \mathbf{w}_1 &= 3.4997 \\ \mathbf{w}_2 &= 1.1996 \\ \mathbf{w}_3 &= 4.6997 \\ \mathbf{w}_4 &= 0.8996 . \end{aligned} \tag{3.33}$$

There have been other procedures developed for finding the centers, radii, and output layer weights in radial basis function networks which are considered in detail in a later section of this chapter. The preceding description, however, gives a basic understanding of the principles of operation in an RBF network.

3.3 Theoretical Capabilities

3.3.1 General

The key reason for using a nonlinear model is to be able to fit nonlinear curves in multidimensional space. Therefore, it is important to understand the capabilities of RBF networks in this context. This book is mainly concerned with the practical uses of neural networks for signal processing applications; however, we briefly review some of the major aspects concerning the theoretical modeling capabilities of RBF networks in the following sections.

3.3.2 Universal Approximation

A major result that has emerged in recent years, with the growth of interest in neural networks, is that a multilayer perceptron (MLP), with a single hidden layer, is capable of approximating any smooth nonlinear input-output mapping to an arbitrary degree of accuracy, provided that a sufficient number of hidden layer neurons is used [1, 9, 12, 17]. This is often referred to as the universal approximation theorem.

For radial basis function networks, universal approximation capabilities have been proven by Park and Sandberg [28, 29]. This property ensures that RBF networks will have at least the same theoretical capabilities as the well known multilayer networks with sigmoidal nonlinearities.

3.3.3 Best Approximation

The universal approximation property is shared by a rather wide range of model types. This property merely indicates that a generating function can be approximated but generally says nothing about the quality of the approximation. It is clear, however, that for solving practical problems, we may be more interested in which model is the best for a given task, as well as other issues such as the ease of training, robustness, memory complexity, or computational complexity.

Girosi and Poggio defined the property of best approximation as an extension of the universal approximation property [13]. In a given set of models, the model which most closely approximates the generating function by some defined distance measure is defined as having the property of best approximation. Thus, best approximation is an important attribute in choosing a model type.

Girosi and Poggio proved that RBF networks which have been derived in a regularization framework have this property. Most importantly, they showed that MLPs do not possess the best approximation property for the class of continuous functions on $\Re^n$, while RBF networks possess this property in a unique sense.

3.3.4 Comparison between RBF Networks and MLPs

Some work has been performed to show the relationship between RBF networks and MLPs. Essentially, if one considers that an MLP is a universal approximator, then it may approximate an RBF network and vice versa [23]. Maruyama, Girosi, and Poggio also showed [23] that for normalized inputs, MLPs can be considered to be RBF networks with irregular basis functions. In a similar vein, Jang and Sun showed the equivalence between RBF networks and fuzzy inference systems [20].

Although these results are of pedagogical interest, it should be kept in mind that, since both types of networks are capable of universation approximation capabilities, the main reason to consider one network over another is its learning performance on particular data sets.

3.4 Learning Algorithms

3.4.1 Overview

Training an RBF network consists of parametrizing the unknown parameters in a particular RBF network. Generally speaking, this means determining (1) the number of basis functions (hidden units), (2) centers and widths of each basis function, and (3) output layer weights. For some algorithms, these steps are carried out separately, while in others, all parameters are found simultaneously. Furthermore, different techniques can be mixed and matched for training the different parameters.

3.4.2 Determination of Centers

Some of the approaches for choosing centers are described below.

3.4.2.1 All Input Data

One of the simplest procedures for selecting the centers for radial basis functions was proposed by Michelli [24]. The approach is based on the notion of using one center for each data point to be approximated. For small data sets, this method is reasonable, but clearly it is not suitable for larger data sets. For finite data sets and where sufficient memory is available, this method may be a useful approach to consider. However, for online signal processing applications where the data increase with time, a more systematic approach to choose the centers is required.

3.4.2.2 Sampled Data

Another relatively simple method for choosing the centers is to randomly sample the data and use the sampled data as centers. By sufficiently oversampling the input space $\Re^n$, good performance may be obtained for some types of problems. In general, however, the success of this approach depends on matching the sampling distribution with the specific requirements of the underlying function to be approximated.

To work well, the sampling should take place in a way which allows the data to be properly approximated. This means more basis functions should be used in regions of the space where the function to be approximated is highly nonlinear or the underlying function has regions of greatest complexity, or on the class boundaries.

If the sampling is inadequate or has incorrect distribution as required to approximate the underlying function, then more units than required are placed in some regions, while too few are placed in others. An additional problem is that if the centers are too close together, then problems of numerical ill-conditioning can occur [7].

It may not be possible to know the required distribution of centers *a priori* to adequately approximate the underlying function. Hence, the performance of this approach is highly problem dependent. To give satisfactory performance, a better approach would be to estimate the centers from the data.

3.4.2.3 Subset Selection

Chen, Cowan, and Grant derived a systematic method of training radial basis functions in the following manner [7]. In contrast to the two-stage approach of selecting the RBF centers and then training the output layer weights, the method they described can be viewed as a one-stage approach. They proposed that choosing the RBF centers can be likened to subset model selection where the aim is to choose a subset of centers from a larger set of candidates. More specifically, they suggested that an orthogonal least squares (OLS) method can be employed as a forward regression procedure by treating the centers as the regressors. The initial set may be the total set of data points or some larger set of centers obtained by some means.

The basic approach to finding the RBF parameters using this approach follows the same initial approach as the least squares method:

1. Determine centers c_i $i = 1 \ldots n$.
2. Form a regression model.

The regression model can be obtained as follows:

$$\mathbf{y} = \mathbf{Z}'\mathbf{w} \tag{3.34}$$

where $\mathbf{Z}$ is the regression matrix given by

$$\mathbf{Z} = \begin{bmatrix} 1 & z_{11} & \cdots & z_{1n_h} \\ \vdots & \vdots & \cdots & \\ 1 & z_{m1} & \cdots & z_{mn_h} \end{bmatrix}. \tag{3.35}$$

The set of equations above permits a least squares approach to solve for the unknown parameter vector $\mathbf{w}$. It is generally assumed that the error vector $\mathbf{e}$ is uncorrelated with the regression matrix $\mathbf{Z}$. However, due to the structure of the model, the elements of the regression vector may be correlated. It is widely recognized that improved performance may be obtained by decorrelating the regression vector in a least squares problem. Methods such as Gram–Schmidt orthogonalization[4] [3] or the

[4]Note that for Gaussian random vectors, orthogonalization is identical to decorrelation.

Housholder transformation [14] can be used to orthogonalize the regression vector.

The orthogonalization process is generally defined by

$$\mathbf{Z} = \mathbf{QS} \tag{3.36}$$

where $\mathbf{Q}$ is an $m + 1 \times n_h$ orthogonal matrix with orthogonal columns $\mathbf{q}_i$ such that

$$\mathbf{G} = \mathbf{Q}'\mathbf{Q} \tag{3.37}$$

and $\mathbf{S}$ is a square $n_h \times n_h$ upper triangular matrix obtained by application of the selected orthogonalization algorithm. The matrix $\mathbf{G}$ is diagonal. Hence, in place of Equation (3.34) we may write a new forward model based on the orthogonal regression vector as

$$\mathbf{y} = \mathbf{Qb}\,. \tag{3.38}$$

The parameter vector $\mathbf{b}$ is given by

$$\mathbf{b} = \mathbf{G}^{-1}\mathbf{Q}'\mathbf{d}\,. \tag{3.39}$$

3.4.2.4 k-means Clustering

Moody and Darken proposed an RBF network in which the basis functions were tuned by k-means clustering [25]. They considered the issue of training the RBF network and compared the conventional back-propagation style training algorithm[5] and a hybrid learning approach.

Moody and Darken found that RBF networks can be trained in a more efficient manner than conventional multilayer networks using the back-propagation algorithm. The reason for this is that instead of using the back-propagation (BP) algorithm to adjust all the weights in the network at each update stage, the locally tuned nature of the RBF network means that it is possible to adjust only a smaller number of RBF units and their associated weights. More specifically, Moody and Darken suggested that the units to be processed at any given update stage can be determined by partitioning the input space using an adaptive grid such as that proposed by Omohundro [27]. Then, only those units with centers which are close to the current input, i.e., within the specified partition, will be updated. Another aspect of training which should be well recognized is that the BP algorithm is a method of nonlinear optimization and is subject to problems of poor convergence properties and high computational and memory cost.

Interestingly, Moody and Darken found that this locally tuned approach can be "defeated" by the back-propagation algorithm. They found that unless a local adaptive algorithm is specifically employed, the use of back-propagation can cause some RBF units which are in a given partition to move out of the partition. In this manner, the local nature of the network is defeated.

In contrast to using the conventional back-propagation algorithm, a hybrid learning algorithm was proposed by Moody and Darken, consisting of the following steps:

1. Determine the centers and widths using a self-organizing (bottom-up) approach such that they are placed maximally over the regions where the data lies. To determine the centers, Moody and Darken propose the k-means clustering algorithm [22]. In this case, the data is clustered into k regions and the centers are determined as the Euclidean centers of each cluster of data. The widths of each basis function can be determined by using a k-nearest-neighbor algorithm.
2. Determine the output weights using the usual LMS rule. Note that the learning function at this stage is linear in the parameters.

---

[5] That is, adjusting the weights of the network in the direction of the instantaneously estimated negative gradient of a specified error function that is the difference between the output(s) of the network and some desired value for the output(s).

3.4.2.5 Constructive Learning

The approach proposed by Moody and Darken offers good performance in many situations; however, in some circumstances, the performance may be less than ideal. In particular, the k-means algorithm will position the centers near the peak density regions of the data. However, some problems require the centers in other areas, such as the boundaries between class types. The data may be quite sparse in the class boundary regions. As such, the resulting network may have poor performance [11].

For classification problems, a better solution than k-means is to use the class labels to determine the centers. An algorithm based on this approach was proposed by Fritzke and was termed "supervised growing cells structures" [11].

The algorithm proceeds as follows:

1. Instantiate a small RBF network.
2. Train the network.
3. Determine where a new RBF unit should be inserted from the errors on the training set.
4. Repeat until errors are small enough.

The insertion of units in the third step will occur in regions of the space where misclassifications occur. Hence, Fritzke suggests the insertion of new units between the unit which corresponds to the maximum error and its nearest topological neighbors. The center c_{new} of the new unit is then given by

$$c_{\text{new}} = \frac{1}{2}(c_i + c_{i+1}) \tag{3.40}$$

where c_i and c_{i+1} correspond to the centers of the two selected units. The output weights of the new unit are obtained by interpolating the existing weights of the neighboring units. The remaining connections are determined to provide minimal disruption to the existing network. In practice, Frizke found that this approach gave good performance and demonstrated it by means of several experiments. For the two-spirals problem, the RBF network learned the required decision boundaries in 180 epochs, and, using a benchmark test set of points [2], 100% classification accuracy was obtained.

Another method of constructive learning for RBF networks was proposed by Platt [30]. He called this method the "resource allocation" network (RAN). In general terms, the RAN classifies each input data vector as easy or hard. For input data vectors which are not near any stored vectors (hard), the network allocates a new unit. Otherwise, the network adjusts the existing parameters. Experimental results showed that this particular type of RBF network was capable of learning to predict the Mackey–Glass time series to a similar degree of accuracy as an RBF network but with about 10 times fewer weights. The RAN learned for this problem was as compact as back-propagation but required much less computation to achieve similar performance.

3.4.2.6 Supervised Learning

One of the primary advantages of RBF networks is the ability to determine the centers by some means other than back-propagation, and, therefore, they only require a simple least squares algorithm to train the output layer weights. However, some researchers have proposed the use of supervised learning to train the centers [31, 42].

Poggio and Girosi proposed the use of gradient descent algorithms to determine the centers of RBF networks and termed the resulting approach generalized radial basis functions (GRBF) [31]. Wettschereck and Dietterich applied the GRBF model with a modified conjugate-gradient version of back-propagation to the classic NETtalk problem [39]. The aim of the NETtalk problem is to learn the mapping from each individual letter in a word to a phoneme and a stress. They found that the use of GRBFs improved the performance significantly compared to the regular RBF network, leading to a direct accuracy improvement of around 17%. To obtain best generalization performance, the use of supervised learning to determine centers appears to have considerable merit. The issue of training time vs. generalization performance is an issue that needs to be considered in practical applications.

3.4.2.7 Support Vector Machines

Support vector machines (SVMs) offer an extremely powerful method of deriving efficient models for multidimensional function approximation and classification [8, 41]. Recently, support vector machines have been proposed for choosing radial basis function centers and weights [6, 38]. The guiding principle behind support vector machines is to fix the empirical risk (or the training set error) associated with an architecture and then minimize the generalization error [40]. This is achieved by obtaining a classifier with minimal VC dimension, which implies low expected probability of generalization errors.

SVMs can be used to classify linearly and nonlinearly separable data. They can be used as nonlinear classifiers and regression machines by mapping the input space to a high-dimensional feature space. The method by which support vector machines can be used for constructing RBF networks requires some explanation, which is given below.

Consider an m-dimensional input vector $\mathbf{x} = [x_1, \ldots, x_m]' \in X \subset \mathcal{R}^m$ and a one-dimensional output $y \in \{-1, 1\}$. Let there exist n training vectors (x_i, y_i) $i = 1, \ldots, n$. A hyperplane capable of performing a linear separation of the training data is described by

$$\mathbf{w}'\mathbf{x} + b = 0 \tag{3.41}$$

where $\mathbf{w} = [w_1 w_2 \ldots w_m]'$, $\mathbf{w} \in W \subset \mathcal{R}^m$.

Suppose we have the following classes,

$$y_i \left[\mathbf{w}'\mathbf{x}_i + b\right] \geq 1 \quad i = 1, \ldots, n \tag{3.42}$$

where $y \in [-1, 1]$. One way in which we can constrain the hyperplane is to observe that on either side of the hyperplane, we may have $\mathbf{w}'\mathbf{x} + b > 0$ or $\mathbf{w}'\mathbf{x} + b < 0$. By considering two points on opposite sides of the hyperplane, the canonical hyperplane is found by maximizing the margin

$$p(\mathbf{w},b) = \min_{i;y_i=1} d(\mathbf{w},b;\mathbf{x}_i) + \min_{j;y_j=1} d\left(\mathbf{w},b;\mathbf{x}_j\right) \tag{3.43}$$

$$= \frac{2}{\|\mathbf{w}\|} . \tag{3.44}$$

This implies that the minimum distance between two classes i and j is at least $\frac{2}{\|\mathbf{w}\|}$ [15, 37]. Hence, an optimization function which must be minimized to obtain canonical hyperplanes is

$$J(\mathbf{w}) = \frac{1}{2} \|\mathbf{w}\|^2 . \tag{3.45}$$

Normally, to find the parameters, we would minimize the training error and place no constraints on $\mathbf{w}, b$. However, in this case, we seek to satisfy the inequality in Equation (3.42). Thus, to obtain a classifier with optimally separating hyperplanes, we introduce the Lagrangian:

$$L(\mathbf{w},b,\alpha) = \frac{1}{2} \|\mathbf{w}\|^2 - \sum_{i=1}^{n} \alpha_i \left(y_i \left[\mathbf{w}'\mathbf{x}_i + b\right] - 1\right) \tag{3.46}$$

where α_i are the Lagrange multipliers and $\alpha_i > 0$. The solution is found by maximizing L with respect to α_i and minimizing it with respect to the primal variables $\mathbf{w}$ and b [37].

To determine the specific coefficients of the optimal hyperplane specified by $(\mathbf{w}_0, b_0)$, we perform some manipulation of the equations to obtain

$$L_D(\mathbf{w},b,\alpha) = \sum_{i=1}^{n} \alpha_i - \frac{1}{2}\sum_{i=1}^{n}\sum_{j=1}^{n} \alpha_i \alpha_j y_i y_j \left(\mathbf{x}_i' \mathbf{x}_j\right) . \tag{3.47}$$

It is necessary to maximize the dual form of the Lagrangian to obtain the required Lagrange multipliers. With reference to Equation (3.42), there will only be some training vectors $(\mathbf{x}_i, y_i)$ for which the equality holds true. These training vectors are called support vectors.

Since we have the Karush–Kühn-Tucker (KKT) conditions that $\alpha_{0i} > 0$, $i = 1, \ldots, n$, and that given by Equation (3.42), from the resulting Lagrangian in Equation (3.46), we may write a further KKT condition

$$\alpha_{0i}\left(y_i\left[\mathbf{w}_0'\mathbf{x}_i + b_0\right] - 1\right) = 0 \quad i = 1, \ldots, n . \tag{3.48}$$

Hence, we have

$$\mathbf{w}_0 = \sum_{i \subset S} \alpha_{0i} \mathbf{x}_i y_i \tag{3.49}$$

where S is the set of all support vectors in the training set.

To obtain the Lagrangian multipliers α_{0i}, we need to maximize Equation (3.47) only over the support vectors, subject to the defined constraints. This is a quadratic programming problem and can be readily solved [40]. Having obtained the Lagrangian multipliers, the weights $\mathbf{w}_0$ can be found from Equation (3.49).

A nonlinear classifier can be obtained using support vector machines by the inner product $\mathbf{x}_i'\mathbf{x}$, where $i \subset S$, the set of support vectors. However, it is not necessary to use the explicit input data to form the classifer. Instead, all that is needed is to use this inner product between the support vectors and the vectors of the feature space [40]. That is, by defining the kernel

$$K\left(\mathbf{x}_i, \mathbf{x}_j\right) = \mathbf{x}_i'\mathbf{x}_j \tag{3.50}$$

a nonlinear decision function can be obtained, which is defined as

$$f(\mathbf{x}) = \text{sgn}\left[\sum_{i=1}^{n_h} y_i \alpha_i \cdot K\left(\mathbf{x}_i, \mathbf{x}_j\right) + b\right] . \tag{3.51}$$

Based on Mercer's theorem, it is possible to introduce a variety of kernel functions, including one for radial basis functions [37, 40]:

$$K\left(\mathbf{x}_i, \mathbf{x}_j\right) = e^{\frac{-\|\mathbf{x}_i - \mathbf{x}_j\|^2}{r_j^2}} . \tag{3.52}$$

The RBF decision function (Equation (3.51)) can be found by maximizing the functional

$$L_D(\mathbf{w},b,\alpha) = \sum_{i=1}^{n} \alpha_i - \frac{1}{2}\sum_{i=1}^{n}\sum_{j=1}^{n} \alpha_i \alpha_j y_i y_j K\left(\mathbf{x}_i, \mathbf{x}_j\right) . \tag{3.53}$$

3.4.3 Selecting the Number of Basis Functions

There are a number of approaches proposed in the literature for selecting the number of basis functions (or hidden units) in an RBF network. Some of them are briefly reviewed here.

3.4.3.1 Orthogononalization and Error Variance Minimization

The OLS method described in Section 3.4.2.3 may also be used to select the number of basis functions used. The approach in this case is to measure the reduction in the error variance by the addition of each additional basis function [7]. Specifically, it was shown that the reduction in error by introducing each additional basis function is given by

$$e_i = \frac{b_i^2 \mathbf{q}_i' \mathbf{q}_i}{\mathbf{d}'\mathbf{d}} \qquad 1 \leq i \leq n_h . \tag{3.54}$$

The Gram–Schmidt algorithm for choosing the output weights of the RBF network is defined below.

To start the procedure, we compute the value of the output weights and the associated initial error variance set $\{e_i^1\}$.

$$b_i = \frac{\mathbf{q}_i' \mathbf{d}}{\mathbf{q}_i' \mathbf{q}_i} . \tag{3.55}$$

An L_1 norm is used to measure the error variance at each step:

$$e^1 = \max e_i \qquad 1 \leq i \leq n_h . \tag{3.56}$$

The basic approach followed next is to orthogonalize $\mathbf{Z}$ by producing one column at each step, orthogonal to the previous ones. The output weight values, $b_i, i = 1, \ldots, n_h$, are computed initially as

$$\begin{aligned} \mathbf{q}_i &= \mathbf{z}_i \\ b_i &= \frac{\mathbf{q}_i' \mathbf{d}}{\mathbf{q}_i' \mathbf{q}_i} \end{aligned}$$

and then, for subsequent orthogonal steps $k = 2, \ldots,$ to a maximum of n_h and for $1 \leq i \leq n_h$ as

$$\begin{aligned} s_{jk} &= \frac{\mathbf{q}_j' \mathbf{z}_i}{\mathbf{q}_j' \mathbf{q}_j} \qquad \leq j < k \\ \mathbf{q}_k &= \mathbf{z}_i - \sum_{j=1}^{k-1} s_{jk} \mathbf{q}_j \\ b_k &= \frac{\mathbf{q}_i' \mathbf{d}}{\mathbf{q}_i' \mathbf{q}_i} . \end{aligned} \tag{3.57}$$

The error measure is computed as

$$1 - \sum_{r=1}^{n_s} e_r < \rho \tag{3.58}$$

where $\rho \in (0, 1)$ is the tolerance and n_s is the number of steps and, hence, the number of basis functions used. When the error variance is reduced to an acceptable level, that subset of basis functions and associated output weights are selected for the model. The tolerance value ρ can be chosen by using criteria such as AIC (Akaike information criteria), BIC (Bayesian information criteria), or MDL (minimum description length).

3.4.3.2 Constructive Learning

Fritzke proposed a constructive algorithm, described above, which permits units to be added iteratively [11]. The issue, then, is to determine when to stop adding units. Again, it is possible to use methods such as AIC, BIC, etc. Alternatively, it is possible to use a simple error criteria on either a training set, or better, a test or validation set.

3.4.4 Determining Output Layer Weights

The determination of output layer weights is relatively simple in comparison to the other parameters in the network. In general, the basic approach to determining the output layer weights can be divided into (1) off-line and (2) online methods. Off-line methods include the usual least squares method, while online methods include the LMS algorithm or RLS (recursive least squares) algorithm. Clearly, many other variations and extensions to these basic algorithms can be introduced at this stage.

3.4.5 Robustness

When training the output layer weights in an RBF, it is important to consider the possible effects of numerical ill-conditioning. Numerical ill-conditioning occurs when one of the columns of $\mathbf{Z}$ is a linear combination of the other columns. The OLS method described above also avoids numerical ill-conditioning through the following simpler observation:

Numerical ill-conditioning implies $\mathbf{q}_k'\mathbf{q}_k = 0$. Hence, a way of avoiding such ill-conditioning is to monitor $\mathbf{q}_k'\mathbf{q}_k$, and if this falls below a small positive value, the corresponding column of $\mathbf{Z}$, z_k is not employed in the model.

Another common approach for improving the reliability in RBF networks which are trained by the simple least-squares algorithm is to use the well known SVD method to choose the output weights. At the same time, this also selects the basis functions.

3.5 Applications

To give some indication of the capabilities of RBF networks, some example applications are provided below. The success of these applications is dependent on the nature of the problem to be solved and the data made available to help solve the problem. Generally speaking, if the problem requires a nonlinear functional mapping and if data are adequately sampled, RBF networks are suitable candidate models to consider. Here, we report on the results of some applications of RBF networks.

3.5.1 Time Series Modeling

Time series models require online estimation of a model

$$y(t) = F(\mathbf{x}(t)) \tag{3.59}$$

where F is the functional map

$$F : \Re^m \to \Re \,. \tag{3.60}$$

RBF networks have been used to model time series by a number of researchers. Kadirkamanathan, Niranjan, and Fallside [21] applied RBF networks to time series prediction.

A popular time series problem is learning to predict the Mackey–Glass time series. The observed data are generated from the Mackey–Glass differential delay equation

$$\frac{dx(t)}{dt} = -bx(t) + a\frac{x(t-\tau)}{1 + x(t-\tau)^{10}} \tag{3.61}$$

where typical parameter values are $\tau = 17$, $a = 0.2$, and $b = 0.1$.

A number of authors have tested RBF networks on learning to predict time series generated by an approximation of the above equation [16, 25, 30]. Moody and Darken tested RBF networks of between 100 and 10,000 units to model the Mackey–Glass time series [25]. They tested methods of selecting basis function centers including nearest neighbors and using one center per basis point, but these are only suitable for finite data sets. For online signal processing applications, they proposed using the k-means clustering algorithm.

Interestingly, when compared with back-propagation, it was found that the RBF network using the above method required around 27 times more data to achieve similar levels of accuracy. This was attributed to the fact that the multilayer back-propagation trained network fits the data in a global sense, while the RBF network uses units in a local sense; hence, it requires more data to train. In computational terms, the RBF network for this problem was around 16 times more efficient than the back-propagation network.

3.5.2 Option Pricing in Financial Markets

The seminal paper by Hutchinson et al. [19] is an excellent example of an application of RBF networks to the well known problem of pricing derivatives in the financial markets.

The Black–Scholes formula [4], while initially derived for very specific conditions, has been extended in a variety of ways. However, in some circumstances, it is not possible to obtain a closed form solution in the form of the original Black–Scholes formula and, in general, it may be a difficult task to rederive a new version of the formula for each situation to be considered.

Neural networks offer an attractive solution to problems of this type which inherently require a nonlinear model, and the degree of difficulty of the problem (or, indeed, the fact that no analytical solution can be derived) means that alternative solutions are required. Hutchinson et al. [19] considered two interesting and related problems. First, they applied RBF networks to the task of learning the Black–Scholes formula from simulated data only. They assumed that the Black–Scholes formula precisely determined the option prices for a representative NYSE stock and then used Monte Carlo simulations to generate the artificial price data. The inputs to the model were taken to be[6]

$$\begin{aligned} S(t) &= \text{stock price at time } t \\ X &= \text{strike price} \\ T - t &= \text{time to maturity} \end{aligned}$$

while the risk-free interest rate r and the volatility σ were excluded due to assuming them as constants throughout the modeling process.

A Monte Carlo simulation approach was adopted to generate a number of daily option and price paths, each of a duration of two years. Artificial price series were generated based on the Black–Scholes assumption of geometric Brownian motion using the following equation

$$S(t) = S(0) \exp\left(\sum_i^t Z(i)\right) \qquad t > 0 \tag{3.62}$$

[6]In fact, the authors made the simplification that the distribution of the stock price returns was independent of the actual stock price; hence, only two inputs to the model were required: $S(t)/X$ and $T - t$.

with the following assumptions:

$$\begin{aligned} S(0) &= \$50.00 \\ \mu &= 10\% \\ \sigma &= 20\% \\ N_d &= 253 \\ Z(t) &= N\left(\mu/N_d, \sigma^2/N_d\right) \end{aligned} \tag{3.63}$$

where μ is the annual continuously compounded expected rate of return, σ is the annual volatility, and N_d is the number of trading days per year.

The Black–Scholes option pricing formula is given by

$$G(t) = S(t)\Psi(d_1) - Xe^{-r(T-t)}\Psi(d_2) \tag{3.64}$$

where $G(t)$ is the price of the option at time t, $\Psi(\cdot)$ is the standard normal cumulative distribution function, σ is the volatility of the continuously compounded stock returns, and

$$d_1 = \frac{\log(S(t)/X) + \left(r + \frac{1}{2}\sigma^2\right)(T-t)}{\sigma\sqrt{T-t}} \tag{3.65}$$

$$d_2 = \frac{\log(S(t)/X) + \left(r - \frac{1}{2}\sigma^2\right)(T-t)}{\sigma\sqrt{T-t}}\,. \tag{3.66}$$

The strike prices X were computed from Chicago Board of Options (CBOE) rules.

The RBF network was trained by forming the following error criterion $J(t)$:

$$\begin{aligned} E(t) &= G(t)/X - \widehat{G/X}(t) \\ J(t) &= \frac{1}{2}E^2(t)\,. \end{aligned} \tag{3.67}$$

The model is then obtained as

$$\widehat{G/X}(t) = F(S(t)/X, T-t) \tag{3.68}$$

where F represents the radial basis function network. Instead of measuring the model's performance by Equation (3.67) directly, Hutchinson et al. used the option prices from the RBF network to institute a delta hedging strategy [18] which is rebalanced until the expiration of the option. The results of this work showed that the RBF network is capable of learning to price options with a reasonable degree of accuracy, as evidenced by the delta hedging performance. For strike prices between \$45 and \$55, it was observed that the RBF network was capable of outperforming the Black–Scholes formula in up to 36% of the cases.

Hutchinson et al. also investigated the performance of RBF networks on pricing and hedging the S&P 500 for the period from 1987 to 1991. They used an approach similar to that described above, but with the additional complexities of having to calculate the Black–Scholes estimated option prices by first estimating the volatility σ and the risk-free interest rate r from actual data. While the authors caution about drawing general inferences from their results, they found that the RBF network (and others they also tested: the MLP and projection pursuit networks) outperformed the standard Black–Scholes formula most of the time.

This example provides some insight into a promising practical use of RBF networks. In contrast to MLP networks, which took around 300 minutes to train, RBF networks required only 7 minutes per network to train. For problems of moderate complexity such as this, RBF networks are very well suited.

3.5.3 Phoneme Classification

In an early practical application, several authors considered the use of RBF networks for phoneme classification [25, 34]. Moody and Darken presented results for the problem of phoneme classification and compared the results to other methods.

The problem considered was to classify ten vowel sounds based on the first and second formant frequencies. The data used for this task were 338 training phonemes and 333 test phonemes. Using the k-means clustering for 100 Gaussian units, a test set error of 18.0% was obtained, the same as the best results obtained in earlier work.

3.5.4 Channel Equalization

The problem of channel equalization was considered by Chen, Cowan, and Grant [7]. Channel equalization is the problem of finding an equalization filter for a channel $C(z)$ defined, for example, as

$$C(z) = \sum_{i=0}^{m} c_i z^{-i} . \tag{3.69}$$

The model is usually defined as

$$y(t) = C(z)s(t) + h(t) \tag{3.70}$$

where $s(t) \in [-1, 1]$ is the input data sequence and $h(t)$ is additive white Gaussian noise. The channel equalization problem is to estimate the inverse filter $F(z, \mathbf{y})$ such that the BER (bit error rate) error is minimized. In the ideal case, this means that

$$\hat{s}(t - \tau) = \text{sgn}\left(F(z, \mathbf{y}(t))\right) \tag{3.71}$$

where τ is a time delay and

$$\text{sgn}(x) = \begin{cases} 1 & x \geq 0 \\ -1 & x < 0 . \end{cases} \tag{3.72}$$

It is widely recognized that the optimum channel equalizer F will be a nonlinear model; hence, an RBF network is well suited to this task. Chen et al. found that for a simple channel described by

$$C(z) = 0.5 + 1.0z^{-1} \tag{3.73}$$

an RBF network with 12 centers was capable of forming decision boundaries which were close to ideal.

They also tested the performance of an RBF network with 70 centers on a more complex channel defined by

$$C(z) = 0.3482 + 0.8704z^{-1} + 0.3482z^{-2} . \tag{3.74}$$

In this case, they found that, with a sufficient number of training data points (600 points were used), the RBF networks could achieve near-optimal performance when coupled with the OLS learning algorithm. When random selection of RBF centers was adopted, the performance was significantly worse.

3.5.5 Symbolic Signal Processing

Frasconi, Gori, Maggini, and Soda proposed a method of recurrent RBF networks that is capable of representing finite state automata [10]. Such networks are of particular interest for developing hybrid systems or symbolic processing systems [26, 36]. Future signal processing applications may benefit strongly from merging symbolic algorithms with more conventional signal processing methods.

3.6 Conclusions

Radial basis function networks can be regarded as a very useful addition to the toolbox of neural networks for signal processing. In general, it can be seen that for many applications, RBF networks can provide a fast and accurate means of approximating a nonlinear mapping based on observed data. Due to the locally acting nature of RBFs, they have a tendency to require more data than a comparable multilayer sigmoidal network. Provided care is taken to overcome issues of numerical ill-conditioning and a suitable algorithm is used to select the radial basis function centers, RBF networks can be readily trained in both online and off-line modes.

References

[1] A.R. Barron. Universal approximation bounds for superpositions of a sigmoidal function. *IEEE Transactions on Information Theory,* 39(3):930–945, 1993.

[2] E.B. Baum and K.J. Lang. Constructing hidden units using examples and queries. In R.P. Lippmann, J. Moody, and D.S. Touretzky, Editors, *Advances in Neural Information Processing Systems,* Morgan Kaufmann Publisher, Inc., San Mateo, CA, 904–910, 1991.

[3] Å. Björck and G.H. Golub. Iterative refinement of linear least squares solutions by Householder transformation. *j-BIT,* 7:322–337, 1967.

[4] F. Black and M. Scholes. The pricing of options and corporate liabilities. *Journal of Political Economy,* 81:637–659, 1973.

[5] D.S. Broomhead and D. Lowe. Multivariable functional interpolation and adaptive networks. *Complex Systems,* 2:321–355, 1988.

[6] C. Burges, F. Girosi, P. Niyogi, T. Poggio, B. Schölkopf, K.K. Sung, and V. Vapnik. Choosing RBF centers with the support vector algorithm. A.I. Memo, MIT Artificial Intelligence Lab., Cambridge, MA, 1995.

[7] S. Chen, C.F.N. Cowan, and P.M. Grant. Orthogonal least squares learning algorithm for radial basis function networks. *IEEE Transactions on Neural Networks,* 2(2):302–309, 1991.

[8] C. Cortes and V. Vapnik. Support vector networks. *Machine Learning,* 20:1–25, 1995.

[9] G. Cybenko. Approximation by superposition of a sigmoidal function. *Mathematical Control Systems Signals,* 2(4):303–314, 1989.

[10] P. Frasconi, M. Gori, M. Maggini, and G. Soda. Representation of finite state automata in recurrent radial basis function networks. *Machine Learning,* 23:5, 1996.

[11] B. Fritzke. Supervised learning with growing cell structures. In J.D. Cowan, G. Tesauro, and J. Alspector, Editors, *Advances in Neural Information Processing Systems,* Volume 6, 255–262. Morgan Kaufmann Publishers, Inc., San Mateo, CA, 1994.

[12] K. Funahashi. On the approximate realization of continuous mappings by neural networks. *Neural Networks,* 2:183–192, 1989.

[13] F. Girosi and T. Poggio. Networks and the best approximation property. Technical Report AIM-1164, Massachusetts Institute of Technology, October 1989.

[14] G.H. Golub and C.F. Van Loan. *Matrix Computations.* 2nd edition. Johns Hopkins University Press, Baltimore, MD, 1989.

[15] S. Gunn. Support vector machines for classification and regression. ISIS technical report, Image Speech and Intelligent Systems Group, University of Southampton, 1997.

[16] S. Haykin and J. Principe. Making sense of a complex world. *IEEE Signal Processing Magazine,* 15(3):66–81, 1998.

[17] K. Hornik, M. Stinchcombe, and H. White. Multilayer feedforward networks are universal approximators. *Neural Networks,* 2(5):359–366, 1989.

[18] J.C. Hull. *Options, Futures, and Other Derivative Securities.* 2nd edition. Prentice-Hall, Englewood Cliffs, NJ, 1993.

[19] J.M. Hutchinson, A. Lo, and T. Poggio. A nonparametric approach to pricing and hedging derivative securities via learning networks. Technical Report AIM-1471, Massachusetts Institute of Technology, April 1994.

[20] J.S. Roger Jang and C.T. Sun. Functional equivalence between radial basis function networks and fuzzy inference systems. *IEEE Transactions on Neural Networks,* 4(1):156–159, 1993.

[21] V. Kadirkamanathan, M. Niranjan, and F. Fallside. Sequential adaptation of radial basis function neural networks and its application to time-series prediction. In R.P. Lippmann, J.E. Moody, and D.S. Touretzky, Editors, *Advances in Neural Information Processing Systems,* Volume 3, 721–727. Morgan Kaufmann Publishers, Inc., San Mateo, CA, 1991.

[22] J. MacQueen. Some methods of classification and analysis of multivariate observations. In L.M. LeCam and J. Neyman, Editors, *Proceedings of the 5th Berkeley Symposium on Mathematics, Statistics and Probability,* 281. University of California Press, Berkeley, 1967.

[23] M. Maruyama, F. Girosi, and T. Poggio. A connection between GRBF and MLP. Technical Memo AIM-1291, Massachusetts Institute of Technology, Artificial Intelligence Laboratory, September 1991.

[24] C.A. Michelli. Interpolation of scattered data: distance matrices and conditionally positive definite functions. *Constructive Approximation,* 2:11–22, 1986.

[25] J. Moody and C. Darken. Fast learning in networks of locally-tuned processing units. *Neural Computation,* 1(2):281–294, 1989.

[26] C.W. Omlin and C.L. Giles. Constructing deterministic finite-state automata in recurrent neural networks. *Journal of the ACM,* 1996.

[27] S. Omohundro. Efficient algorithms with neural network behavior. *Complex Systems,* 1:273, 1987.

[28] J. Park and I.W. Sandberg. Universal approximation using radial-basis-function networks. *Neural Computation,* 3(2):246–257, 1991.

[29] J. Park and I.W. Sandberg. Approximation and radial-basis-function networks. *Neural Computation,* 5(3):305–316, 1993.

[30] J.C. Platt. Leaning by combining memorization and gradient descent. In R.P. Lippmann, J.E. Moody, and D.S. Touretzky, Editors, *Advances in Neural Information Processing Systems*, Volume 3, 714–720. Morgan Kaufmann Publishers, Inc., San Mateo, CA, 1991.

[31] T. Poggio and F. Girosi. A theory of networks for approximation and learning. Technical report, Artificial Intelligence Laboratory, Massachusetts Institute of Technology (MIT), Cambridge, MA, July 1989.

[32] M.J.D. Powell. Radial basis functions for multivariable interpolation: a review. In *Proceedings of the IMA Conference on Algorithms for the Approximation of Functions and Data,* Shrivenham, 1985. RMCS.

[33] M.J.D. Powell. Radial basis functions for multivariable interpolation: a review. In *Algorithms for Approximation,* 143–167. Clarendon Press, Oxford, 1987.

[34] S. Renals and R. Rohwer. Learning phoneme recognition using neural networks. In *Proceedings of the ICASSP 1989,* Glasgow, 1989.

[35] B.D. Ripley. *Pattern Recognition and Neural Networks.* Cambridge University Press, Cambridge, MA, 1995.

[36] C.L. Giles, S. Lawrence, and A.C. Tsoi. Symbolic conversion, grammatical inference and rule extraction for foreign exchange rate prediction. In A.S. Weigend, Y. Abu-Mostafa, and A.P.N. Refenes, Editors, *Proceedings of the Fourth International Conference on Neural Networks in the Capital Market,* Singapore, 1997. World Scientific.

[37] B. Scholkopf. *Support Vector Learning.* Ph.D. thesis, Technical University of Berlin, 1997.

[38] B. Schölkopf, K. Sung, C. Burges, F. Girosi, P. Niyogi, T. Poggio, and V. Vapnik. Comparing support vector machines with Gaussian kernels to radial basis function classifiers. *IEEE Transactions on Signal Processing,* 45:2758–2765, 1997.

[39] T.J. Sejnowski and C.R. Rosenberg. Nettalk: a parallel network that learns to read aloud. Technical Report JHU/EECS-86/01, John Hopkins University, 1986.

[40] V. Vapnik. *The Nature of Statistical Learning Theory.* Springer-Verlag, New York, 1995.

[41] V. Vapnik, S.E. Golowich, and A. Smola. Support vector method for function approximation, regression estimation, and signal processing. In *Advances in Neural Information Processing Systems 9,* 281–287. Morgan Kaufmann Publishers, Inc., San Mateo, CA, 1997.

[42] D. Wettschereck and T. Dietterich. Improving the performance of radial basis function networks by learning center locations. In J.E. Moody, S.J. Hanson, and R.P. Lippmann, Editors, *Advances in Neural Information Processing Systems,* Volume 4, 1133–1140. Morgan Kaufmann Publishers, Inc., San Mateo, CA, 1992.

4

An Introduction to Kernel-Based Learning Algorithms

Klaus-Robert Müller
GMD FIRST and University of Potsdam

Sebastian Mika
GMD FIRST

Gunnar Rätsch
GMD FIRST and University of Potsdam

Koji Tsuda
AIST Computational Biology Research Center

Bernhard Schölkopf
Max-Planck-Insitut für Biologische Kybernetik

This chapter provides an introduction to support vector machines, kernel Fisher discriminant analysis, and kernel PCA as examples for successful kernel-based learning methods. We first give a short background about Vapnik–Chervonenkis (VC) theory and kernel feature spaces and then proceed to kernel-based learning in supervised and unsupervised scenarios, including practical and algorithmic considerations. We illustrate the usefulness of kernel algorithms by finally discussing applications such as OCR and DNA analysis.

4.1 Introduction

In recent years, a number of powerful kernel-based learning machines, e.g., support vector machines (**SVMs**) [12, 22, 110, 111, 142, 143], kernel Fisher discriminant (KFD) [4, 69, 70, 100], and kernel principal component analysis (KPCA) [71, 112, 119], have been proposed. These approaches have shown practical relevance not only for classification and regression problems but also, more recently, in unsupervised learning [71, 75, 112, 114, 119]. Successful applications of kernel-based algorithms have been reported for various fields, for example, in the context of optical pattern and object recognition [11, 21, 25, 61, 97], text categorization [28, 33, 53], time-series prediction

0-8493-2359-2/01/$0.00+$1.50

[66, 75, 76], gene expression profile analysis [18, 41], DNA and protein analysis [46, 52, 152], and many more.[1]

This chapter introduces the main ideas of kernel algorithms and reports applications from OCR (optical character recognition) and DNA analysis. We do not attempt a full treatment of all available literature; rather, we present a somewhat biased point of view illustrating the main ideas by drawing mainly from the work of the authors and providing — to the best of our knowledge — reference to related work for further reading. We hope that it will nevertheless be useful for the reader. It differs from other reviews [20, 24, 111, 126, 142], mainly in the choice of the presented material: we place more emphasis on kernel PCA, kernel Fisher discriminants, and connections to boosting.

This chapter begins by presenting some basic concepts of learning theory in Section 4.2. It then introduces the idea of kernel feature spaces (Section 4.3) and the original *SVM* approach, its implementation, and some variants. Subsequently, the chapter discusses other kernel-based methods for supervised and unsupervised learning in Sections 4.4 and 4.5. Some attention will be devoted to questions of model selection (Section 4.6), i.e., how to properly choose the parameters in SVMs and other kernel-based approaches. Finally, Section 4.7 describes several recent interesting applications.

TABLE 4.1 Notation Conventions Used in This Chapter

i, n	counter and number of patterns
$\mathbf{X}, N$	the input space, $N = \dim(\mathbf{X})$
$\mathbf{x}, y$	a training pattern and the label
$(\mathbf{x} \cdot \mathbf{x}')$	scalar product between $\mathbf{x}$ and $\mathbf{x}'$
$\mathcal{F}$	feature space
Φ	the mapping $\Phi : \mathbf{X} \to \mathcal{F}$
$\mathrm{k}(\cdot, \cdot)$	scalar product in feature space $\mathcal{F}$
F_i	a function class
h	the VC dimension of a function class
d	the degree of a polynomial
$\mathbf{w}$	normal vector of a hyperplane
α_i	Lagrange multiplier/expansion coefficient for $\mathbf{w}$
ξ_i	the "slack-variable" for pattern $\mathbf{x}_i$
ν	the quantile parameter (determines the number of outliers)
$\|\cdot\|_p$	the ℓ_p–norm, $p \in [1, \infty]$
$\|S\|$	number of elements in a set S
Θ	the Heaviside function: $\Theta(z) = 0$ for $z < 0$, $\Theta(z) = 1$ otherwise
$\mathbb{R}_+$	space of non-negative real numbers

4.2 Learning to Classify – Some Theoretical Background

Let us start with a general notion of the learning problems considered in this chapter. The task of classification is to find a rule which, based on external observations, assigns an object to one of several classes. In the simplest case, there are only two different classes. One possible formalization of this task is to estimate a function $f : \mathbb{R}^N \to \{-1, +1\}$ using input-output training data pairs generated identically and independently distributed (i.i.d.) according to an unknown probability distribution $P(\mathbf{x}, y)$

$$(\mathbf{x}_1, y_1), \ldots, (\mathbf{x}_n, y_n) \in \mathbb{R}^N \times Y, \quad Y = \{-1, +1\}$$

such that f will correctly classify unseen examples $(\mathbf{x}, y)$. An example is assigned to class $+1$ if $f(\mathbf{x}) \geq 0$ and to class -1 otherwise. The test examples are assumed to be generated from the same

[1] See also Isabelle Guyon's web page, `http://www.clopinet.com/isabelle/Projects/SVM/applist.html`, on applications of SVMs.

probability distribution $P(\mathbf{x}, y)$ as the training data. The best function f that one can obtain is the one minimizing the expected error (risk):

$$R[f] = \int l(f(\mathbf{x}), y) dP(\mathbf{x}, y) \tag{4.1}$$

where l denotes a suitably chosen loss function, e.g., $l(f(\mathbf{x}), y) = \Theta(-yf(\mathbf{x}))$, where $\Theta(z) = 0$ for $z < 0$ and $\Theta(z) = 1$ otherwise (the so-called 0/1-loss). The same framework can be applied for regression problems, where $y \in \mathbb{R}$. Here, the most common loss function is the squared loss: $l(f(\mathbf{x}), y) = (f(\mathbf{x}) - y)^2$; see the literature [127, 129] for a discussion of other loss functions.

Unfortunately, the risk cannot be minimized directly, since the underlying probability distribution $P(\mathbf{x}, y)$ is unknown. Therefore, we must try to estimate a function that is close to the optimal one based on the available information, i.e., the training sample and properties of the function class F the solution f is chosen from. To this end, we need what is called an induction principle. A particular simple induction principle consists of approximating the minimum of the risk in Equation (4.1) by the minimum of the empirical risk,

$$R_{\text{emp}}[f] = \frac{1}{n} \sum_{i=1}^{n} l\left(f\left(\mathbf{x}_i\right), y_i\right) . \tag{4.2}$$

It is possible to give conditions to the learning machine which ensure that, asymptotically (as $n \to \infty$), the empirical risk will converge towards the expected risk. However, for small sample sizes, large deviations are possible and overfitting might occur (see Figure 4.1). Then, a small gener-

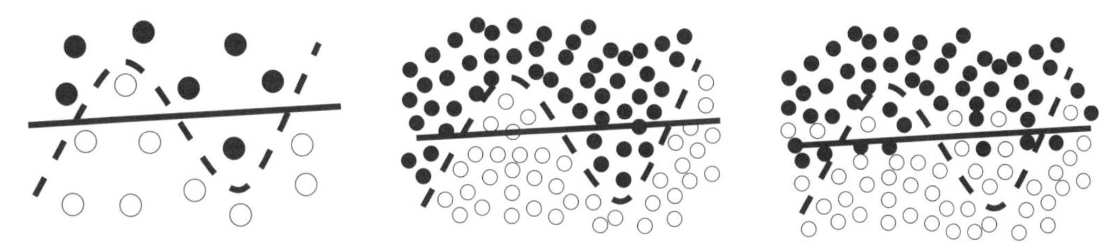

4.1 Illustration of the overfitting dilemma: given only a small sample (left), either the solid or the dashed hypothesis might be true, the dashed one being more complex but also having a smaller training error. Only with a large sample are we able to see which decision more accurately reflects the true distribution. If the dashed hypothesis is correct, the solid would underfit (middle); if the solid were correct, the dashed hypothesis would overfit (right).

alization error can usually not be obtained by simply minimizing the training error (Equation (4.2)). One way to avoid the overfitting dilemma is to restrict the complexity of the function class F from which one chooses the function f [142]. The intuition, which will be formalized in the following, is that a simple (e.g., linear) function that explains most of the data is preferable to a complex one (Occam's razor). Typically, one introduces a regularization term [23, 57, 88, 135] to limit the complexity of the function class F from which the learning machine can choose. This raises the problem of model selection [2, 73, 77, 88], i.e., how to find the optimal complexity of the function (see Section 4.6).

A specific way of controlling the complexity of a function class is given by Vapnik–Chervonenkis (VC) theory and the structural risk minimization (SRM) principle [142, 143, 145]. Here, the concept of complexity is captured by the Vapnik–Chervonenkis (VC) dimension h of the function class F from which the estimate f is chosen. Roughly speaking, the VC dimension measures how many (training) points can be shattered (i.e., separated) for all possible labelings using functions of the class. Constructing a nested family of function classes $F_1 \subset \cdots \subset F_k$ with non-decreasing VC dimension, the SRM principle proceeds as follows. Let $f_1, \ldots, f_k$ be the solutions of the empirical risk minimization (Equation (4.2)) in the function classes F_i. SRM chooses the function class F_i (and the function f_i) such that an upper bound on the generalization error is minimized and can be computed making use of theorems such as the following (see also Figure 4.2).

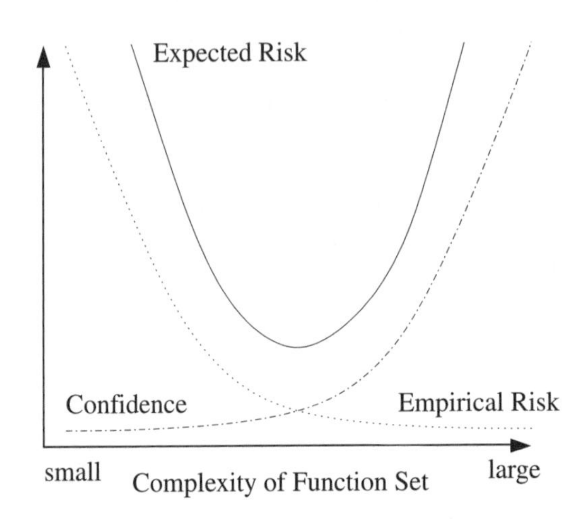

4.2 Schematic illustration of Equation (4.3). The dotted line represents the training error (empirical risk), and the dash-dotted line represents the upper bound on the complexity term (confidence). With higher complexity, the empirical error decreases but the upper bound on the risk confidence becomes worse. For a certain complexity of the function class, the best expected risk (solid line) is obtained. Thus, in practice, the goal is to find the best trade-off between empirical error and complexity.

THEOREM 4.1 *[142, 143] Let h denote the VC dimension of the function class F and let R_{emp} be defined by Equation* (4.2) *using the* $0/1$*-loss. For all $\delta > 0$ and $f \in F$, the inequality bounding the risk*

$$R[f] \leq R_{emp}[f] + \sqrt{\frac{h\left(\ln \frac{2n}{h} + 1\right) - \ln(\delta/4)}{n}} \tag{4.3}$$

holds with probability of at least $1 - \delta$ for $n > h$.

Note that this bound is only an example, and similar formulations are available for other loss functions [143] and other complexity measures, e.g., entropy numbers [151]. Let us discuss Equation (4.3): the goal is to minimize the generalization error $R[f]$, which can be achieved by obtaining a small training error $R_{\text{emp}}[f]$ while keeping the function class as small as possible. Two extremes arise for Equation (4.3): (1) a very small function class (like F_1) yields a vanishing square root term but a large training error might remain, while (2) a huge function class (like F_k) may give a vanishing empirical error but a large square root term. The best class is usually in between (see Figure 4.2), as one would like to obtain a function that explains the data well and have only small risk in obtaining that function. This is analogous to the bias-variance dilemma scenario described for neural networks [42].

4.2.1 VC Dimension in Practice

Unfortunately, in practice, the bound on the expected error in Equation (4.3) is often neither easily computable nor very helpful. Typical problems are that the upper bound on the expected test error might be trivial (i.e., larger than one) or the VC dimension of the function class is either unknown or infinite (in which case, one would need an infinite amount of training data). Although there are different and tighter bounds, most of them suffer from similar problems. Nevertheless, bounds clearly offer helpful theoretical insights into the nature of learning problems.

4.2.2 Margins and VC Dimension

Let us assume, for a moment, that the training sample is separable by a hyperplane (see Figure 4.3), i.e., and we choose functions of the form

$$f(\mathbf{x}) = (\mathbf{w} \cdot \mathbf{x}) + b\,. \tag{4.4}$$

It has been shown [142, 145] that, for the class of hyperplanes, the VC dimension itself can be

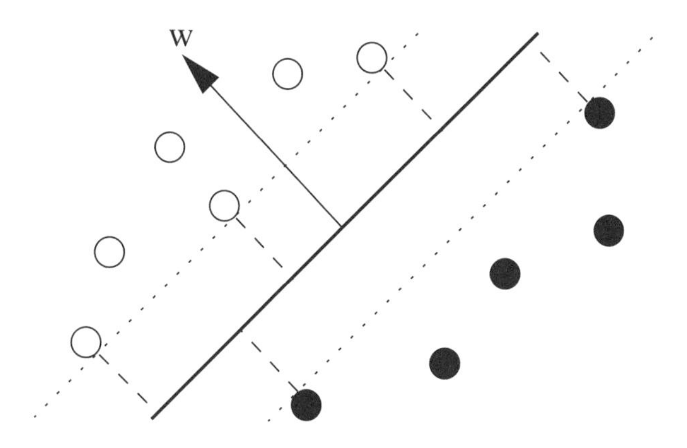

4.3 Linear classifier and margins: a linear classifier is defined by a hyperplane's normal vector $\mathbf{w}$ and an offset b, i.e., the decision boundary is $\{\mathbf{x} | (\mathbf{w} \cdot \mathbf{x}) + b = 0\}$ (thick line). Each of the two halfspaces defined by this hyperplane corresponds to one class, i.e., $f(\mathbf{x}) = \mathrm{sign}((\mathbf{w} \cdot \mathbf{x}) + b)$. The margin of a linear classifier is the minimal distance of any training point to the hyperplane. In this case, it is the distance between the dotted lines and the thick line.

bounded in terms of another quantity, the margin (Figure 4.3). The margin is defined as the minimal distance of a sample to the decision surface. The margin, in turn, depends on the length of the weight vector $\mathbf{w}$ in Equation (4.4): since we assumed that the training sample is separable, we can rescale $\mathbf{w}$ and b such that the points closest to the hyperplane satisfy $|(\mathbf{w} \cdot \mathbf{x}_i) + b| = 1$ (i.e., obtain the so-called canonical representation of the hyperplane). Now consider two samples $\mathbf{x}_1$ and $\mathbf{x}_2$ from different classes with $(\mathbf{w} \cdot \mathbf{x}_1) + b = 1$ and $(\mathbf{w} \cdot \mathbf{x}_2) + b = -1$, respectively. Then, the margin is given by the distance of these two points, measured perpendicular to the hyperplane, i.e., $\left(\frac{\mathbf{w}}{\|\mathbf{w}\|} \cdot (\mathbf{x}_1 - \mathbf{x}_2)\right) = \frac{2}{\|\mathbf{w}\|}$. The result linking the VC dimension of the class of separating hyperplanes to the margin or the length of the weight vector $\mathbf{w}$, respectively, is given by the following inequalities:

$$h \leq \Lambda^2 R^2 + 1 \quad \text{and} \quad \|\mathbf{w}\|_2 \leq \Lambda \tag{4.5}$$

where R is the radius of the smallest ball around the data [142]. Thus, if we bound the margin of a function class from below, e.g., by $\frac{2}{\Lambda}$, we can control its VC dimension.[2] Support vector machines, which we shall deal with more closely in Section 4.4.1, implement this insight.

The choice of linear functions seems to be very limiting (i.e., instead of being likely to overfit, it is now more likely to underfit). Fortunately, there is a way to have both linear models and a very rich set of nonlinear decision functions, by using the tools that will be discussed in the next section.

4.3 Nonlinear Algorithms in Kernel Feature Spaces

Algorithms in feature spaces make use of the following idea: via a nonlinear mapping,

$$\begin{aligned} \Phi : \mathbb{R}^N &\to \mathcal{F} \\ \mathbf{x} &\mapsto \Phi(\mathbf{x}) \end{aligned}$$

the data $\mathbf{x}_1, \ldots, \mathbf{x}_n \in \mathbb{R}^N$ are mapped into a potentially much higher dimensional feature space $\mathcal{F}$. For a given learning problem, one now considers the same algorithm in $\mathcal{F}$ instead of $\mathbb{R}^N$, i.e., one works with the sample

$$(\Phi(\mathbf{x}_1), y_1), \ldots, (\Phi(\mathbf{x}_n), y_n) \in \mathcal{F} \times Y .$$

Given this mapped representation, a simple classification or regression in $\mathcal{F}$ is to be found. This is also implicitly done for (one hidden layer) neural networks, radial basis networks [10, 47, 74, 81], or boosting algorithms [37] where the input data are mapped to some representation given by the hidden layer, the RBF bumps, or the hypotheses space, respectively.

The so-called curse of dimensionality from statistics says, essentially, that the difficulty of an estimation problem increases drastically with the dimension N of the space, since, in principle, as a function of N, one needs exponentially many patterns to sample the space properly. This well known statement creates some doubt about whether it is a good idea to go to a high-dimensional feature space for learning.

However, statistical learning theory says that the opposite can be true: learning in $\mathcal{F}$ can be simpler if one uses a low complexity, i.e., a simple class of decision rules (e.g., linear classifiers). All the variability and richness that one needs to have a powerful function class is then introduced by the mapping Φ. In short, it is not the dimensionality but the complexity of the function class that matters [142]. Intuitively, this idea can be understood from the toy example in Figure 4.4: in two dimensions, a rather complicated nonlinear decision surface is necessary to separate the classes, whereas in a feature space of second order monomials [121],

$$\begin{aligned} \Phi : \mathbb{R}^2 &\to \mathbb{R}^3 \\ (x_1, x_2) &\mapsto (z_1, z_2, z_3) := \left(x_1^2, \sqrt{2}\, x_1 x_2, x_2^2\right) \end{aligned} \tag{4.6}$$

all one needs for separation is a linear hyperplane. In this simple toy example, we can easily control both the statistical complexity (by using a simple linear hyperplane classifier) and the algorithmic complexity of the learning machine, as the feature space is only three-dimensional. However, it becomes rather tricky to control the latter for large real-world problems. For instance, consider images of 16×16 pixels as patterns and 5th order monomials as mapping Φ; then one would map

[2]There are some ramifications to this statement that go beyond the scope of this work. Strictly speaking, VC theory requires the structure to be defined *a priori*, which has implications for the definition of the class of separating hyperplanes [122].

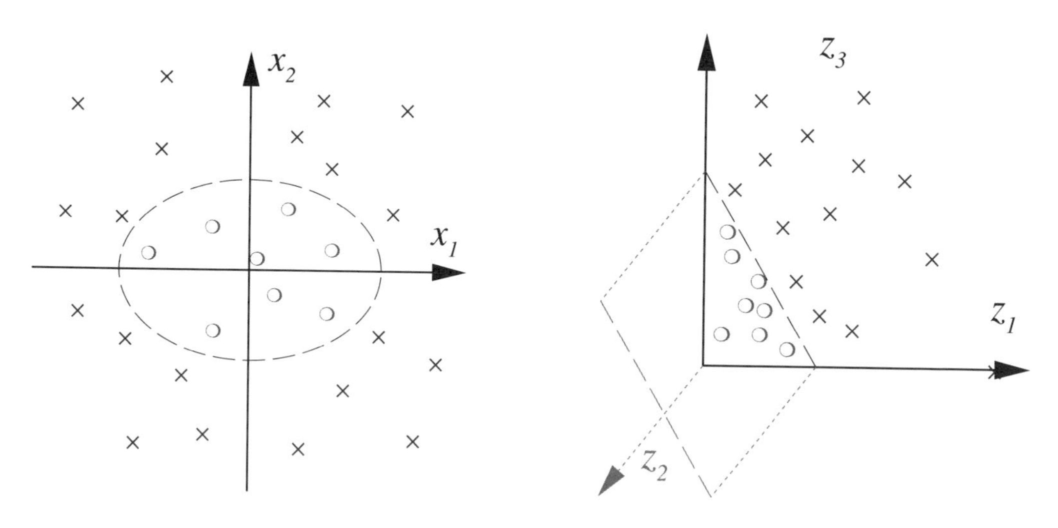

4.4 Two-dimensional classification example. Using the second order monomials x_1^2, $\sqrt{2}x_1x_2$, and x_2^2 as features, a separation in feature space can be found using a linear hyperplane (right). In input space, this construction corresponds to a nonlinear ellipsoidal decision boundary (left) [118].

to a space that contains all 5th order products of 256 pixels, i.e., to a $\binom{5+256-1}{5} \approx 10^{10}$-dimensional space. So, even if one could control the statistical complexity of this function class, one would still run into intractability problems while executing an algorithm in this space.

Fortunately, for certain feature spaces $\mathcal{F}$ and corresponding mappings Φ, there is a highly effective trick for computing scalar products in feature spaces using kernel functions [1, 12, 102, 142]. Let us return to the example from Equation (4.6). There, the computation of a scalar product between two feature space vectors can be readily reformulated in terms of a kernel function k:

$$\begin{aligned}(\Phi(\mathbf{x}) \cdot \Phi(\mathbf{y})) &= \left(x_1^2, \sqrt{2}\, x_1x_2, x_2^2\right)\left(y_1^2, \sqrt{2}\, y_1y_2, y_2^2\right)^\top \\ &= \left((x_1, x_2)\,(y_1, y_2)^\top\right)^2 \\ &= (\mathbf{x} \cdot \mathbf{y})^2 \\ &=: \mathrm{k}(\mathbf{x}, \mathbf{y})\,.\end{aligned}$$

This finding generalizes:

- For $\mathbf{x}, \mathbf{y} \in \mathbb{R}^N$, and $d \in \mathbb{N}$, the kernel function

$$\mathrm{k}(\mathbf{x}, \mathbf{y}) = (\mathbf{x} \cdot \mathbf{y})^d$$

  computes a scalar product in the space of all products of d vector entries (monomials) of $\mathbf{x}$ and $\mathbf{y}$ [119, 142].
- If $k : \mathcal{C} \times \mathcal{C} \to \mathbb{R}$ is a continuous kernel of a positive integral operator on a Hilbert space $L_2(\mathcal{C})$ on a compact set $\mathcal{C} \subset \mathbb{R}^N$, i.e.,

$$\forall f \in L_2(\mathcal{C}) : \quad \int_{\mathcal{C}} \mathrm{k}(\mathbf{x}, \mathbf{y}) f(\mathbf{x}) f(\mathbf{y})\, d\mathbf{x}\, d\mathbf{y} \geq 0$$

  then there exists a space $\mathcal{F}$ and a mapping $\Phi : \mathbb{R}^N \to \mathcal{F}$ such that $\mathrm{k}(\mathbf{x}, \mathbf{y}) = (\Phi(\mathbf{x}) \cdot \Phi(\mathbf{y}))$ [142]. This can be seen directly from Mercer's Theorem [67] which says that any kernel of a positive integral operator can be expanded in its eigenfunctions ψ_j ($\lambda_j > 0$, $N_{\mathcal{F}} \leq \infty$):

$$\mathrm{k}(\mathbf{x}, \mathbf{y}) = \sum_{j=1}^{N_{\mathcal{F}}} \lambda_j \psi_j(\mathbf{x}) \psi_j(\mathbf{y}) .$$

In this case,

$$\Phi(\mathbf{x}) = \left(\sqrt{\lambda_1}\psi_1(\mathbf{x}), \sqrt{\lambda_2}\psi_2(\mathbf{x}), \ldots\right)$$

is a possible realization.

- Note, furthermore, that using a particular SV kernel corresponds to an implicit choice of a regularization operator [44, 88]. For translation invariant kernels, the regularization properties can be expressed conveniently in Fourier space in terms of frequencies [43, 131]. For example, Gaussian kernels (Equation (4.7)) correspond to a general smoothness assumption in all kth order derivatives [131]. Using this correspondence, kernels matching a certain prior condition of the frequency content of the data can be constructed to reflect our prior problem knowledge.

Table 4.2 lists some of the most widely used kernel functions. More sophisticated kernels (e.g., kernels generating splines or Fourier expansions) can be found in some of the literature [46, 110, 127, 131, 133, 143, 152].

TABLE 4.2 Common Kernel Functions

Kernel	Function	
Gaussian RBF	$k(\mathbf{x}, \mathbf{y}) = \exp\left(\frac{-\|\mathbf{x} - \mathbf{y}\|^2}{c}\right)$	(4.7)
Polynomial	$((\mathbf{x} \cdot \mathbf{y}) + \theta)^d$	
Sigmoidal	$\tanh(\kappa(\mathbf{x} \cdot \mathbf{y}) + \theta)$	
Inverse multiquadric	$\frac{1}{\sqrt{\|\mathbf{x} - \mathbf{y}\|^2 + c^2}}$	

Note: Gaussian RBF ($c \in \mathbb{R}$), polynomial ($d \in \mathbb{N}, \theta \in \mathbb{R}$), sigmoidal ($\kappa, \theta \in \mathbb{R}$), and inverse multiquadric ($c \in \mathbb{R}_+$) kernel functions are among the most common ones. While RBF and polynomial are known to fulfill Mercer's condition, this is not strictly the case for sigmoidal kernels [126]. Further valid kernels proposed in the context of regularization networks are multiquadric or spline kernels [44, 88, 131].

4.3.1 Wrapping Up

One interesting point about kernel functions is that the scalar product can be implicitly computed in $\mathcal{F}$ without explicitly using or even knowing the mapping Φ. So, kernels allow the computation of scalar products in spaces where one could otherwise barely perform any computations. A direct consequence of this finding [119] is that every (linear) algorithm that uses only scalar products can implicitly be executed in $\mathcal{F}$ by using kernels, i.e., one can very elegantly construct a nonlinear version of a linear algorithm.[3]

[3] Even algorithms that operate on similarity measures k generating positive matrices $\mathrm{k}(\mathbf{x}_i, \mathbf{x}_j)_{ij}$ can be interpreted as linear algorithms in some feature space $\mathcal{F}$ [110].

The next sections adhere to the following philosophy for supervised and unsupervised learning: by (re-)formulating linear, scalar product-based algorithms that are simple in feature space, one is able to generate powerful nonlinear algorithms which use rich function classes in input space.

4.4 Supervised Learning

This section briefly outlines the algorithms of SVMs and the kernel Fisher discriminant (KFD). It also discusses the boosting algorithm from the kernel feature space point of view and shows a connection to SVMs. Finally, this section points out some recently proposed extensions of these algorithms.

4.4.1 Support Vector Machines

Recall from Section 4.2 that the VC dimension of a linear system, e.g., separating hyperplanes (as computed by a perceptron)

$$y = \operatorname{sign}\left((\mathbf{w} \cdot \mathbf{x}) + b\right)$$

can be upper bounded in terms of the margin (Equation (4.5)). For separating hyperplane classifiers, the conditions for classification without training error are

$$y_i((\mathbf{w} \cdot \mathbf{x}_i) + b) \geq 1, \quad i = 1, \ldots, n .$$

As linear function classes are often not rich enough in practice, we will follow the line of thought of the last section and consider linear classifiers in feature space using dot products. To this end, we substitute $\Phi(\mathbf{x}_i)$ for each training example $\mathbf{x}_i$, i.e., $y = \operatorname{sign}((\mathbf{w} \cdot \Phi(\mathbf{x})) + b)$. In feature space, the conditions for perfect classification are described as

$$y_i \left((\mathbf{w} \cdot \Phi\left(\mathbf{x}_i\right)) + b\right) \geq 1, \quad i = 1, \ldots, n . \tag{4.8}$$

The goal of learning is to find $\mathbf{w} \in \mathcal{F}$ and b such that the expected risk is minimized, however, since we cannot obtain the expected risk itself, we will minimize the bound of Equation (4.3), which consists of the empirical risk and the complexity term. One strategy is to keep the empirical risk at zero by constraining $\mathbf{w}$ and b to the perfect separation case while minimizing the complexity term, which is a monotonically increasing function of the VC dimension h. For a linear classifier in feature space, the VC dimension h is bounded according to $h \leq \|\mathbf{w}\|^2 R^2 + 1$ (Equation (4.5)), where R is the radius of the smallest ball around the training data [142], which is fixed for a given data set. Thus, we can minimize the complexity term by minimizing $\|\mathbf{w}\|^2$. This can be formulated as a quadratic optimization problem

$$\min_{\mathbf{w},b} \quad \frac{1}{2}\|\mathbf{w}\|^2 \tag{4.9}$$

subject to Equation (4.8). However, if the only possible access to the feature space is via dot products computed by the kernel, we cannot solve Equation (4.9) directly since $\mathbf{w}$ lies in that feature space. It turns out that we can get rid of the explicit usage of $\mathbf{w}$ by forming the dual optimization problem. Introducing Lagrange multipliers $\alpha_i \geq 0$, $i = 1, \ldots, n$, one for each of the constraints in Equation (4.8), we get the following Lagrangian:

$$L(\mathbf{w}, b, \boldsymbol{\alpha}) = \frac{1}{2}\|\mathbf{w}\|^2 - \sum_{i=1}^{n} \alpha_i \left(y_i \left((\mathbf{w} \cdot \Phi\left(\mathbf{x}_i\right)) + b\right) - 1\right) . \tag{4.10}$$

The task is to minimize Equation (4.10) with respect to $\mathbf{w}$ and b and to maximize it with respect to α_i. At the optimal point, we have the following saddle point equations:

$$\frac{\partial L}{\partial b} = 0 \quad \text{and} \quad \frac{\partial L}{\partial \mathbf{w}} = 0$$

which translate into

$$\sum_{i=1}^{n} \alpha_i y_i = 0 \quad \text{and} \quad \mathbf{w} = \sum_{i=1}^{\ell} \alpha_i y_i \Phi(\mathbf{x}_i) \ . \tag{4.11}$$

From the right-hand equation of Equation (4.11), we find that $\mathbf{w}$ is contained in the subspace spanned by the $\Phi(\mathbf{x}_i)$. By substituting Equation (4.11) into Equation (4.10) and by replacing $(\Phi(x_i) \cdot \Phi(x_j))$ with kernel functions $\mathrm{k}(\mathbf{x}_i, \mathbf{x}_j)$, we get the dual quadratic optimization problem:

$$\begin{aligned} \max_{\boldsymbol{\alpha}} \quad & \sum_{i=1}^{n} \alpha_i - \frac{1}{2} \sum_{i,j=1}^{n} \alpha_i \alpha_j y_i y_j \, \mathrm{k}\left(\mathbf{x}_i, \mathbf{x}_j\right) \\ \text{subject to} \quad & \alpha_i \geq 0, \ i = 1, \ldots, n, \\ & \textstyle\sum_{i=1}^{n} \alpha_i y_i = 0 \ . \end{aligned}$$

Thus, by solving the dual optimization problem, one obtains the coefficients $\alpha_i, i = 1, \ldots, n$, which one needs to express the $\mathbf{w}$ which solves Equation (4.9). This leads to the nonlinear decision function

$$\begin{aligned} f(\mathbf{x}) &= \operatorname{sgn}\left(\sum_{i=1}^{n} y_i \alpha_i \left(\Phi(\mathbf{x}) \cdot \Phi(\mathbf{x}_i)\right) + b\right) \\ &= \operatorname{sgn}\left(\sum_{i=1}^{n} y_i \alpha_i \, \mathrm{k}(\mathbf{x}, \mathbf{x}_i) + b\right) \ . \end{aligned}$$

Note that, up to now, we have only considered the separable case. This corresponds to an empirical error of zero (see Theorem 4.1). However, for noisy data, this might not be the minimum in the expected risk (see Equation (4.3)), and we might face overfitting effects (see Figure 4.1). Therefore, a "good" trade-off between the empirical risk and the complexity term in Equation (4.3) needs to be found. Using a technique which was first proposed by Bennett and Mangasarian [8] and was later used for SVMs [22], slack variables are introduced to relax the hard-margin constraints:

$$y_i \left((\mathbf{w} \cdot \Phi(\mathbf{x}_i)) + b\right) \geq 1 - \xi_i, \quad \xi_i \geq 0, \qquad i = 1, \ldots, n \ , \tag{4.12}$$

allowing, additionally, for some classification errors. The SVM solution can then be found (1) by keeping the upper bound on the VC dimension small, and (2) by minimizing an upper bound $\sum_{i=1}^{n} \xi_i$ on the empirical risk,[4] i.e., the number of training errors. Thus, one minimizes

$$\min_{\mathbf{w}, b, \boldsymbol{\xi}} \quad \frac{1}{2}\|\mathbf{w}\|^2 + C \sum_{i=1}^{n} \xi_i \ .$$

[4]Other bounds on the empirical error, like $\sum_{i=1}^{n} \xi_i^2$, are also frequently used [22, 63].

where the regularization constant $C > 0$ determines the trade-off between the empirical error and the complexity term. This leads to the dual problem:

$$\max_{\boldsymbol{\alpha}} \quad \sum_{i=1}^{n} \alpha_i - \frac{1}{2} \sum_{i,j=1}^{n} \alpha_i \alpha_j y_i y_j \, \mathrm{k}\left(\mathbf{x}_i, \mathbf{x}_j\right) \tag{4.13}$$

$$\text{subject to} \quad 0 \leq \alpha_i \leq C, \; i = 1, \ldots, n, \tag{4.14}$$

$$\textstyle\sum_{i=1}^{n} \alpha_i y_i = 0 \,. \tag{4.15}$$

From introducing the slack variables ξ_i, one gets the box constraints that limit the size of the Lagrange multipliers: $\alpha_i \leq C, i = 1, \ldots, n$.

4.4.1.1 Sparsity

Most optimization methods are based on the second order optimality conditions, called Karush–Kühn–Tucker (KKT) conditions, which state necessary, and in some cases, sufficient conditions for a set of variables to be optimal for an optimization problem. It comes in handy that these conditions are particularly simple for the dual SVM problem (Equation (4.13)) [141]:

$$\begin{array}{rcll} \alpha_i = 0 & \Rightarrow & y_i f\left(\mathbf{x}_i\right) \geq 1 \quad \text{and} & \xi_i = 0 \\ 0 < \alpha_i < C & \Rightarrow & y_i f\left(\mathbf{x}_i\right) = 1 \quad \text{and} & \xi_i = 0 \\ \alpha_i = C & \Rightarrow & y_i f\left(\mathbf{x}_i\right) \leq 1 \quad \text{and} & \xi_i \geq 0 \,. \end{array} \tag{4.16}$$

They reveal one of the most important property of SVMs: the solution is sparse in $\boldsymbol{\alpha}$, i.e., many patterns are outside the margin area and the optimal α_i is zero. Specifically, the (KKT) conditions show that only such α_i connected to a training pattern $\mathbf{x}_i$, which is either on the margin (i.e., $0 < \alpha_i < C$ and $y_i f(\mathbf{x}_i) = 1$) or inside the margin area (i.e., $\alpha_i = C$ and $y_i f(\mathbf{x}_i) < 1$), are non-zero. Without this sparsity property, SVM learning would hardly be practical for large data sets.

4.4.1.2 ν-SVMs

Several modifications have been proposed to the basic SVM algorithm. One particularly useful modification is ν-SVMs [117], originally proposed for regression. In the case of pattern recognition, ν-SVMs replace the rather nonintuitive regularization constant C with another constant $\nu \in (0, 1]$ and yield, for appropriate parameter choices, identical solutions. Instead of Equation (4.13) one solves

$$\begin{array}{ll} \max\limits_{\boldsymbol{\alpha}} & -\dfrac{1}{2} \sum\limits_{i,j=1}^{n} \alpha_i \alpha_j y_i y_j \, \mathrm{k}\left(\mathbf{x}_i, \mathbf{x}_j\right) \\ \text{subject to} & 0 \leq \alpha_i \leq 1/n, \; i = 1, \ldots, n, \\ & \sum_{i=1}^{n} \alpha_i y_i = 0, \\ & \sum_i \alpha_i \geq \nu \,. \end{array}$$

The advantage is that this new parameter ν has a clearer interpretation than simply “the smaller, the smoother”: under some mild assumptions (data i.i.d. from continuous probability distribution [117]) it is asymptotically (1) an upper bound on the number of margin errors[5] and (2) a lower bound on the number of support vectors.

---

[5] A margin error is a point $\mathbf{x}_i$ which is either misclassified or lies inside the margin area.

4.4.1.3 Computing the Threshold

The threshold b can be computed by exploiting the fact that for all SVs $\mathbf{x}_i$ with $0 < \alpha_i < C$, the slack variable ξ_i is zero. This follows from the Karush–Kühn–Tucker (KKT) conditions (see Equation (4.16)). Thus, for any support vector $\mathbf{x}_i$ with $i \in I := \{i : 0 < \alpha_i < C\}$,

$$y_i \left(b + \sum_{j=1}^{n} y_j \alpha_j \, \mathrm{k}\left(\mathbf{x}_i, \mathbf{x}_j\right) \right) = 1 .$$

Averaging over these patterns yields a numerically stable solution:

$$b = \frac{1}{|I|} \sum_{i \in I} \left(y_i - \sum_{j=1}^{n} y_j \alpha_j \, \mathrm{k}\left(\mathbf{x}_i, \mathbf{x}_j\right) \right) .$$

4.4.1.4 A Geometrical Explanation

This section presents an illustration of the SVM solution to enhance intuitive understandings. Let us normalize the weight vector to 1 (i.e., $\|\mathbf{w}\|_2 = 1$) and fix the threshold $b = 0$. Then, the set of all $\mathbf{w}$ that separate the training samples is completely described as:

$$\mathcal{V} = \{\mathbf{w} | y_i f\left(\mathbf{x}_i\right) > 0; i = 1, \ldots, n, \|\mathbf{w}\|_2 = 1\} .$$

The set $\mathcal{V}$ is called "version space" [80]. It can be shown that the SVM solution coincides with the Tchebycheff center of the version space, which is the center of the largest sphere contained in $\mathcal{V}$ [123]. However, the theoretical optimal point in version space yielding a Bayes optimal decision boundary is the Bayes point, which is known to be closely approximated by the center of mass [89, 146]. The version space is illustrated as a region on the sphere, as shown in Figures 4.5 and 4.6. If the version space is shaped as in Figure 4.5, the SVM solution is near to the optimal point. However, if it has an elongated shape as in Figure 4.6, the SVM solution is far from optimal. To cope with this problem, several researchers [48, 89, 101] proposed a billiard sampling method for approximating the Bayes point. This method can achieve improved results, as shown on several benchmarks in comparison to SVMs.

4.4.1.5 Optimization Techniques for SVMs

To solve the SVM problem, one has to solve the (convex) quadratic programming (QP) problem (Equation (4.13)) under the constraints of Equations (4.14) and (4.15) (Equation (4.13) can be rewritten as maximizing $-\frac{1}{2}\boldsymbol{\alpha}^\top \hat{K} \boldsymbol{\alpha} + \mathbf{1}^\top \boldsymbol{\alpha}$, where $\hat{K}$ is the positive semidefinite matrix $\hat{K}_{ij} = y_i y_j \, \mathrm{k}(\mathbf{x}_i, \mathbf{x}_j)$ and $\mathbf{1}$ is the vector of all ones). Since the objective function is convex, every (local) maximum is already a global maximum. However, there can be several optimal solutions (in terms of the variables α_i) which might lead to different testing performances.

There exists a huge body of literature on solving quadratic programs and several free or commercial software packages [9, 126, 140]. However, the problem is that most mathematical programming approaches are either only suitable for small problems or assume that the quadratic term covered by $\hat{K}$ is very sparse, i.e., most elements of this matrix are zero. Unfortunately, this is not true for the SVM problem and, thus, using standard codes with more than a few hundred variables results in enormous training times and more demanding memory needs. Nevertheless, the structure of the SVM optimization problem allows the derivation of specially tailored algorithms which allow for fast convergence with small memory requirements, even on large problems. The following subsections briefly consider three different approaches. More details and tricks can be found in some of the referenced literature [111, 126].

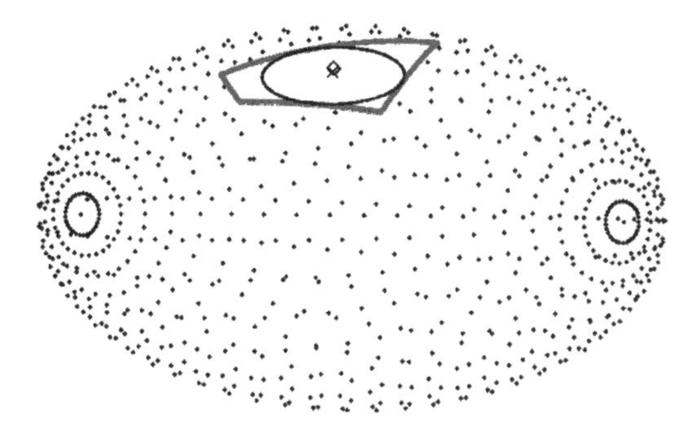

4.5 An example of the version space where the SVM works well. The center of mass ($\diamond$) is close to the SVM solution ($\times$).

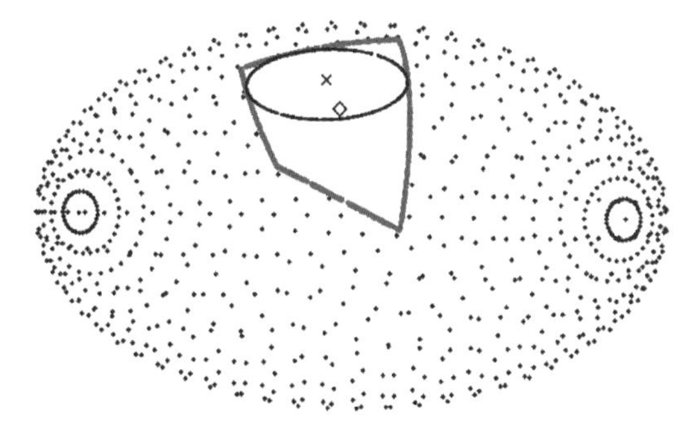

4.6 An example of the version space where SVM works poorly. The version space has an elongated shape and the center of mass ($\diamond$) is far from the SVM solution ($\times$).

4.4.1.5.1 Chunking

A key observation in solving large scale SVM problems is the sparsity of the solution $\boldsymbol{\alpha}$. Depending on the problem, many of the optimal α_i will either be zero or on the upper bound C. If one could know beforehand which α_i were zero, the corresponding rows and columns could be removed from the matrix $\hat{K}$ without changing the value of the quadratic form. Furthermore, a point $\boldsymbol{\alpha}$ can only be optimal for Equation (4.13) if it fulfills the KKT conditions (see Equation (4.16)). Vapnik [141] describes a method called chunking, making use of the sparsity and the KKT conditions. At every step, chunking solves the problem containing all non-zero α_i plus some of the α_i violating the KKT conditions. The size of this problem varies but is finally equal to the number of non-zero coefficients. While this technique is suitable for fairly large problems, it is still limited by the maximal number of support vectors that one can handle and it still requires a quadratic optimizer to solve the sequence of smaller problems. A free implementation can be found, e.g., in Saunders et al. [104].

4.4.1.5.2 Decomposition Methods

These methods are similar in spirit to chunking as they solve a sequence of small QPs as well. But here the size of the subproblems is fixed. Decomposition methods are based on the observations of Osuna et al. [82, 83] that a sequence of QPs which always contains at least one sample violating the KKT conditions will eventually converge to the optimal solution. It was suggested to keep the size of the subproblems fixed and to add and remove one sample in each iteration. This allows the training of arbitrary large data sets. In practice, however, the convergence of such an approach is very slow. Practical implementations use sophisticated heuristics to select several patterns to add and remove from the subproblem plus efficient caching methods. They usually achieve fast convergence even on large data sets with up to several thousands of support vectors. A good quality (free) implementation is $\text{SVM}_{\text{light}}$ [54]. A quadratic optimizer is still required and is contained in the package. Alternatively, the package [104] also contains a decomposition variant.

4.4.1.5.3 Sequential Minimal Optimization (SMO)

This method, proposed by Platt [87], can be viewed as the most extreme case of decomposition methods. In each iteration, it solves a quadratic problem of size two. This can be done analytically and, thus, no quadratic optimizer is required. Here, the main problem is to choose a good pair of variables to optimize in each iteration. The original heuristics presented by Platt [87] are based on the KKT conditions, and there has been some work done [56] to improve them. The implementation of the SMO approach is straightforward (pseudo-code in Platt [87]). While the original work was targeted at an SVM for classification, there are now also approaches which implement variants of SMO for SVM regression [126, 127] and single-class SVMs [114].

4.4.1.5.4 Other Techniques

Further algorithms have been proposed to solve the SVM problem or a close approximation. For instance, the kernel-Adatron [39] is derived from the Adatron algorithm originally proposed by Anlauf and Biehl [3] in a statistical mechanics setting. The kernel-Adatron constructs a large margin hyperplane using online learning. Its implementation is very simple. However, its drawback is that it does not allow for training errors, i.e., it is only valid for separable data sets. Bradley et al. [14] consider a slightly more general approach for data mining problems.

4.4.1.5.5 Codes

A fairly large selection of optimization codes for SVM classification and regression may be found on the Web [132] together with the appropriate references. They range from simple MATLAB implementation to sophisticated C, C++, or FORTRAN programs. Note that most of these implementations are for noncommercial use only.

4.4.2 Kernel Fisher Discriminant

The idea of the kernel Fisher discriminant (KFD) [4, 69, 100] is to solve the problem of Fisher's linear discriminant [36, 40] in a kernel feature space $\mathcal{F}$, thereby yielding a nonlinear discriminant in the input space. In the linear case, Fisher's discriminant aims at finding a linear projection such that the classes are well separated (see Figure 4.7). Separability is measured by two quantities: how far apart the projected means are (should be far) and how big the variance of the data in this direction is (should be small). This can be achieved by maximizing the Rayleigh coefficient:

$$J(\mathbf{w}) = \frac{\mathbf{w}^\top S_B \mathbf{w}}{\mathbf{w}^\top S_W \mathbf{w}} \tag{4.17}$$

of between and within class variance with respect to $\mathbf{w}$, where

$$S_B = (\boldsymbol{m}_2 - \boldsymbol{m}_1)(\boldsymbol{m}_2 - \boldsymbol{m}_1)^\top$$

and

$$S_W = \sum_{k=1,2} \sum_{i \in \mathcal{I}_k} (\mathbf{x}_i - \boldsymbol{m}_k)(\mathbf{x}_i - \boldsymbol{m}_k)^\top .$$

Here, $\boldsymbol{m}_k$ and $\mathcal{I}_k$ denote the sample mean and the index set for class k, respectively. Note that under the assumption that the class distributions are (identically distributed) Gaussians, Fisher's discriminant is Bayes optimal; it can also be generalized to the multiclass case.[6] To formulate the

[6]This can be done with kernel functions as well and has explicitly been carried out [4, 100]. However, most further developments for KFD do not easily carry over to the multiclass case, e.g., resulting in integer programming problems.

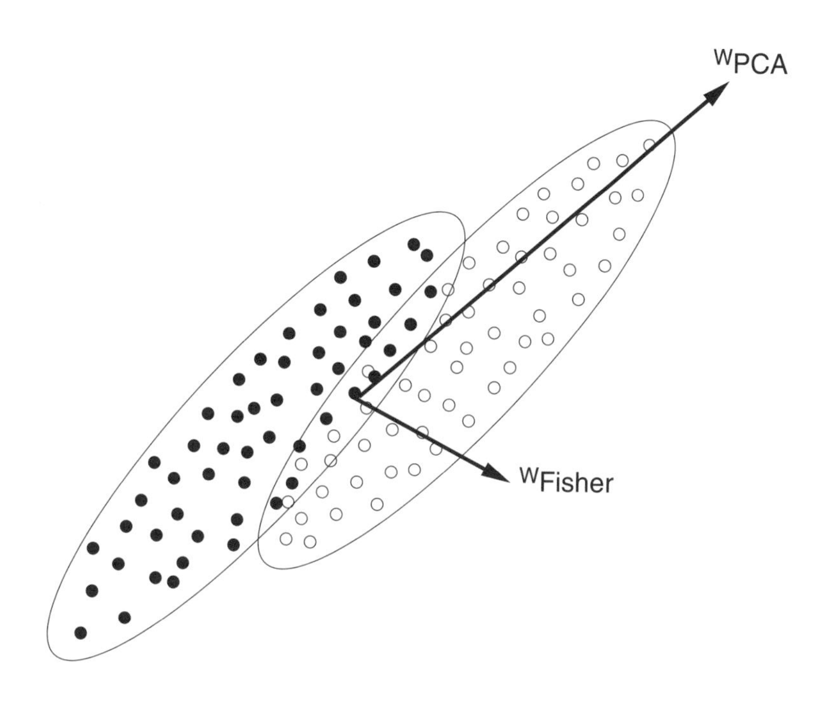

4.7 Illustration of the projections of PCA and Fisher's discriminant for a toy data set. It is clearly seen that PCA is purely descriptive, whereas the Fisher projection is discriminative.

problem in a kernel feature space $\mathcal{F}$, one can make use of an expansion similar to Equation (4.11) in SVMs for $\mathbf{w} \in \mathcal{F}$, i.e., one can express $\mathbf{w}$ in terms of mapped training patterns [69]:

$$\mathbf{w} = \sum_{i=1}^{n} \alpha_i \Phi(\mathbf{x}_i) \ . \tag{4.18}$$

Substituting $\Phi(\mathbf{x})$ for all $\mathbf{x}$ in Equation (4.17) and plugging in Equation (4.18), the optimization problem for the KFD in the feature space can then be written as [70]:

$$J(\boldsymbol{\alpha}) = \frac{(\boldsymbol{\alpha}^\top \boldsymbol{\mu})^2}{\boldsymbol{\alpha}^\top N \boldsymbol{\alpha}} = \frac{\boldsymbol{\alpha}^\top M \boldsymbol{\alpha}}{\boldsymbol{\alpha}^\top N \boldsymbol{\alpha}} \tag{4.19}$$

where $\boldsymbol{\mu}_k = \frac{1}{|\mathcal{I}_k|} K \mathbf{1}_k$, $N = KK^\top - \Sigma_{k=1,2} |I_k| \boldsymbol{\mu}_k \boldsymbol{\mu}_k^\top$, $\boldsymbol{\mu} = \boldsymbol{\mu}_2 - \boldsymbol{\mu}_1$, $M = \boldsymbol{\mu}\boldsymbol{\mu}^\top$, and $K_{ij} = (\Phi(\mathbf{x}_i) \cdot \Phi(\mathbf{x}_j)) = \mathrm{k}(\mathbf{x}_i, \mathbf{x}_j)$. The projection of a test point onto the discriminant is computed by

$$(\mathbf{w} \cdot \Phi(\mathbf{x})) = \sum_{i=1}^{n} \alpha_i \, \mathrm{k}(\mathbf{x}_i, \mathbf{x}) \ .$$

Finally, to use this projection in classification, one needs to find a suitable threshold which can be chosen either as the mean of the average projections of the two classes or, e.g., by training a linear SVM on the projections.

As outlined before, the dimension of the feature space is equal to or higher than the number of training samples n, which makes regularization necessary. Mika et al. [69] proposed adding a multiple of the identity or the kernel matrix K to N, penalizing $\|\boldsymbol{\alpha}\|^2$ or $\|\mathbf{w}\|^2$, respectively [38, 45].

To maximize Equation (4.19) one could either solve the generalized eigenproblem $M\boldsymbol{\alpha} = \lambda N\boldsymbol{\alpha}$, selecting the eigenvector $\boldsymbol{\alpha}$ with maximal eigenvalue λ, or, equivalently, compute $\boldsymbol{\alpha} \equiv N^{-1}(\boldsymbol{\mu}_2 - \boldsymbol{\mu}_1)$. However, as the matrices N and M scale with the number of training samples and the solutions are non-sparse, this is only feasible for a moderate n. One possible solution is to transform the KFD into a convex quadratic programming problem [68], which allows the derivation of a sparse variant of the KFD and a more efficient, sparse-greedy approximation algorithm [72]. Recalling that Fisher's discriminant tries to minimize the variance of the data along the projection while maximizing the distance between the average outputs for each class, the following quadratic program does exactly that:

$$\begin{aligned} \min_{\boldsymbol{\alpha},b,\boldsymbol{\xi}} \quad & \|\boldsymbol{\xi}\|^2 + C\,\mathrm{P}(\boldsymbol{\alpha}) \\ \text{subject to} \quad & K\boldsymbol{\alpha} + \mathbf{1}b = \mathbf{y} + \boldsymbol{\xi} \\ & \mathbf{1}_k^\top \boldsymbol{\xi} = 0 \;\text{ for }\; k = 1, 2 \end{aligned} \tag{4.20}$$

for $\boldsymbol{\alpha}, \boldsymbol{\xi} \in \mathbb{R}^n$ and $b, C \in \mathbb{R}$. Here, P is a regularizer, as mentioned before, and $(\mathbf{1}_k)_i$ is 1 for y_i belonging to class k and zero otherwise. It is straightforward to show that this program is equivalent to Equation (4.19) with the same regularizer added to the matrix N [68]. The proof is based on the facts that (1) the matrix M is rank one, and (2) the solutions $\mathbf{w}$ to Equation (4.19) are invariant under scaling. Thus, one can fix the distance of the means to some arbitrary, positive value, e.g., two, and just minimize the variance. The first constraint, which can be read as $(\mathbf{w} \cdot \mathbf{x}_i) + b = y_i + \xi_i$, $i = 1, \ldots, n$, pulls the output for each sample to its class label. The term $\|\boldsymbol{\xi}\|^2$ minimizes the variance of the error committed, while the constraints $\mathbf{1}_k^\top \boldsymbol{\xi} = 0$ ensure that the average output for each class is the label, i.e., for ± 1 labels, the average distance of the projections is two. For $C = 0$, one obtains the original Fisher algorithm in feature space.

4.4.2.1 Optimization

Besides a more intuitive understanding of the mathematical properties of KFD [68], in particular in relation to SVMs or the relevance vector machine (RVM) [137], the formulation of Equation (4.20) allows the derivation of more efficient algorithms as well. Choosing an ℓ_1-norm regularizer $\mathrm{P}(\boldsymbol{\alpha}) = \|\boldsymbol{\alpha}\|_1$, we obtain sparse solutions (sparse KFD [SKFD]).[7] By going even further and replacing the quadratic penalty on the variables $\boldsymbol{\xi}$ with an ℓ_1–norm as well, we obtain a linear program which can be very efficiently optimized using column generation techniques (linear sparse KFD [LSKFD]) [7]. An alternative optimization strategy arising from Equation (4.20) is to iteratively construct a solution to the full problem, as proposed by Mika et al. [72]. Starting with an empty solution, one adds one pattern in each iteration to the expansion in Equation (4.18). This pattern is chosen such that it (approximately) gives the largest decrease in the objective function (other criteria are possible). When the change in the objective falls below a predefined threshold, the iteration is terminated. The obtained solution is sparse and yields competitive results compared to the full solution. The advantages of this approach are smaller memory requirements and faster training time compared to quadratic programming or the solution of an eigenproblem.

[7] Roughly speaking, one reason for the induced sparseness is the fact that vectors far from the coordinate axes are "larger" with respect to the ℓ_1-norm than with respect to ℓ_p-norms with $p > 1$. For example, consider the vectors $(1, 0)$ and $(1/\sqrt{2}, 1/\sqrt{2})$. For the two norm, $\|(1,0)\|_2 = \|(1/\sqrt{2}, 1/\sqrt{2})\|_2 = 1$, but for the ℓ_1-norm, $1 = \|(1,0)\|_1 < \|(1/\sqrt{2}, 1/\sqrt{2})\|_2 = \sqrt{2}$. Note that using the ℓ_1-norm as a regularizer, the optimal solution is always a vertex solution (or can be expressed as such) and tends to be very sparse.

4.4.3 Connection between Boosting and Kernel Methods

Let us start with a very brief review of boosting methods. For more details see the referenced literature [31, 37, 50, 105, 107, 108]. The first boosting algorithm was proposed by Schapire [106]. This algorithm was able to "boost" the performance of a weak PAC learner [55] such that the resulting algorithm satisfies the strong PAC learning criteria [139].[8] Later, Freund and Schapire [37] found an improved PAC boosting algorithm called AdaBoost, which repeatedly refers to a given "weak learner" $\mathcal{L}$ (also: base learning algorithm) and finally produces a master hypothesis f which is a convex combination of the functions h_j produced by the base learning algorithm, i.e., $f(\mathbf{x}) = \Sigma_{t=1}^{T} \frac{w_t}{\|\mathbf{w}\|_1} h_t(\mathbf{x})$ and $w_t \geq 0$, $t = 1, \ldots, T$. The given weak learner $\mathcal{L}$ is used with different distributions $p = [p_1, \ldots, p_n]$ (where $\Sigma_i p_i = 1$, $p_i \geq 0$, $i = 1, \ldots, n$) on the training set, chosen in such a way that patterns poorly classified by the current master hypothesis are more emphasized than other patterns.

Recently, several researchers [16, 30, 65, 92] have noticed that AdaBoost implements a constraint gradient descent (coordinate-descent) method on an exponential function of the margins. From this, it is apparent that other algorithms can be derived [16, 30, 65, 92].[9] A slight modification of AdaBoost — called Arc-GV — has been proposed by Breiman [17].[10] It can be proven that Arc-GV asymptotically (with the number of iterations) finds a convex combination of all possible base hypotheses that maximize the margin — very closely related to the hard margin SVM mentioned in Section 4.4.1. Let $H := \{h_j \mid j = 1, \ldots, J\}$ be the set of hypotheses from which the base learner can potentially select hypotheses. Then the solution of Arc-GV is the same as the one of the following linear program [17], that maximizes the smallest margin ρ:

$$\begin{aligned} &\max_{\mathbf{w}\in\mathcal{F},\rho\in\mathbb{R}_+} && \rho \\ &\text{subject to} && y_i \sum_{j=1}^{J} w_j h_j(\mathbf{x}_i) \geq \rho \quad \text{for} \quad i = 1, \ldots, n \\ & && \|\mathbf{w}\|_1 = 1\,. \end{aligned} \tag{4.21}$$

Let us recall that SVMs and KFD implicitly compute scalar products in feature space with the help of the kernel trick. Omitting the bias ($b \equiv 0$) for simplicity, the SVM minimization of Equation (4.9) subject to Equation (4.8) can be restated as a maximization of the margin ρ (see Figure 4.3)

$$\begin{aligned} &\max_{\mathbf{w}\in\mathcal{F},\rho\in\mathbb{R}_+} && \rho \\ &\text{subject to} && y_i \sum_{j=1}^{J} w_j \mathrm{P}_j[\Phi(\mathbf{x}_i)] \geq \rho \quad \text{for} \quad i = 1, \ldots, n \\ & && \|\mathbf{w}\|_2 = 1 \end{aligned} \tag{4.22}$$

where $J = \dim(\mathcal{F})$ and P_j is the operator projecting onto the jth coordinate in feature space. The use of the ℓ_2-norm of $\mathbf{w}$ in the last constraint implies that the resulting hyperplane is chosen such that the minimum ℓ_2-distance of a training pattern to the hyperplane is maximized (see Section 4.2.2). More generally, using an arbitrary ℓ_p-norm constraint on the weight vector leads to maximizing the

---

[8] A method that builds a strong PAC learning algorithm from a weak PAC learning algorithm is called a PAC boosting algorithm [31].

[9] See Duffy and Helmbold [31] for an investigation in which potentials lead to PAC boosting algorithms.

[10] A generalization of Arc-GV using slack variables as in Equation (4.12) can be found in Bennett et al. [7] and Rätsch et al. [94].

ℓ_q-distance between hyperplane and training points [62], where $\frac{1}{q} + \frac{1}{p} = 1$. Thus, in Equation (4.21) one maximizes the minimum ℓ_∞-distance of the training points to the hyperplane.

On the level of the mathematical programs of Equations (4.22) and (4.21), one can clearly see the relation between boosting and SVMs. The connection can be made even more explicit by observing that any hypothesis set H implies a mapping Φ by

$$\Phi : \mathbf{x} \mapsto [h_1(\mathbf{x}), \dots, h_J(\mathbf{x})]^\top$$

and, therefore, also a kernel $\mathrm{k}(\mathbf{x}, \mathbf{y}) = (\Phi(y) \cdot \Phi(\mathbf{y})) = \Sigma_{j=1}^{J} h_j(\mathbf{x}) h_j(\mathbf{y})$, which could, in principle, be used for SVM learning. Thus, any hypothesis set H spans a feature space $\mathcal{F}$. Furthermore, for any feature space $\mathcal{F}$ which is spanned by some mapping Φ, the corresponding hypothesis set H can be readily constructed by $h_j = \mathrm{P}_j[\Phi]$.

Boosting, in contrast to SVMs, performs the computation explicitly in feature space. This is well known to be prohibitive if the solution $\mathbf{w}$ is not sparse, as the feature space might be very high-dimensional. As mentioned in Section 4.4.2 (see Footnote 7), using the ℓ_1-norm instead of the ℓ_2-norm, one can expect sparse solutions in $\mathbf{w}$.[11] This might be seen as one important ingredient for boosting, because it relies on the fact that there are only a few hypotheses/dimensions $h_j = \mathrm{P}_j[\Phi]$ needed to express the solution, which boosting tries to find during each iteration. Basically, boosting considers only the most important dimensions in feature space and can therefore be very efficient.

4.4.4 Wrapping Up

SVMs, KFD, and boosting work in very high-dimensional feature spaces. They differ, however, in how they deal with the algorithmic problems that this can cause. One can think of boosting as an SV approach in a high-dimensional feature space spanned by the base hypothesis of some function set H. The problem becomes tractable since boosting effectively uses an ℓ_1-norm regularizer. This induces sparsity; hence, one never really works in the full space, but always in a small subspace. In contrast, one can think of SVMs and KFD as a "boosting approach" in a high-dimensional space. There, the kernel trick is used and, therefore, we never explicitly work in the feature space. Thus, SVMs and KFD get away without having to use ℓ_1-norm regularizers; indeed, they cannot use them on $\mathbf{w}$ because the kernel only allows computation of the ℓ_2-norm in feature space. SVM and boosting both lead to sparse solutions (as does KFD with the appropriate regularizer [68]), albeit in different spaces, and both algorithms are constructed to exploit the form of sparsity they produce. Besides providing insight, this correspondence has concrete practical benefits for designing new algorithms. Almost any new development in the field of SVMs can be translated to a corresponding boosting algorithm using the ℓ_1-norm instead of the ℓ_2-norm and vice versa [91, 93, 94]).

4.5 Unsupervised Learning

In unsupervised learning, only the data $\mathbf{x}_1, \dots, \mathbf{x}_n \in \mathbb{R}^N$ are given, i.e., the labels are missing. Standard questions of unsupervised learning are clustering, density estimation, and data description [10, 29]. As already outlined, the kernel trick can be applied not only in supervised learning scenarios, but also in cases of unsupervised learning, given that the base algorithm can be written in terms of scalar products. The following section reviews one of the most common statistical data analysis algorithm, PCA, and explains its "kernelized" variant: kernel PCA [119]. Subsequently,

[11] Note that the solution of SVMs is, under rather mild assumption, not sparse in $\mathbf{w} = \sum_{i=1}^{n} \alpha_i \Phi(\mathbf{x}_i)$ [95], but is sparse in $\boldsymbol{\alpha}$.

single-class classification is explained. Here, the support of a given data set is being estimated [93, 114, 120, 134]. Recently, single-class SVMs have frequently been used in outlier or novelty detection applications.

4.5.1 Kernel PCA

The basic idea of PCA is depicted in Figure 4.8. For N-dimensional data, a set of orthogonal

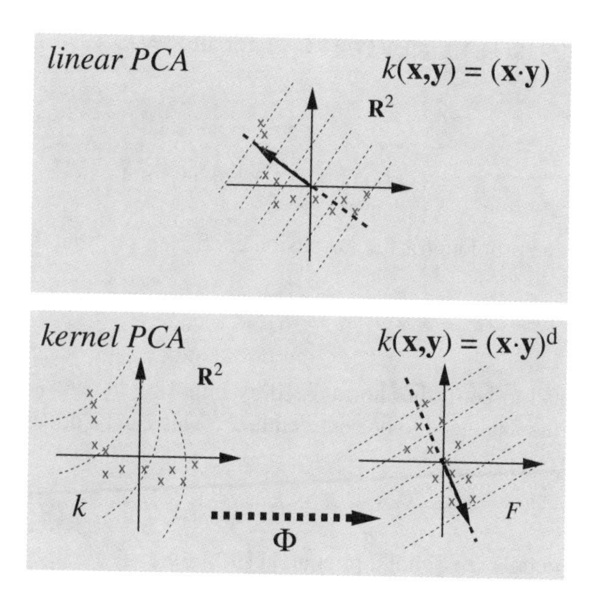

4.8 By using a kernel function, kernel PCA is implicitly performing a linear PCA in some high-dimensional feature space that is nonlinearly related to input space. Linear PCA in the input space (top) is not sufficient to describe the most interesting direction in this toy example. In contrast, using a suitable nonlinear mapping Φ and performing linear PCA on the mapped patterns (kernel PCA), the resulting nonlinear direction in the input space can find the most interesting direction (bottom) [119].

directions capturing most of the variance in the data is computed, i.e., the first k projections ($k = 1, \ldots, N$) allow for reconstruction of the data with minimal quadratic error. In practice, one typically wants to describe the data with reduced dimensionality by extracting a few meaningful components while at the same time retaining most of the existing structure in the data [26]). Since PCA is a linear algorithm, it is clearly beyond its capabilities to extract nonlinear structures in the data as, for example, the one observed in Figure 4.8. It is here where the kernel PCA algorithm sets in. To derive kernel PCA, we first map the data $\mathbf{x}_1, \ldots, \mathbf{x}_n \in \mathbb{R}^N$ into a feature space $\mathcal{F}$ (see Section 4.3) and compute the covariance matrix

$$C = \frac{1}{n}\sum_{j=1}^{n} \Phi\left(\mathbf{x}_j\right) \Phi\left(\mathbf{x}_j\right)^{\top} .$$

The principal components are then computed by solving the eigenvalue problem: find $\lambda > 0$, $\mathbf{V} \neq 0$ with

$$\lambda \mathbf{V} = C\mathbf{V} = \frac{1}{n}\sum_{j=1}^{n} \left(\Phi\left(\mathbf{x}_j\right) \cdot \mathbf{V}\right) \Phi\left(\mathbf{x}_j\right) . \tag{4.23}$$

Furthermore, as can be seen from Equation (4.23) all eigenvectors with non-zero eigenvalue must be in the span of the mapped data, i.e., $\mathbf{V} \in \operatorname{span}\{\Phi(\mathbf{x}_1), \ldots, \Phi(\mathbf{x}_n)\}$. This can be written as

$$\mathbf{V} = \sum_{i=1}^{n} \alpha_i \Phi(\mathbf{x}_i) .$$

By multiplying with $\Phi(\mathbf{x}_k)$, from the left, Equation (4.23) reads:

$$\lambda \left(\Phi(\mathbf{x}_k) \cdot \mathbf{V}\right) = \left(\Phi(\mathbf{x}_k) \cdot C\mathbf{V}\right) \text{ for all } k = 1, \ldots, n .$$

Defining an $n \times n$ matrix,

$$K_{ij} := \left(\Phi(\mathbf{x}_i) \cdot \Phi(\mathbf{x}_j)\right) = \mathrm{k}(\mathbf{x}_i, \mathbf{x}_j) \tag{4.24}$$

one computes an eigenvalue problem for the expansion coefficients α_i that is now solely dependent on the kernel function

$$\lambda \boldsymbol{\alpha} = K \boldsymbol{\alpha} \qquad \left(\boldsymbol{\alpha} = (\alpha_1, \ldots, \alpha_n)^\top\right) .$$

The solutions $(\lambda_k, \boldsymbol{\alpha}^k)$ need to be further normalized by imposing $\lambda_k(\boldsymbol{\alpha}^k \cdot \boldsymbol{\alpha}^k) = 1$ in $\mathcal{F}$. Also, as in every PCA algorithm, the data need to be centered in $\mathcal{F}$. This can be done by simply substituting the kernel matrix K with

$$\hat{K} = K - 1_n K - K 1_n + 1_n K 1_n$$

where $(1_n)_{ij} = 1/n$; for details see Schölkopf et al. [119].

For extracting features of a new pattern $\mathbf{x}$ with kernel PCA, one simply projects the mapped pattern $\Phi(\mathbf{x})$ onto $\mathbf{V}^k$

$$\begin{aligned} \left(\mathbf{V}^k \cdot \Phi(\mathbf{x})\right) &= \sum_{i=1}^{M} \alpha_i^k \left(\Phi(\mathbf{x}_i) \cdot \Phi(\mathbf{x})\right) \\ &= \sum_{i=1}^{M} \alpha_i^k \, \mathrm{k}(\mathbf{x}_i, \mathbf{x}) . \end{aligned} \tag{4.25}$$

Note that in this algorithm for nonlinear PCA, the nonlinearity enters the computation only at two points that do not change the nature of the algorithm: (1) in the calculation of the matrix elements of K (Equation (4.24)), and (2) in the evaluation of the expansion of Equation (4.25). So, for obtaining the kernel PCA components, one only needs to solve a similar linear eigenvalue problem as before for linear PCA, the only difference being that one has to deal with an $n \times n$ problem instead of an $N \times N$ problem. Clearly, the size of this problem becomes problematic for large n. Smola and Schölkopf [130] propose to solve this by using a sparse approximation of the matrix K which still describes the leading eigenvectors sufficiently well. Tipping [136] proposes a sparse kernel PCA approach, set within a Bayesian framework. Finally, the approach given by Smola et al. [128] places an ℓ_1-regularizer into the (kernel) PCA problem with the effect of obtaining sparse solutions as well at a comparably low computational cost. Figures 4.9–4.11 show examples for feature extraction with linear PCA and kernel PCA for artificial data sets. Further applications of kernel PCA for real-world data can be found in Section 4.7.1.1 for OCR or in Section 4.7.3.1 for denoising problems; other applications are found in the referenced literature [71, 98, 111].

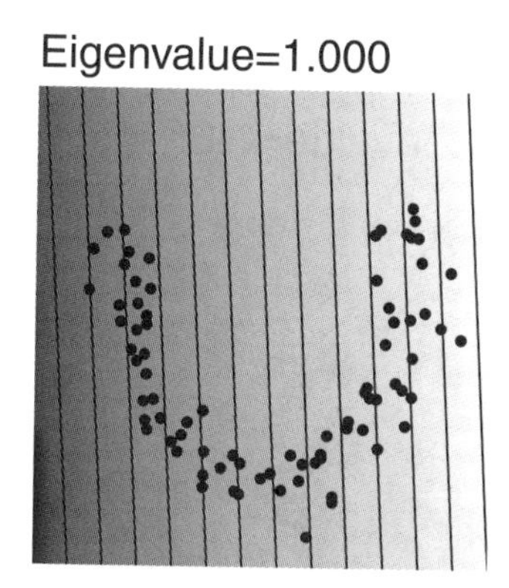

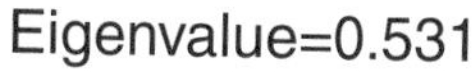

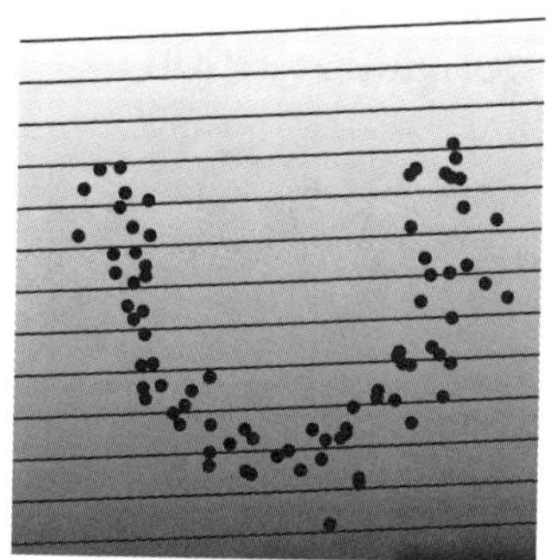

4.9 Linear PCA, or, equivalently, kernel PCA using $k(\mathbf{x}, \mathbf{y}) = (\mathbf{x} \cdot \mathbf{y})$. Plotted are two linear PCA features (sorted according to the size of the eigenvalues) on an artificial data set. Similar gray values denote areas of similar feature value (see Equation (4.25)). The first feature (left) projects to the direction of maximal variance in the data. Clearly, one cannot identify the nonlinear structure in the underlying data using only linear PCA [113].

4.5.2 Single-Class Classification

A classical unsupervised learning task is density estimation. Assuming that the unlabeled observations $\mathbf{x}_1, \ldots, \mathbf{x}_n$ were generated i.i.d. according to some unknown distribution $P(\mathbf{x})$, the task is to estimate its density. However, there are several difficulties involved in this task. First, a density need not always exist — there are distributions that do not possess a density. Second, estimating densities exactly is known to be a difficult task. In many applications, it is enough to estimate the support of a data distribution instead of the full density. Single-class SVMs avoid solving the harder density estimation problem and concentrate on the simpler task [142], i.e., estimating quantiles of the multivariate distribution, such as its support. So far, there are two independent algorithms to solve the problem in a kernel feature space. They differ slightly in spirit and geometric notion [114, 134]. It is, however, not quite clear which of them is preferred in practice (see Figures 4.12 and 4.13). One solution of the single-class SVM problem, proposed by Tax and Duin [134], uses spheres with soft margins to describe the data in feature space, close in spirit to the algorithm of Schölkopf et al. [109]. For certain classes of kernels, such as Gaussian RBF kernels, this sphere single-class SVM algorithm can be shown to be equivalent to the second Ansatz, which is attributed to Schölkopf et al. [114]. For brevity, we will focus on this second approach as it is more in the line of this review because it uses margin arguments. This approach computes a hyperplane in feature space such that a prespecified fraction of the training example will lie beyond that hyperplane, while at the same time, the hyperplane has maximal distance (margin) to the origin. For an illustration, see Figure 4.12. To this end, we solve the following quadratic program [114]:

$$\min_{\mathbf{w} \in F, \boldsymbol{\xi} \in \mathbb{R}^n, \rho \in \mathbb{R}} \quad \frac{1}{2}\|\mathbf{w}\|^2 + \frac{1}{\nu n} \sum_i \xi_i - \rho \tag{4.26}$$

$$\text{subject to} \quad (\mathbf{w} \cdot \Phi(\mathbf{x}_i)) \geq \rho - \xi_i, \ \xi_i \geq 0 \,. \tag{4.27}$$

Here, $\nu \in (0, 1]$ is a parameter akin to the one described above for the case of pattern recognition. Since non-zero slack variables ξ_i are penalized in the objective function, we can expect that if $\mathbf{w}$ and ρ solve this problem, then the decision function $f(\mathbf{x}) = \text{sign}((\mathbf{w} \cdot \Phi(\mathbf{x})) - \rho)$ will be positive for most examples $\mathbf{x}_i$ contained in the training set, while the SV-type regularization term $\|\mathbf{w}\|$ will still be small. The actual trade-off between these two goals is controlled by ν. Deriving the dual problem, the solution can be shown to have an SV expansion (again, patterns $\mathbf{x}_i$ with non-zero α_i

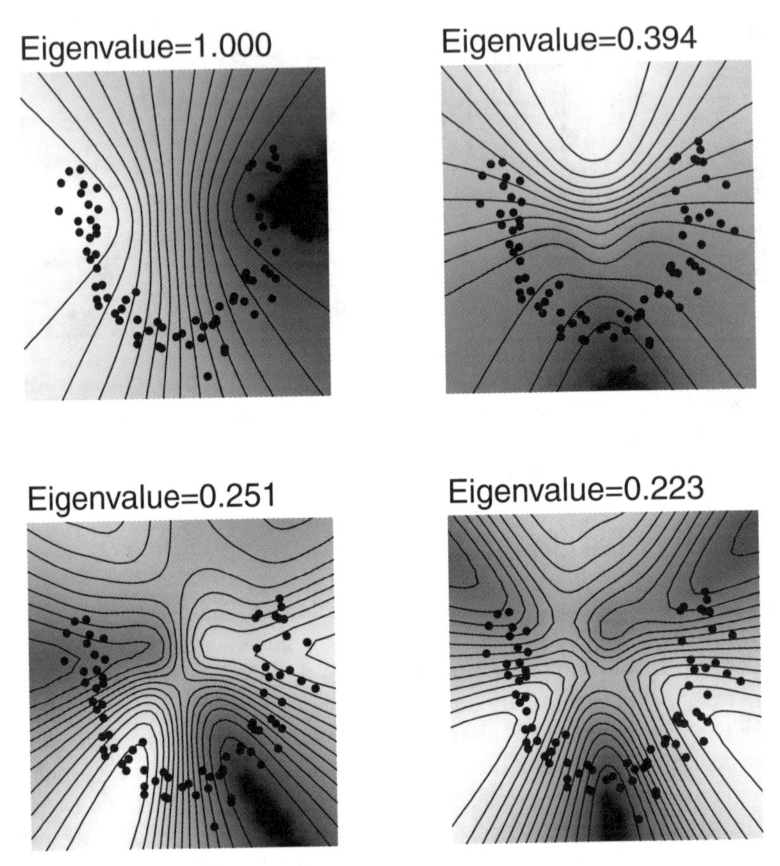

4.10 The first four nonlinear features of kernel PCA using a sigmoidal kernel on the data set from Figure 4.9. The kernel PCA components capture the nonlinear structure in the data, e.g., the first feature (upper left) is better adapted to the curvature of the data than the respective linear feature from Figure 4.9 [113].

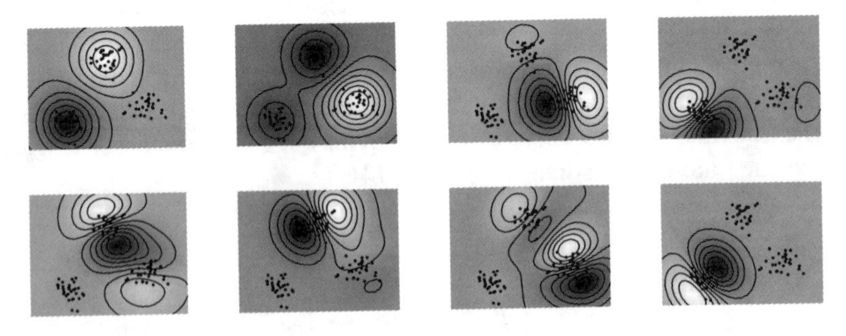

4.11 The first eight nonlinear features of kernel PCA using an RBF kernel on a toy data set consisting of three Gaussian clusters [119]. Upper left: the first and second component split the data into three clusters. Note that kernel PCA is not primarily built to achieve such a clustering. Rather, it tries to find a good description of the data in feature space, and, in this case, the cluster structure extracted has the maximal variance in feature space. The higher components depicted split each cluster in halves (components 3 to 5). Finally, features 6 to 8 achieve orthogonal splits with respect to the previous splits [119].

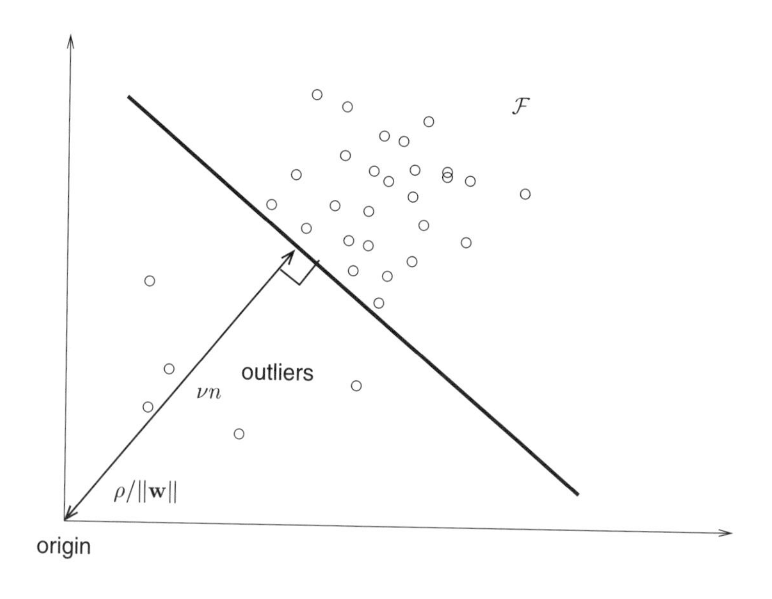

4.12 Illustration of single-class idea. Solving Equation (4.26), a hyperplane in $\mathcal{F}$ is constructed that maximizes the distance to the origin while allowing for ν outliers.

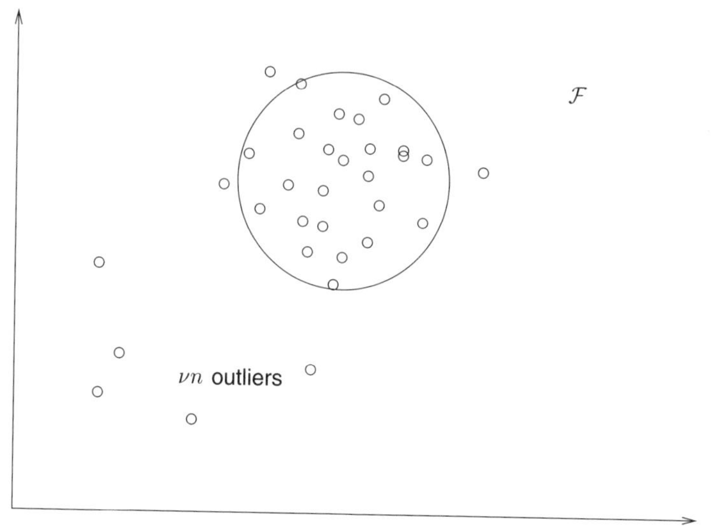

4.13 Illustration of single-class idea. Construction of the smallest soft sphere in $\mathcal{F}$ that contains the data.

are called SVs):

$$f(\mathbf{x}) = \operatorname{sign}\left(\sum_i \alpha_i \operatorname{k}(\mathbf{x}_i, \mathbf{x}) - \rho\right)$$

where the coefficients are found as the solution of the dual problem:

$$\begin{aligned} \min_{\boldsymbol{\alpha}} \quad & \frac{1}{2}\sum_{ij} \alpha_i \alpha_j \operatorname{k}\left(\mathbf{x}_i, \mathbf{x}_j\right) \\ \text{subject to} \quad & 0 \le \alpha_i \le 1/(\nu n), i = 1, \dots, n \\ & \textstyle\sum_{i=1}^{n} \alpha_i = 1\,. \end{aligned} \tag{4.28}$$

This problem can be solved with standard QP routines. It does, however, possess features that set it apart from generic QPs, most notably the simplicity of the constraints. This can be exploited by applying a variant of SMO developed for this purpose [114].

The offset ρ can be recovered by exploiting the fact that for any α_i which is not at the upper or lower bound, the corresponding pattern $\mathbf{x}_i$ satisfies $\rho = (\mathbf{w} \cdot \Phi(\mathbf{x}_i)) = \Sigma_j \alpha_j \, \mathrm{k}(\mathbf{x}_j, \mathbf{x}_i)$.

Note that if ν approaches 0, the upper boundaries on the Lagrange multipliers tend to infinity, i.e., the first inequality constraint in Equation (4.28) becomes void. The problem then resembles the corresponding hard margin algorithm, since the penalization of errors becomes infinite, as can be seen from the primal objective function (Equation (4.26)). It can be shown that if the data set is separable from the origin, this algorithm will find the unique supporting hyperplane with the properties that it separates all data from the origin, and its distance to the origin is maximal among all such hyperplanes. If, on the other hand, ν equals 1, then the constraints alone only allow one solution — the one where all α_i are at the upper bound $1/(\nu n)$. In this case, for kernels with integral 1, such as normalized versions of Equation (4.7), the decision function corresponds to a thresholded Parzen windows estimator. For the parameter ν, one can show that it controls the fraction of errors and SVs (along the lines of Section 4.4.1).

THEOREM 4.2 *[114] Assume that the solution of Equation* (4.27) *satisfies* $\rho \neq 0$. *The following statements hold true: (1)* ν *is an upper bound on the fraction of outliers; (2)* ν *is a lower bound on the fraction of SVs; and (3) Suppose the data were generated independently from a distribution* $P(\mathbf{x})$ *which does not contain discrete components. Suppose, moreover, that the kernel is analytic and non-constant. When the number n of samples goes to infinity, with probability 1,* ν *equals both the fraction of SVs and the fraction of outliers.*

We have, thus, described an algorithm which will compute a region that captures a certain fraction of the training examples. It is a "nice" region, as it will correspond to a small value of $\|\mathbf{w}\|^2$; therefore, the underlying function will be smooth [131]. How about test examples? Will they also lie inside the computed region? This question is the subject of single-class generalization error bounds [114]. Roughly, they state the following: suppose the estimated hyperplane has a small $\|\mathbf{w}\|^2$ and separates part of the training set from the origin by a certain margin $\rho/\|\mathbf{w}\|$. Then, the probability that test examples coming from the same distribution lie outside a slightly larger region will not be much larger than the fraction of training outliers.

Figure 4.14 displays two-dimensional toy examples and shows how the parameter settings influence the solution. For further applications, including an outlier detection task in handwritten character recognition, see Schölkopf [114].

4.6 Model Selection

In the kernel methods discussed so far, the choice of the kernel has a crucial effect on the performance, i.e., if one does not choose the kernel properly, one will not achieve the excellent performance reported in many papers. Model selection techniques provide principled ways to select a proper kernel. Usually, the candidates of optimal kernels are prepared using some heuristic rules, and the one which minimizes a given criterion is chosen. There are three typical methods of model selection with different criteria, each of which is a prediction of the generalization error:

1. **Bayesian evidence framework** — The training of an SVM is interpreted as Bayesian inference, and the model selection is accomplished by maximizing the marginal likelihood (i.e., evidence) [58, 137].
2. **PAC** — The generalization error is upper bounded using a capacity measure depending

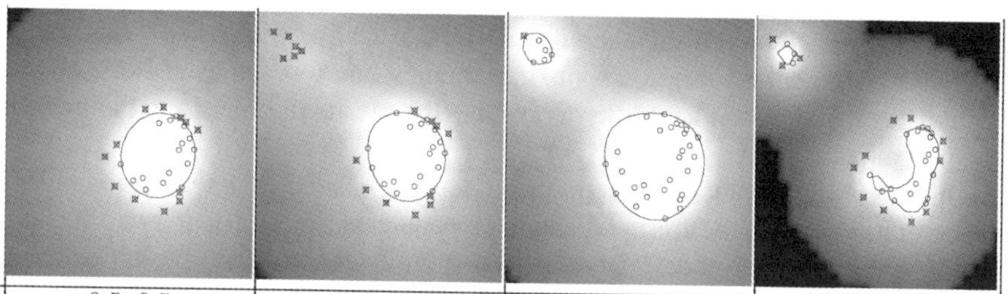

ν, width c	0.5, 0.5	0.5, 0.5	0.1, 0.5	0.5, 0.1
frac. SVs/OLs	0.54, 0.43	0.59, 0.47	0.24, 0.03	0.65, 0.38
margin $\rho/\|\mathbf{w}\|$	0.84	0.70	0.62	0.48

4.14 A single-class SVM using RBF kernels (Equation (4.7)) applied to a toy problem; domain: $[-1, 1]^2$. First two pictures: note how, in both cases, at least a fraction of ν of all examples is in the estimated region (see table). The large value of ν causes the additional data points in the upper left corner to have almost no influence on the decision function. For smaller values of ν, such as 0.1 (third picture), the points can no longer be ignored. Alternatively, one can force the algorithm to take these outliers into account by changing the kernel width (Equation (4.7)): in the fourth picture, using $c = 0.1$, $\nu = 0.5$, the data are effectively analyzed on a different length scale, which leads the algorithm to consider the outliers as meaningful points [114].

both on the weights and the model, and these are optimized to minimize the bound. The kernel selection methods for SVM following this approach are reported in the literature [115, 127, 138].

3. **Cross validation** — Here, the training samples are divided into k subsets, each of which has the same number of samples. Then, the classifier is trained k times: in the ith ($i = 1, \ldots, k$) iteration, the classifier is trained on all subsets except the ith one. Then, the classification error is computed for the ith subset. It is known that the average of these k errors is a rather good estimate of the generalization error [64]. The extreme case, where k is equal to the number of training samples, is called leave-one-out cross validation. Note that bootstrap [34, 35] is also a principled resampling method often used for model selection.

Other approaches, namely asymptotic statistical methods such as AIC [2] and NIC [77] can be used. However, since these methods need a large amount of samples by assumption, they have not been used in kernel methods so far. For methods 1 and 2 above, the generalization error is approximated by expressions that can be computed efficiently. For small sample sizes, these values are sometimes not very accurate, but it is known that, nevertheless, acceptable models are often selected. Among the three approaches, the most frequently used method is cross validation [64], but the problem is that the computational cost is the highest because the learning problem must be solved k times. For SVM, there is an approximate way to evaluate the n-fold cross-validation error (i.e., the leave-one-out classification error) called span bound [144]. If one assumes that the support vectors do not change even when a sample is left out, the leave-one-out classification result of this sample can be computed exactly. Under this assumption, we can obtain an estimate of the leave-one-out error without retraining the SVM many times. Although this assumption is rather crude and not true in many cases, this approach gives a close approximation of the true leave-one-out error in experiments. For KFD, there exists a similar result.

The following describes a particularly efficient model selection method that has often been used [68, 69, 90, 92, 148, 150] in conjunction with the benchmark data sets described in Section 4.7.2. In model selection for SVMs and KFD, we have to determine the kernel parameters (one (RBF) or more (e.g., polynomial kernel)) and the regularization constant C or ν, while for boosting, one needs to choose the model parameters of the base learner, a regularization constant, and the number of boosting iterations. Given a certain benchmark data set, one usually has a number, for example M (e.g., 100), realizations, i.e., splits into training and test set, available (see Section 4.7.2). The different splits are often necessary to average the results in order to get more reliable estimates of the generalization error.

One possibility for model selection would be to consider each realization independently from all others and to perform the cross-validation procedure M times. Then, for each realization, one would end up with different model parameters, as the model selection on each realization will typically have various results.

It is less computationally expensive to have only one model for all realizations of one data set. To find this model, we run a fivefold cross-validation procedure only on a few, for example, five realizations of the data set. This is done in two stages: first, a global search (i.e., over a wide range of the parameter space) is done to find a good guess of the parameter, which becomes more precise in the second stage. Finally, the model parameters are computed as the median of the five estimations and are used throughout the training on all M realizations of the data set. This way of estimating the parameters is computationally still quite expensive, but much less expensive than the full cross-validation approach mentioned above.

4.7 Applications

This section describes selected[12] interesting applications of supervised and unsupervised learning with kernels. It serves to demonstrate that kernel-based approaches achieve competitive results over a whole range of benchmarks with different noise levels and robustness requirements.

4.7.1 Supervised Learning

4.7.1.1 OCR

Historically, the first real-world experiments of SVMs[13] — all done on OCR benchmarks (see Figure 4.15) — exhibited quite high accuracies for SVMs [22, 109, 110, 116] comparable to state-of-the-art results achieved with convolutive multilayer perceptrons [13, 59, 60, 124]. Table 4.3 shows

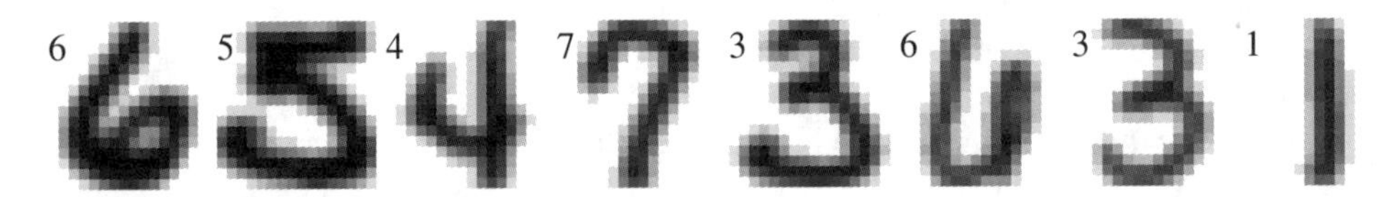

4.15 Typical handwritten digits from the U.S. Postal Service (USPS) benchmark data set with 7291 training and 2007 test patterns (16 × 16 gray scale images).

the classification performance of SVMs in comparison to other state-of-the art classifiers on the U.S. Postal Service (USPS) benchmark. Plain SVMs give a performance very similar to other state-of-the-art methods. However, SVMs can be strongly improved by using prior knowledge. For instance, [110] virtual support vectors have been generated by transforming the set of support vectors with an appropriate invariance transformation and retraining the machine on these vectors. Furthermore,

[12]Note that, for our own convenience, we have biased the selection towards applications pursued by the GMD FIRST IDA group while adding abundant references to other work.
[13]Performed at AT&T Bell Labs.

one can structure kernels such that they induce local invariances like translations, line thickening, or rotations or so that products of neighboring pixels in an image [116], thought to contain more information, are emphasized. So, prior knowledge can be used for engineering a larger data set or problem-specific kernels (see also Section 4.7.1.2 for an application of this idea to DNA analysis). In a two-stage process, we also used kernel PCA to extract features from the USPS data in the first step. A subsequent linear classification on these nonlinear features allows achieving an error rate of 4%, which is better by a factor of two than operating on linear PCA features (8.7%) [119].

TABLE 4.3 Classification Error (in %) for Off-Line Handwritten Character Recognition on the USPS with 7291 Patterns

Linear PCA and linear SVM (Schölkopf et al. [119])	8.7%
k-Nearest Neighbor	5.7%
LeNet1 ([13, 59, 60])	4.2%
Regularized RBF Networks (Rätsch [90])	4.1%
Kernel-PCA and Linear SVM (Schölkopf et al. [119])	4.0%
SVM (Schölkopf et al. [109])	4.0%
Virtual SVM (Schölkopf [110])	3.0%
Invariant SVM (Schölkopf et al. [116])	3.0%
Boosting (Drucker et al. [27])	2.6%
Tangent Distance (Simard et al. [124, 125])	2.5%
Human Error Rate	2.5%

Note: Invariant SVMs are only slightly below the best existing results (parts of the table are from reference [125]). This is even more remarkable since in references [27, 124, 125], a larger training set was used, containing some additional machine-printed digits which have been found to improve accuracy.

A benchmark problem larger than the USPS data set (7291 patterns) was collected by NIST and contains 120,000 handwritten digits. Invariant SVMs achieved the record error rate of 0.6% [25] on this challenging and more realistic data set, better than tangent distance (1.1%) and convolutional neural networks (LeNet 5: 0.9%). With an error rate of 0.7%, an ensemble of LeNet 4 networks that was trained on a vast number of artificially generated patterns (using invariance transformations) almost matches the performance of the best SVM [60].

4.7.1.2 Analyzing DNA Data

The genomic text contains untranslated regions and so-called coding sequences (CDS) that encode proteins. In order to extract protein sequences from nucleotide sequences, it is a central problem in computational biology to recognize the translation initiation sites (TIS) from which coding starts to determine which parts of a sequence will be translated and which will not.

Coding sequences can, in principle, be characterized with alignment methods that use homologous proteins [85] or intrinsic properties of the nucleotide sequence that are learned, for instance, with hidden Markov models [51]. A radically different approach that has turned out to be even more successful is to model the task of finding TIS as a classification problem [86, 152]. A potential start codon is typically an ATG[14] triplet. The classification task is, therefore, to decide whether or not a binary coded (fixed length) sequence window[15] around the ATG indicates a true TIS. The machine learning algorithm, for example, the neural network [86] or the SVM [152], gets a training

[14]DNA has a four-letter alphabet: A,C,G,T.

[15]We define the input space by the same sparse bit-encoding scheme as used by Pedersen and Nielsen (personal communication): each nucleotide is encoded by five bits, exactly one of which is set. The position of the set bit indicates whether the nucleotide is A, C, G, or T, or if it is unknown. This leads to an input space of dimension $n = 1000$ for a symmetric window of size 100 to the left and right of the ATG sequence.

set consisting of an input of binary coded strings in a window around the ATG together with a label indicating true/false TIS. In contrast to alignment methods, both neural networks and the SVM algorithm are finding important structures in the data by learning in the respective feature space to successfully classify from the labeled data.

As indicated in Section 4.7.1.1, one can incorporate prior knowledge to SVMs, e.g., by using a proper feature space $\mathcal{F}$. In particular, in the task of TIS recognition, it turned out to be very helpful to include biological knowledge by engineering an appropriate kernel function [152]. We will give three examples for kernels that are particularly useful for start codon recognition. While certain local correlations are typical for TIS, dependencies between distant positions are of minor importance or are known *a priori* not even to exist. We want the feature space to reflect this. Thus, we modify the kernel utilizing a technique that was originally described for OCR [116]: at each sequence position, we compare the two sequences locally, within a small window of length $2l + 1$ around that position. We count matching nucleotides, multiplied with weights $\mathbf{p}$ increasing from the boundaries to the center of the window. The resulting weighted counts are taken to the d_1^{th} power

$$\text{win}_p(\mathbf{x}, \mathbf{y}) = \left(\sum_{j=-l}^{+l} p_j \ \text{match}_{p+j}(\mathbf{x}, \mathbf{y}) \right)^{d_1}$$

where d_1 reflects the order of local correlations (within the window) that we expect to be of importance. Here, $\text{match}_{p+j}(\mathbf{x}, \mathbf{y})$ is 1 for matching nucleotides at position $p + j$ and 0 otherwise. The window scores computed with win_p are summed over the whole length of the sequence. Correlations between up to d_2 windows are taken into account by applying potentiation with d_2 to the resulting sum:

$$\text{k}(\mathbf{x}, \mathbf{y}) = \left(\sum_{p=1}^{l} \text{win}_p(\mathbf{x}, \mathbf{y}) \right)^{d_2} .$$

We call this kernel locality-improved (contrary to a plain polynomial kernel), as it emphasizes local correlations.

In an attempt to further improve performance, we aimed to incorporate another piece of biological knowledge into the kernel, this time concerning the codon structure of the coding sequence. A codon is a triplet of adjacent nucleotides that codes for one amino acid. By definition, the difference between a true TIS and a pseudo-site is that downstream of a TIS, there is CDS (which shows codon structure), while upstream there is not. CDS and non-coding sequences show statistically different compositions. It is likely that the SVM exploits this difference for classification. We could hope to improve the kernel by reflecting the fact that CDS shifted by three nucleotides still looks like CDS. Therefore, we further modify the locality-improved kernel function to account for this translation invariance. In addition to counting matching nucleotides on corresponding positions, we also count matches that are shifted by three positions. We call this kernel codon-improved. Again, it can be shown to be a valid Mercer kernel function by explicitly deriving the monomial features.

A third direction for the modification of the kernel function is obtained by the Salzberg method, where we essentially represent each data point with a sequence of log odd scores relating, individually for each position, two probabilities: first, how likely the observed nucleotide at that position derives from a true TIS and second, how likely that nucleotide occurs at the given position relative to any ATG triplet. We then proceed analogously to the locality-improved kernel, replacing the sparse bit representation by the sequence of these scores. As expected, this leads to a further increase in classification performance. In a strict sense, this is not a kernel but corresponds to preprocessing.

The results of an experimental comparison of SVMs using these kernel functions with other approaches are summarized in Table 4.4. All results are averaged over six data partitions (about 11,000 patterns for training and 3000 patterns for testing). SVMs are trained on 8000 data points. An optimal set of model parameters is selected according to the error on the remaining training data, and the average errors on the remaining test set are reported in Table 4.4. Note that the windows consist of $2l+1$ nucleotides. The NN results are those achieved by Pedersen and Nielsen [86]. There, model selection seems to have involved test data, which might lead to slightly overoptimistic performance estimates. Positional conditional preference scores are calculated analogously to Salzberg [103], but are extended to the same amount of input data also supplied to the other methods. Note that the performance measure shown depends on the value of the classification function threshold. For SVMs, the thresholds are byproducts of the training process; for the Salzberg method, natural thresholds are derived from prior probabilities by Bayesian reasoning. Overall error denotes the ratio of false predictions to total predictions. The sensitivity vs. specificity trade-off can be controlled by varying the threshold.

TABLE 4.4 Comparison of Classification Errors (Measured on the Test Sets) Achieved with Different Learning Algorithms

Algorithm	Parameter Specificity Setting	Overall Sensitivity Error
Neural network		15.4%
	64.5%	82.4%
Salzberg method		13.8%
	73.7%	68.1%
SVM, simple polynomial	d=1	13.2%
	75.7%	69.2%
SVM, locality-improved kernel	d_1=4, l=4	11.9%
	79.3%	70.0%
SVM, codon-improved kernel	d_1=2, l=3	12.2%
	78.7%	69.0%
SVM, Salzberg kernel	d_1=3, l=1	11.4%
	76.0%	78.4%

In conclusion, all three engineered kernel functions clearly outperform the NN, as devised by Pedersen and Nielsen, or the Salzberg method by reducing the overall number of misclassifications drastically: up to 25% compared to the neural network.

Further successful applications of SVMs have emerged in the context of gene expression profile analysis [18, 41] and DNA and protein analysis [46, 52, 147].

4.7.2 Benchmarks

To evaluate a newly designed algorithm, it is often desirable to have some standardized benchmark data sets. For this purpose, there exist some benchmark repositories, including UCI [78], DELVE [79], and STATLOG [6]. Some of them also provide results of some standard algorithms on these data sets. The problem with these repositories and the given results is that (1) it is unclear how the model selection was performed; (2) it is not always stated how large the training and test samples have been; (3) there is usually no information on how reliable these results are (error bars); (4) the data sometimes need preprocessing; and (5) the problems are often multiclass problems. Some of these factors might influence the result of the learning machine at hand, which makes a comparison with results in other papers difficult.

Thus, another (very clean) repository — the IDA repository [5] — has been created, which contains 13 artificial and real-world data sets collected from the repositories above. The IDA repository is designed to cover a variety of different data sets: from small to high expected error rates, from low- to high-dimensional data, and from small and large sample sizes. For each of the data sets, banana (toy data set [90, 92]), breast cancer,[16] diabetes, german, heart, image segment, ringnorm, flare solar, splice, thyroid, titanic, twonorm, and waveform, the repository includes:

- a short description of the dataset
- 100 predefined splits into training and test samples
- the simulation results for several kernel-based and boosting methods on each split, including the parameters that have been used for each method
- a simulation summary including means and standard deviations on the 100 realizations of the data

To build the IDA repository for problems that are originally not binary classification problems, a random partition into two classes is used.[17] Furthermore, for all sets, preprocessing is performed and 100 different partitions into training and test set (mostly $\approx 60\% : 40\%$) have been generated. On each partition, a set of different classifiers is trained, the best model is selected by cross validation, and then its test set error is computed. Some of the results are stated in Table 4.5. This repository has been used so far to evaluate kernel and boosting methods [50, 68, 69, 90, 92, 148, 150].

TABLE 4.5 Comparison among Support Vector Machines, the Kernel Fisher Discriminant (KFD), a Single Radial Basis Function Classifier (RBF), AdaBoost (AB), and Regularized AdaBoost (AB_R) on 13 Different Benchmark Datasets [70].

	SVM	KFD	RBF	AB	AB_R
Banana	11.5±0.07	**10.8±0.05**	**10.8±0.06**	12.3±0.07	*10.9±0.04*
B. Cancer	*26.0±0.47*	**25.8±0.46**	27.6±0.47	30.4±0.47	26.5±0.45
Diabetes	*23.5±0.17*	**23.2±0.16**	24.3±0.19	26.5±0.23	23.8±0.18
German	**23.6±0.21**	*23.7±0.22*	24.7±0.24	27.5±0.25	24.3±0.21
Heart	**16.0±0.33**	*16.1±0.34*	17.6±0.33	20.3±0.34	16.5±0.35
Image	*3.0±0.06*	3.3±0.06	3.3±0.06	**2.7±0.07**	**2.7±0.06**
Ringnorm	1.7±0.01	**1.5±0.01**	1.7±0.02	1.9±0.03	*1.6±0.01*
F. Sonar	**32.4±0.18**	*33.2±0.17*	34.4±0.20	35.7±0.18	34.2±0.22
Splice	10.9±0.07	10.5±0.06	*10.0±0.10*	10.1±0.05	**9.5±0.07**
Thyroid	4.8±0.22	**4.2±0.21**	4.5±0.21	*4.4±0.22*	4.6±0.22
Titanic	**22.4±0.10**	23.2±0.20	23.3±0.13	*22.6±0.12*	*22.6±0.12*
Twonorm	3.0±0.02	**2.6±0.02**	2.9±0.03	3.0±0.03	*2.7±0.02*
Waveform	*9.9±0.04*	*9.9±0.04*	10.7±0.11	10.8±0.06	**9.8±0.08**

Best result in bold face, second best in italics.

Table 4.5 shows experimental comparisons between SVM, RBF, KFD, and AdaBoost variants [70]. Due to the careful model selection performed in the experiments, all kernel-based methods exhibit a similarly good performance. Note that we can expect such a result since all such methods use similar implicit regularization concepts by employing the same kernel [131]. The remaining differences arise from their different loss functions which induce different margin optimization strategies: KFD maximizes the average margin, whereas SVM maximizes the soft margin (ultimately the minimum margin). In practice, KFD or RVM has the advantage that, if required (e.g., medical application, motion tracking), it can also supply a confidence measure for a decision. Furthermore, the solutions for KFD with a sparsity regularization are as sparse as for RVM [137] (i.e., much higher sparsity than for SVMs can be achieved), yet take less computing time than the RVM [68].

[16] The breast cancer domain was obtained from the University Medical Center, Institute of Oncology, Ljubljana, Yugoslavia. Thanks to M. Zwitter and M. Soklic for providing the data.

[17] A random partition generates a mapping m of n to two classes. For this, a random ± 1 vector $\mathbf{m}$ of length n is generated. The positive classes (and the negative, respectively) are then concatenated.

4.7.2.1 Miscellaneous Applications

The high-dimensional problem of text categorization seems to be another application where SVMs have been performing particularly well. A popular benchmark is the Reuters-22173 text corpus, where Reuters collected 21,450 news stories from 1997 and partitioned and indexed them into 135 different categories to simplify the access. The feature typically used to classify Reuters documents is 10,000-dimensional vectors containing word frequencies within a document. With such a coding, SVMs have been achieving excellent results [32, 54].

Further applications of SVMs include object and face recognition tasks as well as image retrieval [15, 84]. SVMs have also been successfully applied to solve inverse problems [143, 149].

4.7.3 Unsupervised Learning

4.7.3.1 Denoising

Kernel PCA as a nonlinear feature extractor has proven powerful as a preprocessing step for classification algorithms. But considering it as a natural generalization of linear PCA, the question arises of how to use nonlinear features for data compression, reconstruction, and denoising — applications common in linear PCA. This is a nontrivial task, as the results provided by kernel PCA live in the high-dimensional feature space and need not have an exact representation by a single vector in input space. In practice, this issue has been alleviated by computing approximate pre-images [71, 112, 136].

Formally, one defines a projection operator P_k, which for each test point $\mathbf{x}$ computes the projection onto the first k (nonlinear) principal components, i.e.,

$$\mathrm{P}_k\, \Phi(\mathbf{x}) = \textstyle\sum_{i=1}^{k} \beta_i \mathbf{V}^i$$

where $\beta_i := (\mathbf{V}^i \cdot \Phi(\mathbf{x})) = \Sigma_{j=1}^{n} \alpha_j^i\, \mathrm{k}(\mathbf{x}, \mathbf{x}_j)$. Assume that the eigenvectors $\mathbf{V}$ are ordered with decreasing eigenvalue size. It can be shown that these projections have optimality properties similar to linear PCA [71], making them good candidates for the following applications:

4.7.3.1.1 Denoising

Given a noisy $\mathbf{x}$, map it into $\Phi(\mathbf{x})$, discard higher components to obtain $\mathrm{P}_k\, \Phi(\mathbf{x})$, and then compute a pre-image $\mathbf{z}$. Here, the hope is that the main structure in the data set is captured in the first k directions, and the remaining components mainly pick up the noise. In this sense, $\mathbf{z}$ can be thought of as a denoised version of $\mathbf{x}$.

4.7.3.1.2 Compression

Given the eigenvectors $\boldsymbol{\alpha}^i$ and a small number of features β_i of $\Phi(\mathbf{x})$, but not $\mathbf{x}$, compute a pre-image as an approximate reconstruction of $\mathbf{x}$. This is useful if k is smaller than the dimensionality of the input data.

4.7.3.1.3 Interpretation

Visualize a nonlinear feature extractor $\mathbf{V}^i$ by computing a pre-image. This can be achieved by computing a vector $\mathbf{z}$ satisfying $\Phi(\mathbf{z}) = \mathrm{P}_k\, \Phi(\mathbf{x})$. The hope is that, for the kernel used, such a $\mathbf{z}$ will be a good approximation of $\mathbf{x}$ in input space. However, such a $\mathbf{z}$ will not always exist and, if it exists, it need not be unique [71, 112]. When the vector $\mathrm{P}_k\, \Phi(\mathbf{x})$ has no pre-image $\mathbf{z}$, one can approximate it by minimizing

$$\rho(\mathbf{z}) = \|\Phi(\mathbf{z}) - \mathrm{P}_k\, \Phi(\mathbf{x})\|^2 \qquad (4.29)$$

which can be seen as a special case of the reduced set method [19, 112]. The optimization of Equation (4.29) can be formulated using kernel functions. Especially for RBF kernels (see Equation (4.7)) there exists an efficient fixed-point iteration. For further details of how to optimize Equation (4.29) and for details of the experiments reported below, refer to Schölkopf et al. [112].

Example The example cited here [71] was carried out with Gaussian kernels, minimizing Equation (4.29). Figure 4.16 illustrates the pre-image approach in an artificial denoising task on the USPS database. In these experiments, linear and kernel PCA were trained with the original data. To the test set, additive Gaussian noise with zero mean and standard deviation $\sigma = 0.5$, or "speckle" noise, where each pixel is flipped to black or white with probability $p = 0.2$, was added. For the noisy test sets, projections onto the first k linear and nonlinear components were computed, and the reconstruction was carried out for each case. The results were compared by taking the mean squared distance of each reconstructed digit of the noisy test set to its original counterpart.

For the optimal number of components in linear and kernel PCA, the nonlinear approach did better by a factor of 1.6 for the Gaussian noise and by a factor of 1.2 for the speckle noise (the optimal number of components were 32 in linear PCA, and 512 and 256 in kernel PCA, respectively). Taking identical numbers of components in both algorithms, kernel PCA becomes up to 8 times better than linear PCA. Recently, a similar approach was used together with sparse kernel PCA on real-world images, showing far superior performance compared to linear PCA [136].

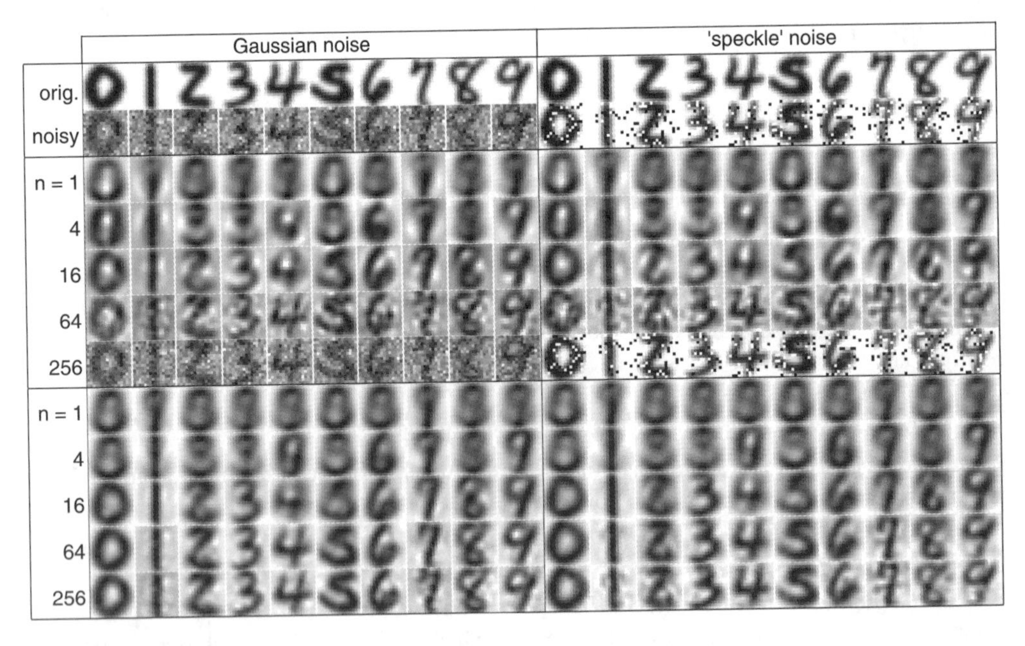

4.16 Denoising of USPS data (see text). The left half shows (top): the first occurrence of each digit in the test set, (second row): the upper digit with additive Gaussian noise ($\sigma = 0.5$); (following five rows): the reconstruction for linear PCA using $k = 1, 4, 16, 64, 256$ components; and, (last five rows): the results of the approximate pre-image approach using the same number of components. The right half shows the same but for speckle noise with probability $p = 0.2$ [71].

Other applications of kernel PCA can be found for object detection [96], and for preprocessing in regression and classification tasks [98, 99, 110].

4.8 Conclusions and Discussion

The goal of this chapter was to give a simple introduction to the exciting field of kernel-based learning methods. We only briefly touched upon learning theory and feature spaces — omitting many details of VC theory [143] — and instead focused on how to use and work with the algorithms. In the supervised learning section, we dealt with classification; however, a similar reasoning leads to algorithms for regression with KFD [68], boosting [95], or SVMs [126].

We proposed a conceptual framework for KFD, boosting, and SVMs as algorithms that essentially differ in how they handle the high dimensionality of kernel feature spaces. One can think of boosting as a "kernel algorithm" in a space spanned by the basis hypotheses. The problem becomes only tractable since boosting uses an ℓ_1-norm regularizer, which induces sparsity, i.e., we essentially only work in a small subspace. In SVMs and KFD, on the other hand, we use the kernel trick only implicitly to work in feature spaces. The three methods use different optimization strategies, each well suited to maximize the (average) margin in the respective feature space and to achieve sparse solutions.

The unsupervised learning section reviewed (1) kernel PCA, a nonlinear extension of PCA for finding projections that give useful nonlinear descriptors of the data, and (2) the single-class SVM algorithm that estimates the support (or, more generally, quantiles) of a data set and is an elegant approach to the outlier detection problem in high dimensions. Similar unsupervised single-class algorithms can also be constructed for boosting [93] or KFD.

Selected real-world applications served to exemplify that kernel-based learning algorithms are indeed highly competitive on a variety of problems with different characteristics.

To conclude, we would like to encourage the reader to follow the presented methodology of (re-)formulating linear, scalar product-based algorithms into nonlinear algorithms to obtain further powerful kernel-based learning machines.

Acknowledgments

We thank A. Smola, A. Zien, and S. Sonnenburg for valuable discussions. Moreover, we gratefully acknowledge partial support from DFG (JA 379/9-1, MU 987/1-1), EU (IST-1999-14190–BLISS), and travel grants from DAAD, NSF, and EU (Neurocolt II). SM thanks for warm hospitality during his stay at Microsoft Research in Cambridge. Furthermore, GR would like to thank UC Santa Cruz and CRIEPI for warm hospitality. Thanks also to the reviewers for giving valuable comments that improved this chapter.

References

[1] M. Aizerman, E. Braverman, and L. Rozonoer. Theoretical foundations of the potential function method in pattern recognition learning. *Automation and Remote Control,* 25, 821–837, 1964.

[2] H. Akaike. A new look at the statistical model identification. *IEEE Transactions on Automation Control,* 19(6), 716–723, 1974.

[3] J.K. Anlauf and M. Biehl. The adatron: an adaptive perceptron algorithm. *Europhysics Letters,* 10, 687–692, 1989.

[4] G. Baudat and F. Anouar. Generalized discriminant analysis using a kernel approach. *Neural Computation,* 12(10), 2385–2404, 2000.

[5] `http://ida.first.gmd.de/~raetsch/data/benchmarks.htm` (IDA Benchmark repository used in several boosting, KFD, and SVM papers).

[6] `ftp://ftp.ncc.up.pt/pub/statlog` (benchmark repository used for the STATLOG competition).

[7] K.P. Bennett, A. Demiriz, and J. Shawe-Taylor. A column generation algorithm for boosting. In P. Langley, Editor, *Proceedings, 17th ICML,* Morgan Kaufmann, San Francisco, 2000, 65–72.

[8] K.P. Bennett and O.L. Mangasarian. Robust linear programming discrimination of two linearly inseparable sets. *Optimization Methods and Software,* 1, 23–34, 1992.

[9] D.P. Bertsekas. *Nonlinear Programming.* Athena Scientific, Belmont, MA, 1995.

[10] C.M. Bishop. *Neural Networks for Pattern Recognition.* Oxford University Press, New York, 1995.

[11] V. Blanz, B. Schölkopf, H. Bülthoff, C.J.C. Burges, V.N. Vapnik, and T. Vetter. Comparison of view-based object recognition algorithms using realistic 3D models. In C. von der Malsburg, W. von Seelen, J.C. Vorbrüggen, and B. Sendhoff, Editors, *Artificial Neural Networks — ICANN'96,* Springer-Verlag, Berlin, 1996, 251–256.

[12] B.E. Boser, I.M. Guyon, and V.N. Vapnik. A training algorithm for optimal margin classifiers. In D. Haussler, Editor, *Proceedings of the 5th Annual ACM Workshop on Computational Learning Theory,* ACM Press, Pittsburgh, 1992, 144–152.

[13] L. Bottou, C. Cortes, J.S. Denker, H. Drucker, I. Guyon, L.D. Jackel, Y.A. LeCun, U.A. Müller, E. Säckinger, P.Y. Simard, and V.N. Vapnik. Comparison of classifier methods: a case study in handwritten digit recognition. In *Proceedings of the 12th International Conference on Pattern Recognition and Neural Networks, Jerusalem,* IEEE Computer Society Press, 1994, 77–87.

[14] P.S. Bradley, U.M Fayyad, and O.L Mangasarian. Mathematical programming for data mining: formulations and challenges. *Journal of Computing,* 1998.

[15] B. Bradshaw, B. Schölkopf, and J. Platt. Kernel methods for extracting local image semantics. Unpublished manuscript, private communication, 2000.

[16] L. Breiman. Arcing the edge. Technical Report 486, Statistics Department, University of California, June 1997.

[17] L. Breiman. Prediction games and arcing algorithms. Technical Report 504, Statistics Department, University of California, December 1997.

[18] M.P.S. Brown, W.N. Grundy, D. Lin, N. Cristianini, C. Sugnet, T.S. Furey, M. Ares, and D. Haussler. Knowledge-based analysis of microarray gene expression data using support vector machines. *Proceedings of the National Academy of Sciences,* 97(1), 262–267, 2000.

[19] C.J.C. Burges. Simplified support vector decision rules. In L. Saitta, Editor, *Proceedings ICML'96,* Morgan Kaufmann, San Mateo, CA, 1996, 71–77.

[20] C.J.C. Burges. A tutorial on support vector machines for pattern recognition. *Knowledge Discovery and Data Mining,* 2(2), 121–167, 1998.

[21] C.J.C. Burges and B. Schölkopf. Improving the accuracy and speed of support vector learning machines. In M. Mozer, M. Jordan, and T. Petsche, Edtors, *Advances in Neural Information Processing Systems 9,*, MIT Press, Cambridge, MA, 1997, 375–381.

[22] C. Cortes and V.N. Vapnik. Support vector networks. *Machine Learning,* 20, 273–297, 1995.

[23] D.D. Cox and F. O'Sullivan. Asymptotic analysis of penalized likelihood and related estimates. *The Annals of Statistics,* 18(4), 1676–1695, 1990.

[24] N. Cristianini and J. Shawe-Taylor. *An Introduction to Support Vector Machines.* Cambridge University Press, Cambridge, UK, 2000.

[25] D. DeCoste and B. Schölkopf. Training invariant support vector machines. *Machine Learning,* to appear.

[26] K.I. Diamantaras and S.Y. Kung. *Principal Component Neural Networks.* John Wiley & Sons, New York, 1996.

[27] H. Drucker, R. Schapire, and P.Y. Simard. Boosting performance in neural networks. *International Journal of Pattern Recognition and Artificial Intelligence,* 7, 705–719, 1993.

[28] H. Drucker, D. Wu, and V.N. Vapnik. Support vector machines for span categorization. *IEEE Transactions on Neural Networks,* 10(5), 1048–1054, 1999.

[29] R.O. Duda and P.E. Hart. *Pattern Classification and Scene Analysis.* John Wiley & Sons, New York, 1973.

[30] N. Duffy and D.P. Helmbold. A geometric approach to leveraging weak learners. In P. Fischer and H.U. Simon, Editors, *Computational Learning Theory: 4th European Conference (EuroCOLT '99),* Springer–Verlag, Berlin, March 1999, 18–33.

[31] N. Duffy and D.P. Helmbold. Potential boosters? In S.A. Solla, T.K. Leen, and K.R. Müller, Editors, *Advances in Neural Information Processing Systems 12,* MIT Press, Cambridge, MA, 2000, 258–264.

[32] S. Dumais. Using SVMs for text categorization. *IEEE Intelligent Systems,* 13(4), 1998.

[33] S. Dumais, J. Platt, D. Heckerman, and M. Sahami. Inductive learning algorithms and representations for text categorization. In *7th International Conference on Information and Knowledge Management,* 1998.

[34] B. Efron and R.J. Tibshirani. *An Introduction to the Bootstrap.* Chapman and Hall, New York, 1994.

[35] B. Efron and R.J. Tibshirani. Improvements on cross-validation: the .632+ bootstrap method. *Journal of the American Statistical Association,* 92, 548–560, 1997.

[36] R.A. Fisher. The use of multiple measurements in taxonomic problems. *Annals of Eugenics,* 7, 179–188, 1936.

[37] Y. Freund and R.E. Schapire. A decision-theoretic generalization of online learning and an application to boosting. *Journal of Computer and System Sciences,* 55(1), 119–139, 1997.

[38] J.H. Friedman. Regularized discriminant analysis. *Journal of the American Statistical Association,* 84(405), 165–175, 1989.

[39] T.T. Fried, N. Cristianini, and C. Campbell. The kernel adatron algorithm: A fast and simple learning procedure for support vector machines. In J. Shavlik, Editor, *Proceedings ICML'98,* Morgan Kaufmann Publishers, San Mateo, CA, 1998, 188–196.

[40] K. Fukunaga. *Introduction to Statistical Pattern Recognition,* 2nd edition. Academic Press, San Diego, CA, 1990.

[41] T. Furey, N. Cristianini, N. Duffy, D. Bednarski, M. Schummer, and D. Haussler. Support vector machine classification and validation of cancer tissue samples using microarray expression data. *Bioinformatics,* to appear.

[42] S. Geman, E. Bienenstock, and R. Doursat. Neural networks and the bias/variance dilemma. *Neural Computation,* 4(1), 1–58, 1992.

[43] F. Girosi. An equivalence between sparse approximation and support vector machines. A.I. Memo No. 1606, MIT, 1997.

[44] F. Girosi, M. Jones, and T. Poggio. Priors, stabilizers and basis functions: from regularization to radial, tensor and additive splines. Technical Report A.I. Memo No. 1430, MIT, June 1993.

[45] T.J. Hastie, A. Buja, and R.J. Tibshirani. Penalized discriminant analysis. *Annals of Statistics,* 23, 73–102, 1995.

[46] D. Haussler. Convolution kernels on discrete structures. Technical Report UCSC-CRL-99-10, UC Santa Cruz, July 1999.

[47] S. Haykin. *Neural Networks: A Comprehensive Foundation.* Macmillan, New York, 1994.

[48] R. Herbrich and T. Graepel. Large scale Bayes point machines. In T.K. Leen, T.G. Dietterich, and V. Tresp, Editors, *Advances in Neural Information System Processing 13,* MIT Press, Cambridge, MA, 2001, 528–534.

[49] R. Herbrich, T. Graepel, and C. Campbell. Bayesian learning in reproducing kernel Hilbert spaces. Technical report, Technical University of Berlin, 1999. TR 99-11.

[50] `http://www.boosting.org` (boosting web-site: a collection of references, software, and Web pointers concerned with boosting and ensemble learning methods).

[51] C. Iseli, C.V. Jongeneel, and P. Bucher. ESTScan: a program for detecting, evaluating, and reconstructing potential coding regions in EST sequences. In T. Lengauer, R. Schneider, P. Bork, D. Brutlag, J. Glasgow, H.W. Mewes, and R. Zimmer, Editors, *ISMB'99,* AAAI Press, Menlo Park, CA, 1999, 138–148.

[52] T.S. Jaakkola, M. Diekhans, and D. Haussler. A discriminative framework for detecting remote protein homologies. Unpublished, available at `http://www.cse.ucsc.edu/~research/compbio/research.html`.

[53] T. Joachims. Text categorization with support vector machines: learning with many relevant features. In C. Nédellec and C. Rouveirol, Editors, *Proceedings of the European Conference on Machine Learning,* Springer-Verlag, Berlin, 1998, 137–142.

[54] T. Joachims. Making large-scale SVM learning practical. In B. Schölkopf, C.J.C. Burges, and A.J. Smola, Editors, *Advances in Kernel Methods — Support Vector Learning,* MIT Press, Cambridge, MA, 1999, 169–184.

[55] M. Kearns and L. Valiant. Cryptographic limitations on learning Boolean formulae and finite automata. *Journal of the ACM,* 41(1), 67–95, 1994.

[56] S.S. Keerthi, S.K. Shevade, C. Bhattacharyya, and K.R.K. Murthy. Improvements to Platt's SMO algorithm for SVM classifier design. Technical Report CD-99-14, National University of Singapore, 1999. http://guppy.mpe.nus.edu.sg/~mpessk.

[57] G.S. Kimeldorf and G. Wahba. Some results on Tchebycheffian spline functions. *Journal of Mathematical Analysis and Applications,* 33, 82–95, 1971.

[58] J. Kwok. Integrating the evidence framework and the support vector machine. In M. Verleysen, Editor, *Proceedings, ESANN'99,* Brussels, 1999, 177–182.

[59] Y.A. LeCun, B. Boser, J.S. Denker, D. Henderson, R.E. Howard, W. Hubbard, and L.J. Jackel. Backpropagation applied to handwritten zip code recognition. *Neural Computation,* 1, 541–551, 1989.

[60] Y.A. LeCun, L.D. Jackel, L. Bottou, A. Brunot, C. Cortes, J.S. Denker, H. Drucker, I. Guyon, U.A. Müller, E. Säckinger, P.Y. Simard, and V.N. Vapnik. Comparison of learning algorithms for handwritten digit recognition. In F. Fogelman-Soulié and P. Gallinari, Editors, *Proceedings ICANN'95 — International Conference on Artificial Neural Networks,* volume 2, EC2, Nanterre, France, 1995, 53–60.

[61] Y.A. LeCun, L.D. Jackel, L. Bottou, A. Brunot, C. Cortes, J.S. Denker, H. Drucker, I. Guyon, U.A. Müller, E. Säckinger, P.Y. Simard, and V.N. Vapnik. Learning algorithms for classification: a comparison on handwritten digit recognition. *Neural Networks,* 261–276, 1995.

[62] O.L. Mangasarian. Arbitrary-norm separating plane. *Operation Research Letters,* 24(1), 15–23, 1999.

[63] O.L. Mangasarian and D.R. Musicant. Lagrangian support vector machines. *Journal of Machine Learning Research,* 1, 161–177, 2001.

[64] J.K. Martin and D.S. Hirschberg. Small sample statisics for classification error rates I: error rate measurements. Technical Report 96-21, Department of Information and Computer Science, UC Irvine, 1996.

[65] L. Mason, J. Baxter, P.L. Bartlett, and M. Frean. Functional gradient techniques for combining hypotheses. In A.J. Smola, P.L. Bartlett, B. Schölkopf, and D. Schuurmans, Editors, *Advances in Large Margin Classifiers,* MIT Press, Cambridge, MA, 2000, 221–247.

[66] D. Mattera and S. Haykin. Support vector machines for dynamic reconstruction of a chaotic system. In B. Schölkopf, C.J.C. Burges, and A.J. Smola, Editors, *Advances in Kernel Methods — Support Vector Learning,* MIT Press, Cambridge, MA, 1999, 211–242.

[67] J. Mercer. Functions of positive and negative type and their connection with the theory of integral equations. *Philosophical Transactions of the Royal Society of London,* A 209, 415–446, 1909.

[68] S. Mika, G. Rätsch, and K.R. Müller. A mathematical programming approach to the Kernel Fisher algorithm. In T.K. Leen, T.G. Dietterich, and V. Tresp, Editors, *Advances in Neural Information System Processing 13,* MIT Press, Cambridge, MA, 2001, 591–597.

[69] S. Mika, G. Rätsch, J. Weston, B. Schölkopf, and K.R. Müller. Fisher discriminant analysis with kernels. In Y.H. Hu, J. Larsen, E. Wilson, and S. Douglas, Editors, *Neural Networks for Signal Processing IX,* IEEE, 1999, 41–48.

[70] S. Mika, G. Rätsch, J. Weston, B. Schölkopf, A.J. Smola, and K.R. Müller. Invariant feature extraction and classification in kernel spaces. In S.A. Solla, T.K. Leen, and K.R. Müller, Editors, *Advances in Neural Information Processing Systems 12,* MIT Press, Cambridge, MA, 2000, 526–532.

[71] S. Mika, B. Schölkopf, A.J. Smola, K.R. Müller, M. Scholz, and G. Rätsch. Kernel PCA and de–noising in feature spaces. In M.S. Kearns, S.A. Solla, and D.A. Cohn, Editors, *Advances in Neural Information Processing Systems 11,* MIT Press, Cambridge, MA, 1999, 536–542.

[72] S. Mika, A.J. Smola, and B. Schölkopf. An improved training algorithm for kernel Fisher discriminants. In T. Jaakkola and T. Richardson, Editors, *Proceedings AISTATS 2001,* Morgan Kaufmann, San Mateo, CA, 2001, 98–104.

[73] J. Moody. The *effective* number of parameters: an analysis of generalization and regularization in non-linear learning systems. In S.J. Hanson, J. Moody, and R.P. Lippman, Editors, *Advances in Neural Information Processings Systems 4,* Morgan Kaufman, San Mateo, CA, 1992, 847–854.

[74] J. Moody and C. Darken. Fast learning in networks of locally-tuned processing units. *Neural Computation,* 1(2), 281–294, 1989.

[75] S. Mukherjee, E. Osuna, and F. Girosi. Nonlinear prediction of chaotic time series using a support vector machine. In J. Principe, L. Gile, N. Morgan, and E. Wilson, Editors, *Neural Networks for Signal Processing VII — Proceedings of the 1997 IEEE Workshop,* IEEE, New York, 1997, 511–520.

[76] K.-R. Müller, A.J. Smola, G. Rätsch, B. Schölkopf, J. Kohlmorgen, and V.N. Vapnik. Predicting time

series with support vector machines. In W. Gerstner, A. Germond, M. Hasler, and J.D. Nicoud, Editors, *Artificial Neural Networks — ICANN'97,* Springer-Verlag, Berlin, 1997, 999–1004.

[77] N. Murata, S. Amari, and S. Yoshizawa. Network information criterion — determining the number of hidden units for an artificial neural network model. *IEEE Transactions on Neural Networks,* 5, 865–872, 1994.

[78] University of California at Irvine. `http://www.ics.uci.edu/~mlearn` (UCI benchmark repository — a huge collection of artificial and real-world data sets).

[79] University of Toronto. `http://www.cs.utoronto.ca/~delve/data/datasets.html` (DELVE benchmark repository — a collection of artificial and real-world data sets).

[80] M. Opper and D. Haussler. Generalization performance of Bayes optimal classification algorithm for learning a perceptron. *Physical Review Letters,* 66, 2677, 1991.

[81] G. Orr and K.R. Müller, Editors. *Neural Networks: Tricks of the Trade,* volume 1524. Springer-Verlag, Berlin, 1998.

[82] E. Osuna, R. Freund, and F. Girosi. Support vector machines: training and applications. A.I. Memo AIM-1602, MIT A.I. Lab, 1996.

[83] E. Osuna, R. Freund, and F. Girosi. An improved training algorithm for support vector machines. In J. Principe, L. Gile, N. Morgan, and E. Wilson, Editors, *Neural Networks for Signal Processing VII — Proceedings of the 1997 IEEE Workshop,* IEEE, New York, 1997, 276–285.

[84] E. Osuna, R. Freund, and F. Girosi. Training support vector machines: an application to face detection. In *Proceedings CVPR'97,* 1997.

[85] W.R. Pearson, T. Wood, Z. Zhang, and W. Miller. Comparison of DNA sequences with protein sequences. *Genomics,* 46(1), 24–36, 1997.

[86] A.G. Pedersen and H. Nielsen. Neural network prediction of translation initiation sites in eukaryotes: perspectives for EST and genome analysis. In *ISMB'97,* volume 5, 1997, 226–233.

[87] J. Platt. Fast training of support vector machines using sequential minimal optimization. In B. Schölkopf, C.J.C. Burges, and A.J. Smola, Editors, *Advances in Kernel Methods — Support Vector Learning,* MIT Press, Cambridge, MA, 1999, 185–208.

[88] T. Poggio and F. Girosi. Regularization algorithms for learning that are equivalent to multilayer networks. *Science,* 247, 978–982, 1990.

[89] T. Graepel, R. Herbrich, and C. Campbell. Bayes point machines: estimating the Bayes point in kernel space. In *Proceedings of IJCAI Workshop Support Vector Machines,* pages 23–27, 1999.

[90] G. Rätsch. Ensemble learning methods for classification. Master's thesis, Department of Computer Science, University of Potsdam, April 1998. In German.

[91] G. Rätsch, A. Demiriz, and K. Bennett. Sparse regression ensembles in infinite and finite hypothesis spaces. NeuroCOLT2 Technical Report 85, Royal Holloway College, London, September 2000, *Machine Learning,* to appear.

[92] G. Rätsch, T. Onoda, and K.R. Müller. Soft margins for AdaBoost. *Machine Learning,* 42(3), 287–320, 2001.

[93] G. Rätsch, B. Schölkopf, S. Mika, and K.R. Müller. SVM and boosting: one class. Technical Report 119, GMD FIRST, Berlin, November 2000.

[94] G. Rätsch, B. Schölkopf, A.J. Smola, S. Mika, T. Onoda, and K.R. Müller. Robust ensemble learning. In A.J. Smola, P.L. Bartlett, B. Schölkopf, and D. Schuurmans, Editors, *Advances in Large Margin Classifiers,* MIT Press, Cambridge, MA, 2000, 207–219.

[95] G. Rätsch, M. Warmuth, S. Mika, T. Onoda, S. Lemm, and K.R. Müller. Barrier boosting. In *Proceedings, COLT,* Morgan Kaufmann, San Mateo, CA, 2000, 170–179.

[96] S. Romdhani, S. Gong, and A. Psarrou. A multiview nonlinear active shape model using kernel PCA. In *Proceedings of BMVC,* Nottingham, UK, 1999, 483–492.

[97] D. Roobaert and M.M. Van Hulle. View-based 3d object recognition with support vector machines. In Y.-H. Hu, J. Larsen, E. Wilson, and S. Douglas, Editors, *Neural Networks for Signal Processing IX,* IEEE, 1999.

[98] R. Rosipal, M. Girolami, and L. Trejo. Kernel PCA feature extraction of event–related potentials for human signal detection performance. In Malmgren, Borga, and Niklasson, Editors, *Proceedings of Intlernational Conference on Artificial Neural Networks in Medicine and Biology,* Springer-Verlag, Berlin, 2000, 321–326.

[99] R. Rosipal, M. Girolami, and L. Trejo. Kernel PCA for feature extraction and de–noising in non–linear regression. Submitted, see `http://www.researchindex.com`.

[100] V. Roth and V. Steinhage. Nonlinear discriminant analysis using kernel functions. In S.A. Solla, T.K. Leen, and K.R. Müller, Editors, *Advances in Neural Information Processing Systems 12*, MIT Press, Cambridge, MA, 2000, 568–574.

[101] P. Ruján. Playing billiard in version space. *Neural Computation*, 9, 197–238, 1996.

[102] S. Saitoh. *Theory of Reproducing Kernels and its Applications*. Longman Scientific & Technical, Harlow, England, 1988.

[103] S.L. Salzberg. A method for identifying splice sites and translational start sites in eukaryotic mRNA. *Computational Applied Bioscience*, 13(4), 365–376, 1997.

[104] C. Saunders, M.O. Stitson, J. Weston, L. Bottou, B. Schölkopf, and A.J. Smola. Support vector machine reference manual. Technical Report CSD-TR-98-03, Royal Holloway University, London, 1998.

[105] R.E. Schapire. The strength of weak learnability. *Machine Learning*, 5(2), 197–227, 1990.

[106] R.E. Schapire. The Design and Analysis of Efficient Learning Algorithms. Ph.D. thesis, MIT, 1992.

[107] R.E. Schapire. A brief introduction to boosting. In *Proceedings of the Sixteenth International Joint Conference on Artificial Intelligence*, 1999.

[108] R.E. Schapire, Y. Freund, P.L. Bartlett, and W.S. Lee. Boosting the margin: a new explanation for the effectiveness of voting methods. In *Proceedings of the 14th International Conference on Machine Learning*, Morgan Kaufmann, San Mateo, CA, 1997, 322–330.

[109] B. Schölkopf, C.J.C. Burges, and V.N. Vapnik. Extracting support data for a given task. In U.M. Fayyad and R. Uthurusamy, Editors, *Proceedings, First International Conference on Knowledge Discovery and Data Mining*. AAAI Press, Menlo Park, CA, 1995.

[110] B. Schölkopf. *Support Vector Learning*. Oldenbourg Verlag, Munich, 1997.

[111] B. Schölkopf, C.J.C. Burges, and A.J. Smola. *Advances in Kernel Methods — Support Vector Learning*. MIT Press, Cambridge, MA, 1999.

[112] B. Schölkopf, S. Mika, C.J.C. Burges, P. Knirsch, K.R. Müller, G. Rätsch, and A.J. Smola. Input space vs. feature space in kernel-based methods. *IEEE Transactions on Neural Networks*, 10(5), 1000–1017, 1999.

[113] B. Schölkopf, K.R. Müller, and A.J. Smola. Lernen mit Kernen. *Informatik Forschung und Entwicklung*, 14, 154–163, 1999.

[114] B. Schölkopf, J. Platt, J. Shawe-Taylor, A.J. Smola, and R.C. Williamson. Estimating the support of a high-dimensional distribution. TR 87, Microsoft Research, Redmond, WA, 1999. To appear in *Neural Computation*.

[115] B. Schölkopf, J. Shawe-Taylor, A.J. Smola, and R.C. Williamson. Kernel dependent support vector error bounds. In D. Willshaw and A. Murray, Editors, *Proceedings of ICANN'99*, volume 1, IEEE Press, New York, 1999, 103–108.

[116] B. Schölkopf, P.Y. Simard, A.J. Smola, and V.N. Vapnik. Prior knowledge in support vector kernels. In M. Jordan, M. Kearns, and S. Solla, Editors, *Advances in Neural Information Processing Systems 10*, MIT Press, Cambridge, MA, 1998, 640–646.

[117] B. Schölkopf, A.J. Smola, R.C. Williamson, and P.L. Bartlett. New support vector algorithms. *Neural Computation*, 12, 1207–1245, 2000.

[118] B. Schölkopf and A.J. Smola. *Learning with Kernels*. MIT Press, Cambridge, MA, 2001, in press.

[119] B. Schölkopf, A.J. Smola, and K.R. Müller. Nonlinear component analysis as a kernel Eigenvalue problem. *Neural Computation*, 10, 1299–1319, 1998.

[120] B. Schölkopf, R.C. Williamson, A.J. Smola, J. Shawe-Taylor, and J.C. Platt. Support vector method for novelty detection. In S.A. Solla, T.K. Leen, and K.R. Müller, Editors, *Advances in Neural Information Processing Systems 12*, MIT Press, Cambridge, MA, 2000, 582–588.

[121] J. Schürmann. *Pattern Classification: A Unified View of Statistical and Neural Approaches*. John Wiley & Sons, New York, 1996.

[122] J. Shawe-Taylor, P.L. Bartlett, R.C. Williamson, and M. Anthony. A framework for structural risk minimization. In *Proceedings, COLT*. Morgan Kaufmann, San Mateo, CA, 1996.

[123] J. Shawe-Taylor and R.C. Williamson. A PAC analysis of a Bayesian estimator. Technical Report NC2-TR-1997-013, Royal Holloway, University of London, 1997.

[124] P.Y. Simard, Y.A. LeCun, and J.S. Denker. Efficient pattern recognition using a new transformation distance. In S.J. Hanson, J.D. Cowan, and C.L. Giles, Editors, *Advances in Neural Information Processing Systems 5,* Morgan Kaufmann, San Mateo, CA, 1993, 50–58.

[125] P.Y. Simard, Y.A. LeCun, J.S. Denker, and B. Victorri. Transformation invariance in pattern recognition — tangent distance and tangent propagation. In G. Orr and K.R. Müller, Editors, *Neural Networks: Tricks of the Trade,* volume 1524, Springer-Verlag, Berlin, 1998, 239–274.

[126] A.J. Smola and B. Schölkopf. A tutorial on support vector regression. *Statistics and Computing,* 2001, to appear.

[127] A.J. Smola. Learning with kernels. Ph.D. thesis, Technische Universität Berlin, 1998.

[128] A.J. Smola, O.L. Mangasarian, and B. Schölkopf. Sparse kernel feature analysis. Technical Report 99-04, University of Wisconsin, Data Mining Institute, Madison, 1999.

[129] A.J. Smola and B. Schölkopf. On a kernel-based method for pattern recognition, regression, approximation and operator inversion. *Algorithmica,* 22, 211–231, 1998.

[130] A.J. Smola and B. Schölkopf. Sparse greedy matrix approximation for machine learning. In P. Langley, Editor, *Proceedings, ICML'00,* Morgan Kaufmann, San Mateo, CA, 2000, 911–918.

[131] A.J. Smola, B. Schölkopf, and K.R. Müller. The connection between regularization operators and support vector kernels. *Neural Networks,* 11, 637–649, 1998.

[132] `http://www.kernel-machines.org` (a collection of literature, software and Web pointers dealing with SVM and Gaussian processes).

[133] M. Stitson, A. Gammerman, V.N. Vapnik, V. Vovk, C. Watkins, and J. Weston. Support vector regression with ANOVA decomposition kernels. Technical Report CSD-97-22, Royal Holloway, University of London, 1997.

[134] D. Tax and R. Duin. Data domain description by support vectors. In M. Verleysen, Editor, *Proceedings, ESANN,* D. Facto Press, Brussels, 1999, 251–256.

[135] A.N. Tikhonov and V.Y. Arsenin. *Solutions of Ill-posed Problems.* W.H. Winston, Washington, D.C., 1977.

[136] M. Tipping. Sparse kernel principal component analysis. In T.K. Leen, T.G. Dietterich, and V. Tresp, Editors, *Advances in Neural Information System Processing 13,* MIT Press, Cambridge, MA, 2001, 633–639.

[137] M.E. Tipping. The relevance vector machine. In S.A. Solla, T.K. Leen, and K.R. Müller, Editors, *Advances in Neural Information Processing Systems 12,* MIT Press, Cambridge, MA, 2000, 652–658.

[138] K. Tsuda. Optimal hyperplane classifier based on entropy number bound. In D. Willshaw and A. Murray, Editors, *Proceedings of ICANN'99,* volume 1, IEEE Press, New York, 1999, 419–424.

[139] L.G. Valiant. A theory of the learnable. *Communications of the ACM,* 27(11), 1134–1142, 1984.

[140] R.J. Vanderbei. Interior-point methods: algorithms and formulations. *ORSA Journal on Computing,* 6(1), 32–34, 1994.

[141] V.N. Vapnik. *Estimation of Dependences Based on Empirical Data.* Springer-Verlag, Berlin, 1982.

[142] V.N. Vapnik. *The Nature of Statistical Learning Theory.* Springer-Verlag, New York, 1995.

[143] V.N. Vapnik. *Statistical Learning Theory.* John Wiley & Sons, New York, 1998.

[144] V.N. Vapnik and O. Chapelle. Bounds on error expectation for support vector machines. *Neural Computation,* 12(9), 2013–2036, 2000.

[145] V.N. Vapnik and A.Y. Chervonenkis. *Theory of Pattern Recognition* [in Russian]. Nauka, Moscow, 1974.

[146] T. Watkin. Optimal learning with a neural network. *Europhysics Letters,* 21, 871–877, 1993.

[147] C. Watkins. Dynamic alignment kernels. In A.J. Smola, P.L. Bartlett, B. Schölkopf, and D. Schuurmans, Editors, *Advances in Large Margin Classifiers,* MIT Press, Cambridge, MA, 2000, 39–50.

[148] J. Weston. LOO-Support Vector Machines. In A.J. Smola, P.L. Bartlett, B. Schölkopf, and D. Schuurmans, Editors, *Proceedings of IJCNN'99,* 1999.

[149] J. Weston, A. Gammerman, M. Stitson, V.N. Vapnik, V. Vovk, and C. Watkins. Support vector density estimation. In B. Schölkopf, C.J.C. Burges, and A.J. Smola, Editors, *Advances in Kernel Methods — Support Vector Learning,* MIT Press, Cambridge, MA, 1999, 293–305.

[150] J. Weston and R. Herbrich. Adaptive margin support vector machines. In A.J. Smola, P.L. Bartlett, B. Schölkopf, and D. Schuurmans, Editors, *Advances in Large Margin Classifiers,* MIT Press, Cambridge, MA, 2000, 281–296.

[151] R.C. Williamson, A.J. Smola, and B. Schölkopf. Generalization performance of regularization networks and support vector machines via entropy numbers of compact operators. NeuroCOLT Technical Report NC-TR-98-019, Royal Holloway College, University of London, UK, 1998. To appear in *IEEE Transactions on Information Theory.*

[152] A. Zien, G. Rätsch, S. Mika, B. Schölkopf, T. Lengauer, and K.R. Müller. Engineering support vector machine kernels that recognize translation initiation sites. *BioInformatics,* 16(9), 799–807, 2000.

5

Committee Machines

Volker Tresp
Siemens AG, Corporate Technology

This chapter describes some of the most important architectures and algorithms for committee machines. We discuss three reasons for using committee machines. The first is that a committee can achieve a test set performance unobtainable by a single committee member. As typical representative approaches, we describe simple averaging, bagging, and boosting. Second, with committee machines, one obtains modular solutions, which is advantageous in many applications. The prime example given here is the mixture of experts (ME) approach, the goal of which is to autonomously break up a complex prediction task into subtasks which are modeled by the individual committee members. The third reason for using committee machines is a reduction in computational complexity. In the presented Bayesian committee machine, the training data set is partitioned into several smaller data sets, and the different committee members are trained on the different sets. Their predictions are then combined using a covariance-based weighting scheme. The computational complexity of the Bayesian committee machine approach grows only linearly with the size of the training data set, independent of the learning systems used as committee members.

5.1 Introduction

In committee machines, an ensemble of estimators — consisting typically of neural networks or decision trees — is generated by means of a learning process, and the prediction of the committee for a new input is generated in the form of a combination of the predictions of the individual committee members. Committee machines can be useful in many ways. First, the committee might exhibit a test set performance unobtainable by an individual committee member on its own. The reason for this is that the errors of the individual committee members cancel out to some degree when their predictions are combined. The surprising discovery of this line of research is that even

0-8493-2359-2/01/$0.00+$1.50

if the committee members were trained on data derived from the same data set, the predictions of the individual committee members might be sufficiently different such that this averaging process takes place and is beneficial. This line of research is described in Section 5.2. A second reason for using committee machines is modularity. It is sometimes beneficial if a mapping from input to target is not approximated by one estimator but by several estimators, where each estimator can focus on a particular region in input space. The prediction of the committee is obtained by a locally weighted combination of the predictions of the committee members. It could be shown that, in some applications, the individual members self-organize in such a way that the prediction task is modernized in a meaningful way. The most important representatives of this line of research are the mixture of experts approach and its variants, which are described in Section 5.3. The third reason for using committee machines is a reduction in computational complexity. Instead of training one estimator using all training data, it is computationally more efficient for some types of estimators to partition the data set into several data sets, train different estimators on the individual data sets, and then combine the predictions of the individual estimators. Typical examples of estimators for which this procedure is beneficial are Gaussian process regression, kriging, regularization neural networks, smoothing splines, and the support vector machine, since for those systems, training time increases drastically with increasing training data set size. By using a committee machine approach, the computational complexity increases only linearly with the size of the training data set. Section 5.4 shows how the estimates of the individual committee members can be combined so that the performance of the committee is not substantially degraded compared to the performance of one system trained on all data.

The interest of the machine learning community in committee machines began around the middle of the 1990s, and this field of research is still very active. A recent compilation of important work can be found in Sharkey's work [1], and two Web sites dedicated to the issue of committee machines can be found at http://melone.tussy.uni-wh.de/~chris/ensemble and http://www.boosting.org. In the addition to the activities in the machine learning community, there has been considerable work performed on committee machines in the area of economic forecasting [2]. One should also emphasize that traditional Bayesian averaging can be interpreted as a committee machine approach. Assume that a statistical model allows the inference about the variable y in the form of the predictive probability density $P(y|w)$, where w is a vector of model parameters. Furthermore, assume that we have a data set D which contains information about the parameter vector w in the form of the probability density $P(w|D)$. We then obtain

$$P(y|D) = \int P(y|w)P(w|D)dw \approx \frac{1}{M}\sum_{i=1}^{M} P(y|w_i)$$

where M samples $\{w_i\}_{i=1}^{M}$ are generated from the distribution $P(w|D)$. The last approximation tells us that for Bayesian inference, one should average the predictions of a committee of estimators. This form of Bayesian averaging will not be discussed further in this chapter; interested readers should consult the literature on Bayesian statistics, e.g., the book by Bernardo and Smith [4].

5.2 Averaging, Bagging, and Boosting

5.2.1 Introduction

The basic idea is to train a committee of estimators and combine the individual predictions with the goal of achieving improved generalization performance as compared to the performance achievable with a single estimator. As estimators, most researchers use either neural networks or decision trees, generated with CART or C4.5 [5].

In regression, the committee prediction for a test input x is calculated by forming a weighted sum of the predictions of the M committee members:

$$\hat{t}(x) = \sum_{i=1}^{M} g_i f_i(x)$$

where $f_i(x)$ is the prediction of the ith committee member at input x and g_i are weights which are often required to be positive and to sum to one.

In classification, the combination is typically implemented as a voting scheme. The committee assigns the pattern to the class that obtains the majority of the (possibly weighted) vote:

$$\widehat{class(x)} = \arg\max_j \sum_{i=1}^{M} g_i f_{i,class=j}(x)$$

where $f_{i,class=j}(x)$ is the output of the classifier i for class j. The output typically either corresponds to the posterior class probability $f_{i,class=j}(x) \in [0,1]$ or to a binary decision $f_{i,class=j}(x) \in \{0,1\}$.

Committee machines can be generalized in various directions. Sections 5.3 and 5.4 use non-constant weights, i.e., weighting functions which reflect the relevance of a committee member given the input. Also, it might not be immediately obvious, but, as explored in Section 5.4, predictions of the committee members at other inputs can help improve the prediction at a given x.

The motivation for pursuing committee methods can be understood by analyzing the prediction error of the combined system, which is particularly simple if we use a squared error cost function. The expected squared difference between the prediction of a committee member f_i and the true but unknown target t (for simplicity, we do not denote the dependency on x in most parts of this section explicitly),

$$\begin{aligned} E\,(f_i - t)^2 &= E\,(f_i - m_i + m_i - t)^2 \\ &= E\,(f_i - m_i)^2 + E\,(m_i - t)^2 + 2E\,((f_i - m_i)(m_i - t)) \\ &= var_i + b_i^2 \end{aligned} \tag{5.1}$$

decomposes into the variance $var_i = E(f_i - m_i)^2$ and the square of the bias $b_i = m_i - t$ with $m_i = E(f_i)$. $E(\cdot)$ stands for the expected value, which is calculated with respect to different data sets of the same size and possible variations in the training procedure such as different initializations of the weights in a neural network. As stated earlier, we are interested in estimating t by forming a linear combination of the f_i:

$$\hat{t} = \sum_{i=1}^{M} g_i f_i = g' f$$

where $f = (f_1, \ldots, f_M)'$ is the vector of the predictions of the committee members and $g = (g_1, \ldots, g_M)'$ is the vector of weights. The expected error of the combined system is [6, 7]

$$\begin{aligned} E\,(\hat{t} - t)^2 &= E\left(g'f - E\left(g'f\right)\right)^2 + E\left(E\left(g'f\right) - t\right)^2 \\ &= E\left(g'(f - E(f))\right)^2 + E\left(g'm - t\right)^2 \\ &= g'\Omega g + \left(g'm - t\right)^2 \end{aligned} \tag{5.2}$$

where Ω is an $M \times M$ covariance matrix with

$$\Omega_{ij} = E\left[(f_i - m_i)\left(f_j - m_j\right)\right]$$

and $m = (m_1, \ldots, m_M)'$ is the vector of the expected values of the predictions of the committee members. Here, $g'\Omega g$ is the variance of the committee and $g'm - t$ is the bias of the committee.

If we simply average the predictors, i.e., set $g_i = 1/M$, the last expression simplifies to

$$E\left(\hat{t} - t\right)^2 = \frac{1}{M^2}\sum_{i=1}^{M}\Omega_{ii} + \frac{1}{M^2}\sum_{i=1}^{M}\sum_{j=1, j\neq i}^{M}\Omega_{ij} + \frac{1}{M^2}\left(\sum_{i=1}^{M}(m_i - t)\right)^2 . \tag{5.3}$$

If we now assume that the mean $m_i = mean$, the variance $\Omega_{ii} = var$, and the intermember covariances $\Omega_{ij} = cov$ are identical for all members, we obtain

$$E\left(\hat{t} - t\right)^2 = \frac{1}{M}var + \frac{M^2 - M}{M^2}cov + (mean - t)^2 .$$

It is apparent that the bias of the combined system $(mean - t)$ is identical to the bias of each member and is not reduced. Therefore, estimators should be used which have low bias, and regularization — which introduces bias — should be avoided. Secondly, the estimators should have low covariance, since this term in the error function cannot be reduced by increasing M. The good news is that the term which results from the variances of the committee members decreases as $1/M$. Thus, if we have estimators with low bias and low covariance between members, the expected error of the combined system is significantly less than the expected errors of the individual members. So in some sense, a committee can be used to reduce both bias and variance: bias is reduced in the design of the members by using little regularization, and variance is reduced by the averaging process which takes place in the committee. Unfortunately, things are not quite as simple in practice, and we are faced with another version of the well-known bias-variance dilemma (see also Section 5.2.3).

In regression, $t(x)$ corresponds to the optimal regression function and $f_i(x)$ corresponds to the prediction of the ith estimator. Here, the squared error is commonly used and the bias-variance decomposition described in this section is applicable. In (two-class) classification, $t(x)$ might correspond to the probability for class one, $1 - t(x)$ to the probability for class two, and $f_i(x)$ is the estimate of the ith estimator for $t(x)$. Although it is debatable if the squared error is the right error measure for posterior class possibilities, the previously described decompositions are applicable as well. In contrast, if we consider as the output of a classifier a decision, i.e., the assigned class, the previously described bias-variance decomposition cannot be applied. A number of alternative bias-variance decompositions for this case have been described in the literature. In particular, Breiman describes a decomposition in which the role of the variance is played by a term named spread [8]. In the same paper, that author showed that the spread can be dramatically reduced by bagging, a committee approach introduced in Section 5.2.3.

5.2.2 Simple Averaging and Simple Voting

In this approach, committee members are typically neural networks. The neural networks are all trained on the complete training data set. A decorrelation among the neural network predictions is typically achieved by varying the initial conditions in training the neural networks such that different neural networks converge into different local minima of the cost function. Despite its simplicity, this procedure is surprisingly successful and turns an apparent disadvantage, local minima in training neural networks, into something useful. This approach was initialized by the work of Perrone [9] and drew a lot of attention to the concept of committee machines. Using the Cauchy inequality, Perrone could show that even for correlated and biased predictors, the squared prediction error of the committee machine (obtained by averaging) is equal to or less than the mean squared prediction error of the committee members, i.e.,

$$\left(\hat{t} - t\right)^2 \leq \frac{1}{M} \sum_{i=1}^{M} (f_i - t)^2 .$$

Loosely speaking, this means that as long as the committee members have good prediction performance, averaging cannot really make things worse; it is as good as the average model or better. This can also be understood from the work of Krogh and Vedelsby [10]. Again applied to the special case of averaging (i.e., $g_i = 1/M$), they show that (using the notation of Section 5.2.1)

$$\left(\hat{t} - t\right)^2 = \frac{1}{M} \sum_{i=1}^{M} (f_i - t)^2 - \frac{1}{M} \sum_{i=1}^{M} \left(f_i - \hat{t}\right)^2 \tag{5.4}$$

which means that the generalization error of the committee is equal to the average of the generalization error of the members minus the average variance of the committee members (the ambiguity), which immediately leads to the previous bound. In highly regularized neural networks, the ensemble ambiguity is typically small and the generalization error is essentially equal to the average generalization error of the committee members. If neural networks are not strongly regularized, the ensemble ambiguity is high and the generalization error of the committee should be much smaller than the average generalization error of the committee members. Note that the last equation is valid for a given committee. The expected value of the right side is identical to the right side of Equation (5.3).

5.2.3 Bagging

Despite the success of the procedures described in the previous section, it quickly became clear that if the training procedure is disturbed such that the correlation between the estimators is reduced, the generalization performance of the combined systems can be further improved. The most important representative of this approach was introduced by Breiman under the name of bagging (from bootstrap aggregation) [8]. The idea behind bagging can be understood in the following way. Assume that each committee member is trained on a different data set. Then, surely, the covariance between the predictions of the individual members is zero. Unfortunately, we typically have to work with a fixed training data set. Although it is then impossible to obtain a different training data set for each member, we can at least mimic this process by training each member on a bootstrap sample of the original data set. Bootstrap data sets are generated by randomly drawing K data points from the original data set of size K with replacements. This means that some data points will appear more than once in a given new data set, and some will not appear at all. We repeat this procedure M times and obtain M nonidentical data sets which are then used to train the estimators. The output of the committee is then obtained by simple averaging (regression) or by voting (classification).

Experimental evidence suggests that bagging typically outperforms simple averaging and voting. Breiman makes the point that committee members should be unstable for bagging to work. By unstable, it is meant that the estimators should be sensitive to changes in the training data set, e.g., neural networks should not be strongly regularized. But recall that well regularized neural networks generally perform better than underregularized neural networks, and we are faced with another version of the well-known bias-variance dilemma: if we use underregularized neural networks, we start with suboptimal committee members, but bagging improves performance considerably. If we start with well-regularized neural networks, we start with well-performing committee members, but bagging does not significantly improve performance. Experimental evidence indicates that regularization improves bagging results [7]. Breiman mostly works with CART decision trees as committee members.

There are other ways of perturbing the training data set besides using bootstrap samples for training (e.g., adding noise, flipping classification labels) [11, 12] which, in some cases, also work well. Raviv and Intrator [13] report good results by adding noise on bootstrap samples to increase the decorrelation between committee members, in combination with a sensible regularization of the committee members.

5.2.4 Boosting

This section discusses only the classification case. The difference from the previous approaches is that in boosting, committee members are trained sequentially, and the training of a particular committee member is dependent on the training and the performance of previously trained members. Also in contrast to the previous approaches, boosting is able to reduce both variance and bias in the prediction [14]. This is due to the fact that more emphasis is put on data points which are misclassified by previously trained committee members.

The original boosting approach, boosting by filtering, is attributed to Schapire [15]. Here, three neural networks are used, and the existence of an oracle which can produce an arbitrary number of training data points is assumed. The first neural network is trained on K training data points. Then, the second neural network is also trained on K training data points. These training data are selected from the pool of training data (or the oracle) such that half of them are classified correctly and half of them are classified incorrectly by the first neural network. The third network is trained only on data on which networks one and two disagree. The classification is then achieved by a majority vote of the three neural networks. Note that the second network obtains 50% of training patterns which were misclassified by network one and that network three only obtains critical patterns in the sense that network one and two disagree on those patterns. The original motivation for boosting came out of PAC-learning theory (PAC stands for probably approximately correct). The theory requires only that the committee members are weak learners, i.e., that the learners with high probability produce better results than random classification.

Boosting by filtering requires an oracle or, at least, a very large training data set: one needs, for example, a large training data set to obtain K patterns on which networks one and two disagree. AdaBoost (from adaptive boosting) is a combination of the ideas behind boosting and bagging and does not have a demand on a large training data set [16]. Many variants of AdaBoost have been suggested in the literature. Here, we present the algorithm in the form described by Breiman [8], which is an instance of boosting by subsampling:

Let $\{P(1), \ldots, P(K)\}$ *be a set of probabilities defined for each training pattern.*
Initialized with $P(j) = 1/K$.
FOR $i = 1, \ldots, M$

1. *Train the* i*th member by taking bootstrap samples from the original training data set with replacement following probability distribution* $\{P(1), \ldots, P(K)\}$.
2. *Let* $d(j) = 1$ *if the* j*th pattern was classified incorrectly and let it equal zero otherwise.*
3. *Let*
$$\epsilon_i = \sum_{j=1}^{K} d(j)p(j) \qquad \text{and} \qquad \beta_i = (1 - \epsilon_i)/\epsilon_i \,.$$
4. *The updated probabilities are*
$$P(j) = cP(j)\beta_i^{d(j)}$$
where c normalizes the probabilities.

END.

The committee output is calculated as a majority vote

$$\widehat{class(x)} = \arg\max_j \sum_{i=1}^{M} \log(\beta_i)\, f_{i,class=j}(x)$$

with weight $\log(\beta_i)$.

As in bagging, committee members are trained using bootstrap samples, but here, the probability of selecting a sample depends on previously trained classifiers. If a pattern j was misclassified by the previous classifier ($d(j) = 1$), it will be picked with higher probability for training the following classifier. Also, if the previous classifier generally performed well (indicated by a large β_i), the probabilities will be shifted more stringently to favor misclassified samples. Finally, the weight of the ith classifier in the committee voting is $\log \beta_i$, putting more emphasis on committee members that perform well.

Table 5.1 shows results from Breiman [8]. Committee members consisted of CART decision trees. It can be seen that AdaBoost typically outperforms bagging except when a significant overlap in the classes exists, as in the diabetes data set. Here, AdaBoost tends to assign significant resources to learn to predict outliers. This is in accordance with results reported by Dietterich [11]. There, it was shown that AdaBoost provides better performance in settings with little classification noise, but that bagging is superior when class labels are ambiguous.

TABLE 5.1 Test Set Error (in %)

Data Set	AdaBoost	Bagging
heart	1.1	2.8
breast cancer	3.2	3.7
ionosphere	6.4	7.9
diabetes	26.6	23.9
glass	22.0	23.2
soybean	5.8	6.8
letters	3.4	6.4
satellite	8.8	10.3
shuttle	0.007	0.014
DNA	4.2	5.0
digit	6.2	10.5

Source: Breiman, L., Combining predictors, in *Combining Artificial Neural Nets,* Sharkey, A.J.C., Ed., Springer-Verlag, New York, NY, 1999.

Another variant of AdaBoost is boosting by reweighting. In this deterministic version, the $\{P(1), \ldots, P(K)\}$ are not used for resampling but are used as weights for data points. In Friedman et al. [14], several variants of this deterministic version are described. Furthermore, AdaBoost can be used in context with classifiers which produce "confidence-rates" predictions (e.g., class probabilities) and can also be applied to regression [17].

Recent research shows that there is a connection between AdaBoost and large margin classifiers (i.e., the support vector machine (SVM); see the corresponding chapter): both methods find a linear combination in a high-dimensional space which has a large margin on the instances in the sample [18, 19]. A large margin provides superior generalization in the case that classes do not overlap. For noisy data, Rätsch et al. have introduced regularized AdaBoost [20] and ν-Arc [21]. Both are boosting algorithms which tolerate outliers in classification and display improved performance for cases with overlapping classes.

It was also recently shown that AdaBoost can be seen as performing gradient descent in an error function with respect to the margin, respectively, that AdaBoost can be interpreted as an approximation to additive modeling by performing gradient descent on certain cost-functionals [14], [17], [22]–[24].[1]

5.2.5 Concluding Remarks

The generalization performance for the various committee machines is certainly impressive. Committee machines improve performance when the individual members have low bias and are decorrelated. The particular feature of boosting is that it reduces both bias and variance. Due to its superior performance, boosting (in the form of AdaBoost) is currently the most frequently used algorithm of the ones described.

Finally, we also would like to mention stacking, which is one of the earliest approaches to committee machines. In stacking, the weights g_i are determined after training the committee members, typically by using leave-one-out cross validation. Stacking was introduced by Wolpert [25] and extended by Breiman. The general perception is that results obtained using stacking are somewhat mixed.

5.3 The Mixture of Experts and its Variants

5.3.1 Mixtures of Experts

The initial motivation for developing the mixture of experts (ME) approach was to design a system in which different neural networks are responsible for modeling different regions in input space. This modularity leads to greater modeling capability and, potentially, to a meaningful and interpretable segmentation of the map. In the ME approach, the weights become input-dependent weighting functions [26],

$$\hat{t}(x) = \sum_{i=1}^{M} g_i(x) f_i(x) \; . \tag{5.5}$$

The committee members $f_i(x)$ are "expert" neural networks and the $g_i(x)$ — which are positive and sum to one — are generated using a gating network. The gating network determines which expert is responsible for the different regions in input space. Figure 5.1 illustrates how the gating network and the expert neural networks interact.

The most important training algorithm for the ME is derived using the following probabilistic assumptions. Given an input x, expert network i is selected with probability $g_i(x)$. An output is generated by adding Gaussian noise with variance $\sigma_i(x)^2$ to the output of the expert network $f_i(x)$. Since it is unknown in the data which expert network produced the output, the probability of an output given the input is a mixture distribution of the form

$$P(y|x) = \sum_{i=1}^{M} g_i(x) \, G\left(y;\, f_i(x), \sigma_i(x)^2\right)$$

[1]The population version of AdaBoost (Friedman et al. [14]) builds an additive logistic regression model via Newton-like updates for minimizing $E(e^{-y\hat{t}(x)})$ where E is the expectation taken over the population.

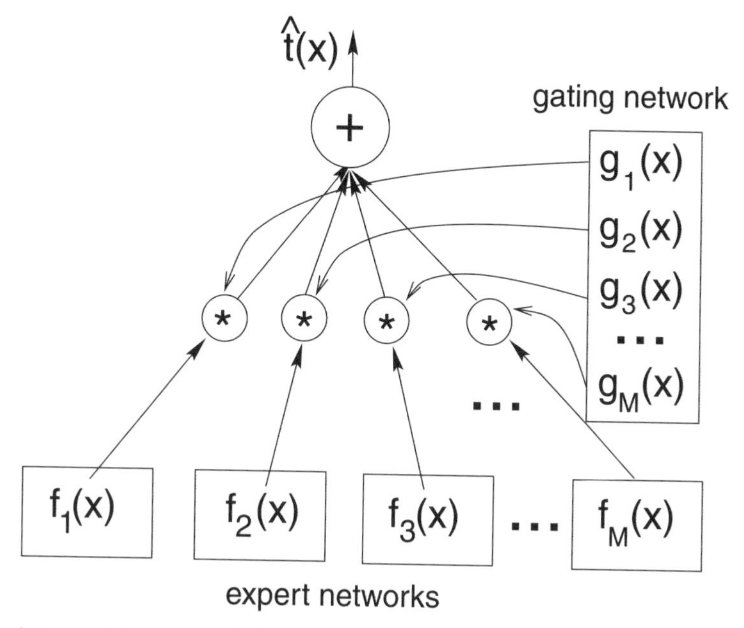

5.1 The ME architecture. The outputs of the gating network modulate the outputs of the expert neural networks.

which yields

$$E(y|x) = \sum_{i=1}^{M} g_i(x)\ f_i(x)$$

where $G\left(y;\ f_i(x), \sigma_i(x)^2\right)$ is the notation for a Gaussian probability density centered at $f_i(x)$, with variance $\sigma_i(x)^2$, evaluated at y. By looking at the previous equations, it becomes clear that the ME can also be considered a flexible model for conditional probability densities [27, 28]. Note that in this most general formulation, the outputs of the gating network, the expert neural networks, and the noise variance are functions of the input. To ensure that the $g_i(x)$ are positive and sum to one and that the standard deviation is positive, one parameterizes

$$g_i(x) = \frac{\exp h_i(x)}{\sum_{j=1}^{M} \exp h_j(x)} \quad \text{and} \quad \sigma_i(x) = \exp\left(s_i(x)\right)$$

where the functions $h_i(x)$ and $s_i(x)$ are typically modeled as neural networks. For training the ME system, a maximum likelihood error function is used. The contribution of the jth pattern to the log-likelihood function is

$$l_j = \log \sum_{i=1}^{M} g_i\left(x_j\right) G\left(y_j;\ f_i\left(x_j\right), \sigma_i\left(x_j\right)^2\right) .$$

Following the derivation in Bishop [28], the gradients of l_j with respect to the outputs of the various networks become

$$\frac{\partial l_j}{\partial f_i\left(x_j\right)} = P\left(i|x_j, y_j\right)\frac{y_j - f_i\left(x_j\right)}{\sigma_i\left(x_j\right)^2}$$

$$\frac{\partial l_j}{\partial h_i\left(x_j\right)} = P\left(i|x_j, y_j\right) - g_i\left(x_j\right)$$

$$\frac{\partial l_j}{\partial s_i\left(x_j\right)} = P\left(i|x_j, y_j\right)\left(\frac{\left(y_j - f_i\left(x_j\right)\right)^2}{\sigma_i\left(x_j\right)^2} - 1\right)$$

where the probability that the ith expert generated data point (x_j, y_j) is calculated as

$$P\left(i|x_j, y_j\right) = \frac{g_i\left(x_j\right)\ G\left(y_j; f_i\left(x_j\right), \sigma_i\left(x_j\right)^2\right)}{\sum_{i=1}^{M} g_i\left(x_j\right)\ G\left(y_j; f_i\left(x_j\right), \sigma_i\left(x_j\right)^2\right)}$$

using the current parameter estimates.

The adaptation rules simplify if both $h_i(x)$ and $f_i(x)$ are linear functions of the inputs [29]. Tresp [30] describes a variant in which both $h_i(x)$ and $f_i(x)$ are modeled using Gaussian processes. For the $f_i(x)$, Gaussian processes with different bandwidths are used such that, input dependent, the expert with the appropriate bandwidth is selected by the gating network.

5.3.2 Extensions to the ME Approach

5.3.2.1 Hierarchical Mixtures of Experts

The hierarchical mixtures of experts (HMEs) have two (or more) layers of gating networks, and their output is calculated as

$$\hat{t}(x) = \sum_{i=1}^{M} g_i(x) \sum_{j=1}^{N(i)} g_{i,j}(x) f_{i,j}(x) \tag{5.6}$$

where

$$g_{i,j}(x) = \frac{\exp h_{i,j}(x)}{\sum_{j=1}^{N(i)} \exp h_{i,j}(x)} .$$

In the HME, a weighted combination of the outputs of M ME networks is formed. $N(i)$ is the number of experts in the ith ME network. In the HME approach, $h_i(x)$, $h_{i,j}(x)$, and $f_i(x)$ are typically linear functions. By using several layers of gating networks in the HME, one obtains large modeling flexibility despite the simple linear structure of the expert networks. On the other hand, by using linear models, the HME can be trained using an expectation maximization (EM) algorithm which exhibits fast convergence.

The HME can be seen as a soft decision tree, and (hard) decision tree learning algorithms, such as the CART algorithm, can be used to initialize the HME. The HME was developed by Jordan and Jacobs [31]. An extensive discussion of the HME is found in Haykin [29].

5.3.2.2 Alternative Training Procedures

A number of variations of the architecture and the training procedure for the ME have been reported. The learning procedure of the last section produces competing MEs in the sense that the committee members compete for the responsibility for the data. The cooperating MEs are achieved if the squared difference $\sum_{j=1}^{K}(y_j - \hat{t}(x_j))^2$, between output data and predictions, i.e., $\Sigma_{j=1}^{K}(y_j - \hat{t}(x_j))^2$ is minimized. Here, the solutions are typically less modular and the model has a larger tendency to overtrain.

Another variant starts from the joint probability model,

$$P(i)P(x|i)P(y|x, i)$$

where $P(i)$ is the prior probability of expert i, $P(x|i)$ is the probability density of input x for expert i, and $P(y|x, i)$ is the probability density of y given x and expert i. If we assume that the latter is modeled as before, we obtain Equation (5.5) with

$$g_i(x) = P(i|x) = \frac{P(i)P(x|i)}{\sum_{j=1}^{M} P(j)P(x|j)} . \tag{5.7}$$

In some applications, the experts are trained *a priori* on different data sets. In that case, we can estimate $P(i)$ as the fraction of data used to train expert i, and $P(x|i)$ as the input density of the data used to train expert i. Tresp and Taniguchi [33] suggested modeling the latter as a mixture of Gaussians. Tresp et al. and Xu et al. [34, 35] described approaches to generating the HME model based on joint probability models.

A very simple ME variant is obtained by modeling the joint input-output probability of $(x, y)'$ as a mixture of Gaussians. If we calculate the expected value of y given x, we obtain an ME network with linear experts and the gating network of Equation (5.7) where all conditional probability densities are Gaussians. The advantage of this simple variant is that it can be described in terms of simple probabilistic rules which can be formulated by a domain expert. Various combinations of the ME network with domain expert knowledge are described by Tresp et al. [32, 34].

5.3.3 Concluding Remarks

The ME is typically not used if the only goal is prediction accuracy, but it is applied in cases where its unique modeling properties, interpretability, and fast learning (in the case of the HME) are of interest. The capability of the ME to model a large class of conditional probability densities is useful in the estimation of risk [28], in optimal control and portfolio management [27], and in graphical models [36]. In some applications, the ME has been shown to lead to interesting segmentations of the map, as in the cognitive modeling of motor control [37].

Of the many generalizations of the ME approach, we want to mention the work of Jacobs and Tanner [38], who generalized the ME approach to a wider class of statistical mixture models, i.e., mixtures of distributions of the exponential family, mixtures of hidden Markov models, mixtures of marginal models, mixtures of Cox models, mixtures of factor models, and mixtures of trees.

5.4 A Bayesian Committee Machine

Consider the case that a large training data set is available. It is not obvious that a neural network trained on such a large data set makes efficient use of all the data. It might make more sense to divide the data set into M data sets, train M neural networks on the data sets, and then combine their predictions using a committee machine (see Figure 5.2). This approach is even more appropriate if the estimators are kernel-based systems such as Gaussian process regression systems, smoothing splines, or support vector machines. Parameter estimation for those systems requires operations whose computational complexity grows quickly with the size of the training data set such that those systems are not well suited for large data sets. An obvious solution would be to split the training data set into M data sets, train individual estimators on the partitioned data sets, and then combine

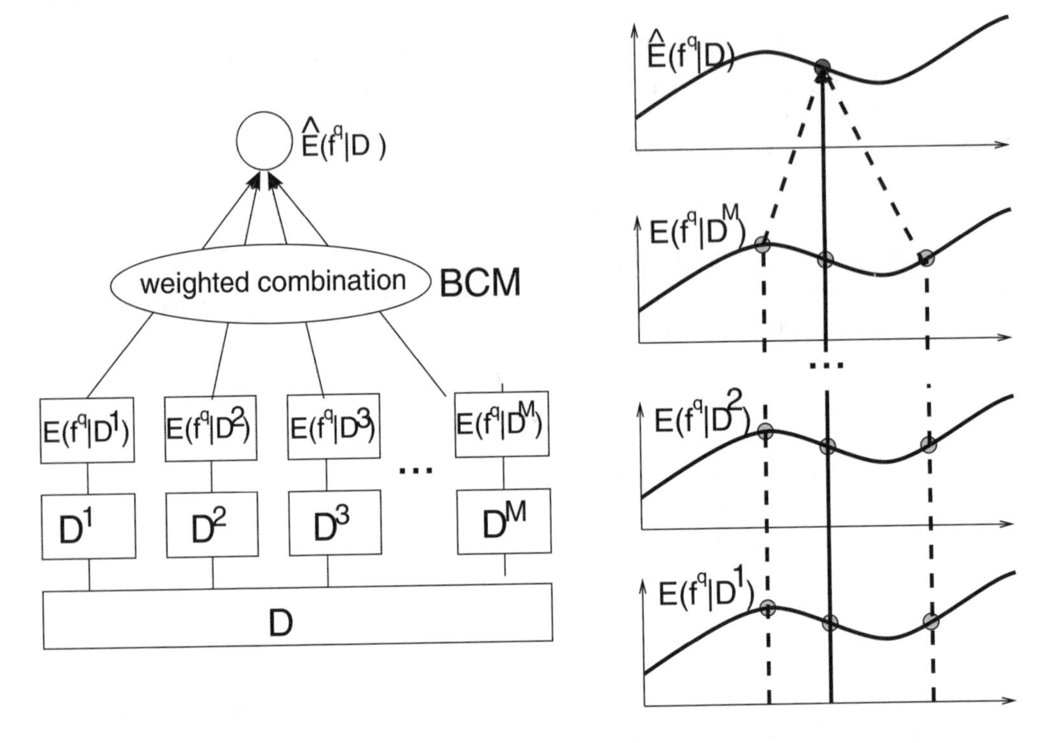

5.2 Left: Bayesian committee machine (BCM), data sets are partitioned and the committee members estimate the targets based on the partitioned data sets. The prediction of the committee is formed by a weighted combination of the predictions. Right: in most committee machines, the prediction at a given input is calculated by a combination of the predictions of the committee members at the same input (vertical continuous line). In the BCM, predictions at other inputs are also used (vertical dashed lines).

their predictions. The computational complexity of such an approach grows only linearly with the size of the training data set if M grows proportional to the size of the training data set. Important questions are (1) does one lose prediction performance by this procedure, and (2) what is a good combination scheme? This section analyzes this approach from a Bayesian point of view. It turns out that the optimal combining weights can be calculated based on the covariance structure and that for the optimal prediction of the committee at a given input x, the prediction of the members at inputs other than x can be exploited. Note that in previous sections, only predictions at x were used in the committee machines. A main result of this work is that the quality of the predictions depends critically on the number of different inputs which contribute to the prediction. If this number is identical to the effective number of parameters, then the performance of the committee machine is very close to the performance of one system trained on all data.

This section is different in character from the previous sections. Whereas previous sections provided an overview of the state-of-the-art of the respective topics, this section almost exclusively presents recent results of the author [39, 40].

5.4.1 Theoretical Foundations

Let x be a vector of input variables and let y be the output variable. We assume that, given a function $f(x)$, the output data are (conditionally) independent with conditional density $P(y|f(x))$.

Furthermore, let $X^q = \{x_1^q, \ldots, x_{N_Q}^q\}$ denote a set of N_Q test points (where q represents query) and let $f^q = (f_1^q, \ldots, f_{N_Q}^q)$ be the vector of the corresponding unknown response variables. Note that we query the system at a set of query points (or test points) at the same time, which will be important later on.

As indicated in the introduction, we now assume a setting where, instead of training one estimator using all the data, we split up the data into M data sets $D = \{D^1, \ldots, D^M\}$ (typically of approximately the same size) and train M estimators on the partitioned training data sets. Let $\bar{D}^i = D \setminus D^i$ denote the data which are not in D^i.

Then we have, in general,[2]

$$P\left(f^q|\bar{D}^i, D^i\right) \propto P\left(f^q\right) P\left(\bar{D}^i|f^q\right) P\left(D^i|\bar{D}^i, f^q\right) .$$

Now we would like to approximate

$$P\left(D^i|\bar{D}^i, f^q\right) \approx P\left(D^i|f^q\right) . \tag{5.8}$$

This is not true in general unless f^q contains the targets at the input locations of all the training data; only then are all outputs in the training data independent. The approximation in Equation (5.8) becomes more accurate when (1) N_Q is large, since then f^q determines f everywhere; (2) the correlation between the outputs in $\bar{D}^i$ and D^i is small, for example, if inputs in those sets are spatially separated from each other; and (3) the size of the data set in D^i is large, since then those data become more independent on average.

Using the approximation and applying Bayes' formula, we obtain

$$P\left(f^q|\mathcal{D}^{i-1}, D^i\right) \approx const \times \frac{P\left(f^q|\mathcal{D}^{i-1}\right) P\left(f^q|D^i\right)}{P\left(f^q\right)} \tag{5.9}$$

such that we can achieve an approximate predictive density

$$\hat{P}\left(f^q|D\right) = const \times \frac{\prod_{i=1}^M P\left(f^q|D^i\right)}{P\left(f^q\right)^{M-1}} \tag{5.10}$$

where *const* is a normalizing constant. The posterior predictive probability densities are simply multiplied. Note that since we multiply posterior probability densities, we have to divide by the priors $M-1$ times. This general formula can be applied to the combination of any suitable Bayesian estimator.

5.4.2 The BCM

In the case that the predictive densities $P(f^q|D^i)$ and the prior densities are Gaussian (or can be approximated reasonably well by a Gaussian), Equation (5.9) takes on an especially simple form. Assume that the *a priori* predictive density at the N_Q query points is a Gaussian with zero mean and covariance Σ^{qq}, and the posterior predictive density for each committee member is a Gaussian with mean $E(f^q|D^i)$ and covariance $cov(f^q|D^i)$. In that case, we achieve ($\hat{E}$ and $\widehat{cov}$ are calculated with respect to the approximate density $\hat{P}$) [39]:

$$\hat{E}\left(f^q|D\right) = \frac{1}{C} \sum_{i=1}^{M} cov\left(f^q|D^i\right)^{-1} E\left(f^q|D^i\right) \tag{5.11}$$

[2] We assume that inputs are given.

with

$$C = \widehat{cov}\left(f^q|D\right)^{-1} = -(M-1)\left(\Sigma^{qq}\right)^{-1} + \sum_{i=1}^{M} cov\left(f^q|D^i\right)^{-1}. \tag{5.12}$$

We recognize that the predictions of each committee member i are weighted by the inverse covariance of its prediction. But note that we do not compute the covariance between the committee members but the covariance at the N_Q query points. This means that predictive densities at all query points contribute to the prediction of the Bayesian committee machine (BCM — a way of combining predictions of committee members) at a given query point (see Figure 5.2). An intuitive appealing effect is that by weighting the predictions of the committee members by the inverse covariance, committee members uncertain about their predictions are automatically weighted less than committee members that are certain about their predictions.

5.4.3 Experiments

In the experiments, we applied the BCM to Gaussian process regression. Gaussian process regression is particularly suitable since prior and posterior densities are Gaussian distributed, and the covariance matrices required for the BCM are easily calculated. A short introduction into Gaussian process regression can be found in the Appendix at the end of this chapter.

Figure 5.3 shows results of applying the BCM to Gaussian process regression for a large artificial data set [39]. Note that the BCM with $K = 60{,}000$ training data points achieves results unobtainable with simple Gaussian process regression, which is limited to a training data set of approximately $K = 1000$.

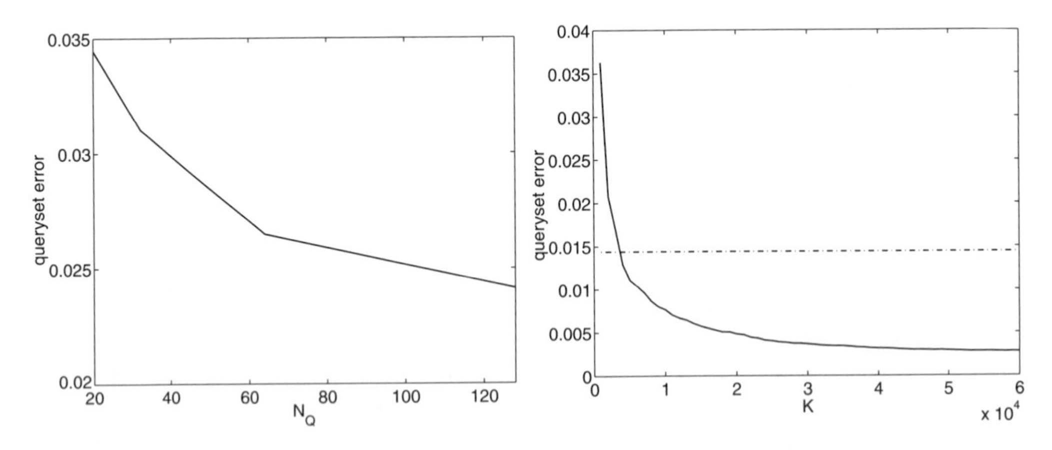

5.3 Left: the mean squared query-set error as a function of the number of query points N_Q with $K = 1000$ training data points and for $K/M = 100$ data points in the training data set of each committee member. Note that for small N_Q, the performance deteriorates. Right: The test of the BCM algorithm using an artificial data set. The continuous line is the mean squared query-set error for $N_Q = 1000$ and $K/M = 1000$ as a function of the size of the training data set K. The dash dotted line shows the error of Gaussian process regression ($M = 1$) with $K = 1000$, approximately the largest training data size suitable for Gaussian process regression. Note the great improvement with the BCM, which can use the larger data sets.

5.4.4 Concluding Remarks

The previous discussion on the BCM focused on regression. In the form of the generalized BCM (GBCM), the approach has been extended towards classification, the prediction of counts, the prediction of lifetimes, and other applications which can be derived from the exponential family of distributions [40]. The support vector machine is closely related to Gaussian processes and can also be used in the BCM [41]. Furthermore, it is possible to derive online Kalman filter versions of the BCM, which only require one path through the data set and the storage of a matrix of the dimension of the number of query or test points [39]. After training, the prediction at additional test points only requires resources dependent on the number of query points, but it is independent of the size of the training data set. An interesting question is how many query points are ideally required. It turns out that the number of query points should be equal to or larger than the effective number of parameters of the map. If this is the case, the query points uniquely define the map (if appropriately chosen), and the approximation in Equation (5.8) becomes an equality (see Figure 5.3) [39].

Since the BCM has the form of a committee machine, it might be possible to further improve performance by connecting it with ideas from Section 5.2. The issue of boosting the BCM is a focus of current work.

Finally, it is also possible to derive the BCM solution from a non-Bayesian perspective where the covariance matrices are derived from variations over repeated experiments (i.e., variations over data sets). The goal is to form a linear combination of the predictions at the query points

$$\hat{f}_i^q = \sum_{k=1}^{M} \sum_{j=1}^{N_Q} g_{i,k}\left(x_j\right) f_k^q\left(x_j\right)$$

such that the expected error is minimum. Here, $\hat{f}_i^q$ is the estimate of the committee for input x_i, $g_{i,k}(x_j)$ is the weight of query point j of committee member k to predict query point i, and $f_k^q(x_j)$ is the prediction of committee member k for input x_j. We use the assumption that the individual committee members are unbiased and enforce the constraint that the combined system is unbiased by requiring that

$$\sum_{k=1}^{M} g_{i,k}\left(x_i\right) = 1 \quad \text{and} \quad \sum_{k=1}^{M} g_{i,k}\left(x_j\right) = 0 \quad \forall\, j \neq i\,.$$

As a solution, we obtain the BCM with $(\Sigma^{qq})^{-1} \rightarrow 0$ (negligible prior). Details can be found in Tresp [39].

5.5 Conclusions

The research on committee machines is still very young but has already produced a number of interesting architectures and algorithms. Due to the limited space, we naturally could not provide a comprehensive overview covering all aspects of committee machines. As examples, boosting has been analyzed from the perspectives of PAC-learning, game theory, and "conventional" statistics. Furthermore, committee machines have been applied to density estimation [42, 43], hidden Markov models, and a variety of statistical mixture models. Also, we completely left out approaches to committee machines originating from statistical physics and modular approaches for sensory fusion and control. Finally, there are interesting common aspects between committee machines and biological systems. Committee machines, in general, are very tolerant vs. the breakdown of any of their components, and, similar to biological systems, system performance only deteriorates dramatically if a large number of committee members are malfunctioning.

In their many facets, committee machines have made important contributions to various branches of neural computation, machine learning, and statistics and are becoming increasingly popular in the KDD community. They have opened up a new dimension in machine learning since committees can be formed using virtually any prediction system. As demonstrated by the numerous contributions from various communities, committee machines can be understood and analyzed from a large number of different viewpoints, often revealing new interesting insights. We can expect numerous novel architectures, algorithms, applications, and theoretical insights for the future.

5.6 Appendix: Gaussian Process Regression

In contrast to the usual parameterized approach to regression, in Gaussian process regression, we specify the prior model directly in function space. In particular, we assume that, *a priori,* f is Gaussian distributed (in fact it would be an infinite-dimensional Gaussian) with zero mean and a covariance $cov(f(x_1), f(x_2)) = \sigma_{x_1,x_2}$. We assume that we can only measure a noisy version of f

$$y(x) = f(x) + \epsilon(x)$$

where $\epsilon(x)$ is independent Gaussian distributed noise with zero mean and variance $\sigma_\psi^2(x)$.

Let $(\Sigma^{mm})_{ij} = \sigma_{x_i^m, x_j^m}$ be the covariance matrix of the measurements, $\Psi^{mm} = \sigma_\psi^2(x)I$ be the noise variance of the outputs, $(\Sigma^{qq})_{ij} = \sigma_{x_i^q, x_j^q}$ be the covariance matrix of the query points, and $(\Sigma^{qm})_{ij} = \sigma_{x_i^q, x_j^m}$ be the covariance matrix between training data and query data. I is the K-dimensional unit matrix. Let y^m be the vector of training targets.

Under these assumptions, the conditional density of the response variables at the query points is Gaussian distributed with mean

$$E\left(f^q|D\right) = \Sigma^{qm}\left(\Psi^{mm} + \Sigma^{mm}\right)^{-1} y^m \tag{5.13}$$

and covariance

$$cov\left(f^q|D\right) = \Sigma^{qq} - \Sigma^{qm}\left(\Psi^{mm} + \Sigma^{mm}\right)^{-1}\left(\Sigma^{qm}\right)' . \tag{5.14}$$

Note that for the ith query point, we obtain

$$E\left(f_i^q|D\right) = \sum_{j=1}^{K} \sigma_{x_i^q, x_j^m}\, v_j \tag{5.15}$$

where v_j is the jth component of the vector $(\Psi^{mm} + \Sigma^{mm})^{-1} y^m$. The last equation describes the weighted superposition of kernel functions $b_j(x_i^q) = \sigma_{x_i^q, x_j^m}$, which are defined for each training data point and are equivalent to some solutions obtained for kriging, regularization neural networks, and smoothing splines. The experimenter has to specify the positive definite covariance matrix. A common choice is that $\sigma_{x_i,x_j} = \exp(-1/(2\gamma^2)||x_i - x_j||^2)$ with $\gamma > 0$ such that we obtain Gaussian basis functions, although other positive definite covariance functions are also used.

Acknowledgments

Valuable comments by Salvatore Ingrassia and Michal Skubacz are gratefully acknowledged.

References

[1] Sharkey, A.J.C., *Combining Artificial Neural Nets,* Springer-Verlag, New York, 1999.
[2] Rehfuss, S., Wu, L., and Moody, J., Trading with committees: a comparative study, in *Neural Networks in the Capital Markets,* Refenes, A., Abu-Mostafa, Y., Moody, J., and Weigend, A., Eds., World Scientific, London, 1996.
[3] Granger, C.W.J., Combining forecasts twenty years later, *Journal Forecasting,* 8, 167, 1989.
[4] Bernardo, J.M. and Smith, A.F.M., *Bayesian Theory,* John Wiley & Sons, New York, 1993.
[5] Quinlan, J.R., *Thirteenth National Conference on Artificial Intelligence (AAAI-96),* AAAI Press, 1996.
[6] Meir, R., Bias, variance and the combination of least squares estimators, in *Advances in Neural Information Processing Systems 7,* Tesauro, G., Touretzky, D.S., and Leen, T.K., Eds., MIT Press, Cambridge, MA, 1995, 295.
[7] Taniguchi, M. and Tresp, V., Averaging regularized estimators, *Neural Computation,* 9, 1163, 1997.
[8] Breiman, L., Combining predictors, in *Combining Artificial Neural Nets,* Sharkey, A.J.C., Ed., Springer-Verlag, New York, 1999, 31.
[9] Perrone, M.P., Improving regression estimates: averaging methods for variance reduction with extensions to general convex measure optimization, Ph.D. thesis, Brown University, 1993.
[10] Krogh, A. and Vedelsby, J., Neural network ensembles, cross validation, and active learning, in *Advances in Neural Information Processing Systems 7,* Tesauro, G., Touretzky, D.S., and Leen, T.K., Eds., MIT Press, Cambridge, MA, 1995, 231.
[11] Dietterich, T.G., An experimental comparison of three methods for constructing ensembles of decision trees: bagging, boosting and randomization, *Machine Learning,* 40, 130, 2000.
[12] Breiman, L., Randomizing outputs to increase prediction accuracy, *Machine Learning,* 40, 229, 2000.
[13] Raviv, Y. and Intrator, N., Variance reduction via noise and bias constraints, in *Combining Artificial Neural Nets,* Sharkey, A.J.C., Ed., Springer-Verlag, New York, 1999, 31.
[14] Friedman J., Hastie T., and Tibshirani, R., Additive logistic regression: a statistical view of boosting, *Annals of Statistics,* 38(2):337, 2000.
[15] Schapire, R.E., The strength of weak learnability, *Machine Learning,* 5, 197, 1990.
[16] Freund, Y. and Schapire, R.E., Experiments with a new boosting algorithm, in *Machine Learning: Proceedings of the Thirteenth International Conference,* 148, 1996.
[17] Zemel, R.S. and Pitassi, T., A gradient-based boosting algorithm for regression problems, in *Advances in Neural Information Processing Systems 13,* Leen, T.K., Dietterich, T.G., and Tresp, V., Eds., MIT Press, Cambridge, MA, 2001, 696.
[18] Schapire, R.E., Freund, Y., Bartlett, P., and Lee, W.S. Boosting the margin: a new explanation for the effectiveness of voting methods, *The Annals of Statistics,* 26(2):1651, 1998.
[19] Drucker, H., Boosting neural networks, in *Combining Artificial Neural Nets,* Sharkey, A.J.C., Ed., Springer-Verlag, New York, 1999, 51.
[20] Rätsch, G., Onoda, T., and Müller, K.R., Regularizing AdaBoost, in *Advances in Neural Information Processing Systems 11,* Kearns, M.S., Solla, S.A., and Cohn, D.A., Eds., MIT Press, Cambridge, MA, 1999, 564.
[21] Rätsch, G., Schölkopf, B., Smola, A., Müller, K.R., Onoda, T., and Mika, A., ν-Arc: ensemble learning in the presence of noise, in *Advances in Neural Information Processing Systems 12,* Solla, S.A., Leen, T.K., and Müller, K.R., Eds., MIT Press, Cambridge, MA, 2000, 561.
[22] Schapire, R.E. and Singer, Y., Improved boosting algorithms using confidence-rated predictions, in *Proceedings of the Eleventh Annual Conference on Computational Learning Theory,* 1998.
[23] Breiman, L., Predicting games and arcing algorithms, TR. 504, Statistics Department, University of California, December, 1997.
[24] Mason, L., Baxter, J., Bartlett, P., and Frean, M., Boosting algorithms as gradient descent, in *Advances in Neural Information Processing Systems 12,* Solla, S.A., Leen, T.K., and Müller, K.R., Eds., MIT Press, Cambridge, MA, 2000, 512.
[25] Wolpert, D.H., Stacked generalization, *Neural Networks,* 5, 241, 1992.
[26] Jacobs, R.A., Jordan, M.I., Nowlan, S.J., and Hinton, J.E., Adaptive mixtures of local experts, *Neural Computation,* 3, 79, 1991.

[27] Neuneier, R.F., Hergert, W., Finnof, W., and Ormoneit, D., Estimation of conditional densities: a comparison of approaches, *Proceedings of ICANN*94,* 1, 689, 1994.
[28] Bishop, C.M., *Neural Networks for Pattern Recognition,* Clarendon Press, Oxford, UK, 1995.
[29] Haykin, S., *Neural Networks, a Comprehensive Foundation,* 2nd ed., Prentice-Hall, Englewood Cliffs, NJ, 1999.
[30] Tresp, V., Mixtures of Gaussian processes, in *Advances in Neural Information Processing Systems 13,* Leen, T.K., Dietterich, T.G., and Tresp, V., Eds., MIT press, Cambridge, MA, 2001, 654.
[31] Jordan, M.I. and Jacobs, R.A., Hierarchical mixtures of experts and the EM algorithm, *Neural Computation,* 6, 181, 1994.
[32] Tresp, V., Hollatz, J., and Ahmad, S., Network structuring and training using rule-based knowledge, in *Advances in Neural Information Processing Systems 5,* Giles, C.L., Hanson, S.J., and Cowan J.D., Eds., Morgan Kaufman, San Mateo, CA, 1993, 871.
[33] Tresp, V. and Taniguchi, M., Combining estimators using non-constant weighting functions, in *Advances in Neural Information Processing Systems 7,* Tesauro, G., Touretzky, D.S., and Leen, T.K., Eds., MIT Press, Cambridge, MA, 1995, 419.
[34] Tresp, V., Hollatz, J., and Ahmad, S., Representing probabilistic rules with networks of Gaussian basis functions, *Machine Learning,* 27, 173, 1997.
[35] Xu, L., Jordan, M.I., and Hinton, G.E., An alternative model for mixtures of experts, in *Advances in Neural Information Processing Systems 7,* Tesauro, G., Touretzky, D.S., and Leen, T.K., Eds., MIT Press, Cambridge, MA, 1995, 633.
[36] Hofmann, R. and Tresp, V., Discovering structure in continuous variables using Bayesian networks, in *Advances in Neural Information Processing Systems 8,* Touretzky, D.S., Mozer, M.C., and Hasselmo, M.E., Eds., MIT Press, Cambridge, MA, 1996, 500.
[37] Brashers-Krug, T., Shadmehr, R., Todorov, E., and Jacobs, R., Catastrophic inference in human motor learning, in *Advances in Neural Information Processing Systems 7,* Tesauro, G., Touretzky, D.S., and Leen, T.K., Eds., MIT Press, Cambridge, MA, 1995, 19.
[38] Jacobs, R. and Tanner, M., Mixtures of X, in *Combining Artificial Neural Nets,* Sharkey, A.J.C., Ed., Springer-Verlag, New York, NY, 1999, 267.
[39] Tresp, V., The Bayesian committee machine, *Neural Computation,* 12, 2000.
[40] Tresp, V., The generalized Bayesian committee machine, *Proceedings of the Sixth ACM SIGKDD International Conference on Knowledge Discovery and Data Mining, KDD-2000,* 130, 2000.
[41] Schwaighofer, A. and Tresp, V., The Bayesian committee support vector machine, *Proceedings of the Eleventh International Conference on Artificial Intelligence,* ICANN, 2001.
[42] Ormoneit, D. and Tresp, V., Averaging, maximum penalized likelihood and Bayesian estimation for improving Gaussian mixture probability density estimates, *IEEE Transactions on Neural Networks,* 9, 639, 1998.
[43] Smyth, P. and Wolpert, D., Stacked density estimation, in *Advances in Neural Information Processing Systems 10,* Jordan, M.I., Kearns, M.J., and Solla, A.S., Eds., MIT Press, Cambridge, MA, 1998, 668.

6

Dynamic Neural Networks and Optimal Signal Processing

Jose C. Principe
University of Florida

The major purpose of this chapter is to further our understanding of optimal signal processing by integrating concepts from function approximation, linear and nonlinear regression, dynamic modeling, and delay operators using the concepts from approximations of causal shift-invariant processes. We seek an integrating view of all these subjects with an emphasis on the choice of the basis functions. We review proofs of the uniform approximation properties of dynamic networks created by a cascade of linear filters and static nonlinearities. We conclude by presenting a general class of linear operators that can implement the finite memory kernels required to approximate nonlinear operators with approximate finite memory.

6.1 Introduction

The theory of optimal signal processing has a long history that began with the seminal work of Norbert Wiener [1] and was later made practical by many advances, from which Bernard Widrow's LMS algorithm [2] is singled out here. What is less known is that optimal filtering is a special case of the much older problem of function approximation which has been extensively studied in mathematics since the 18th century [3]. When seen from the function approximation point of view, there are many apparently unrelated topics in optimal information processing, such as least squares, linear and nonlinear regression, classification, optimal linear and nonlinear filtering, and nonlinear dynamical modeling, that become very much related. What changes are the spaces (vector or functional spaces),

0-8493-2359-2/01/$0.00+$1.50

the metric (Minskowski, Borel), and the type of approximant (linear or nonlinear). The view just presented allows many interesting insights and, in particular, is able to unify optimal linear filtering and dynamic neural network modeling, two areas that unfortunately live in almost disjoint worlds. This framework further shows the commonality of the problems faced, which are directly related to function approximation: how to choose bases and how to estimate optimal weights and optimal orders. It also shows how the old ideas of seeking extrema of functions permeate all these solutions, first in an analytic form (the least squares) and then in its iterative embodiment (gradient descent learning for nonlinear systems).

The problem concerning the choice of bases is the least addressed in the signal processing literature. Although we agree that, under a linear signal model, the bases are somewhat predetermined, they are a key player in nonlinear signal processing. This is the reason we emphasize the choice of bases in functional spaces and show how the bank of linear filters followed by static nonlinearities creates networks that are universal approximators for the class of nonlinear functions with approximately finite memory. This type of network is called a dynamic neural network and is illustrated by the time delay neural network (TDNN). Unfortunately, the proofs are existence proofs, which means that the designer still needs to decide parsimonious architectures to achieve good results that are insensitive to noise and generalize well. In this context, this chapter also treats a set of delay operators that generalize the ideal delay operator almost exclusively utilized in digital signal processing. Due to the breadth of topics covered and the limited space, we omit most problems related to training networks and the selection of model order.

6.2 Function Approximation and Adaptive Systems

6.2.1 Function Approximation

Function approximation seeks to describe the behavior of complicated functions by ensembles of simpler functions. Very important results have been established in this branch of mathematics. For instance, Legendre and Gauss used polynomials to approximate functions, Chebyshev developed the concept of best uniform approximation, and Weierstrass proved that polynomials can approximate arbitrarily well any continuous real function in an interval. The core advantage of polynomials is that only multiplications and additions are necessary to implement them. We will start by formalizing the concept of function approximation.

Let $f(x)$ be a continuous real function in $\Re^n \to \Re$, i.e., a function of a real-valued vector $\boldsymbol{x} = [x_1, x_2, \ldots, x_n]^T$ that is square integrable over the real numbers. Most real-world data can be modeled by such conditions. We restrict this study to the linear projection theorem. The goal of function approximation is to describe the behavior of $f(x)$, in a compact area S of the input space, by a combination of simpler functions $\phi_i(x)$:

$$\hat{f}(x) = \sum_{i=1}^{N} w_i \phi_i(\boldsymbol{x}) \tag{6.1}$$

where w_i are real-valued entries of the coefficient vector $\boldsymbol{w} = [w_1\; w_2\; w_N]^T$ such that

$$\left| f(x) - \hat{f}(x) \right| < \varepsilon \tag{6.2}$$

and where ε can be made arbitrarily small. The function $\hat{f}(x)$ is called an approximant to $f(x)$ in S. The block diagram of Figure 6.1 describes this formulation. We clearly see that function approximation can be practically implemented by classes of parameteric models given by Equation (6.1).

Let us examine Equations (6.1) and (6.2). A real function is a map from the input vector space to real numbers, $\Re^n \to \Re$. This expression states that one obtains the value of the function when x is

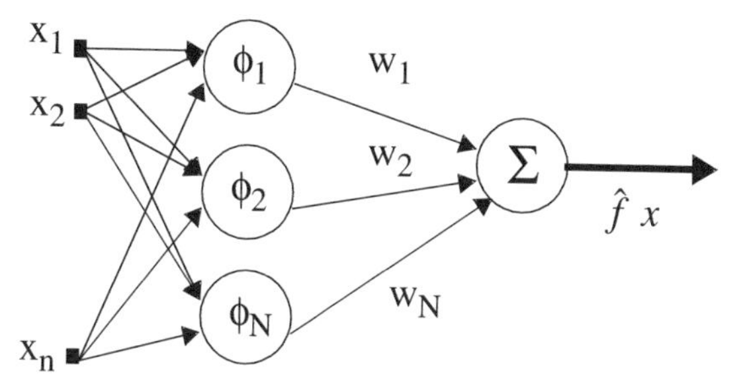

6.1 Function approximation by a linear combination of bases.

in S by using an intermediate set of simpler functions, $\{\phi_i(x)\}$, called the elementary functions, and then linearly combining them (Figure 6.1).

When one can find coefficients w_i and $\phi_i(x)$ that make ε arbitrarily small for any function $f(.)$ over the domain of interest, we say that the function $\hat{f}(x)$ has the property of universal approximation for the class of functions $f(.)$, or that the set of elementary functions $\{\phi_i(x)\}$ is complete. From Equation (6.1) we see that there are three basic tasks in function approximation:

1. the choice of elementary functions $\phi_i(x)$
2. how to compute the weights w_i
3. how to select the number of elementary functions N.

Therefore, function approximation involves finding an element of the class of functions that minimizes Equation (6.2). Although we need to solve for the three items when approximating unknown functions $f(x)$, their role and importance varies. The essential role of the basis is to "cover" the space of the range of the function. If the bases span the space of the functional values, then it is just a matter of finding a way to compute the weights and choosing the most appropriate size of the space to guarantee the quality of the approximation. If the basis is not a spanning basis, there are no weight values that guarantee arbitrarily small approximation error. Unfortunately, the choice of a basis set is not straightforward because it depends on the type of function we want to approximate (which, most of the time, we do not know), and, in many instances, there are many choices. This is the reason an "axiomatic" approach to choose the bases is normally preferred, and mathematical arguments are normally utilized to show that a given basis set is able to provide universal approximation for the class of functions under analysis.

Under the linear signal model (linear functional $f(x)$), affine transforms of the input space axes are normally appropriate. In the case of nonlinear functions, polynomials have been the de facto default choice because of their well known properties [4], but splines also have a well established niche [5]. However, the recent advances in neural network theory may very well enchance these choices.

The second problem is how to compute the coefficients w_i, which depends on how the difference or discrepancy between $f(x)$ and $\hat{f}(x)$ is measured. Equation (6.2) is formulated as an L_1 metric, which makes the mathematics rather difficult, and it is normally not utilized. However, if we define the error with an L_2 metric (the mean square error), the method of least squares [6] can solve for w_i analytically. This metric corresponds to the minimization of the mean square error defined as

$$J = \int \left(f(x) - \hat{f}(x) \right)^2 dx \tag{6.3}$$

which leads to the normal equations

$$\begin{bmatrix} p_1 \\ \cdots \\ p_N \end{bmatrix} = \begin{bmatrix} r_{11} & \cdots & r_{1N} \\ \cdots & \cdots & \cdots \\ r_{N1} & \cdots & r_{NN} \end{bmatrix} \begin{bmatrix} w_1 \\ \cdots \\ w_N \end{bmatrix}$$

and the solution becomes

$$w = R^{-1} p \,. \tag{6.4}$$

In Equation (6.4), w is a vector with the coefficients, p is a vector of the inner products (cross-correlation) between the function evaluated at a certain number of points in the domain and the basis functions $p_j = \langle f, \phi_j \rangle = \int f(x)\phi_j(x)\, dx$, and R is a matrix with entries given by the values of the inner products (autocorrelation) of the elementary functions at each of the points in the domain $r_{jk} = \langle \phi_j, \phi_k \rangle = \int \phi_j(x)\phi_k\, dx$. An important condition that must be placed on the elementary functions is that the inverse of R must exist, which practically means that the set of $\{\phi_i(x)\}$ are linearly independent. With a complete orthonormal basis, the weights of the decomposition become very simple to compute [4]. It can be easily shown that in this case, $w_i = \langle f(x), \phi_i(x) \rangle$. There is a very powerful geometric interpretation of the mean square error solution that goes as follows: the value of $\hat{f}(x)$ is the orthogonal projection of $f(x)$ in the space spanned by the bases $\{\phi_i(x)\}$ [7]. Normally, however, we have a set of $M > N$ samples in the domain $f(x)|_{x=x_i}$, and Equation (6.3) becomes

$$J = \frac{1}{M} \sum_{i=1}^{M} \left(f(x_i) - \hat{f}(x_i) \right)^2 \tag{6.5}$$

effectively transforming function approximation into interpolation. However, the solution is basically unchanged if the samples sufficiently cover the domain of interest.

The third item is the determination of the dimension, N, of the space. This is not as straightforward as it may seem. If the basis set is complete, in principle, the larger the N, the smaller the approximation error, eventually reaching zero. However, this increase in N may not be practical for two reasons: first, the data may be noisy, and a large N will start to represent the noise with no net gain; second, we may not have enough data samples to continue to increase N. This can be inferred from Equations (6.1) and (6.4), where we see that a larger N requires the calculation of a larger matrix inverse that becomes progressively less accurate.

6.2.2 Regression and Classification

Linear regression and classification are special cases of the function approximation problem just described. One major difference is that the problem is formulated in a vector space with a probability measure, that is, x is a random variable. We will follow the approach of Vapnik [8] in this formulation.

Let us assume that there is an unknown generator for the observed L pairs of random input and target variables (x, y) (called the training set) consistent with some unknown but fixed joint distribution function $F(x, y)$. These pairs are assumed to be identically and independently distributed (i.i.d.). The role of the learning machine is to construct an operator that predicts (approximates) the value of y by observing x, i.e., the goal is to approximate the conditional distribution function $F(y|x)$ with an appropriate metric (Figure 6.2).

The construction of the operator is accomplished by selecting a parametric form for the learning machine and finding the best possible set of parameters. Referring to Equation (6.1), the learning machine implements the approximant $\hat{f}(x)$. The issue is how to measure the discrepancy between

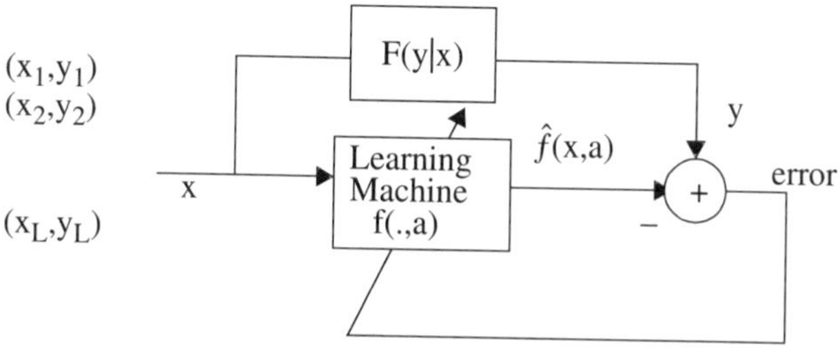

6.2 The problem of linear regression and classification from samples.

two random variables. Let us define the risk functional as

$$R(a) = \int L\left(y, \hat{f}(x, a)\right) dF(y) \tag{6.6}$$

where $x \in \Re^n$, a is a parameter vector, and the function $L(.)$ is called a loss function that measures the discrepancy between y and the value of $\hat{f}(x, a)$. The problem is then one of minimizing the risk functional with respect to the parametric function $\hat{f}(x, a)$. Note, however, that we cannot evaluate this integral since we do not know $F(y)$; we only know a set of M i.i.d. observations of $F(x, y)$. Instead of Equation (6.6), let us define the empirical risk functional

$$R_{\text{emp}}(a) = \frac{1}{M} \sum_{i=1}^{M} L\left(y_i, f\left(x_i, a\right)\right) . \tag{6.7}$$

One of the fundamental theorems of statistics [9] shows that when L increases, the empirical distribution function converges to the true distribution, and so R_{emp} approaches $R(a)$. Normally, the loss function is the L_2 norm, and Equation (6.7) reduces to evaluating the mean square error.

6.2.2.1 Regression

Now we are ready to discuss the regression and classification problems. Regression is the problem of estimating $F(y|x)$; however, it is sufficient to estimate the regression function

$$r(x) = \int y dF(y|x) \tag{6.8}$$

which, under mild conditions [8], is equivalent to minimizing

$$R(a) = \int \left(y - \hat{f}(x, a)\right)^2 dF(x, y) \tag{6.9}$$

or simply

$$R_{\text{emp}}(a) = \frac{1}{M} \sum_{i=1}^{M} \left(y_i - \hat{f}\left(x_i, a\right)\right)^2 . \tag{6.10}$$

Notice how close this expression is to Equation (6.3). The most common application of Equation (6.10) is in linear regression, where the basis functions are simply the input space axes, i.e., $\phi_i(x) = x_i$ with a bias to yield

$$\hat{f}(x) = \sum_{i=1}^{N} w_i x_i + b . \tag{6.11}$$

Hence, the solution of linear regression is Equation (6.4), where the cross-correlation is computed between the inputs x_i and the targets y_i, and the autocorrelation function pertains to the input data pairs x_i and x_j. Instead of using the analytic solution of Equation (6.4), we can use gradient descent learning or the LMS algorithm [10]. Linear regression is applicable when we assume that the data model is an affine transform of the input and the error is Gaussian distributed.

In nonlinear regression, we have reason to believe that the data model is nonlinear, so fitting a hyperplane through the data is not going to be an optimal solution. For nonlinear regression, the choice of the basis functions becomes very important. In the neural network literature, the learning machine is either a multilayer perceptron (MLP) or a radial basis function (RBF) network [11]. A one hidden layer MLP with a linear output or an RBF implements exactly the structure of Figure 6.1. In the MLP, the approximant is

$$\hat{f}(x) = \sum_{i=1}^{N_2} w_i \phi_i(x) \qquad \phi_i(x) = \sigma\left(\sum_{j=1}^{N_1} a_{ij} x_j\right) \tag{6.12}$$

where σ is a sigmoidal nonlinearity such as the logistic function or the tanh [10]. The bases functions are, in fact, global because they respond with a large value to all input spaces. Note that the outputs of the hidden layer processing elements (PEs) become the basis set for the approximation.

In the case of the RBF network, the bases are the multidimensional Gaussian function

$$\phi_i(x) = \exp\left(\frac{-(x - x_i)^T \sum^{-1} (x - x_i)}{2}\right) \tag{6.13}$$

where Σ is the covariance function of the kernel components. Notice that in this case, the basis responds primarily to the area around the sample x_i, and, therefore, the basis is called local. Having made these choices, the pertinent question is whether the basis sets of these two neural topologies are appropriate for approximating functions in $\Re^n$. It is no surprise to verify that extensive work on the mapping capabilities of the MLP (and the RBF) has been conducted in the literature. Now we know that both of these networks are universal approximators of continuous functions in vector spaces [12, 13], so they are alternatives to polynomial approximators presenting advantages in high-dimensional spaces in terms of convergence rates (see Barron [14]) and smoothness [15], respectively.

Training of the MLP can be done using the back-propagation algorithm [18]. Training of the RBF is normally divided into a clustering step to select the centers of the Gaussians, followed by a least squares operation (or LMS) to train the weights w_i [16].

6.2.2.2 Classification

The case of classification can also be easily framed as function approximation by utilizing what has been called a special type of conditional distribution based on indicator functions [8]. In classification, we assume that the input data belong to a finite number of k classes $c \in \{1, 2, \ldots k\}$. The task is to discover the partnership of each one of the input samples x_i according to $F(c|x)$. So, we minimize the risk functional

$$R(a) = \int L\left(c, \hat{f}(x, a)\right) dF(c, x) \tag{6.14}$$

on the set of parametric functions $\hat{f}(x, a)$. In terms of the empirical risk, we create a training set $\{x_i, c_i\}$ and minimize

$$R_{\text{emp}}(a) = \frac{1}{M} \sum_{i=1}^{M} L\left(c_i, \hat{f}(x_i, a)\right) \tag{6.15}$$

Notice that here the goal is to minimize the number of errors. Therefore, the loss function need not be the MSE, although in practice, most of the work in neural networks uses MSE. Networks trained with MSE have the appeal of estimating the *a posteriori* probability of the class given the data, which is known to be optimal in Bayesian terms [11]. However, other possible criteria include the crossentropy criterion [17] and Vapnik's structural risk minimization [8]. The networks for classification tasks are invariably nonlinear, either an MLP with a sigmoidal or softmax output, or an RBF. The most common choice for parameter adaptation is gradient descent learning (back-propagation) [18]. There are many issues in the appropriate training of classifiers and how to set the size of the networks, but we will not address them here. We refer the reader to Haykin [18] or Bishop's [11] extensive treatments of these topics.

6.2.3 Optimal Linear Filtering

Up until now, we have treated static problems, i.e., the approximant $\hat{f}(x)$ was only a function of the present (possibly multidimensional) input; for example, the approximation problem was done in vector spaces $f(x) : \Re^n \rightarrow \Re$. In digital signal processing, we are interested in the analysis of time series that are continuous real functions of the time variable. This radically changes the structure of the space where the approximation is conducted. Instead of a vector space, it now is a function space. $C(\Re)$ denotes the space of all continuous real valued functions $: \Re \rightarrow \Re$ with an appropriate norm $\|f\| = \sup_{t \in R} |f(t)|$.

A time series by definition carries information in its time structure, so instantaneous mappers such as the regressor, the MLP, and the RBF are not appropriate for time series analysis. How can these concepts of function approximation and regression apply to time series modeling. Due to the different assumptions, optimal linear filters were independently developed from regressors; however, there are many similarities outlined below. Thus far, we have started by presenting first the deterministic case and then extended the reasoning to random variables. However, for historical reasons, we will switch the order of presentation in subsequent sections.

Optimal linear filtering was originally developed by Wiener in continuous time for stochastic processes (a family of random variables over time) [1]. The digital counterpart of Wiener's theory using the finite impulse response (FIR) filter utilizes the same mathematical tools of least squares. Let us assume that the time series is the output of an unknown linear system, $U(z)$, excited by a white stochastic process (white noise). The idea in time series modeling with FIRs is to approximate the next sample of the time series by a linear combination of its N past samples,

$$\hat{f}(x(n)) = \sum_{i=1}^{N} w_i x(n-i) \tag{6.16}$$

according to the block diagram of Figure 6.3.

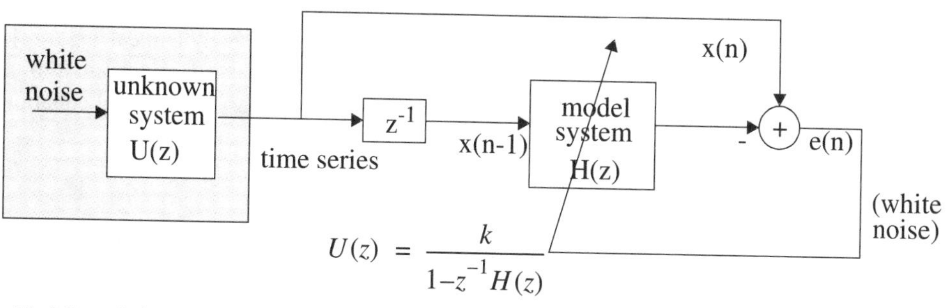

6.3 Modeling of a linear stochastic process.

We can immediately see the analogy of this figure with Figures 6.1 and 6.2, which depict function approximation and regression. Here, the model system is a finite impulse response (FIR) filter, as shown in Figure 6.4.

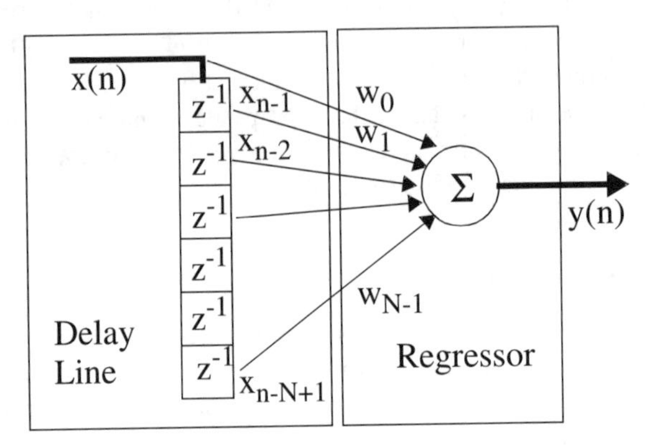

6.4 The FIR as a cascade of a delay line and regressor.

The goal of optimal linear filtering is to adapt the coefficients of the filter such that the MSE between the filter output and a desired response is minimized, i.e., define $e(n) = x(n) - \hat{f}(x(n))$ and minimize

$$J = \sum_{n=1}^{M} e^2(n) . \tag{6.17}$$

It is easy to see that this problem defaults to the normal equations of Equation (6.4) with the optimal solution given by Equation (6.5), except that now the cross-correlation vector and the autocorrelation matrix involve the time cross-correlation and autocorrelation functions, respectively. Hence, we conclude that time series modeling is a special case of function approximation where the basis functions are the input signal vector and its delayed versions $\phi_i(n) = x(n-i)$.

As long as the output error $e(n)$ is white, the system model will approach the inverse of the unknown linear system. The FIR filter structure is just one of three possibilities (the others being an all-pole model or a pole-zero model [19]) to model the unknown linear system. These choices effectively correspond to the choice of the basis to perform the approximation. In the above discussion, the desired response was the next sample of the time series, which leads to modeling. But other desired signals are possible (such as a noiseless and delayed version of the input time series) that lead to the general case of optimal filtering [19].

6.2.4 Dynamic Modeling

If the time series is modeled as the output of an autonomous deterministic system instead of the stochastic model of Figure 6.3, then its generator has to be a nonlinear dynamical system [21]; otherwise, the estimated signal will decay to zero or will be a sinusoidal waveform. A Kth order autonomous dynamical system can be represented by a set of Kth ordinary differential equations:

$$\frac{d}{dt}\mathbf{s}(t) = \Phi(\mathbf{s}(t)) \tag{6.18}$$

where $\mathbf{s}(t) = [s_1(t), s_2(t), \ldots, s_K(t)]$ is a vector of system states, and Φ is called the vector field. Bold letters represent vectors. The system state can, at any time, be specified in a K-dimensional space. The vector field maps a manifold M to a tangent space T. If Φ is a nonlinear function of the system state, the system is called nonlinear. Assume there is a closed form solution to Equation (6.18) $\varphi_t : M \to M$. For a given initial condition s_0, the function $\varphi_t(s_0)$ represents a state-space trajectory of the system (the mapping φ is called the flow). If the vector field is continuously differentiable, then the system flow and its inverse exist for any finite time. This implies that the trajectories of an autonomous system never intersect each other.

The FIR structure is not the most appropriate solution to approximate Φ because it is a linear operator and we just argued that the system that generated the time series must be nonlinear. However, the delay line portion of the FIR structure implements a very special transformation called a time-delay embedding [25]. The delay line can be thought of as a structure that maps the time series to a vector space of size N that we call the signal space. Each N-tuple in time becomes a point in the N-dimensional signal space, where the first time series sample becomes the coordinate ϕ_1, the second sample becomes the coordinate ϕ_2, and the Nth sample becomes the coordinate ϕ_N of the first point in signal space. When time ticks, this point evolves in signal space and creates a trajectory (Figure 6.5).

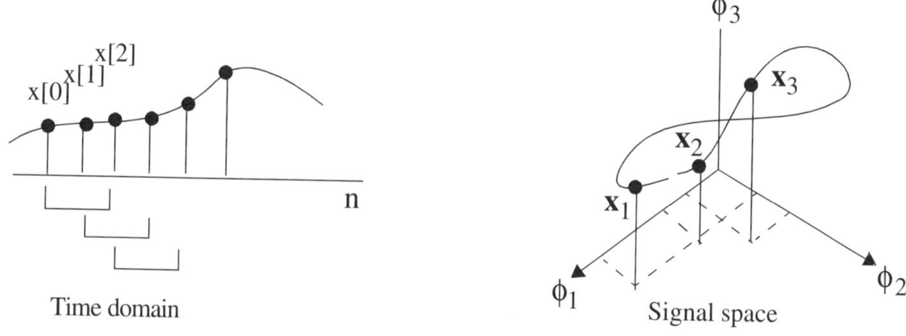

6.5 Constructing the trajectory in a three-dimensional signal space from the time series.

There is a fundamental theorem about embeddings that has been proven by Takens [26]. Takens showed that if the size N of the signal space is twice as large the dimensionality K of the dynamical system that generated the time series ($N > 2K$), then there is a one-to-one smooth map Ψ with a smooth inverse from the Kth dimensional manifold M of the original system to the Euclidean reconstruction space $\Re^N$. Such mapping is called an embedding and the theorem is known as Takens' embedding theorem. According to this theorem, when $N > 2K$, a map $F : \Re^N \to \Re^N$ exists that transforms the current reconstructed state $\boldsymbol{x}(n)$ to the next state $\boldsymbol{x}(n+\tau)$, where τ is the normalized delay. For simplicity, we will set $\tau = 1$, which means

$$\boldsymbol{x}(n+1) = F(\boldsymbol{x}(n)) \tag{6.19}$$

or

$$\begin{bmatrix} x(n+1) \\ \cdots \\ x(n-N+2) \end{bmatrix} = F\left(\begin{bmatrix} x(n) \\ \cdots \\ x(n-N+1) \end{bmatrix}\right) .$$

Note that Equation (6.19) specifies a multiple input-multiple output system F built from several (nonlinear) filters and a nonlinear predictor [56]. The predictive mapping is the centerpiece of modeling since, once determined, F can be obtained from the predictive mapping by simple matrix operations. The predictive mapping $f : \Re^N \to \Re$ can be expressed as

$$x(n+1) = f(\boldsymbol{x}(n)) . \tag{6.20}$$

Equation (6.20) defines a deterministic nonlinear autoregressive (NAR) model of the signal. The existence of this predictive model lays a theoretical basis for dynamic modeling in the sense that it opens the possibility to build a model from a vector time series to approximate the mapping f. The result and steps in dynamical modeling are depicted in Figure 6.6.

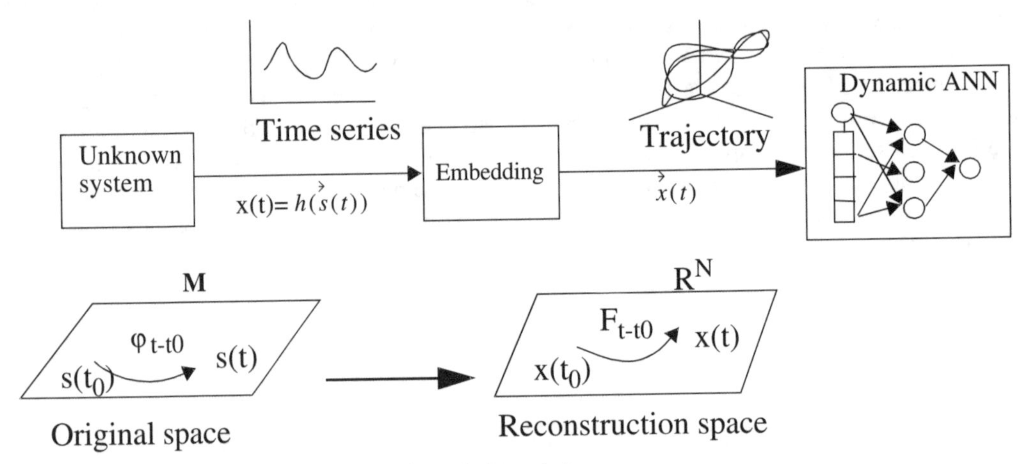

6.6 Nonlinear modeling steps and their mathematical translation.

Dynamic modeling implies a two-step process [24]. The first step is to transform the observed time series into a trajectory in the signal space by using one of the embedding techniques [28]. The most common is a time delay embedding which can practically be implemented with a delay line (also called a memory structure in neurocomputing) with a size specified by Takens' embedding theorem. The dimension K of the attractor can be estimated by the correlation dimension algorithm [29], but other methods exist [30]. The second step in dynamic modeling is to build the predictive model of Equation (6.20) from the trajectory in reconstruction space [27].

With this argument, we can immediately ask the following question: do we know a topology that can implement an NAR model? Using the arguments from the previous section, we can easily substitute the linear regressor of Figure 6.4 by an MLP or an RBF network to implement a nonlinear filter that, when trained with steepest descent, leads to an optimum nonlinear filter (Figure 6.7).

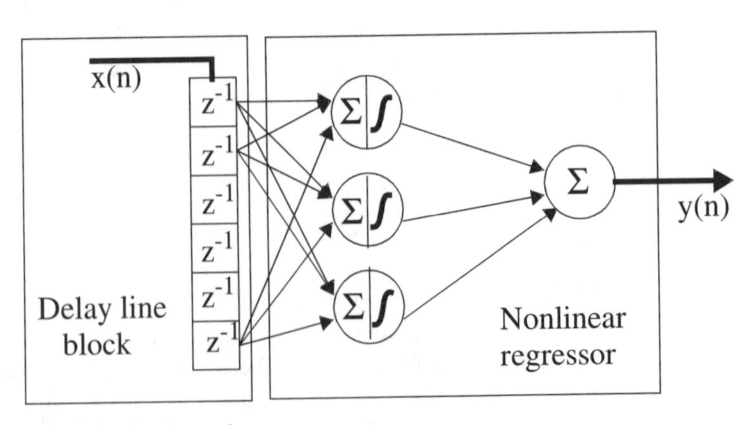

6.7 A nonlinear model for the time series.

There are other possibilities to create nonlinear models of time series, but we will not pursue this discussion here. The interested reader is referred to the referenced literature [22, 23, 31].

This solution of coupling a delay line to the PEs of the MLP was proposed many years ago by Waibel [33] and was called the time delay neural network (TDNN). The most common TDNN (called the focused TDNN) is shown in Figure 6.7 and can be considered a nonlinear (static) combination of adaptive linear FIR filters. The results reported by many researchers (Narendra [34], Mozer [23], Lapedes and Farber [35], and Principe and Kuo [27], among others) with focused TDNNs were very exciting and provide a living proof that the arrangement of linear filters followed by static nonlinearities is appropriate for dynamic modeling.

If the time series is modeled by a stochastic process, as done by Wiener, this topological equivalence between time series and trajectories in signal space becomes less formal (we do not know of any result that proves the embedding theorem for random processes). However, the plausibility of the topological equivalence is still present. Although random processes may require an infinite-dimensional signal space, the truth of the matter is that real-world time series have a time structure that can be captured by a finite state Markov chain [36]. This means that there is a vanishing dependency over time in real time series. If this is the case, then random processes can practically be embedded in finite-dimensional spaces, and we can also expect that the information between the time series is mapped entirely into signal space. But can we be sure that the basis sets utilized in the TDNN are complete in functional spaces?

6.3 Topological Approximation with Static Nonlinear Combinations of Linear Finite Memory Operators

In optimal nonlinear filtering, we are interested in approximating the class of continuous real valued functions or its discrete counterparts. Therefore, we are interested in functionals. Wiener was one of the pioneers to study linear and nonlinear approximations in functional spaces. However, here we are interested in approximating nonlinear dynamical systems with stochastic inputs by either a continuous time parametric model or its discrete counterpart. Before the recent interest in neural networks, the Volterra series was the established procedure to study nonlinear function approximation [37, 38]. The Volterra series expansion is a generalization of the convolution description of linear time invariant systems given by

$$y(t) = h(t) + \int_0^t h_1(t; t_1)\, x(t_1)\, dt_1 + \frac{1}{2!}\int_0^t \int_0^t h_2(t; t_1, t_2)\, x(t_1)\, x(t_2)\, dt_1 dt_2 + \ldots \quad (6.21)$$

where $x(t)$ is the input, $y(t)$ is the output, and $h_k : \Re^{k+1} \to \Re$ are multivariate kernels. For linear systems, only the first two terms are different from zero and they provide the well-known zero-input response and the convolution operation (zero state response). When seen as an operator, the Volterra series provides an approximation to a large class of causal, time invariant nonlinear operators in compact sets and for finite time [38]. Experience has shown that they are not very practical due to computational problems (multiple integrals, many parameters), and the quality of the approximation also suffers for low orders, providing only reasonably good approximations at or near an operating point.

In the early 1980s Figueiredo proposed a methodology for nonlinear system identification based on a weighted Fock space framework, which is a reproducing kernel Hilbert space of Volterra functionals [40]. Effectively, his approach leads to a bank of linear filters (made up of Volterra kernels) combined by static nonlinearities, but his work was largely unnoticed by the neural network community. Boyd and Chua, in the mid 1980s [42], enhanced the Volterra series framework with the constraint of fading memory in the operator and showed that it can approximate nonlinear time invariant operators over infinite time intervals. The same idea of a bank of filters followed by a layer of memoryless nonlinearities was proposed. More recently, in the early 1990s, Sandberg [44] showed specifically that a focused TDNN is a universal approximator for an important class of functions (which he called myopic maps), formalizing once and for all the intuitive and experimental arguments outlined above. As an historical note, the constraint of fading memory was mentioned by Volterra [37] and Wiener [39], but it was never fully utilized by them in the approximation machinery. This concept makes a lot of engineering sense, stating that the effect of the output of a system is mostly determined by the short term past of the input.

This chapter now necessarily becomes more formal to show that the focused TDNN (and other structures built from finite memory kernels followed by static nonlinearities) are, in fact, universal approximators in functional spaces for the class of functions with approximately finite memory, which is important in engineering practice. The basis of our presentation is centered on Sandberg's results, but we emphasize the role of shift operators in the approximation. We conclude the chapter with a general class of linear operators that can be used instead of linear FIR filters to implement the approximately finite memory operators.

6.3.1 The Concept of Approximately Finite Memory (Myopic)

Sandberg proved the following very powerful theorem [45]: Any shift-invariant myopic dynamic map can be uniformly approximated by a structure consisting of finite sums of the form

$$\sum_i c_i \sigma \left[\sum_j a_{ij} Q_j(.) + b_i \right] \tag{6.22}$$

where a, b, c are real constants, σ is a sigmoidal nonlinearity, and $Q(.)$ is a linear function. Note that this expression can be implemented by a bank of linear filters nonlinearly combined by a set of static nonlinearity with a linear output, as shown in the one hidden layer focused TDNN of Figure 6.7. It is remarkable that such a large class of functions can be approximated by such a simple topology. The important concept and probably the most interesting to signal processing specialists is the approximation power achieved by shift evaluations of a given operator and the concept of approximately finite memory maps. We elaborate only on these two topics here. For a full proof of Sandberg's results, see Sandberg and Xu [45].

Boyd [43] defined fading memory mathematically as a weighting function in the definition of a continuous operator in the space of continuous functions.

DEFINITION 6.1 $C(\Re)$ denotes the space of all continuous real valued functions : $\Re \rightarrow \Re$ with the norm $\|u\| = \sup_{t \in R} |u(t)|$.

DEFINITION 6.2 (Boyd). An operator T has fading memory on a subset X of $C(\Re)$ if there is a decreasing function $w : \Re_+ \rightarrow (0, 1)$, $\lim_{t \rightarrow \infty} w(t) = 0$ such that for each $u \in X$ and $\varepsilon > 0$, there is a $\delta > 0$ such that for all $v \in X$,

$$\sup_{t \leq 0} \left| u(t) - v(t) \right| w(-t) < \delta \rightarrow |T(u)(0) - T(v)(0)| < \varepsilon \,. \tag{6.23}$$

This definition can also be included in the norm of the topological space in the following way:

DEFINITION 6.3 On $C(\Re)$, define the weighted norm:

$$\|u\|_w = \|u(t)w(-t)\| = \sup_{t \le 0} |u(t)w(-t)| \tag{6.24}$$

then, T has finite memory on X if and only if a functional F is continuous with respect to the norm $\| \|_w$. With this weighted norm on $C(\Re)$, T is compact. It is interesting to note that Figueiredo utilized the same procedure when he defined the weighted Fock space [40]. The impact of the finite memory constraint in the structure of the space is enormous. First, it does not imply that signals in X are time limited. It also means that X is not necessarily a compact subset of $C(\Re)$, but it guarantees that we can obtain approximations valid for all time on noncompact sets [42].

Sandberg's approach to the finite memory definition is slightly different and extends Boyd's definition. We start with the concept of shift invariant operator, which is a simple extension of the definition given in signal processing textbooks. We will discuss only the case of causal systems. Let $S = \{x \in l(Z) | x(t) = 0 \text{ for } t \le 0\}$, where Z is the set of integers. Define the unit step function $u : Z \to \Re$ by

$$u(t) = \begin{cases} 1 & \text{if } t \ge 0 \\ 0 & \text{otherwise.} \end{cases} \tag{6.25}$$

Suppose $x \in S$ and $n \in Z$. The translate function of x by n, $x_n : Z \to \Re$, is defined by

$$x_n(t) = u(t)x(t-n) \tag{6.26}$$

for $t \in Z$. If $n > 0$, x_n is a right shift of x. The shift operator $R_n : S \to S$ is defined by $R_n(x) = x_n$ for $x \in S$. Note that R_n is a linear operator.

DEFINITION 6.4 A transformation $T : S \to S$, not necessarily linear, is right shift invariant provided that for every $n \in Z^+$, $T \bullet R_n = R_n \bullet T$. That is, for every $x \in S$ and $n \in Z^+$, $T(x_n)(t) = T(x)(t-n)$, for all $t \in Z$.

Suppose $a, n \in Z$ with $a > 0$. The window operator of length a located at n, $w_{n,a}$ is defined by

$$w_{n,a}(x)(t) = \begin{cases} x(t) & n \le t \le n+a \\ 0 & \text{otherwise} \end{cases} \tag{6.27}$$

for $x \in S$. A transformation $T : S \to S$ is causal provided that, for every $x \in S$ and $t \in Z$, $T(x)(t) = T(w_{0,t}(x))(t)$.

DEFINITION 6.5 T is said to be approximated by shift evaluations provided that, for every $\varepsilon > 0$, there exists n such that $|T(x)(t) - T(x_{n-t})(n)| < \varepsilon$ for all $x \in S$ and $t \in Z$.

DEFINITION 6.6 (Sandberg). A transformation $T : S \to S$ has approximately finite memory provided that, for every $\varepsilon > 0$, there exists $n \in Z^+$ such that

$$\left| T(x)(t) - T\left(w_{t-n,n}(x)\right)(t) \right| < \varepsilon \tag{6.28}$$

for all $x \in S$ and $t \in Z$. An example of such a transformation is implemented by shift invariant causal linear systems provided the system is bounded input, bounded output stable. An important relation between approximately finite memory operators and the quality of the approximation achieved by shift operators is detailed next.

PROPOSITION 6.1 Suppose $T : S \to S$ is right shift invariant. Then T is causal and approximated by shift evaluations if and only if T has approximately finite memory.

LEMMA 6.1 If $n, a \in Z$ and $a > 0$, then $R_n \bullet w_{0,a} = w_{n,a} \bullet R_n$.

PROOF 6.1 Proof of Lemma: Suppose $x \in S$ and $t \in Z$. Then,

$$\begin{aligned}\left(R_n \bullet w_{0,a}(x)\right)(t) &= \left(w_{0,a}(x)\right)_n(t) = u(t)\left(w_{0,a}(x)\right)(t-n)\\ &= \begin{cases} u(t)x(t-n) & \text{if } 0 \le t-n \le a \\ 0 & \text{otherwise.}\end{cases}\end{aligned} \tag{6.29}$$

Likewise,

$$\left(w_{0,a} \bullet R_n(x)\right)(t) = w_{n,a}\left(x_n\right)(t) = \begin{cases} x_n(t) = u(t)x(t-n) & \text{if } n \le t \le n+a \\ 0 & \text{otherwise.}\end{cases} \tag{6.30}$$

Since $n \le t \le n+a$ if and only if $0 \le t-n \le a$, this proves the lemma.

PROOF 6.2 Proof of Proposition: First note that, if $k \in Z^+$, then $(x_k)_{-k} = x$ for all $x \in S$. We see this as follows:

$$\left(x_k\right)_{-k}(t) = u(t)x_k(t+k) = u(t)u(t+k)x(t+k-k)\ . \tag{6.31}$$

Since $k \ge 0, t+k < 0$ implies $t < 0$. Thus, $u(t+k)u(t) = u(t)$, and the right-hand side above reduces to $x(t)$. Suppose that T is right shift invariant causal approximated by shift evaluation on S. Suppose $\varepsilon > 0$. Then there is an $n \in Z^+$ such that Equation (6.28) holds true for all $x \in S$ and $t \in Z$:

$$\begin{aligned}T\left(w_{t-n,n}(x)\right)(t) &= T\left(w_{t-n,n}\left(\left(x_{n-t}\right)\right)_{t-n}\right)(t)\\ &= T\left(w_{0,n}\left(\left(x_{n-t}\right)\right)_{t-n}\right)(t)\\ &= T\left(w_{0,n}\left(\left(x_{n-t}\right)\right)\right)(t-(t-n))\\ &= T\left(w_{0,n}\left(x_{n-t}\right)\right)(n) = T\left(x_{n-t}\right)(n)\ .\end{aligned} \tag{6.32}$$

The last equality follows from T being causal. Thus,

$$\left|T(x)(t) - T\left(w_{t-n,n}(x)\right)(t)\right| = \left|T(x)(t) - T\left(x_{n-t}\right)(n)\right| < \varepsilon \tag{6.33}$$

for all $x \in S$ and $t \in Z$. This result is one of the key components in proving the universal approximation properties of the TDNN and tells about the importance of shift invariance operators for the representation of time information. The terminology myopic map is preferred to approximately finite memory because these results can be extended to noncausal systems, where memory loses meaning [45].

6.3.2 Topological Approximation Using the Stone–Weierstrass Theorem

This section outlines a proof of the universal approximation of TDNNs for the class of myopic maps, using causal shift-invariance processes within the framework of the Stone–Weierstrass theorem.

THEOREM 6.1 *If X is a topological space, we denote the set of all continuous real valued functions on X by $C(X, \Re)$. If X is a compact Hausdorff space, we may define a metric on $C(X, \Re)$ by*

$$d(f(x), g(x)) = \sup_{x \in X} |f(x) - g(x)| \tag{6.34}$$

which denotes the uniform norm of uniform metric. The lattice operations V and Λ are defined on $C(X, \Re)$ by

$$\begin{aligned}(f \vee g)(x) &= \max\ d(f(x), g(x)) \\ (f \wedge g)(x) &= \min\ d(f(x), g(x))\end{aligned} \tag{6.35}$$

for $f, g \in C(X, \Re)$ and all $x \in X$. We note that both of these operations are commutative and that $C(X, \Re)$ is a lattice, in the sense that it is closed under both V and Λ. A subset $L \subseteq C(X, \Re)$ is a sublattice of $C(X, \Re)$, provided that L is closed under both V and Λ. One formulation of the Stone-Weierstrass theorem is the following [46]:

THEOREM 6.2 *Suppose X is a nondegenerate compact Hausdorff space and L is a sublattice of $C(X, \Re)$ such that, for all $x, y \in X$ with $x \neq y$ and all $a, b \in \Re$, there exists $f \in L$ with $f(x) = a$ and $f(y) = b$. Then, the uniform closure of L is $\bar{L} = C(X, \Re)$.*

Throughout the remainder of this section, we assume that X is a nondegenerate compact Hausdorff space. If $A \subseteq C(X, \Re)$, the lattice generated by A, $L(A)$, is the smallest sublattice of $C(X, \Re)$ which contains A. The collection $L(A)$ consists of all functions (necessarily in $C(X, \Re)$) which can be constructed from functions in A by finitely many lattice operations. Let us formalize what we mean by this construction. We do so recursively, with the recursive construction for a particular lattice map corresponding to the parenthetization of the lattice expression.

For $n \in Z^+$, a mapping $L : \Re^n \to \Re$ is a lattice map provided that (1) $L =$ identity if $n = 1$, and (2) either $L = f \vee g$ or $L = f \wedge g$ for $f : \Re^i \to \Re$, $g : \Re^j \to \Re$ lattice maps with $i + j = n$ for $n > 1$.

Denote the collection of lattice maps from $\Re^n \to \Re$ by Λ_n. Note that $\Lambda_n \subseteq C(\Re^n, \Re)$ for all $n \in Z^+$. If $A \subseteq C(X, \Re)$, the statement previously made concerning $L(A)$ can now be rephrased formally as

$$\begin{aligned}L(A) = \big\{ l : X \to \Re | \exists n \in Z^+, L \in \Lambda_n, \text{ and } \alpha_1, \alpha_2, \ldots \alpha_n \in A \text{ such that} \\ l(x) = L(\alpha_1(x), \alpha_2(x), \ldots \alpha_n(x)) \text{ for all } x \in X \big\} .\end{aligned} \tag{6.36}$$

A subset $B \subseteq C(X, \Re)$ is said to separate points of X provided that, for all $x, y \in X$ with $x \neq y$, there is a function $f \in B$ such that $f(x) \neq f(y)$. We can now state the specialization of the Stone–Weierstrass theorem that we will use here.

THEOREM 6.3 *(Stone–Weierstrass). Suppose that $B \subseteq C(X, \Re)$ separates points of X. Let*

$$A = \{\alpha \in C(X, \Re) | \exists \beta \in B,\ w, c \in \Re \text{ such that } \alpha(x) = w\beta(x) + c, \text{ for } x \in X\} . \tag{6.37}$$

That is, A is the collection of all compositions of maps from B and simple affine transforms from $\Re \to \Re$. Then, $L(A)$ is dense in $C(X, \Re)$.

PROOF 6.3 Suppose $x, y \in X$ with $x \neq y$, and $a, b \in \Re$. Since B separates points of X, there is a function $\beta \in B$ such that $\beta(x) \neq \beta(y)$ (and therefore, $\beta(x) - \beta(y) \neq 0$). Let

$$w = \frac{a - b}{\beta(x) - \beta(y)}, \quad c = b - \beta(y)\frac{a - b}{\beta(x) - \beta(y)} \tag{6.38}$$

and let $\alpha \in A$ be defined as $\alpha(x) = w\beta(x) + c$. Then,

$$\alpha(x) = \frac{a-b}{\beta(x)-\beta(y)}\beta(x) + b - \beta(y)\frac{a-b}{\beta(x)-\beta(y)} = a \tag{6.39}$$
$$\alpha(y) = \frac{a-b}{\beta(x)-\beta(y)}\beta(y) + b - \beta(y)\frac{a-b}{\beta(x)-\beta(y)} = b\,.$$

Therefore, by Theorem 6.2, $\overline{L(A)} = C(X, \Re)$.

We now use a theorem enunciated by Hornik, Stinchcombe, and White (HSW) [12] to reformulate our previous results. Let $\sigma : \Re \to [0, 1]$ be an increasing (non-decreasing) continuous function such that $\lim_{x\to\infty} \sigma(x) = 1$ and $\lim_{x\to-\infty} \sigma(x) = 0$. The idea of applying their theorem to our formulation is straightforward, as shown in the diagram below:

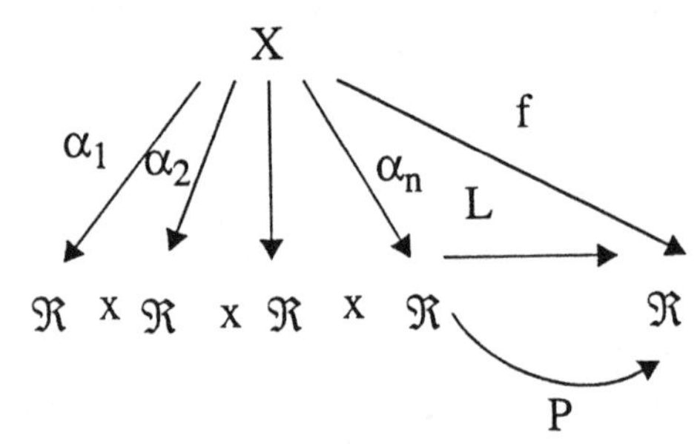

The theorem from HSW shows that mappings $f : \Re^n \to \Re$ of the form

$$f(y_1, y_2, \ldots, y_n) = \sum_{i=1}^{m} c_i \sigma \left(\sum_{j=1}^{n} a_{ij} y_j + b_j \right) \tag{6.40}$$

are uniformly dense on compact subsets of $\Re^n$ in $C(X, \Re)$. The existence of the mappings $\alpha_1, \alpha_2, \ldots, \alpha_n \in \Re$ and $L \in L(A)$ comes from our previous theorem, and the map $P \in P(\Re)$ is from the HWS theorem.

THEOREM 6.4 *Suppose $B \in C(X, \Re)$ is a separating collection and that A, the set of affine maps produced from B, is defined as in the previous theorem. Then $P(\Re)$ is uniformly dense in $C(X, \Re)$.*

PROOF 6.4 Suppose $f \in C(X, \Re)$ and $\varepsilon > 0$. Then, by the Stone–Weierstrass theorem, $\exists n \in Z^+, \alpha_1, \alpha_2, \ldots, \alpha_n \in \Re$, and $L : \Re^n \to \Re$ with L representing a lattice function such that, for every $x \in X$,

$$|f(x) - L(\alpha_1(x), \alpha_2(x), \ldots, \alpha_n(x))| < \frac{\varepsilon}{2}\,. \tag{6.41}$$

Since $L : \Re^n \to \Re$ is continuous, $L(X)$ is compact. Thus, by the HWS theorem, there exists $m \in Z^+, c_i, b_i \in \Re$ for $i = 1, \ldots, m$, $a \in \Re$, $i = 1, \ldots, m$, $j = 1, \ldots, n$ such that

$$\left| L(y_1, y_2, \ldots, y_n) - \sum_{i=1}^{m} c_i \sigma \left(\sum_{j=1}^{n} a_{ij} y_i + b_i \right) \right| < \frac{\varepsilon}{2} \tag{6.42}$$

for all $(y_1, y_2, \ldots, y_n) \in L(x)$. Therefore,

$$\left| f(x) - \sum_{i=1}^{m} c_i \sigma \left(\sum_{j=1}^{n} a_{ij} y_i + b_i \right) \right| < \frac{\varepsilon}{2} \tag{6.43}$$

for all $x \in X$. Since the mapping $g : X \to \Re$, defined by

$$g(x) = \sum_{i=1}^{m} c_i \sigma \left(\sum_{j=1}^{n} a_{ij} y_i + b_i \right) \tag{6.44}$$

is in $P(A)$, we have that $P(A)$ is dense in $C(X, \Re)$. This completes our alternate proof.

One of the aspects that is not apparent from this (nor Sandberg) derivation is how to construct the myopic maps. They can be implemented by linear shift-invariant stable filters (finite memory), but neither their order nor their shape is constrained in the proofs.

6.4 Construction of Linear Approximately Finite Memory Operators

The previous sections studied the power of the combination of a bank of linear filters followed by a static nonlinearity for universal approximation of nonlinear systems. However, many problems still need to be faced to design practical systems. Some of the more serious are how to decide the size of the topologies and how to adapt their coefficients. Here we address only the size of the topologies by designing appropriate delay operators. We saw how important the concept of finite memory operators is for universal approximations of nonlinear systems. But we remark that this definition never implied finite extent operators such as we normally implement with the FIR filter.

Unfortunately, in signal processing, we still almost exclusively use the delay operator, z^{-1}, which is not a suitable operator for short term sampling intervals because it has too short a memory (just one sample) [49]. By using delay operators with longer regions of support (eventually infinite), the number of stages in the cascade can be reduced for a given approximation error. This will make our dynamic neural networks much more parsimonious and will improve generalization. This fact has been remarked by several researchers [47, 48]. We will start by providing an intuitive view of alternate delay operators and then present the class of Kautz functions, which is a set of orthogonal rational transfer functions that implements arbitrary linear delay operators [50].

6.4.1 Delay Operators in Optimal Filtering

Consider the problem of approximating an unknown linear system with a rational transfer function $H(z)$ by a causal finite impulse response filter (FIR). This can be accomplished by expanding the transfer function in a Laurent series around the point $z = 0$ (also called a power series) [51]:

$$H(z) = \sum_{k=0}^{\infty} w_k \cdot z^{-k} . \tag{6.45}$$

Of course, for any practical implementation, we must truncate the infinite series to a finite length

$$\tilde{H}(z) \approx \sum_{k=0}^{K} w_k \cdot z^{-k} \tag{6.46}$$

which we immediately recognize as being a Kth order FIR filter, which can be implemented with a tapped-delay line and a series of feed-forward weights w_k. For example, consider the following low pass IIR linear system:

$$H(z) = \frac{1 + 0.25z^{-2}}{1 - z^{-1} + 0.5z^{-2}} \tag{6.47}$$

which has two zeros at $\pm 0.5j$, two poles at $0.5 \pm 0.5j$, and a region of convergence (ROC) for $z > 0.707$. The pole-zero locations and frequency and impulse responses are shown in Figure 6.8.

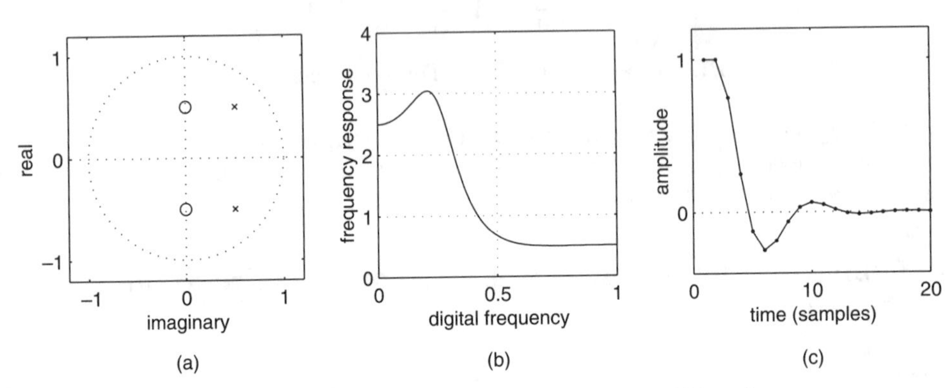

6.8 Example filter properties: (a) pole-zero locations; (b) frequency response; (c) impulse response.

If we expand this in a Laurent series up to fourth order,

$$\tilde{H}(z) \approx 1 + z^{-1} + 0.75z^{-2} + 0.25z^{-3} - 0.125z^{-4} + O\left(z^{-5}\right) \tag{6.48}$$

there results the FIR filter shown in Figure 6.9.

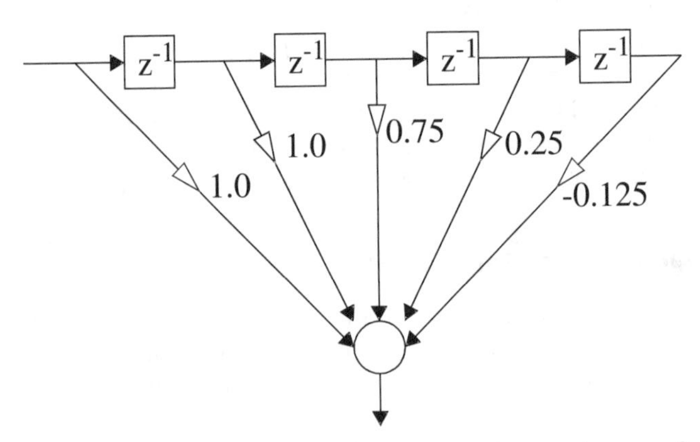

6.9 Approximation of IIR system: truncated Laurent series expansion about a pole at $z = 0$.

6.4.2 The Gamma Delay Operator

Note that the power series is effectively an expansion about a pole at the origin. In fact, we have the freedom to perform the expansion about any point in the z-plane that belongs to the region of convergence of $H(z)$, and the results should be identical according to the theory of complex functions [51]. Therefore, let us consider expanding about the real pole at $z = a$:

$$H(z) = \sum_{k=0}^{\infty} w_k \cdot (z - a)^{-k} \tag{6.49}$$

where $|a| \leq 1$ to ensure stability. Once again, in any practical implementation, we must truncate the series to a finite number of terms:

$$\tilde{H}(z) = \sum_{k=0}^{K} w_n \cdot (z-a)^{-k} . \tag{6.50}$$

This is no longer an FIR filter. In fact, it is a weighted sum of a cascade of identical first order IIR filters which we have called the gamma filter [57]. To see this, let us define the gamma kernel function

$$G(z) = \frac{1}{(z-a)} \tag{6.51}$$

and then rewrite Equation (6.49) as

$$\tilde{H}(z) = \sum_{k=0}^{K} w_k \cdot G^k(z) . \tag{6.52}$$

Through recursion of powers of the kernel function, we can represent the transfer function at each stage in terms of the previous stage:

$$G^k(z) = G^{k-1}(z) \cdot G(z) . \tag{6.53}$$

Equation (6.53) represents a cascade of identical IIR sections. Note that this includes the pure tapped-delay line as a special case when $a = 0$. Returning to our example, expanding $H(z)$ up to fourth order about $z = a$ results in

$$\begin{aligned}\tilde{H}(z) \approx\; & 1 + (z-a)^{-1} + (0.75 - a)(z-a)^{-2} + \left(0.25 - 1.5a + a^2\right)(z-a)^{-3} \\ & + \left(-0.25 - 0.75a + 2.25a^2 - a^3\right)(z-a)^{-4} + O\left((z-a)^{-5}\right)\end{aligned} \tag{6.54}$$

which is shown in Figure 6.10.

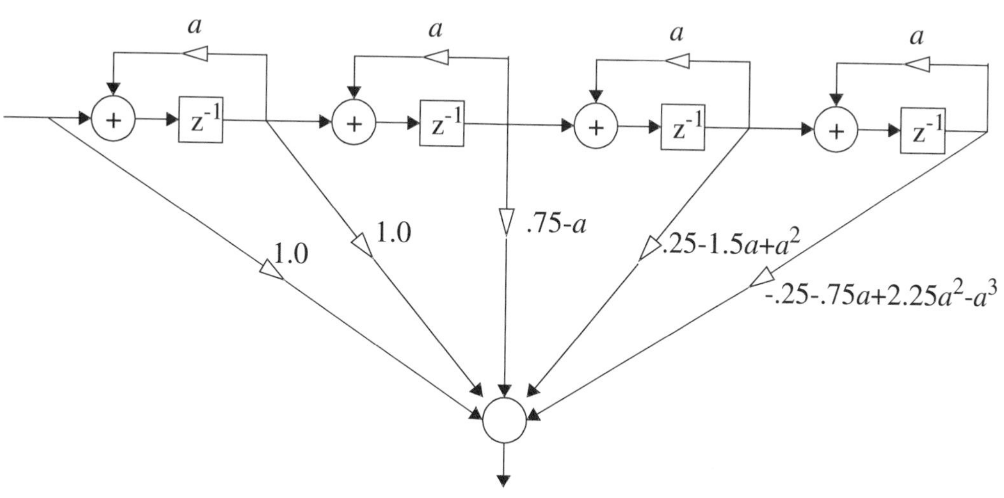

6.10 Approximation of IIR system: truncated Laurent expansion about a pole at $z = a$.

Unlike the FIR case, the feed-forward weights now depend on the feedback parameter a. Have we gained anything by this added complexity? The answer is yes if we can show that the expansion about the pole at $z = a$ is a better approximation than the FIR expansion, given the same number of expansion terms. First, we need a suitable metric to compare the original transfer function with the approximations. We can use the Itakuro–Saito distance between two power spectra [52]

$$D_{ij} = \frac{1}{2\pi} \int_{-\pi}^{\pi} \left[\frac{S_i(f) - S_j(f)}{S_j(f)} \right] df \, . \tag{6.55}$$

This has the nice interpretation of being the normalized difference between the power spectra of the two filters. Note that this distance measure does not take phase into account.

We took the expansion about the pole at $z = a$ for orders of 1, 2, 3, and 4, and then compared the power spectra of the expansion with that of the original transfer function for all stable values of the feedback parameter. The results are shown in Figure 6.11.

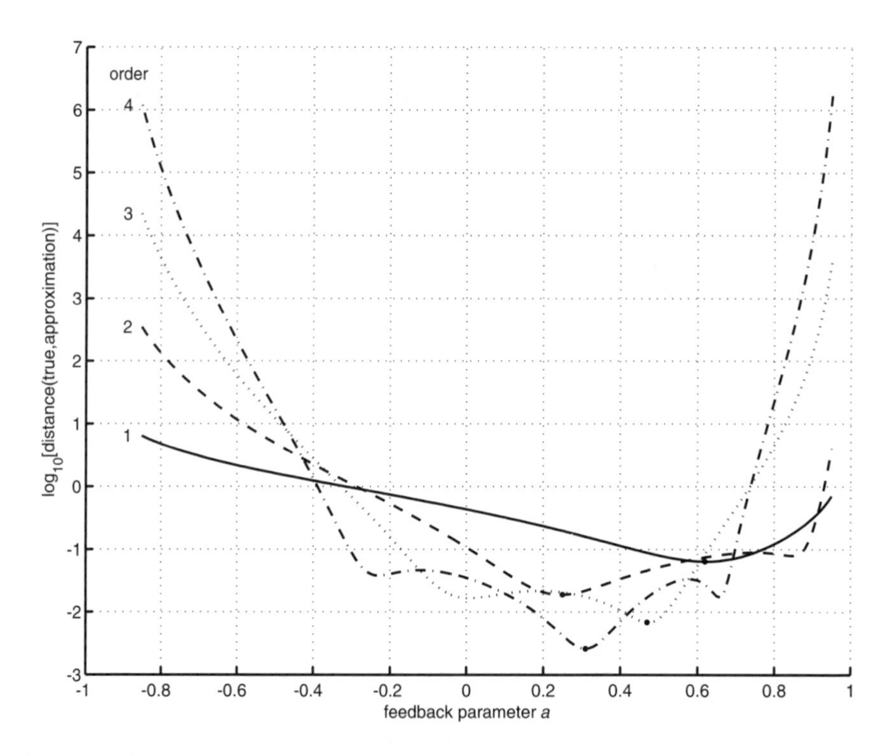

6.11 Itakuro–Saito distance between true and truncated expansion power spectrums for order 1 (solid), 2 (dash), 3 (dot), and 4 (dash-dot).

Several points must be noted: (1) for this problem, the global minimum never occurs at the FIR equivalent of $a = 0$; (2) the location of the global minimum depends on expansion order; and (3) there are multiple local minima but only one global minimum that improves with the order. For each order expansion, we then took the optimal value of the feedback parameter (shown by the dot in the curves), computed the frequency response, and compared both it and the FIR expansion to the true frequency response. The results are shown in Figure 6.12.

The FIR filter can only do spectral shaping through the placement of zeros, while the expansion about the pole at $z = a$ has the additional freedom of the placement of a single pole (with multiplicity given by the filter order). Continuing the example, the magnitude of the frequency response of the FIR expansion and the expansion about $z = a$ for various orders are shown in Figure 6.12. This

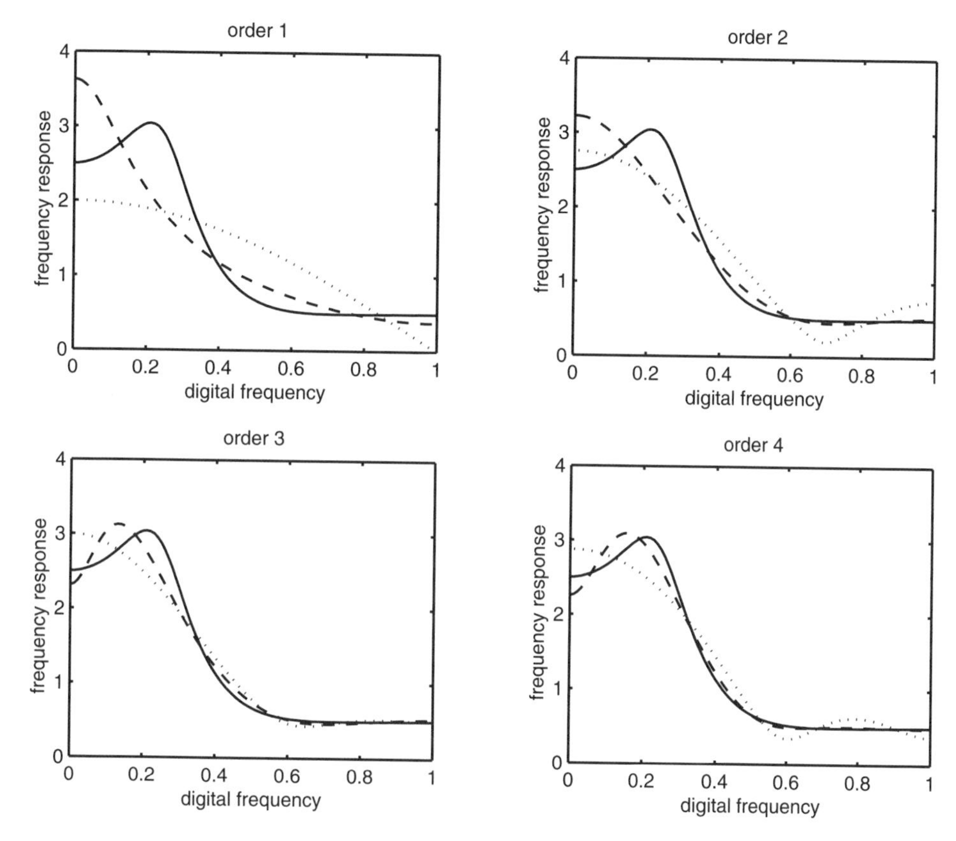

6.12 Frequency response for the true filter (solid), FIR expansion (dotted), and optimal expansion about $z = a$ (dashed) for various expansion orders.

simple example shows that there are practical advantages in using alternative delay operators in our optimal filtering work. Principe et al. [57] showed how to adapt the gamma filter parameters using gradient descent. Note that the adaptation involves the feedback parameter, but it is still easy to guarantee stability.

It is interesting to provide the equivalent time domain view of the delay operators in terms of memory kernels. As we know from adaptive filtering [53] or system identification [54], the selection of the model order is crucial for good results. On one hand, the order of the model should be comparable to the extent of the impulse response of the unknown system to allow for the identification of the time dependencies. On the other hand, if the plant has a long impulse response, this means that many delays are needed, which may produce over-parameterization (too many parameters) with high noise sensitivity and poor generalization. We will now show that the gamma filter, which is a cascade of lowpass filters, has an extra degree of freedom to provide a better compromise between the extent of the impulse response and the number of free parameters. The impulse response for the input to the kth gamma memory kernel is given by [57]:

$$g_k(n) = \binom{n-1}{k-1} (1-a)^k a^{n-k} \tag{6.56}$$

which is depicted in Figure 6.13 for different orders and the same feedback parameter, $a = 0.3$. Notice that, in the figure, the time axis has been scaled uniformly by $(1 - a)$; in other words, for a given filter order, we can still increase or decrease the extent of the impulse response by selecting the feedback parameter.

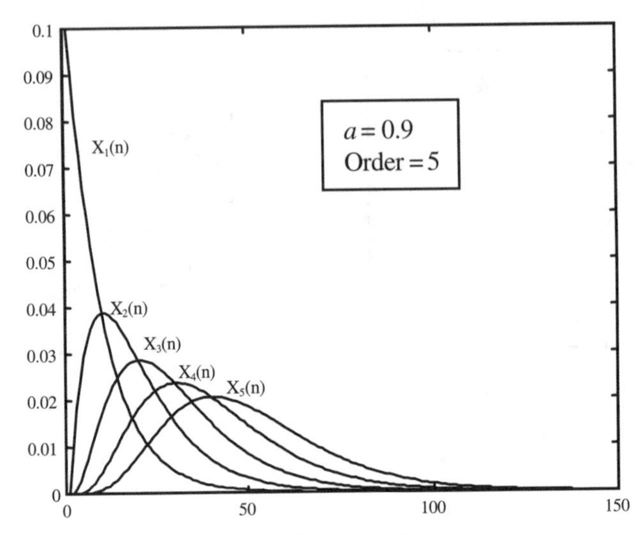

6.13 The impulse response from the input to successive gamma kernel outputs.

Let us define the mean memory depth D of a Kth long gamma memory as

$$D = \sum_{n=0}^{\infty} n g_K(n) = \frac{K}{1-a} \,. \tag{6.57}$$

We see that the memory depth of the gamma memory kernel of length K is scaled by $(1-a)$. Notice that the memory depth of the FIR of order K is K (since $a = 0$). Therefore, a Kth order gamma filter can have essentially any memory depth. De Vries and Principe [47] developed a procedure to find the best memory depth online and applied the procedure in the gamma neural model. We showed excellent results in the modeling of dynamical systems [58], and classification of temporal patterns for word spotting [59]. Sandberg proved that the gamma neural network, i.e., a TDNN where the delay operators are substituted by $G(z)$, is also a universal approximator [55]. Even without a formal proof, we expect that the rate of convergence of the approximation with the gamma neural network will be superior to that of the TDNN for the same number of nonlinear PEs and the same number of delays. The reason for this is the more versatile structure of the memory kernels that are able to capture longer time dependencies with fewer stages.

6.4.3 Kautz Models

Although it is a straightforward extension of the FIR filter, the gamma filter can be improved further. One of the drawbacks of the gamma filter is that the basis functions (the impulse responses shown in Figure 6.13) are not orthogonal, so the adaptation is slow and, practically, only relatively short filters can be implemented (since each stage is a lowpass filter). We now present a general model that extends the gamma filter and the FIR to the general class of orthogonal filter structures linear in the parameters (linear models). The eigenfunctions of linear systems are the complex exponentials [60]. Therefore, we seek orthogonal expansions of complex exponentials. Kautz elegantly solved, in the 1950s, the orthogonalization of the set of continuous time exponential functions, hence the name Kautz models [50]. We present here the results for discrete problems. See Wahlberg [62] or Oliveira e Silva [63] for a complete treatment.

The sequence of functions $\{\Psi_j(z)\}$ defined by

$$\begin{aligned}\Psi_{2k+1}(z) &= C_1^{(k)}\left(1 - a_1^{(k)}z\right)\Gamma^{(k)}(z) \\ \Psi_{2k}(z) &= C_2^{(k)}\left(1 - a_2^{(k)}z\right)\Gamma^{(k)}(z)\end{aligned} \tag{6.58}$$

where

$$\Gamma^{(k)}(z) = \frac{\prod_{j=1}^{k-1}\left(1-\beta_j z\right)\left(1-\beta^*{}_j z\right)}{\prod_{j=1}^{k}\left(z-\beta_j\right)\left(z-\beta^*{}_j\right)} \tag{6.59}$$

and

$$\begin{aligned}C_1^{(k)} &= \left(\frac{\left(1-\beta_k^2\right)\left(1-\beta_k^{*2}\right)\left(1-\beta_k\beta_k^*\right)}{\left(1+a_1^{(k)2}\right)\left(1+\beta_k\beta_k^*\right)-2a_1^{(k)}\left(\beta_k+\beta_k^*\right)}\right)^{\frac{1}{2}} \\ C_2^{(k)} &= \left(\frac{\left(1-\beta^2 k\right)\left(1-\beta_k^{*2}\right)\left(1-\beta_k\beta_k^*\right)}{\left(1+a_2^{(k)2}\right)\left(1+\beta_k\beta_k^*\right)-2a_2^{(k)}\left(\beta_k+\beta_k^*\right)}\right)^{\frac{1}{2}}\end{aligned} \tag{6.60}$$

with

$$\left(1+a_1^{(k)}a_2^{(k)}\right)\left(1+\beta_k\beta_k^*\right)-\left(a_1^{(k)}+a_2^{(k)}\right)\left(\beta_k+\beta_k^*\right)=0 \tag{6.61}$$

forms an orthogonal set. Here $\{\beta_k\}$ are complex numbers in the region $|\beta_k| < 1$ and a_1 and a_2 are real constants. Figure 6.14 shows the block diagram that implements an adaptive filter based on the Kautz functions:

$$H(z) = \sum_{i=0}^{N-1} w_i \Psi_i(z)\,. \tag{6.62}$$

The discrete Kautz functions $\{\Psi_j(z)\}$ implement a cascade of second order pole-zero delay kernels (also called lattice filters) that are orthogonal for delta function inputs. As is well known, if one desires an orthogonal basis for an arbitrary signal, then the lattices have to be adaptive [64]. The Kautz kernels are the closest we can get to an orthogonal basis without adapting the coefficients of the lattice. Due to the special structure of the Kautz kernels, it is still possible to adapt this IIR filter with an easy check for stability. However, the performance surface of Kautz filters is nonconvex [63].

The general case of the Kautz functions places poles anywhere in the z domain. Equations (6.58)-(6.61) were written to provide real quantities inside the filter when the input is real. But even in this case, the designer has the freedom of placing the pairs of complex poles anywhere in the unit circle and in a position that best approximates the power spectrum of the input time series. This is the most general case of practical interest. Many interesting results have been achieved in approximations with Kautz functions [62]. For our work with dynamic neural networks, Kautz functions implement the most general approximately finite memories.

Kautz functions provide, as special cases, well known system identification structures. Let us give a few examples. First, consider that $\beta_k = a$ are all the same and real with $|a| < 1$. Set

$$a_1^{(k)} = a,\, a_2^{(k)} = \frac{1}{a},\, C_1^{(k)} = \sqrt{1-a^2},\, C_2^{(k)} = \sqrt{\left(1-a^2\right)a} \tag{6.63}$$

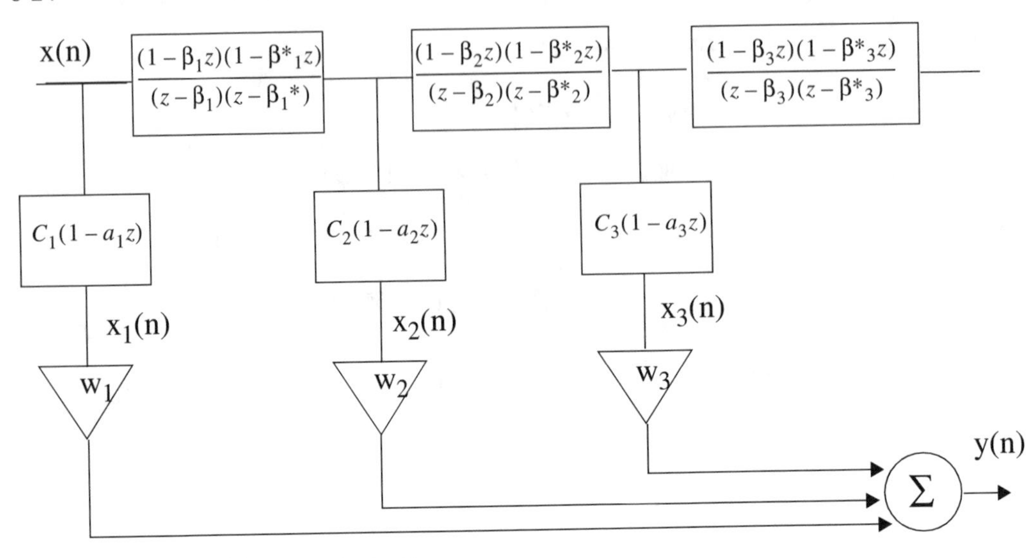

6.14 Block diagram of the Kautz adaptive filter.

and we will obtain the Laguerre functions [61]:

$$L_j(z, a) = \frac{\sqrt{1-a^2}}{z-a}\left(\frac{1-az}{z-a}\right)^{j-1} \tag{6.64}$$

Laguerre functions have been widely used for linear system identification and dynamic neural models (Wiener and Lee [66] proposed their use to implement the optimal filter in continuous time). They are an orthonormal set of bases which is dense in the disc of functions, analytic inside the unit circle, and continuous on the unit circle. If we set $a = 0$, we obtain the conventional FIR filter. The delay operator in the Laguerre filter is an all-pass function with a pole at $z = a$ and a zero at $z = 1/a$. If the zero is moved to the origin, we get the gamma delay operator. In fact Celebi and Principe [67] showed that the Laguerre delay operator is closely related to the gamma delay operator, orthogonalizing the gamma space. Both decompositions have the same real poles.

6.5 Conclusions

This chapter discussed the area of optimal nonlinear signal processing from a different perspective. Instead of starting by extending linear optimum filtering, we presented optimal nonlinear filtering as an approximation problem. As such, we first discussed the approximation with linear operators in vector spaces and then treated the stochastic case by introducing a probabilistic metric in $\Re^n$. We went beyond the linear operator case by presenting the multilayer perceptron (MLP) and the radial basis function (RBF) networks. This chapter also called attention to the primordial role that the basis functions take to obtain uniform approximation.

Through the introduction of the delay operator as a time-to-space mapping, we treated the case of optimum linear and nonlinear filtering for both deterministic and stochastic signals. But the lack of formal proof for an embedding for stochastic signals leads us to present some results of approximation theory in functional spaces, which clearly show that networks created by a bank of linear filters followed by static nonlinearities are capable of uniform approximation in a class of functionals of interest in engineering (the class of finite memory operators). This is, however, an existence proof, so the work left for the practitioner is to find parsimonious topologies to achieve the goal.

With this view, we presented the Kautz filters as the most versatile class of linear operators at our disposal to create practical, approximately finite memory linear maps. We showed that some of the conventional delay kernels such as the tap delay line, the gamma, or the Laguerre kernels are special cases of the Kautz kernel.

This chapter is intended as a integration of concepts normally found in different areas of the information processing literature. Due to length constraints, we did not cover some of the practical aspects of creating optimal filters from data, such as how to set the size of the filter topologies and, more importantly, how to adapt the filter parameters in a robust way. These aspects can be found in other books such as those by Bishop [11] and Haykin [18].

There are still very important issues to be researched in the area of optimal nonlinear signal processing. The first is to pursue asymptotic convergence results, which has not been done in functional spaces. This work should mimic the development of Vapnik in probability spaces for regression and classification. Hopefully, there will be ways to relate the size of the topologies and the convergence rate of the approximation. A close second is how to extend these results to the class of time-varying continuous maps. There are many practical problems in which the input–output map changes over time. The types of time-varying maps of interest in engineering are the ones that are created by feedback; these normally produce dynamic changes on a much longer time scale than the feed-forward dynamics. There is evidence that dynamic neural networks with feedback have remarkable system identification capabilities, as illustrated in control applications [68] and in dynamic modeling of chaotic time series [32]. Presently, we do not have a theory to study the mapping capabilities of such networks.

Lastly, dynamic neural networks must work with real data. Here, adaptation of these topologies surfaces as the most important of the bottlenecks. First-order search methods such as real time recurrent learning or back-propagation through time are not powerful enough to train these dynamic neural networks. There is the problem of long term dependencies [69], which slows down the training; higher order search methods, such as the multiple streaming DEKF; (decoupled Kalman filter) [68] are required, but they still do not seem to solve all the problems. Therefore, we have to be resourceful enough to go beyond the gradient descent learning and incorporate unsupervised and supervised learning. A timid first step is reported by Euliano and Principe [70].

Acknowledgments

The author would like to acknowledge the work of his former students, Bert deVries, Samel Celebi, James Kuo, James Tracey, Douglas Jones, Ludong Wang, Mark Motter, Neil Euliano, Craig Fancourt, and James Davis, who helped develop the gamma model and the insights expressed in this chapter. This work was supported across nine years by three grants from the National Science Foundation (NeuroEngineering program) ECS-9208789, ECS-9510715, and ECS-9900394.

References

[1] Wiener, N., *Extrapolation, Interpolation and Smoothing of Stationary Time Series, with Engineering Applications,* John Wiley & Sons, New York, 1949.
[2] Widrow, B. and Stearns, S.D. *Adaptive Signal Processing,* Prentice-Hall, Englewood Cliffs, NJ, 1985.
[3] Behnke, H., Bachmann, F., Fladt, K., and Suss, W., *Fundamentals of Mathematics,* Vol. III, MIT Press, Cambridge, MA, 1983.
[4] Szego, G., *Orthogonal polynomials,* Vol. XXII, *American Mathematical Society Colloquium,* 1939.
[5] Whaba, G., Splines for observational data, *SIAM,* 1990.
[6] Rao, C., *Linear Statistical Inference and its Applications,* John Wiley & Sons, New York, 1965.

[7] Kolmogorov, A., Sur l'interpolation et extrapolation des suites stationaires, *Compte rendus de l'Acad. Sci.,* Vol. 208, 2043–2045, 1939.
[8] Vapnik, V., *The Nature of Statistical Learning Theory,* Springer-Verlag, New York, 1995.
[9] Glivenko, V., Sulla determinazione empirica di probabilita, *G. Inst. Ital. Attuari,* 4, 1933.
[10] Principe, J., Euliano, N., and Lefebvre, C., *Neural Systems: Fundamentals through Simulations,* CD-ROM textbook, John Wiley & Sons, New York, 2000.
[11] Bishop, C., *Neural Networks for Pattern Recognition,* Oxford Press, Oxford, UK, 1995.
[12] Hornik, K., Stinchcombe, M., and White, H., MLPs are universal approximators, *Neural Networks,* 2, 359–366, 1989.
[13] Park, J. and Sandberg, E., Universal approximation using radial basis function networks, *Neural Computation,* 3, 303–314, 1989.
[14] Barron, A., Universal approximation bounds for superposition of sigmoid functions, *IEEE Transactions on Information Theory,* 39(3), 930–945, 1993.
[15] Poggio, T. and Girosi, F., Networks for approximation and learning, *Proceedings of the IEEE,* 78, 1990.
[16] Moody, J. and Darken, C., Fast learning in networks of locally tuned processing units, *Neural Computation,* 1, 281–294, 1989.
[17] Hertz, J., Krogh, A., and Palmer, R., *Introduction to the Theory of Neural Computation,* Addison-Wesley, Reading, MA, 1991.
[18] Haykin, S., *Neural Networks: A Comprehensive Foundation,* Macmillan College Publishing, New York, 1994.
[19] Box, G.E.P. and Jenkins, G.M., *Time Series Analysis: Forecasting and Control,* Holden-Day, 1976.
[20] Kailath, T., A view of three decades of linear filtering theory, *IEEE Transactions on Information Theory,* IT-20, 146–181, 1974.
[21] Casdagli, M., Nonlinear prediction of chaotic time series, *Physics D 35,* 335, 1989.
[22] Wan, E., Time series prediction by using a connectionist network with internal delay lines, in *Times Series Prediction: Forecasting the Future and Understanding the Past,* (Eds. Weigend and Gerschenfeld), Addison-Wesley, Reading, MA, 1994, 195–217.
[23] Mozer, M., Neural architectures for temporal sequence processing, in *Predicting the Future and Understanding the Past,* (Eds. Weigend and Gerschenfeld), Addison-Wesley, Reading, MA, 1994.
[24] Principe, J.C., Wang, L., and Kuo, J.M., Chaotic time series modeling with neural networks, *Signal Analysis and Prediction,* (Eds. Prochazka et al.), Birkhauser, 1998, 275–289.
[25] Packard, N.H., Crutchfield, J.P., Farmer, J.D., and Shaw, R.S., Geometry from a time series, *Physics Review Letters,* 45, 712, 1980.
[26] Takens, F., Detecting strange attractors in turbulence, in *Dynamical Systems and Turbulence,* (Eds. D.A. Rand and L.S. Yang), Springer-Verlag, Berlin, 1981, 365–381.
[27] Kuo, J.M. and Principe, J., Noise reduction in state space using the focused gamma model, *Proceedings ICASSP94,* 2, 533–536, 1994.
[28] Sauer, T., Yorke, J.A., and Casdagli, M., Embedology, *Journal of Statistical Physics,* 65, (3/4), 579–616, 1991.
[29] Grassberger, P. and Procaccia, I., Measuring the strangeness of strange attractors, *Physica 9D,* 189–208, 1983.
[30] Abarbanel, H.D.I., Brown, R., Sidorowich, J.J., and Tsimring, L.S., The analysis of observed chaotic data in physical systems, *Review of Modern Physics,* 65(4), 1331, 1993.
[31] Principe, J., Wang, L., and Motter, M., Local dynamic modeling with self-organizing feature maps and applications to nonlinear system identification and control, Special Issue on Intelligent Signal Processing, *IEEE Proceedings,* 86(11), 2240–2258, 1998.
[32] Haykin, S. and Principe, J., Dynamic modeling of chaotic time series with neural networks, *IEEE DSP Magazine,* May, 1998.
[33] Waibel, A., Hanazawa, T., Hinton, G., Shikano, K., and Lang, K., Phoneme recognition using time-delay neural networks, *IEEE Transactions of the ACSSP,* 37(3), 328–339, 1989.
[34] Narendra, K.S. and Mukhopadhyay, S., Adaptive control using neural networks and approximate models, in *IEEE Transactions on Neural Networks,* 8(3), 475–485, 1997.

[35] Lapedes, A. and Farber, R., Nonlinear signal processing using neural networks: prediction and system modeling, Tech. Rep. LA-UR-87-2662, Los Alamos Natl. Lab., Los Alamos, NM, 1987.

[36] Singer, A.C., Wornell, G., and Oppenheim, A., Codebook prediction: a nonlinear signal modeling paradigm, *IEEE ICASSP*, 5, 325, 1992.

[37] Volterra, V., *Theory of Functionals and of Integral and Integro-Differential Equations*, Dover, New York, 1959.

[38] Rugh, W., *Nonlinear System Theory: The Volterra/Wiener Approach*, John Hopkins University Press, Baltimore, MD, 1981.

[39] Wiener, N., Nonlinear problems in random theory, MIT RLE Tech Report #355, 1959.

[40] Figueiredo, R. and Dwyer, T., A best approximation framework and implementation for simulation of large scale nonlinear systems, *IEEE Transactions on Circuits and Systems*, CAS-27:11, 1005–1014, 1980.

[41] Mhaskar, N., Approximation properties for a multilayer feedforward artificial neural network, *Ad. Comp. Math.*, 1, 61–80, 1993.

[42] Boyd, S. and Chua, L, Fading memory and the problem of approximating nonlinear operators with Volterra series, *IEEE Transactions on Circuits and Systems*, CAS:11, 1150–1161, 1985.

[43] Boyd, S., Volterra Series: Engineering Fundamentals, Ph.D. dissertation, University of California, Berkeley, 1985.

[44] Sandberg, I., Structure theorems for nonlinear systems, *Multidimensional Systems and Signal Processing*, 2, 267–286, 1991.

[45] Sandberg, I. and Xu, L., Uniform approximation of multidimensional myopic maps, *IEEE Transactions on Circuits and Systems*, 44, 477–485, 1997a.

[46] Stone, M., A generalized weierstrass approximation theorem, in *Studies of Modern Analysis*, Vol. 1, Prentice-Hall, Englewood Cliffs, NJ, 1962.

[47] De Vries, B. and Principe, J.C., The gamma model — a new neural model for temporal processing, *Neural Networks*, 5(4), 565–576, 1992.

[48] Tsoi, A. and Back, A., Locally recurrent globally feedforward networks: a critical review of architectures, *IEEE Transactions on Neural Networks*, 5(2), 229–239, 1994.

[49] Middleton, R. and Goodwin, G., *Digital Estimation an Control: A Unified Approach*, Prentice-Hall, Englewood Cliffs, NJ, 1990.

[50] Kautz, W., Transient synthesis in the time domain, *IRE Transactions on Circuit Theory*, 1, 29–39, 1954.

[51] Churchill, R., *Introduction to Complex Variables and Applications*, McGraw-Hill, New York, 1948.

[52] Itakura, F. and Saito, S., Digital filtering techniques for speech analysis and synthesis, *Proceedings of the 7th International Congress on Acoustics*, Budapest, 1971.

[53] Haykin, S., *Adaptive Filter Theory*, Prentice-Hall, Englewood Cliffs, NJ, 1991.

[54] Goodwin, G.C. and Sin, K.S., *Adaptive Filtering, Prediction and Control*, Prentice-Hall, Englewood Cliffs, NJ,1984.

[55] Sandberg, I., and Xu, L., Uniform approximation and gamma neural networks, *Neural Networks*, 10, 781–784, 1997b.

[56] Principe, J.C. and Kuo, J.M., Dynamic modeling of chaotic time series with neural networks, *Proceedings of Neural Information Processing Systems*, 7, 311–318, 1995.

[57] Principe, J., deVries, B., and Guedes de Oliveira, P., The gamma filters: a new class of adaptive IIR filters with restricted feedback, *IEEE Transactions on Signal Processing*, 41(2), 649–656, 1993.

[58] Principe, J., Kuo, J.M., and Celebi, S., An analysis of short term memory structures in dynamic neural networks, in *IEEE Transactions on Neural Networks*, special issue on dynamic nets, 5(2), 331–337, 1995.

[59] Principe, J. and Tracey, J., Isolated word speech recognition using the gamma model, *Journal of Artificial Neural Networks*, 1(14), 481–489, 1994.

[60] Papoulis, A., *Probability, Random Variables, and Stochastic Processes*, McGraw-Hill, New York, 1984.

[61] Oliveira e Silva, T., On the determination of the optimal pole position of Laguerre filters, *IEEE Transactions on Signal Processing*, 43(9), 2079–2087, 1995.

[62] Wahlberg, B., System identification using Laguerre models, *IEEE Transactions on Automatic Control*, 36(5), 551–562, 1991.

[63] Oliveira e Silva, T., Optimality conditions for truncated Kautz networks with two periodically repeating complex conjugate poles, *IEEE Transactions on Automatic Control,* 40(2), 342–346, 1995.

[64] Makhoul, J., Stable and efficient lattice methods for linear prediction, *IEEE Transactions on Acoustics, Speech and Signal Processing,* ASSP-25, 423–428, 1977.

[65] Principe, J., Celebi, S., deVries, B., and Harris, J., Locally recurrent networks: the gamma operator, properties and extensions, in *Neural Networks and Pattern Recognition,* (Eds. Omidvar and Dayhoff), Academic Press, New York, 1996, 311–344.

[66] Lee, Y., *Statistical Theory of Communication,* John Wiley & Sons, New York, 1960.

[67] Celebi, S. and Principe, J., Parametric least squares approximation using gamma bases, *IEEE Transactions on Signal Processing,* 43(3), 781–784, 1995.

[68] Feldkamp, L. and Puskorius, G., A signal processing framework based on dynamic neural networks with applications to the problems in adaptation, filtering, and classification, *Proceedings of the IEEE,* 86, 2259–2277, 1998.

[69] Bengio, Y., Simard, P., and Fransconi, P., Learning long term dependencies with gradient descent is difficult, *IEEE Transactions on Neural Networks,* 5, 157–166, 1994.

[70] Euliano, N. and Principe, J., Dynamic subgrouping in RTRL provides a faster $O(N^2)$ algorithm, *Proceedings of ICASSP,* 2000.

7

Blind Signal Separation and Blind Deconvolution

Scott C. Douglas
Southern Methodist University

7.1 Introduction

7.1.1 What is Blind Signal Separation?

In signal separation, multiple streams of information are extracted from linear mixtures of these signal streams. This process is blind if examples of the source signals, along with their corresponding mixtures, are unavailable for training. Blind signal separation (BSS) is sometimes used interchangeably with independent component analysis (ICA), although, technically, BSS and ICA are different tasks. BSS is most appropriate in situations where a linear mixture model is plausible.

Interest in blind signal separation has recently developed for three reasons: (1) the development of statistical frameworks for understanding the BSS task, (2) a corresponding development of several useful BSS methods, and (3) the identification of many potential applications of BSS. We provide brief descriptions of three such applications below.

Array processing in wireless communications — In modern-day wireless communications networks, several wireless devices attempt to communicate with a base station. The base station employs multiple antennas to better receive and isolate the various users' signals within the spectral bandwidth of the communications channel. When the devices' transmitted signals overlap in time and

0-8493-2359-2/01/$0.00+$1.50

frequency, BSS can be applied to the antenna measurements to separate and enhance the various transmitted signals without knowing the devices' positions relative to the base station and without knowing the exact forms of the transmitted signals [1].

Signal enhancement in medicine — Many noninvasive medical sensing technologies (e.g., EEG and MRI) characterize bodily processes through multichannel recordings. Due to the complicated propagation properties of human body tissue, these multichannel recordings can be difficult to decipher. BSS offers the potential of extracting coherent and identifiable signal features that can be more easily tied to specific bodily functions or ailments [2].

Speech separation in acoustics — Speech signals that are collected by distant microphones in room environments can be hard to understand, particularly if multiple conversations are ongoing. BSS can be used to separate individual speech signals from the microphones' signals, thereby making them more intelligible and listenable [3].

The above three BSS applications differ in the type of mixing generated by the measurement process. Generally, two types of mixing conditions are possible: (1) instantaneous or spatial mixing, in which the mixtures are weighted sums of the individual source signals without dispersion or time delay, and (2) convolutive or spatio-temporal mixing, in which the mixtures contain filtered, delayed, and reverberated versions of the individual signals due to multipath effects. In the examples described above, narrowband array processing in wireless communications involves spatial mixing conditions, whereas multi-microphone speech separation involves spatio-temporal mixing conditions. Generally, BSS algorithms for convolutive mixtures are much more difficult to develop and implement than BSS algorithms for instantaneous mixtures. Even if one's interest is in the convolutive mixing case, however, it is quite useful to study the instantaneous BSS task to grasp the fundamental issues and limitations surrounding various classes of BSS methods.

7.1.2 What is Blind Deconvolution?

Deconvolution describes a discrete-time filtering process that attempts to transform a sampled signal into one whose samples are statistically independent. Such a process assumes that the signal being deconvolved is a filtered version of a statistically independent sequence of symbols. This process is blind if one or more training signal pairs containing the independent symbol sequence and the filtered version of this sequence are unavailable. Blind deconvolution is sometimes used interchangeably with blind equalization, although blind equalization usually applies to situations in which the symbol sequence is discrete-valued.

Blind deconvolution has a number of potential applications in various fields, a few of which are described below.

Channel equalization in digital communications — When a communications device transmits bit or symbol information through a physical medium, dispersive effects of the medium can "smear" the transmitted information, creating inter-symbol interference (ISI) in the received signal waveform. In situations where the physical nature of the channel remains fixed for long periods, blind deconvolution can be used to remove ISI in the received waveform, thus simplifying the detection of the transmitted symbols [4].

Seismic data analysis in geophysical exploration — Geophysicists in search of oil and gas within the earth use manmade acoustic signals to probe and determine the earth's local geological structure. Blind deconvolution procedures can be applied to the received acoustic signals to locate the fuel deposits more accurately. If a layered-earth acoustic channel model can be assumed, simple linear predictive procedures are more appropriate [5].

Image enhancement in astrophysical exploration — When collecting optical images of stellar objects from a terrestrial telescope, the resolution limits of the imaging system and the effects of the earth's atmosphere can degrade image quality. Two-dimensional blind deconvolution procedures can be used to enhance the collected images and resolve new features of the object under study [6].

Blind deconvolution and blind signal separation are clearly related tasks. Blind signal separation attempts to enforce spatial independence of two or more signal streams, and blind deconvolution attempts to enforce temporal independence of a single signal stream. The combination of these two goals yields the problem of multichannel blind deconvolution. In this task, multiple signal streams are processed by a multiple-input–multiple-output filtering system to obtain parallel output signal streams that are approximately independent from sample to sample and from output to output. Multichannel blind deconvolution is similar to spatio-temporal blind signal separation in that multichannel temporal filtering is required; however, the goals of the two problems are different. The multichannel blind deconvolution problem figures prominently in wideband antenna arrays for wireless communications, in which both spatial separation and temporal equalization of the received symbol streams from multiple users are desired.

7.1.3 Purpose of Chapter

The goal of this chapter is threefold:

1. to introduce basic concepts, criteria, and algorithms for BSS and blind deconvolution
2. to draw relationships between the BSS and blind deconvolution tasks
3. to consider open issues and challenges within these related fields

As for mathematical notation, all quantities are assumed to be real-valued, although complex-valued extensions of results are indicated where appropriate. Scalar, vector, and matrix quantities are indicated by lowercase italic, lowercase bold, and uppercase bold letters, respectively. All signals are assumed to be sampled discrete-time random processes with time index k.

7.2 Blind Signal Separation of Instantaneous Mixtures

To simplify the overall presentation of concepts and methods, we first consider the problem of BSS for instantaneously mixed sources, in which no dispersive or convolutive effects are present. The problem of BSS for convolutive mixing conditions is considered in Section 7.4.

7.2.1 Problem Formulation

Figure 7.1 shows the structure of BSS for instantaneously mixed sources. At the left is the unknown source signal vector at time k, given by

$$\mathbf{s}(k) = [s_1(k)\ s_2(k) \ldots s_m(k)]^T \tag{7.1}$$

where $s_i(k)$ is the ith source signal. These m source signals are linearly mixed by the $(n \times m)$ unknown mixing matrix $\mathbf{A}$ with entries a_{ij}, yielding the n-dimensional measured or observed signal vector $\mathbf{x}(k)$ as

$$\mathbf{x}(k) = \mathbf{A}\mathbf{s}(k) + \boldsymbol{\nu}(k) \tag{7.2}$$

where $\boldsymbol{\nu}(k)$ is an n-dimensional noise vector sequence that is unrelated to the source signal sequence $\mathbf{s}(k)$. In typical BSS applications, the source signals contain useful but unknown information, and

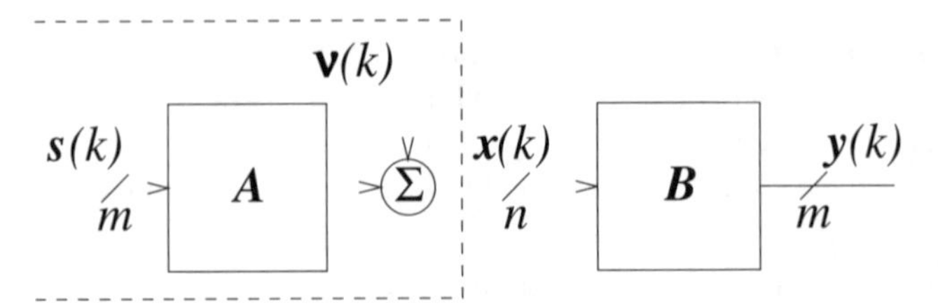

7.1 Block diagram of the blind signal separation (BSS) task.

the mixing model describes the undesirable smoothing and propagation effects inherent in some physical measurement process. The inclusion of noise within the model accounts for any sensor noise at the measuring devices. For our discussion, we assume that $\boldsymbol{\nu}(k)$ contains uncorrelated and jointly Gaussian-distributed elements that are independent of the elements of $\mathbf{s}(k)$, a common assumption in many signal processing formulations.

An important feature of the BSS model is the relative values of m and n. We can distinguish three important cases:

1. When $m = n$, the number of independent sources is equal to the number of measurement sensors.
2. When $m < n$, the number of independent sources is fewer than the number of measurement sensors.
3. When $m > n$, the number of independent sources is more than the number of measurement sensors.

The case of $m = n$ is most often assumed in theoretical formulations to the BSS tasks, in order to simplify the derivation of BSS algorithms. In practice, however, it can be unreasonable to assume that the number of sources is always equal to the number of sensors. In array processing for wireless communications, for example, sources can "come and go" depending on the current network state and transmitter use. Of the remaining two situations, the case where $m < n$ is more desirable in practice, as then all of the sources $s_j(k)$ in $\mathbf{s}(k)$ can be extracted from $\mathbf{x}(k)$ if rank$[\mathbf{A}] = m$ using a linear system of the form

$$\mathbf{y}(k) = \mathbf{B}(k)\mathbf{x}(k) \tag{7.3}$$

in the noise-free case, where $\mathbf{B}(k)$ is an $(m \times n)$ adjustable demixing matrix. In other words, when the mixing conditions are linear and $m \leq n$, a linear demixing system is sufficient to isolate each source signal $s_i(k)$ in a separate output $y_j(k)$ in $\mathbf{y}(k)$. Such a separation structure is illustrated in Figure 7.1. It is much more difficult to develop separation solutions for the case where $m > n$, because then it is impossible to exactly extract more sources than there are sensors in the noise-free case with a linear separating system. For this reason, we shall focus on the cases where $m \leq n$ in the discussions that follow.

The quality of the source estimates in $\mathbf{y}(k)$ can be measured in two ways:

1. A zero-forcing solution removes all source signal crosstalk in the extracted outputs. Such a solution attempts to adapt the demixing matrix such that

$$\lim_{k\to\infty} \mathbf{B}(k)\mathbf{A} = \mathbf{\Phi}\mathbf{D} \tag{7.4}$$

where $\mathbf{\Phi}$ is an $(m \times m)$ permutation matrix with one unity entry in any row or column and $\mathbf{D}$ is a diagonal nonsingular scaling matrix. If such is the case, then

$$y_i(k) = d_{jj}s_j(k) + \sum_{l=1}^{n} b_{il}(k)\eta_l(k) \tag{7.5}$$

for some non-replicative assignment $j \rightarrow i$ for $1 \leq i \leq m$ and $1 \leq j \leq m$. Thus, each element of $\mathbf{y}(k)$ is the sum of a single unique source in $\mathbf{s}(k)$ and a noise term.

2. A minimum mean-squared error solution attempts to minimize the average squared error between the estimated outputs and the true source signals, such that the cost function

$$\mathcal{J}_{MSE}(\mathbf{B}(k)) = E\left\{||\mathbf{\Phi D s}(k) - \mathbf{y}(k)||^2\right\} \tag{7.6}$$

is minimized.

When there is no noise ($\boldsymbol{\nu}(k) = \mathbf{0}$), the above two solutions are identical.

To date, most BSS algorithms have been designed to work in the no-noise situation, effectively assuming that $\boldsymbol{\nu}(k) = \mathbf{0}$. For this reason, we shall focus on the no-noise case in the following sections. Recently, several algorithms have been developed to perform minimum MSE BSS; see Bose and Friedlander [7] and Douglas [8] for a presentation of these methods.

7.2.2 Blind Criteria for BSS

The procedure for adjusting the entries of $\mathbf{B}(k)$ depends on what is assumed about the sources in $\mathbf{s}(k)$. Generally, two formulations of the BSS task have been extensively explored: (1) those that use spatial independence and non-Gaussianity, and (2) those that use spatial decorrelation and temporal correlation. Recently, a third formulation employing signal nonstationarity has been proposed and used for BSS [9]—[11]. Our discussion limits its focus to signals with stationary statistics, so that the former two methods are most appropriate. We first introduce the underlying signal conditions assumed in these methods before exploring each problem genre more fully.

7.2.2.1 Signal Separation Using Spatial Independence

In this class of BSS methods, each $s_i(k)$ is assumed to be statistically independent of $s_j(k)$ for $1 \leq i < j \leq n$. In addition, the marginal probability density functions (PDFs) of at least $(m-1)$ of the sources must be non-Gaussian. Taken together, these two assumptions imply that the joint PDFs of $\mathbf{s}(k)$ is of the form

$$p_{\mathbf{s}}(s_1, \ldots, s_m) = p_{s_1}(s_1) \times p_{s_2}(s_2) \times \cdots \times p_{s_m}(s_m) \tag{7.7}$$

where $p_{s_i}(s_i)$, the marginal PDF of $s_i(k)$, cannot be the Gaussian kernel for more than one value of i. The non-Gaussianity of the sources is due to certain identifiability conditions that must be satisfied for this BSS formulation to work properly.

BSS methods that employ this formulation rely on some knowledge of the higher-order or lower-order amplitude statistics of the source signals to perform separation.

7.2.2.2 Signal Separation Using Temporal Correlation

In this class of BSS methods, each $s_i(k)$ is assumed to be uncorrelated with $s_j(k-l)$ for $1 \leq i < j \leq n$ and all l. In addition, each $s_i(k)$ must exhibit a different level of correlation with $s_i(k-l)$ for some $l \neq 0$, such that the values of the normalized correlation coefficients

$$\rho_i(l) = \frac{E\{s_i(k)s_i(k-l)\}}{\sqrt{E\{s_i^2(k)\}E\{s_i^2(k-l)\}}} \tag{7.8}$$

are distinct for all $1 \leq i \leq m$ and at least one value of $l \neq 0$. The additional constraint on the correlation statistics of the sources is again due to certain identifiability conditions that must be satisfied for this formulation to work properly.

BSS methods that employ this formulation rely on some knowledge of the second-order statistics of the source signals to perform separation.

7.2.3 BSS Algorithms Using Spatial Independence

Approaches for BSS using spatial independence can be classified into one of two types: (1) those that use density matching of the sources, and (2) those that use contrast function optimization. We explore the two BSS formulations separately. In each case, we describe a popular algorithm that has been developed for the particular formulation.

7.2.3.1 Density Matching BSS Using Natural Gradient Adaptation

Density matching BSS methods rely heavily on concepts in information theory, a half-century-young field with applications in numerous fields including communications, economics, neuroscience, and physics [12]. Information theory is useful for BSS because with it one can characterize the amount of shared information in a set of signals. Intuitively, separation is obtained when no common information can be found between any two output signal subsets.

The basic idea behind density matching can be simply stated as follows: adjust $\mathbf{B}(k)$ so that the joint PDF of $\mathbf{y}(k)$, denoted as $p_{\mathbf{y}}(\mathbf{y})$, is as close as possible to some model distribution $\widehat{p}_{\mathbf{y}}(\mathbf{y})$. Although many different formulations to this type of density-match approach can be developed [13, 14], Cardoso has shown that all of these formulations can be unified using the Kullback–Leibler divergence measure given by [15]:

$$D\left(p_{\mathbf{y}}||\widehat{p}_{\mathbf{y}}\right) = \int p_{\mathbf{y}}(\mathbf{y}) \log \left(\frac{p_{\mathbf{y}}(\mathbf{y})}{\widehat{p}_{\mathbf{y}}(\mathbf{y})}\right) d\mathbf{y} \tag{7.9}$$

where $p_{\mathbf{y}}(\mathbf{y})$ and $\widehat{p}_{\mathbf{y}}(\mathbf{y})$ are the actual and model distributions, respectively, of the output signal vector. Equation (7.9) measures the "distance" between $p_{\mathbf{y}}(\mathbf{y})$ and $\widehat{p}_{\mathbf{y}}(\mathbf{y})$, although this measure is asymmetric.

The choice of $\widehat{p}_{\mathbf{y}}(\mathbf{y})$ is governed by the assumptions on and *a priori* knowledge of $\mathbf{s}(k)$. If all $s_i(k)$ are identically distributed, a reasonable choice is

$$\widehat{p}_{\mathbf{y}}(\mathbf{y}) = C \prod_{i=1}^{m} p_s\left(y_i\right) \tag{7.10}$$

where C is an integration constant chosen such that $\widehat{p}_{\mathbf{y}}(\mathbf{y})$ integrates to unity. This choice of density model yields a maximum-likelihood (ML) estimate of the demixing matrix $\mathbf{B}(k)$ for the given signal statistics. Alternatively, by estimating the marginal PDFs $\widehat{p}_{y_i}(y_i)$ for the current $\mathbf{B}(k)$ and setting $\widehat{p}_{\mathbf{y}}(\mathbf{y}) = \prod_{i=1}^{m} \widehat{p}_{y_i}(y_i)$, one obtains a minimum mutual information (MI) approach to BSS [15].

The main advantage of Equation (7.9) as a cost function is its statistical efficiency. With a "good" choice of model $\widehat{p}_{\mathbf{y}}(\mathbf{y})$, one can make good use of the source signal characteristics, e.g., to obtain more accurate source signal estimates for a given data set size. The main drawback to Equation (7.9) is the practical need to choose a model. The most general choice (MI) is computationally demanding to compute, whereas the most restrictive choice (ML) can actually lead to algorithm failure if the marginal PDFs used within $\widehat{p}_{\mathbf{y}}(\mathbf{y})$ differ too much from the actual distributions of the extracted $y_i(k)$. See Amari et al. [16] for a discussion of the stability conditions that the marginal PDFs within $\widehat{p}_{\mathbf{y}}(\mathbf{y})$ must satisfy for local convergence. Moreover, it should be noted that Equation (7.9) has not been proven to possess only separating minima for any arbitrary density model choice. As such, separation is not guaranteed with this cost function, although numerous simulations have indicated that ill-convergence is extremely rare for even gross marginal approximations within $\widehat{p}_{\mathbf{y}}(\mathbf{y})$.

Once a cost function has been chosen, any locally convergent optimization procedure can be used to adjust the elements of $\mathbf{B}(k)$. In what follows, we develop simple gradient procedures for Kullback–Leibler divergence minimization. For simplicity, assume that each $s_i(k)$ is identically distributed and $m = n$. An instantaneous cost function whose expected value matches the value of $D(p_{\mathbf{y}}(\mathbf{y})||\widehat{p}_{\mathbf{y}}(\mathbf{y}))$ up to a constant is

$$\widehat{\mathcal{J}}(\mathbf{B}) = -\log\left(|\det \mathbf{B}|\prod_{i=1}^{m} p_s(y_i(k))\right) \tag{7.11}$$

where $\det \mathbf{B}$ is the determinant of $\mathbf{B}$. Using simple calculus, a stochastic gradient descent procedure can be derived from this cost function as

$$\begin{aligned}
\mathbf{B}(k+1) &= \mathbf{B}(k) - \mu(k)\frac{\partial \widehat{\mathcal{J}}(\mathbf{B}(k))}{\partial \mathbf{B}} && (7.12)\\
&= \mathbf{B}(k) + \mu(k)\left[\mathbf{B}^{-T}(k) - \mathbf{f}(\mathbf{y}(k))\mathbf{x}^T(k)\right] && (7.13)
\end{aligned}$$

where $\mathbf{f}(\mathbf{y}) = [f(y_1) \ \cdots \ f(y_m)]^T$, $f(y) = -\partial \log p_s(y)/\partial y$, and $\mu(k)$ is a small positive step size. Moreover, although derived for identically distributed source signals, Equation (7.13) can perform BSS even for simple choices of $f(y)$. For example, choosing $f(y) = y^3$ allows Equation (7.13) to separate negative-kurtosis source signals (i.e., $E\{s_i^4\} - 3E^2\{s_i^2\} < 0$), whereas the choice $f(y) = \text{sgn}(y)$ is effective for instantaneously mixed speech signals. The main drawbacks of Equation (7.13) are (1) its computational complexity, as $\mathbf{B}^{-T}(k)$ must be computed, and (2) its slow convergence speed when $\mathbf{A}$ is ill-conditioned.

It is widely accepted that stochastic gradient descent suffers from slow convergence in many practical problems due to dependencies in the data being processed. The oft-proposed remedy for this situation is a Newton-based update, such as that provided by least squares methods in linear regression tasks [17]. Such a procedure makes sense when the error surface being searched is nearly quadratic. In BSS, however, the cost function is not quadratic. Fortunately, a modification to Equation (7.13) has been developed that largely removes all effects of an ill-conditioned mixing matrix $\mathbf{A}$. Termed the natural gradient by Amari [18] and the relative gradient by Cardoso [15], this modification is

$$\begin{aligned}
\mathbf{B}(k+1) &= \mathbf{B}(k) - \mu(k)\frac{\partial \widehat{\mathcal{J}}(\mathbf{B}(k))}{\partial \mathbf{B}}\mathbf{B}^T(k)\mathbf{B}(k) && (7.14)\\
&= \mathbf{B}(k) + \mu(k)\left[\mathbf{I} - \mathbf{f}(\mathbf{y}(k))\mathbf{y}^T(k)\right]\mathbf{B}(k)\,. && (7.15)
\end{aligned}$$

To see how Equation (7.15) behaves, define the combined system matrix $\mathbf{C}(k)$ as

$$\mathbf{C}(k) = \mathbf{B}(k)\mathbf{A}\,. \tag{7.16}$$

Clearly, we desire $\mathbf{C}(k) \to \mathbf{\Phi D}$ over time, from Equation (7.4). If we post-multiply both sides of Equation (7.15) by $\mathbf{A}$ and recognize that $\mathbf{y}(k) = \mathbf{C}(k)\mathbf{s}(k)$, we can write the update in Equation (7.15) as

$$\mathbf{C}(k+1) = \mathbf{C}(k) + \mu(k)\left[\mathbf{I} - \mathbf{f}(\mathbf{C}(k)\mathbf{s}(k))\mathbf{s}^T(k)\mathbf{C}^T(k)\right]\mathbf{C}(k)\,. \tag{7.17}$$

Notice that this expression depends only on the combined system matrix $\mathbf{C}(k)$, the source signal vector sequence, and $\mu(k)$; the mixing matrix $\mathbf{A}$ has been absorbed as an initial condition into

$\mathbf{C}(0) = \mathbf{B}(0)\mathbf{A}$. Thus, the deterministic evolutionary behavior of the combined system $\mathbf{C}(k)$ is not fundamentally limited by $\mathbf{A}$, as long as $\mathbf{C}(k)$ can easily escape from "bad" initial conditions, and simulations indicate that $\mathbf{C}(k)$ escapes from "poor" initial conditions even for small values of $\mu(k)$. The adaptive performance of the algorithm is further aided by the "good" statistical properties of the sequence $\mathbf{s}(k)$ (e.g., its independent elements). For all of these reasons, Equation (7.15) possesses excellent adaptation behavior. The uniform performance provided by Equation (7.15) is due to the so-called equivariance property provided by the natural/relative gradient BSS update [15]. Amazingly, this performance improvement comes with an added benefit: the algorithm is made simpler because $\mathbf{B}^{-T}(k)$ need not be computed. For more details regarding the natural gradient and its properties, see Douglas and Amari [19].

7.2.3.2 Contrast Function Optimization for BSS Using Constrained Adaptation

The concept of a contrast function for blind signal separation was introduced by Comon in his seminal 1994 paper [20]. A contrast function is a non-quadratic cost function that depends on a single extracted output signal. This function is used in a constrained minimization or maximization procedure over the demixing matrix elements to extract independent sources from their linear mixtures. Like density matching, BSS methods that use contrast functions rely on the spatial independence and non-Gaussianity of the source signals to perform separation. Unlike density-based methods, however, contrast-based BSS methods do not require significant knowledge about the natures of the source signal PDFs in order to perform separation.

The structure of a typical contrast-based BSS system is shown in Figure 7.2. This system contains

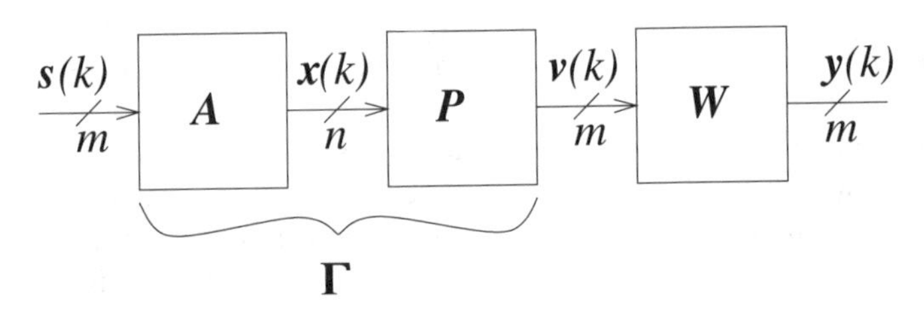

7.2 Block diagram of the contrast-based BSS task.

two processing stages ($m \leq n$):

1. a prewhitening stage, in which an $(m \times n)$ prewhitening matrix $\mathbf{P}$ is used to compute a prewhitened signal vector sequence as

$$\mathbf{v}(k) = \mathbf{P}\mathbf{x}(k) \tag{7.18}$$

2. a separation stage, in which an $(m \times m)$ separation matrix $\mathbf{W}$ is used to extract the individual sources from $\mathbf{v}(k)$ as

$$\mathbf{y}(k) = \mathbf{W}(k)\mathbf{v}(k)\ . \tag{7.19}$$

Comparing Figures 7.1 and 7.2, it is clear that $\mathbf{B}(k)$, $\mathbf{W}(k)$, and $\mathbf{P}$ are related by

$$\mathbf{B}(k) = \mathbf{W}(k)\mathbf{P}\ . \tag{7.20}$$

Unlike density matching approaches, however, $\mathbf{P}$ and $\mathbf{W}(k)$ are not jointly adapted; each matrix is optimized separately under its own criterion.

The goal of the prewhitening stage is to calculate a prewhitened signal sequence $\mathbf{v}(k)$ whose covariance matrix is

$$E\left\{\mathbf{v}(k)\mathbf{v}^T(k)\right\} \approx \mathbf{I}\,. \tag{7.21}$$

In other words, elements of the prewhitened signal vector sequence are spatially uncorrelated and of unit variance. If block processing is employed, any one of a number of different procedures can be used to calculate the matrix $\mathbf{P}$ from the measured sequence $\mathbf{x}(k)$, e.g., using an eigenvalue decomposition of the deterministic autocorrelation matrix of $\mathbf{x}(k)$ over the data block. Many adaptive prewhitening procedures are also available; two such procedures are

$$\mathbf{P}(k+1) = \mathbf{P}(k) + \mu\left[\mathbf{I} - \mathbf{v}(k)\mathbf{v}^T(k)\right]\mathbf{P}(k) \tag{7.22}$$

$$\mathbf{P}(k+1) = \mathbf{P}(k) + \mu\left[\mathbf{I} - \mathbf{v}(k)\mathbf{v}^T(k)\right]. \tag{7.23}$$

See Douglas and Cichocki [21] for a description and analysis of these approaches. The reason for the prewhitening stage in contrast-based BSS methods becomes clear when one considers the combined mixing-plus-prewhitening matrix that relates $\mathbf{v}(k)$ to $\mathbf{s}(k)$, as given by

$$\mathbf{\Gamma} = \mathbf{PA}\,. \tag{7.24}$$

It is straightforward to show that, if $\mathbf{P}$ is a prewhitening matrix, $\mathbf{\Gamma}$ is orthonormal; that is, $\mathbf{\Gamma}\mathbf{\Gamma}^T = \mathbf{\Gamma}^T\mathbf{\Gamma} = \mathbf{I}$. Hence, the separation matrix $\mathbf{W}(k)$ in the second processing stage can also be constrained to be orthonormal. The key feature of such a constraint is the uniqueness of each of the rows of $\mathbf{W}(k)$; that is, once a source has been extracted by the ith row of $\mathbf{W}(k)$, its solution can be effectively "ignored" in solving for the other rows of $\mathbf{W}(k)$ by making these other rows orthogonal to the ith row. Such a constraint can be imposed in one of many different ways, such as Gram–Schmidt orthogonalization or a singular-value decomposition.

The optimization procedure used to calculate any one row of $\mathbf{W}(k)$ in this formulation of the BSS task has the general form

$$\text{maximize or minimize} \quad \mathcal{J}_C\left(\mathbf{w}_i(k)\right) = \phi\left[y_i(k)\right] \tag{7.25}$$

$$\text{such that} \quad \mathbf{w}_i^T(k)\mathbf{w}_j(k) = \delta_{ij}, \qquad 1 \le j \le m \tag{7.26}$$

where $\mathbf{W}(k) = [\mathbf{w}_1(k) \ \cdots \ \mathbf{w}_m(k)]^T$ and $\phi[y_i(k)]$ is a contrast function that depends on the ith output signal sequence $y_i(k) = \mathbf{w}_i^T(k)\mathbf{v}(k)$. The constraint in Equation (7.26) makes effective use of the prewhitening conditions while providing an additional benefit: the potential solutions for each $\mathbf{w}_i(k)$ are, by definition, bounded.

The choice of the contrast function $\phi[y_i(k)]$ is the critical component in contrast-based BSS methods. This function must identify separating solutions at extremal values for the particular amplitude statistics of the sources in $\mathbf{s}(k)$. The best known and most popular choice of contrast function is the squared kurtosis contrast given by

$$\phi_\kappa\left[y_i(k)\right] = \left|\kappa\left[y_i(k)\right]\right|^2 \tag{7.27}$$

$$\kappa\left[y_i(k)\right] = E\left\{|y_i(k)|^4\right\} - 3E^2\left\{|y_i(k)|^2\right\} \tag{7.28}$$

where $\kappa[y_i(k)]$ is the kurtosis of the output signal $y_i(k)$. It can be shown in the noise-free case that $\phi_\kappa[\mathbf{y}(k)]$ achieves its maximum value in each $\mathbf{w}_i(k)$ corresponding to a separating solution

$$\mathbf{W}(k)\mathbf{\Gamma} = \mathbf{\Phi}\mathbf{D} \tag{7.29}$$

if the orthogonality constraints in Equation (7.26) are satisfied and if $\kappa[s_i(k)] \neq 0$. The latter condition is satisfied by most source signals; a notable exception are Gaussian sources, which have $\kappa[s_i(k)] = 0$. In practice, one requires that at least $(m-1)$ sources have non-zero kurtosis for this procedure to work, as the zero-kurtosis source can be extracted using the orthogonality constraints in Equation (7.26). The calculation of $\mathbf{w}_i(k)$ to solve the contrast BSS task in Equations (7.25) and (7.26) can take one of many different forms. Since $\phi[y_i(k)]$ is non-quadratic in $\mathbf{w}_i(k)$, iterative procedures for $\mathbf{w}_i(k)$ are most often used. One of the most popular procedures for contrast-based BSS is the fastICA algorithm developed by Hyvärinen and Oja [22]. This method is a block-based procedure for maximizing the kurtosis-based contrast in Equation (7.27); as such, it uses block averaging to approximate the statistical expectations in Equation (7.27). The updates for a given N-sample block of data are

$$\widetilde{\mathbf{w}}_i(k) = \left[\sum_{l=0}^{N-1} y_i^3(k+l)\mathbf{v}(k+l)\right] - 3\mathbf{w}_i(k) \tag{7.30}$$

$$\mathbf{w}_i(k+N) = \frac{\widetilde{\mathbf{w}}_i(k)}{||\widetilde{\mathbf{w}}_i(k)||}. \tag{7.31}$$

The update in Equation (7.30) can be shown to be an approximate Newton step for maximizing the kurtosis contrast function in Equation (7.27), whereas the second step maintains the unit-length constraint on $\mathbf{w}_i(k)$ imposed by Equation (7.26) for $i = j$. To extract several sources in parallel, an orthogonalization procedure can be applied to each $\mathbf{w}_i(k)$ either during or after the coefficient updating step. If the mixing conditions remain fixed over the data set, the same block of data can be used to compute each block average, such that $\mathbf{v}(l) = \mathbf{v}(l+N)$ for all l. In such cases, the convergence of this procedure can be quite fast, often occurring in ten iterations or less.

The fastICA algorithm described above uses the kurtosis within its contrast function. It is possible to choose other contrast functions $\phi[y_i(k)]$ within the constrained optimization procedure. As in density matching, the performance of the separation method can be improved by careful matching of the form of the contrast to the source signal statistics. It should be noted, however, that other choices of contrast function can generate spurious non-separating solutions for each $\mathbf{w}_i(k)$. For simple polynomial-based output contrasts, only kurtosis-based contrast functions appear to uniquely identify the class of separating solutions satisfying Equation (7.4) for arbitrary signal statistics [23]. This area is the subject of much current research, however, and new contrasts that separate a wide class of source distributions may appear in the future.

7.2.4 BSS Algorithms Using Temporal Correlation

The use of temporal correlation properties of the sources for BSS was pioneered by the work of Molgedey and Schuster [24] and later refined by Belouchrani et al. [25]. These approaches rely on a different set of signal properties as compared to the approaches described previously. In particular, spatial independence of the sources is not required; rather, the sources need only be spatially uncorrelated such that

$$E\left\{s_i(k)s_j(k+l)\right\} = 0 \text{ for } i \neq j \text{ and all } l. \tag{7.32}$$

This condition is weaker than spatial independence, and it also can include nearly Gaussian-distributed sources. In addition to this condition, the sources must be temporally correlated such that the normalized cross-correlation matrix

$$\overline{\mathbf{R}}_{\mathbf{ss}}(l) = \left[E\{\mathbf{s}(k)\mathbf{s}^T(k)\}\right]^{-1} E\left\{\mathbf{s}(k)\mathbf{s}^T(k+l)\right\} \tag{7.33}$$

has m unique eigenvalues for some value of $l \neq 0$. This condition is identical to the uniqueness of the $\rho_i(l)$ values in Equation (7.8) due to the diagonal nature of both matrices on the right-hand side of Equation (7.33).

To see how the above condition yields a separating solution, consider the corresponding normalized cross-correlation matrix of the input signals

$$\begin{aligned} \overline{\mathbf{R}}_{\mathbf{xx}}(l) &= \left[E\left\{\mathbf{x}(k)\mathbf{x}^T(k)\right\}\right]^{-1} E\left\{\mathbf{x}(k)\mathbf{x}^T(k+l)\right\} && (7.34) \\ &= \left[\mathbf{A}E\left\{\mathbf{s}(k)\mathbf{s}^T(k)\right\}\mathbf{A}^T\right]^{-1} \mathbf{A}E\left\{\mathbf{s}(k)\mathbf{s}^T(k+l)\right\}\mathbf{A}^T . && (7.35) \end{aligned}$$

Without loss of generality, assume that each source signal has unit variance, such that $E\{\mathbf{s}(k)\mathbf{s}^T(k)\} = \mathbf{I}$, and $m = n$. Then, we have

$$\begin{aligned} \overline{\mathbf{R}}_{\mathbf{xx}}(l) &= \mathbf{A}^{-T} E\left\{\mathbf{s}(k)\mathbf{s}^T(k+l)\right\}\mathbf{A}^T && (7.36) \\ &= \mathbf{A}^{-T}\overline{\mathbf{R}}_{\mathbf{ss}}(l)\mathbf{A}^T . && (7.37) \end{aligned}$$

Define the eigenvalue decomposition of $\overline{\mathbf{R}}_{\mathbf{xx}}(l)$ as

$$\overline{\mathbf{R}}_{\mathbf{xx}}(l) = \mathbf{Q}\boldsymbol{\Lambda}(l)\mathbf{Q}^{-1} . \quad (7.38)$$

Then, we have

$$\boldsymbol{\Lambda}(l) = \boldsymbol{\Phi}\overline{\mathbf{R}}_{\mathbf{ss}}(l)\boldsymbol{\Phi}^T \quad \text{and} \quad \mathbf{Q} = \mathbf{A}^{-T}\boldsymbol{\Phi}^T \quad (7.39)$$

such that the demixing matrix $\mathbf{B}$ can be calculated as

$$\mathbf{B} = \mathbf{Q}^T . \quad (7.40)$$

Thus, all that is required is an eigenvalue decomposition of a normalized cross-correlation matrix.

In practice, most BSS methods that use temporal correlation identify the demixing system by solving the following nonlinear system of m^2 equations for the m^2 entries of $\mathbf{B} = [\mathbf{b}_1 \ \dots \ \mathbf{b}_m]^T$ when $m = n$:

$$\begin{aligned} \mathbf{b}_i^T E\left\{\mathbf{x}(k)\mathbf{x}^T(k)\right\}\mathbf{b}_j &= \delta_{ij}, \qquad 1 \le i \le j \le m && (7.41) \\ \mathbf{b}_i^T E\left\{\mathbf{x}(k)\mathbf{x}^T(k+l)\right\}\mathbf{b}_j &= 0, \qquad 1 \le i < j \le m . && (7.42) \end{aligned}$$

Procedures that solve this type of task are referred to as joint diagonalization procedures, as they search for a matrix whose rows are the eigenvectors of at least two different structured data matrices. Alternatively, a two-stage approach similar to contrast optimization can be used, whereby the first prewhitening stage yields a prewhitened sequence $\mathbf{v}(k)$ whose eigenvectors are the orthogonal separating matrix through

$$\mathbf{W}^T E\left\{\mathbf{v}(k)\mathbf{v}^T(k+l)\right\}\mathbf{W} = \mathbf{I} . \quad (7.43)$$

Solutions of the above type can be found in Diamantaras [26]. BSS using temporal decorrelation has the distinct advantage of requiring only second-order statistics to be estimated. Thus, there is likely to be a numerical advantage when finite-length data records are used to estimate the data-dependent quantities needed within the separation method. These methods have the drawback, however, of requiring a rather artificial constraint on the normalized cross-correlation values $\rho_i(l)$ in Equation (7.8). The performance of this class of methods deteriorates when the normalized cross-correlations become close to one another for the chosen lag value l. For this reason, it is a good idea to use several cross-correlation matrices for different values of l in a joint diagonalization criterion, as recommended by Belouchrani et al. [25], to increase the odds of good identifiability.

7.3 Single-Channel Blind Deconvolution

This section introduces the mathematical notation for the blind deconvolution task. We also indicate the relationships between this task and BSS for instantaneous mixtures, showing how these BSS algorithms can be translated to the blind deconvolution task.

7.3.1 Problem Formulation

Figure 7.3 indicates the structure of the blind deconvolution task. An unknown signal, given by $s(k)$,

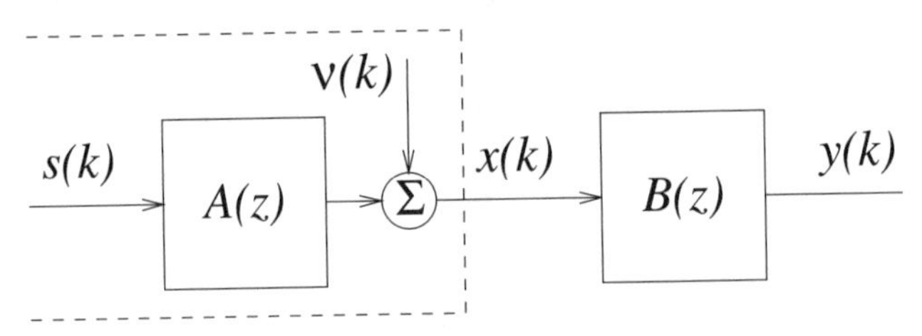

7.3 Block diagram of the blind deconvolution task.

passes through an unknown linear time-invariant filter with impulse response a_i, $-\infty < i < \infty$. The resulting noisy received signal $x(k)$ is given by

$$x(k) = \sum_{i=-\infty}^{\infty} a_i s(k-i) + \nu(k) \tag{7.44}$$

where $\nu(k)$ is a zero-mean Gaussian random process that is independent of the source signal $s(k)$. In typical applications, the source signal contains useful but unknown information, and the unknown filter describes the smoothing effects of a physical system. The measurement noise $\nu(k)$ models any sensor and channel noise inherent in the measurement process.

The goal of the blind deconvolution task is to extract an estimate of the source signal sequence $s(k)$ from the measured sequence $x(k)$ using a linear filter of the form

$$y(k) = \sum_{l=0}^{L} b_l(k)x(k-l) \tag{7.45}$$

where $b_l(k)$ for $0 \le l \le L$ are the coefficients of the system and L is a filter length parameter. In this model, we have assumed a causal finite-impulse-response (FIR) filter for the deconvolution model. FIR models are ideal candidates for adaptive filters, as they are both computationally simple and bounded-input–bounded-output stable for bounded coefficients. As in the BSS task, the quality of the signal estimates can be measured using one of two criteria:

1. The zero-forcing solution attempts to attain the following condition:

$$\lim_{k\to\infty} \sum_{l=0}^{L} b_l(k)a(i-l) \approx d\delta_{i-\Delta} \tag{7.46}$$

   where d is a scalar constant and Δ is a positive integer delay. If this is the case, then $y(k)$ is the sum of a scaled, time-shifted version of $s(k)$ and a noise term, or

$$y(k) = ds(k-\Delta) + \sum_{l=0}^{L} b_l(k)\nu(k-l) . \tag{7.47}$$

In other words, a single unique sample of the source sequence contributes to each sample of the output sequence. Note that the FIR form of the deconvolution model prevents the exact extraction of the source signal sequence; however, such a condition can be nearly attained for suitably large values of L and Δ.

2. The minimum MSE solution calculates $b_l(k)$, $0 \leq l \leq L$ to minimize the criterion

$$\mathcal{J}_{MSE}\left(\{b_l(k)\}\right) = E\left\{|ds(k-\Delta) - y(k)|^2\right\} . \tag{7.48}$$

The solution to this problem is a special case of the well-known Wiener–Hopf solution in linear estimation [27].

When there is no noise ($\nu(k) = 0$), the above two solutions are identical. As in the case of BSS, we ignore the effects of $\nu(k)$ in the discussion that follows; however, it should be noted that this noise can be significant in many applications, such as in channel equalization for wireless communications.

7.3.2 Relationships between Blind Deconvolution and BSS

Comparing Figures 7.1 and 7.3, it is not hard to see that blind deconvolution and blind signal separation are similar tasks. Both problems involve blindly estimating the inverse of a linear system from measurements of the system's output. Therefore, it should not be surprising that blind signal separation methods can be easily translated to solve blind deconvolution tasks. The technique for performing this translation is now described. Additional details about this process can be found in Douglas and Haykin [28].

Consider the BSS task in Figure 7.1 under the assumption that $m = n$ and the mixing matrix $\mathbf{A}$ is circulant. A circulant matrix has entries

$$a_{ij} = a_{[i-j]_m} \tag{7.49}$$

where $[q]_m$ denotes the modulo-m or remainder operation on the integer q. A circulant matrix is completely specified by any one row or column, as the other rows or columns of the matrix are simply modulo-shifted versions of this row or column. For example, the first column of $\mathbf{A}$ is $[a_0\ a_1 \ldots a_{m-1}]^T$, the second column of $\mathbf{A}$ is $[a_{m-1}\ a_0 \ldots a_{m-2}]^T$, and so on. The assumption of a circulant mixing matrix is completely artificial; practically no physical mixing system exhibits this structure. As we shall see, however, the circulant form of this BSS task yields a simple connection with the blind deconvolution task.

Under circulant mixing conditions, the observed mixture $\mathbf{x}(k)$ has the form of a cyclic convolution of the elements of $\mathbf{s}(k)$ and the elements of any one row of $\mathbf{A}$, as

$$x_i(k) = \sum_{j=1}^{m} a_{[i-j]_m} s_j(k), \qquad 1 \leq i \leq m . \tag{7.50}$$

Since the mixing matrix is circulant, the demixing matrix $\mathbf{B}(k)$ can also be assumed to be circulant, such that

$$b_{ij} = b_{[i-j]_m} . \tag{7.51}$$

The resulting output signal vector $\mathbf{y}(k)$ is computed using a circular convolution as

$$y_i(k) = \sum_{j=1}^{m} b_{[i-j]_m} x_j(k), \qquad 1 \le i \le m \,. \tag{7.52}$$

The goal of the BSS task in this scenario is to adjust the elements of $b_i(k)$ such that

$$\lim_{k\to\infty} \sum_{j=0}^{m-1} b_j(k) a_{i-j} = d\delta_{[i-\Delta]_m}, \qquad 0 \le i \le m-1 \,. \tag{7.53}$$

Such a solution yields a scaled and modulo-shifted version of the elements of $\mathbf{s}(k)$ in $\mathbf{y}(k)$.

Comparing the forms of Equations (7.50), (7.52), and (7.53) with the corresponding equations for blind deconvolution in Equations (7.44), (7.45), and (7.46), we see that they are quite similar in form if we assign

$$s_j(k) = s(k-j), \quad x_j(k) = x(k-j), \quad y_j(k) = y(k-j), \qquad \text{and } m = L+1 \,. \tag{7.54}$$

The only differences are (1) the limits of the sums and (2) the modulo operations within the circular convolutions. Since the BSS task for circulant mixtures is in the exact form of a BSS task, however, one can derive algorithms for separating circulant mixtures using similar derivations and assumptions as in the regular BSS case. Once these updates have been obtained, they can be translated to the blind deconvolution task using the following three-step procedure:

1. Let $m \to \infty$, such that circular convolutions become linear convolutions [29].
2. Truncate the length of any filters within the separation system to FIR form.
3. Insert delays within any filtering and/or coefficient update operations such that all calculations become causal.

The resulting blind deconvolution algorithms have abilities that correspond to their spatial BSS counterparts in terms of the underlying source signal statistics as well. This translation procedure can generally be applied to any BSS method, as long as the statistical assumptions on the source signals make sense within the translation.

7.3.2.1 Density Matching Blind Deconvolution Using Natural Gradient Adaptation

Douglas Haykin [28] applied the aforementioned translation procedure to the density-matching BSS algorithm in Equation (7.15) for complex-valued signals and coefficients. The resulting blind deconvolution algorithm updates each coefficient $b_l(k)$, $0 \le l \le L$ in the deconvolution filter as

$$b_l(k+1) = b_l(k) + \mu \left[b_l(k) - f(y(k-L)) u^*(k-l) \right] \tag{7.55}$$

where $*$ denotes complex-conjugate and the filtered output signal $u(k)$ is computed as

$$u(k) = \sum_{i=0}^{L} b_{L-i}^*(k) y(k-i) \,. \tag{7.56}$$

This algorithm employs approximately four complex multiply/adds per filter tap per sample, making it a remarkably simple adaptive procedure. In addition, it can deconvolve a wide range of source signal sequences depending on the chosen nonlinearity $f(y)$. See Douglas and Haykin [28] for a simulation example involving complex-valued quadrature-amplitude-modulated (QAM) source signals.

7.3.2.2 Contrast Function Optimization for Blind Deconvolution Using Constrained Adaptation

The aforementioned derivation method can also be applied to the fastICA algorithm in Equations (7.30) and (7.31). This derivation results in the following changes to the fastICA algorithm [30]:

- The prewhitening step is implemented using a prewhitening filter of the form

$$v(k) = \sum_{i=0}^{M} p_i x(k-i) \tag{7.57}$$

  where $p_i, 0 \leq i \leq M$ are the coefficients of the prewhitening filter. The values of p_i can be calculated in any one of a number of different ways, such as a forward linear predictor or using the temporal extensions of the prewhitening algorithms in Equations (7.22) or (7.23) [30].
- The unit-norm constraint on the rows of $\mathbf{W}(k)$ becomes an allpass constraint on the frequency response of the deconvolution filter. An allpass or phase-only filter has a unity magnitude frequency response.

One way to approximate the allpass constraint using an FIR filter is to normalize the overall frequency response of the deconvolution filter using the discrete Fourier transform after each block update. The algorithm obtained from this procedure shall be called the fastdeconv algorithm for purposes of discussion. The updates of this algorithm for an N-sample block of complex-valued data are

$$\widetilde{w}_l(k) = \left[\sum_{i=0}^{N-1} \left|y^2(k+i)\right| y(k+i)v^*(k+i-l)\right] - 3w_l(k) \tag{7.58}$$

$$\widetilde{\mathcal{W}}_l(k) = \sum_{p=0}^{L} \widetilde{w}_p(k) e^{-j2\pi pl/(L+1)} \tag{7.59}$$

$$\mathcal{W}_l(k) = \frac{\widetilde{\mathcal{W}}_l(k)}{|\widetilde{\mathcal{W}}_l(k)|} \tag{7.60}$$

$$w_l(k+N) = \frac{1}{L+1} \sum_{q=0}^{L} \mathcal{W}_q(k) e^{j2\pi lq/(L+1)} \tag{7.61}$$

where $j = \sqrt{-1}$. In addition, if $(L+1)$ is a power of two, this method can be further simplified by using the fast Fourier transform to implement the discrete Fourier transform calculations in the normalization step. Similar frequency-domain normalization methods can be used for gradient-based contrast optimization; see Douglas and Kung [30] for more details on these procedures.

7.4 Spatio-Temporal Extensions

We now consider the spatio-temporal extensions of BSS and blind deconvolution, namely, the multichannel blind deconvolution and convolutive BSS tasks, respectively. Both of these extensions involve the same overall mixture model and separation structure, but they differ from one another in terms of their goals and underlying assumptions on the source signals.

7.4.1 Common Problem Formulation

Figure 7.4 shows the common mixture model for the multichannel blind deconvolution and convolutive BSS tasks. In this model, an m-dimensional signal vector sequence $\mathbf{s}(k)$ passes through

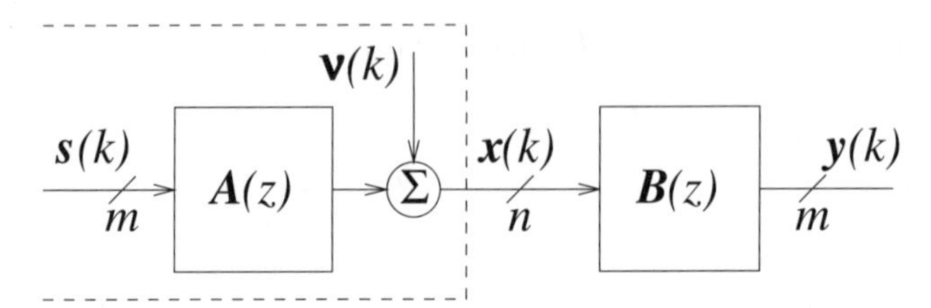

7.4 The common block diagram of the multichannel blind deconvolution and convolutive BSS tasks.

an unknown linear time-invariant $(n \times m)$ multichannel filter with matrix impulse response $\mathbf{A}_i$, $-\infty < i < \infty$. The resulting noisy received signal vector sequence $\mathbf{x}(k)$ is given by

$$\mathbf{x}(k) = \sum_{i=-\infty}^{\infty} \mathbf{A}_i \mathbf{s}(k-i) + \boldsymbol{\nu}(k) \tag{7.62}$$

where $\boldsymbol{\nu}(k)$ is a zero-mean Gaussian vector random process that is independent of the source signal $\mathbf{s}(k)$. In both applications, $\mathbf{s}(k)$ contains m unknown signals that are spatially independent from one another, and the unknown multichannel filter describes the mixing and smoothing effects of some multiterminal physical system. The measurement noise vector sequence $\boldsymbol{\nu}(k)$ models any sensor and channel noise inherent in the measurement process.

Solutions for both the multichannel blind deconvolution and convolutive BSS tasks attempt to extract an estimate of the source signal sequence $\mathbf{s}(k)$ from the measured sequence $\mathbf{x}(k)$ using a multichannel linear filter of the form

$$\mathbf{y}(k) = \sum_{l=0}^{L} \mathbf{B}_l(k)\mathbf{x}(k-l) \tag{7.63}$$

where $\mathbf{B}_l(k)$, $0 \le l \le L$ are the $(m \times n)$ matrix coefficients of the separation system and L is a filter length parameter. Again, we have assumed a causal FIR filter for the multichannel separation model, as FIR models are ideal candidates for adaptive procedures.

The desired solutions for the multichannel blind deconvolution and convolutive BSS tasks are generally different. Despite this fact, we can develop a common notation for measuring the qualities of the signal estimates in the output sequence $\mathbf{y}(k)$ in both tasks:

- The zero-forcing solution attempts to attain the following condition:

$$\lim_{k\to\infty} \sum_{l=0}^{L} \mathbf{B}_l(k)\mathbf{A}(i-l) \approx \mathbf{\Phi}\mathbf{D}(i) \tag{7.64}$$

  where $\mathbf{\Phi}$ is an $(m \times m)$ permutation matrix and $\mathbf{D}$ is a sequence of $(m \times m)$ diagonal matrices whose diagonal entries are denoted by $d_{jj}(i)$, $1 \le j \le m$. If this condition is met, then

$$y_i(k) = \sum_{l=-\infty}^{\infty} d_{jj}(l)s_j(k-l) + \sum_{l=0}^{L}\sum_{p=1}^{n} b_{ipl}(k)\nu_p(k-l) \tag{7.65}$$

for some non-replicative assignment $j \rightarrow i$ for $1 \leq i \leq m$ and $1 \leq j \leq m$, where $b_{ijl}(k)$ is the (i, j)th entry of $\mathbf{B}_l(k)$. Thus, each sequence $y_i(k)$ in the vector sequence $\mathbf{y}(k)$ contains a single unique, filtered source sequence $s_j(k)$ in $\mathbf{s}(k)$, along with a noise term.

- The minimum MSE solution calculates $\mathbf{B}_l(k)$, $0 \leq l \leq L$ to minimize the criterion

$$\mathcal{J}_{MSE}(\{\mathbf{B}_l(k)\}) = E\left\{\left|\boldsymbol{\Phi}\left[\sum_{i=-\infty}^{\infty} \mathbf{D}(i)\mathbf{s}(k-i)\right] - \mathbf{y}(k)\right|^2\right\}. \tag{7.66}$$

  The solution to this problem is the multichannel equivalent of the well-known Wiener–Hopf solution in linear estimation [27].

As in previous discussions, both the zero-forcing and minimum MSE solutions for $\mathbf{B}_l(k)$ are identical when the noise $\boldsymbol{\nu}(k)$ is absent, and we shall ignore the effects of $\boldsymbol{\nu}(k)$ in what follows.

7.4.2 Multichannel Blind Deconvolution

7.4.2.1 Assumptions and Goals

The multichannel blind deconvolution task is the logical union of the BSS and blind deconvolution tasks. As such, the underlying assumptions and goals for this task are closely related to those described for these similar tasks.

As for the underlying signal assumptions in multichannel blind deconvolution, each signal $s_i(k)$ is assumed to be temporally as well as spatially independent, such that $s_i(k)$ does not carry any information about $s_j(l)$ when $i \neq j$ or when $k \neq l$. This assumption is the logical union of the spatial and temporal independence assumptions used in BSS and blind deconvolution, respectively. Such an assumption is reasonable in certain scenarios, such as in wideband array processing for multiterminal wireless communications scenarios.

The goal of the multichannel blind deconvolution task in the noise-free case is given by Equation (7.64) for $\nu_j(k) = 0$, where the diagonal entries of $\mathbf{D}(i)$ have the form

$$d_{jj}(i) = d_{jj}\left(\Delta_j\right)\delta\left(i - \Delta_j\right) \tag{7.67}$$

where $\Delta_1, \Delta_2, \ldots, \Delta_m$ are all integers in the range $[0, L]$. If such is the case, then in the noise-free case, the zero-forcing and minimum MSE solutions yield the output sequences

$$y_i(k) = d_{jj}\left(\Delta_j\right)s_j\left(k - \Delta_j\right) \tag{7.68}$$

for some non-replicative assignment $j \rightarrow i$ for $1 \leq i \leq m$ and $1 \leq j \leq m$. In other words, each $y_i(k)$ in the vector sequence $\mathbf{y}(k)$ contains a single unique, possibly delayed source sequence in $\mathbf{s}(k)$. Thus, multichannel blind deconvolution attempts to make each sample in every extracted output vector $\mathbf{y}(k)$ independent of all other samples in the current, previous, and past output vectors.

7.4.2.2 Algorithms for Multichannel Blind Deconvolution

It is possible to transform BSS algorithms for instantaneous mixtures into multichannel blind deconvolution algorithms. The transformation process involves following three simple rules that make associations between matrices in the BSS task, such as $\mathbf{A}$, $\mathbf{B}(k)$ and $\mathbf{f}(\mathbf{y}(k))\mathbf{x}^T(k)$, and matrix sequences in the multichannel blind deconvolution task, such as $\mathbf{A}_l$, $\mathbf{B}_l(k)$ and $\mathbf{f}(\mathbf{y}(k))\mathbf{x}^T(k-l)$. These rules can be summarized as follows [28, 39]:

1. Multiplication of two matrices in instantaneous BSS is equivalent to convolution of their associated matrix sequences in multichannel blind deconvolution.

2. Addition of two matrices in instantaneous BSS is equivalent to element-by-element addition of their associated matrix sequences in multichannel blind deconvolution.
3. Transposition of a matrix in instantaneous BSS is equivalent to element-by-element transposition and time-reversal of its associated matrix sequence in multichannel blind deconvolution.

In addition, it may be necessary to employ approximations, such as sequence truncation and insertion of delay, in order to arrive at an implementable algorithm. Similar approximations have been used in deriving the blind deconvolution algorithms in Section 7.3.2.

The above procedure can be applied to the density matching BSS algorithm using natural gradient adaptation in Equation (7.15). The resulting coefficient updates for $\mathbf{B}_l(k)$, $0 \leq l \leq L$, are [31]

$$\mathbf{B}_l(k+1) = \mathbf{B}_l(k) + \mathbf{M}(k)\left[\mathbf{B}_l(k) - \mathbf{f}(\mathbf{y}(k-L))\mathbf{u}^T(k-l)\right] \tag{7.69}$$

$$\mathbf{u}(k) = \sum_{i=0}^{L} \mathbf{B}_{L-i}^T(k)\mathbf{y}(k-i) \tag{7.70}$$

where $\mathbf{y}(k)$ is as defined in Equation (7.63) and $\mathbf{M}(k)$ is a diagonal matrix of step size values $\mu_i(k)$, $1 \leq i \leq m$. The separation capabilities of this algorithm for a given set of nonlinearities in $\mathbf{f}(\mathbf{y})$ mirror those in the original algorithm for instantaneous BSS; see Amari et al. [16] for the local stability conditions.

The above procedure can also be applied to contrast function optimization for instantaneous BSS algorithms. The resulting methods employ two stages of processing. The first processing stage implements a multichannel prewhitening filter. The second processing stage involves another multichannel filter whose coefficients are optimized according to a constrained optimization procedure. The sets of constraints on the impulse response $\mathbf{W}_l(k)$, $0 \leq l \leq L$, of this system can be approximately described as

$$\sum_{l=0}^{L} \mathbf{W}(l)\mathbf{W}^T(i+l) \approx \mathbf{I}\delta(i), \qquad -L \leq i \leq L\,. \tag{7.71}$$

Equation (7.71) describes the impulse response of a paraunitary filter. Paraunitary filters are useful for numerous problems, particularly in multirate systems and coding applications [32]. Moreover, adaptive algorithms for adjusting the coefficients to maintain approximate paraunitariness of the overall system impulse response have recently been derived [33]. See Sun and Douglas [34] for examples of algorithms that are based on this approach.

7.4.3 BSS of Convolutive Mixtures

7.4.3.1 Assumptions and Goals

The convolutive BSS task is similar to the multichannel blind deconvolution task in that the sensor measurements follow the same model as in Equation (7.62). The goal, however, is not to "separate" in both space and time; rather, spatial separation is the overall goal. Thus, the sources need only be spatially independent, such that $s_i(k)$ is independent of $s_j(k+l)$ for $i \neq j$ and all l. Moreover, the desired solution in the noise-free case is given by Equation (7.64), where each impulse response $d_{jj}(i)$ has non-zero gain at all discrete-time frequencies ω in the range $|\omega| \leq \pi$. In effect, the temporal characteristics of the sources are ignored in the separation task, and the system's outputs can only achieve zero crosstalk among the individual sources.

In acoustics, the convolutive BSS task is most easily understood as the "cocktail party problem," whereby the goal is to extract m individual talkers' speech as recorded by n microphones in a multichannel audio recording system. Clearly, the intelligibility of the speech is only partially affected by temporal filtering, and such intelligibility can be improved using post-processing of the individually extracted signals.

7.4.3.2 Algorithms for BSS of Convolutive Mixtures

Several algorithms that are specifically designed for separating two-channel convolutive mixtures of spatially independent sources (e.g., a stereo audio recording of two talkers) have been described in the literature [35]–[38]. These estimation-based methods rely heavily on the two-channel nature of the underlying problem, and their performances are greatly enhanced when separating single source dominant mixtures, in which each of the unknown sources is the loudest in only one of the signal mixtures. In such cases, successful separation has been achieved using least squares-type approaches, which inherently rely on second-order statistical properties of the signals [35]. There are surprisingly few algorithms specifically designed for BSS of convolutive mixtures of more than two source signals. The difficulty in this task is the use of temporal information, as the correlation properties of the unknown source signals are nuisance parameters in the design of the multichannel separation filter coefficients. Although the general m-source, n-sensor convolutive BSS problem appears to be challenging, many researchers have noted that multichannel blind deconvolution algorithms can give quite adequate separation performance in the convolutive BSS task. In other words, an algorithm that is designed for separating spatially and temporally independent signals from spatio-temporal mixtures can often do a reasonable job of separating spatio-temporal mixtures of temporally dependent signals. One such example is the natural gradient algorithm for multichannel blind deconvolution in Equations (7.69) and (7.70), of which various algorithm forms have been applied extensively to audio recordings [39]–[42]. Not surprisingly, these methods tend to flatten the spectral content of the sources in the extracted outputs, although this "whitening" effect is not an exact second-order whitening operation. For speech signals, the extracted signals are quite intelligible despite their thin acoustic character. For music signals, the deconvolution properties of the method can significantly alter the extracted source signals; such results are discussed in the following section on simulation.

7.5 Simulation Examples

This section illustrates the performance of several of the algorithms described in this chapter through simulations. In every case, we have used MATLAB, the popular signal analysis and manipulation software package, to implement and simulate each algorithm. For the instantaneous BSS and single-channel blind deconvolution examples, the relevant programs are provided in figures at the end of this chapter to enable readers to conduct experiments of their own.

7.5.1 BSS for Instantaneous Mixtures

We first explore the behaviors of two algorithms for instantaneous BSS. In both cases, we have implemented a three-input, three-output ($m = n = 3$) separation system. The three source distributions were uniform, binary, and Gaussian, respectively, all with zero means and unit variances. The mixing matrix was arbitrarily chosen as

$$\mathbf{A} = \begin{bmatrix} -0.8 & 0.1 & 0.6 \\ 0.3 & 0.5 & -0.7 \\ 0.4 & -0.9 & 0.2 \end{bmatrix}. \tag{7.72}$$

In each simulation run, we evaluated the performance metric

$$\rho(k) = \frac{1}{m-1}\left[m - \frac{1}{2}\sum_{i=1}^{m}\left(\frac{\max\limits_{1\le j\le m}|c_{ij}(k)|^2}{\sum\limits_{j=1}^{m}|c_{ij}(k)|^2} + \frac{\max\limits_{1\le j\le m}|c_{ji}(k)|^2}{\sum\limits_{j=1}^{m}|c_{ji}(k)|^2}\right)\right]. \tag{7.73}$$

This dimensionless performance metric measures the deviation of the combined system from a diagonally scaled permutation matrix. In fact, the performance metric has the following features:

- $0 \le \rho(k) \le 1$ for all matrices $\mathbf{C}(k)$
- $\rho(k) = 1$ if and only if $|c_{ij}(k)|^2 = |c_{pq}(k)|^2$ for all i, j, p, and q in the range $[1, m]$ (i.e., maximally mixed sources in the system outputs)
- $\rho(k) = 0$ if and only if $\mathbf{C}(k) = \mathbf{\Phi D}$ (i.e., separated sources in the system outputs)

Figure 7.5 shows the evolution of $\rho(k)$ for four different simulation runs of the density matching BSS algorithm using the natural gradient in Equation (7.15) for the nonlinearity choice $f_i(y) = y^3$, $1 \le i \le m$. Such a choice allows this algorithm to separate mixtures of negative-kurtosis

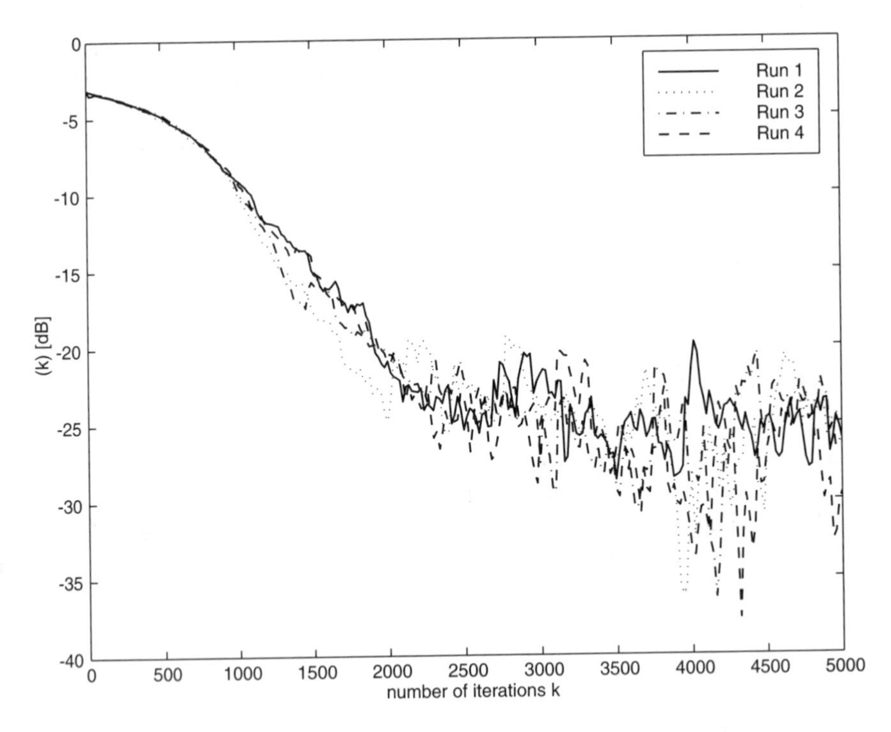

7.5 Evolutions of $\rho(k)$ for four different runs of the natural gradient BSS algorithm (Figure 7.6 contains the MATLAB code for this figure).

sources [16]. In each case, we have chosen $\mathbf{B}(0) = \mathbf{I}$ and $\mu = 0.002$. The MATLAB program `natgradBSSex.m` used to generate this figure is provided in Figure 7.6. As can be seen, the performance factor $\rho(k)$ converges to a small value — approximately -22dB — for each of the simulation runs, indicating that the algorithm accurately separates the source signals from their linear mixtures.

```
function [msg] = natgradBSSex();
mu = 0.002; ntr = 5000; A = [-8 1 6; 3 5 -7; 4 -9 2]/10;
s = zeros(3,ntr); rho = zeros(5,ntr/20+1); m = 0:20:ntr;
for j=1:4;
     s(1,:) = sign(randn(1,ntr));
     s(2,:) = sqrt(3)*(2*rand(1,ntr)-1);
     s(3,:) = randn(1,ntr);
     [B,y,r] = natgradBSS(mu,A,s);
     rho(j,:) = r(m+1);
end; plot(m,rho(1,:),'-',m,rho(2,:),':',m,rho(3,:),'-.',
          m,rho(4,:),'--');
xlabel('number of iterations k'); ylabel('\rho(k) [dB]');
legend('Run 1','Run 2','Run 3','Run 4'); msg = 'Done!';


%%%%%%%%%%%%%%%%%%%%%%%%%%%%%%%%%%%%%%%%%%%%%%%%%%%%%%%%%%%%%%%%%%%

function [B,y,rho] = natgradBSS(mu,A,s);
[m,ntr] = size(s); [n,m] = size(A);
x = A*s;
B = eye(m,n); y = zeros(m,ntr); rho = zeros(1,ntr+1);
C = B*A; C2 = C.^2;
rho(1) = 10*log10((m-sum(max(C2)./sum(C2)+
                         max(C2')./sum(C2'))/2)/(m-1));
for i=1:ntr;
     Y = B*x(:,i);
     muF = mu*Y.^3;
     U = B'*Y;
     B = (1+mu)*B - muF*U';
     C = B*A; C2 = C.^2;
     rho(i+1) = 10*log10((m-sum(max(C2)./sum(C2)+max(C2')./
                     sum(C2'))/2)/(m-1));
end;
```

7.6 MATLAB code for density modeling BSS using the natural gradient algorithm.

Figure 7.7 shows the evolution of $\rho(Ni)$ for four different simulation runs of one implementation of the fastICA algorithm in Equations (7.30) and (7.31), where $\mathbf{W}(0) = \mathbf{I}$. In each case, we have used a single block of $N = 5000$ samples to compute all coefficient updates for the given run, where $\mathbf{x}(k + Ni) = \mathbf{x}(k)$ for all integer values $i \geq 0$ and $0 \leq k \leq N - 1$. The MATLAB program `fasticaBSSex.m` used to generate this figure is provided in Figure 7.8. As can be seen, the algorithm takes between three and five epochs to converge. Depending on the simulation run, the performance factor varies from −31dB to −44dB due to random differences in the source signals. The accuracy of the method generally improves for increasing values of block length N. It should be noted that, although all sources have non-negative kurtosis in the simulations, the fastICA algorithm successfully separates mixtures of non-zero kurtosis sources, and, in this sense, the algorithm is applicable to a wider range of source signal types than is the density-based natural gradient BSS algorithm in Equation (7.15) for fixed nonlinearities $f_i(y)$.

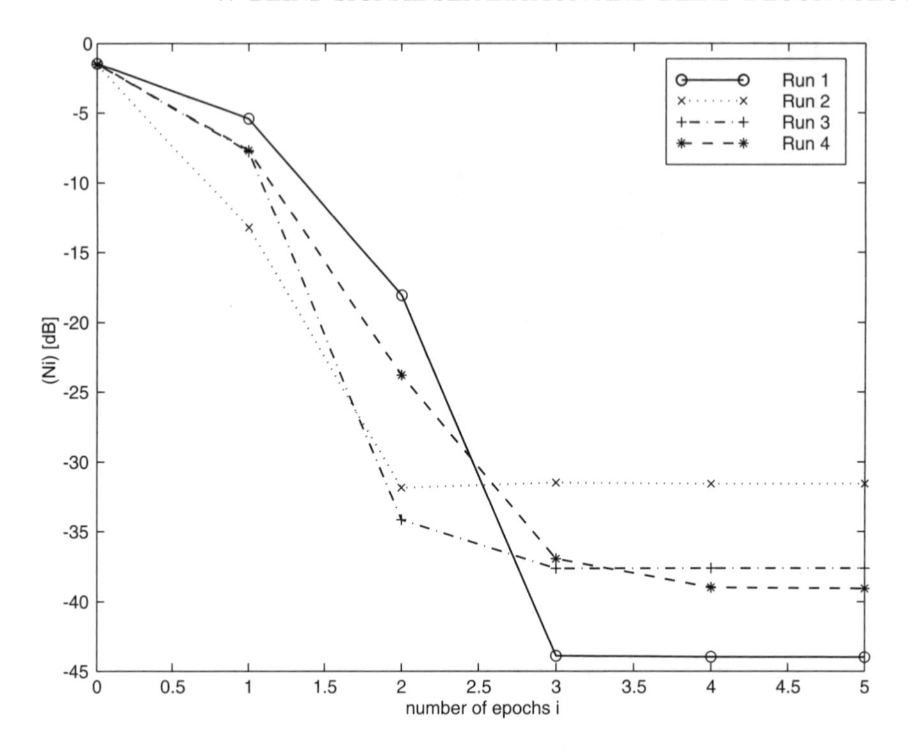

7.7 Evolutions of $\rho(Ni)$ for four different runs of the fastICA BSS algorithm (Figure 7.8 contains the MATLAB code for this figure).

7.5.2 Blind Deconvolution

We now illustrate the behavior of the fastdeconv algorithm for single-channel blind deconvolution. In these simulations, we have chosen a 16-QAM complex-valued communications source signal whose instantaneous probability mass function (PMF) is

$$p_s(s) = \begin{cases} \dfrac{1}{16} & \text{if } s \in \mathcal{S} \\ 0 & \text{otherwise} \end{cases} \tag{7.74}$$

and the sixteen-element set $\mathcal{S}$ contains all values of $s_R + js_I$ with $s_R \in \{-3, -1, 1, 3\}$ and $s_I \in \{-3, -1, 1, 3\}$. The mixing filter used in these simulations is described by the difference equation

$$x(k) = -\alpha x(k-1) + \alpha^* s(k) + s(k-1) \tag{7.75}$$

where $\alpha = 0.7e^{j\pi/3}$. It is easy to show that the above system is an allpass filter. As such, we may set $v(k) = x(k)$ as no prewhitening filter is required. The deconvolution filter's impulse response was initialized using a "center spike" strategy, in which

$$w_l(0) = \begin{cases} 1 & \text{if } l = L/2 \\ 0 & \text{otherwise} . \end{cases} \tag{7.76}$$

```
function [msg] = fasticaBSSex();
nepoch = 5; ntr = 5000; A = [-8 1 6; 3 5 -7; 4 -9 2]/10;
s = zeros(3,ntr); rhoN = zeros(4,nepoch+1); m = 0:nepoch;
for j=1:4;
     s(1,:) = sign(randn(1,ntr));
     s(2,:) = sqrt(3)*(2*rand(1,ntr)-1);
     s(3,:) = randn(1,ntr);
     x = A*s;
     [Q,Lam] = eig(x*x'); P = sqrt(ntr)*Lam^(-1/2)*Q';
     v = P*x;
     Gam = P*A;
     [W,y,rhoN(j,:)] = fasticaBSS(nepoch,Gam,v);
end;
plot(m,rhoN(1,:),'o-',m,rhoN(2,:),'x:',m,rhoN(3,:),'+-.',
     m,rhoN(4,:),'*--');
xlabel('number of epochs i'); ylabel('\rho(Ni) [dB]');
legend('Run 1','Run 2','Run 3','Run 4'); msg = 'Done!';

%%%%%%%%%%%%%%%%%%%%%%%%%%%%%%%%%%%%%%%%%%%%%%%%%%%%%%%%%%%%%%%%

function [W,y,rhoN] = fasticaBSS(numiter,Gam,v);
[m,ntr] = size(v);
W = eye(m); y = zeros(m,ntr); rhoB = zeros(1,numiter+1);
C = W*Gam; C2 = C.^2;
rhoN(1) = 10*log10((m-sum(max(C2)./sum(C2)
                     +max(C2')./sum(C2'))/2)/(m-1));
for i=1:numiter;
     for j=1:m
          y(j,:) = W(j,:)*v;
          f = y(j,:).^3;
          W(j,:) = (1/ntr)*f*v' - 3*W(j,:);
          Wnew = W(j,:) - (W(j,:)*W(1:j-1,:)')*W(1:j-1,:);
          W(j,:) = Wnew/norm(Wnew);
     end;
     C = W*Gam; C2 = C.^2;
     rhoN(i+1) = 10*log10((m-sum(max(C2)./sum(C2)+max(C2')./
                    sum(C2'))/2)/(m-1));
end;
```

7.8 MATLAB code for contrast function optimization BSS using the fastICA algorithm.

To evaluate the algorithm's deconvolution performance, we computed the performance metric

$$\rho_f(k) = \frac{M+1}{M}\left[1 - \left(\frac{\max\limits_{0\le l\le M} |c_l(k)|^2}{\sum\limits_{l=0}^{M} |c_l(k)|^2}\right)\right] \tag{7.77}$$

where $c_l(k)$ is the truncated impulse response of the combined mixing/separation system given by

$$c_l(k) = -\alpha c_{l-1}(k) + \alpha^* w_l(k) + w_{l-1}(k), \qquad 0 \leq l \leq M \tag{7.78}$$

and $M = 3L$. This performance metric measures the deviation of the combined system from a scaled unit impulse. In fact, it can be shown that

- $0 \leq \rho_f(k) \leq 1$ for all impulse responses $c_l(k)$.
- $\rho_f(k) = 1$ if and only if $|c_i(k)|^2 = |c_j(k)|^2$ for all i and j in the range $[0, M]$ (i.e., a maximally convolved source sequence in the system's output).
- $\rho_f(k) = 0$ if and only if $c_i(k) = d\delta(i - \Delta)$ for some non-zero constant d and integer delay Δ in the range $[0, M]$ (i.e., a deconvolved source sequence in the system's output).
- For finite-energy impulse responses $c_l(k)$, $\rho_f(k)$ tends to a fixed value as $M \to \infty$.

Figure 7.9 shows the evolution of $\rho(Ni)$ for four different simulation runs of the fastdeconv algorithm. In each case, we have used a single block of $N = 5000$ samples to compute all coefficient

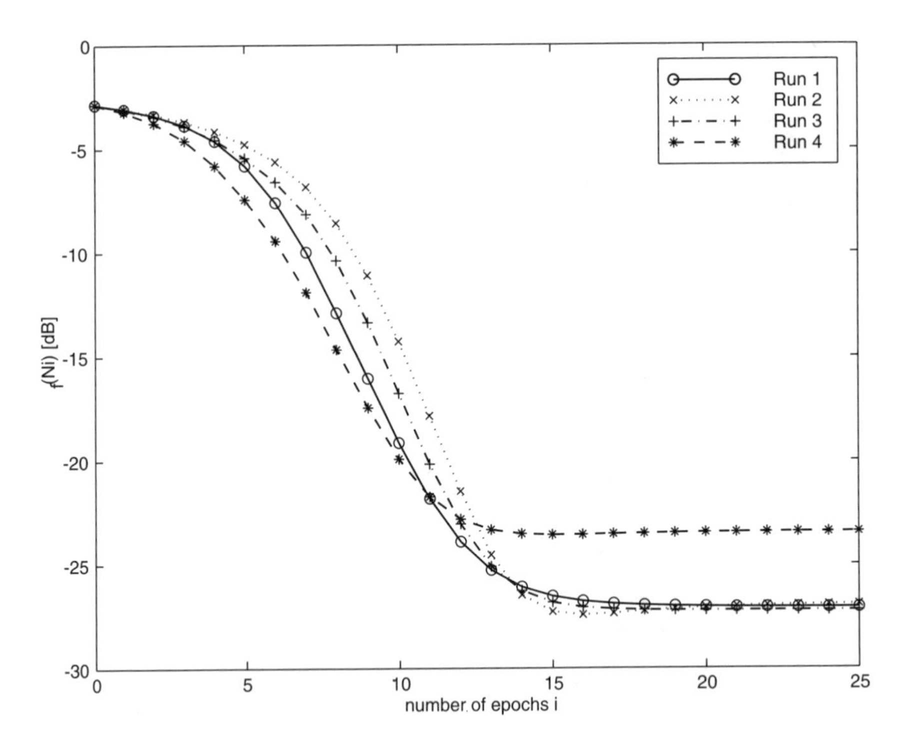

7.9 Evolutions of $\rho_f(k)$ for four different runs of the fastdeconv blind deconvolution algorithm. (Figure 7.10 contains the MATLAB code for this figure.)

updates for the given run, where $\mathbf{x}(k + Ni) = \mathbf{x}(k)$ for all integer values $i \geq 0$ and $0 \leq k \leq N - 1$. The MATLAB program `fastdeconvex.m` used to generate this figure is provided in Figure 7.10. As can be seen, the algorithm takes about twenty epochs to converge. Depending on the simulation run, the steady-state value of the performance factor varies from −24dB to −27dB due to random differences in the source signal sequences across each run. Figure 7.11 shows the signal constellations of the source sequence $s(k)$, the mixed signal sequence $v(k)$, and the extracted output sequence $y(k)$ for the fourth simulation run. Clearly, the source signal distribution has been nearly restored at

```
function [msg] = fastdeconvex();
nepoch = 25; ntr = 5000; L = 24; alpha = 0.7*exp(j*pi/3);
rhoN = zeros(4,nepoch+1); m = 0:nepoch;
for i=1:4;
     t1 = rand(1,ntr); t2 = rand(1,ntr);
     s = (-3 + 2*(t1>0.25) + 2*(t1>0.5) + 2*(t1>0.75));
     s = s + j*(-3 + 2*(t2>0.25) + 2*(t2>0.5) + 2*(t2>0.75));
     v = filter([conj(alpha) 1],[1 alpha],s); v = v/std(v);
     [W,y,rhof(i,:)] = fastdeconv(nepoch,L,alpha,v);
end;
figure(1);
plot(m,rhof(1,:),'o-',m,rhof(2,:),'x:',m,rhof(3,:),'+-.',
     m,rhof(4,:),'*--');
xlabel('number of epochs i'); ylabel('\rho_f(Ni) [dB]');
legend('Run 1','Run 2','Run 3','Run 4');
figure(2);
subplot(2,2,1); plot(s(L:ntr),'o'); xlabel('Re\{s(k)\}');
ylabel('Im\{s(k)\}');
axis('square'); axis([-4 4 -4 4]);
subplot(2,2,2); plot(v(L:ntr),'.'); xlabel('Re\{v(k)\}');
ylabel('Im\{v(k)\}');
axis('square'); axis([-3 3 -3 3]);
subplot(2,1,2); plot(y(L:ntr),'.'); xlabel('Re\{y(k)\}');
ylabel('Im\{y(k)\}');
axis('square'); axis([-2 2 -2 2]);
msg = 'Done!';
%%%%%%%%%%%%%%%%%%%%%%%%%%%%%%%%%%%%%%%%%%%%%%%%%%%%%%%%%%
function [W,y,rhof] = fastdeconv(nepoch,L,alpha,v);
ntr = length(v); M = 3*L;
W = zeros(L+1,1); W(round(L/2)) = 1;
y = zeros(1,ntr); rhof = zeros(1,nepoch+1);
ll = 1:L; llp1 = ll+1; V = zeros(L+1,1);
C = filter([conj(alpha) 1],[1 alpha],
           [W;zeros(M-L,1)]); C2 = C.*conj(C);
rhof(1) = 10*log10((M+1)*(1 - max(C2)/sum(C2))/M);
for i=1:nepoch;
     y = filter(W,1,v);  FV = zeros(L+1,1);
     for j=1:ntr;
          V(llp1) = V(ll);
          V(1) = v(j);
          FV = FV + abs(y(j))^2*y(j)*conj(V);
     end;
     W = (1/ntr)*FV - 3*W;
     W = ifft(sign(fft(W)));
     C = filter([conj(alpha) 1],[1 alpha],[W;zeros(M-L,1)]);
     C2 = C.*conj(C);
     rhof(i+1) = 10*log10((M+1)*(1 - max(C2)/sum(C2))/M);
end;
```

7.10 MATLAB code for contrast function optimization blind deconvolution using the fastdeconv algorithm.

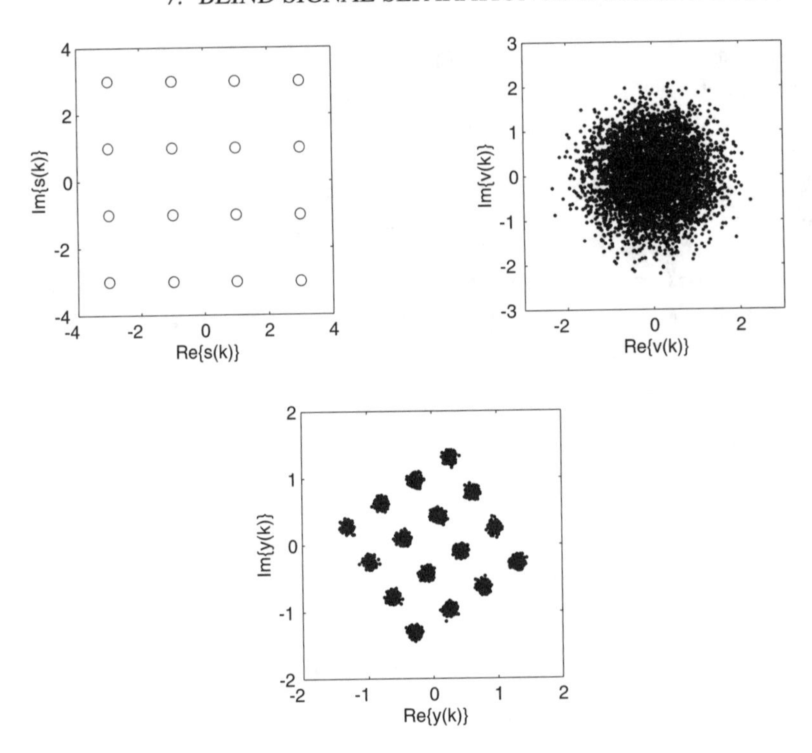

7.11 Scatter plots of the complex data values in (a) $s(k)$, (b) $x(k)$, and (c) $y(k)$ after convergence of the fastdeconv algorithm for a single simulation run.

the deconvolution filter's output, up to a complex-valued scale factor. It should be noted that the fastICA algorithm can be applied to the blind deconvolution task, whereby the coefficient vector $[w_0(k)\ w_1(k) \ldots w_L(k)]^T$ is normalized to unit length after each adjustment. This approach only produces a steady-state value of the performance factor between -13dB and 21dB for the same data, however. The fastdeconv algorithm provides superior performance due to its use of the allpass filter constraint for prewhitened signal mixtures.

7.5.3 BSS for Convolutive Mixtures

One possible application of BSS for convolutive mixtures is the separation of musical instrument sounds in multichannel audio recordings. Such processing methods could be used to isolate individual musical performances for analysis (e.g., through automated pitch recognition [43]), or they could be a first processing step towards the removal of individual musical performances (e.g., for creating karaoke-type recordings). We now describe some preliminary experiments that explore the behavior of a version of the natural gradient multichannel blind deconvolution algorithm in Equations (7.69) and (7.70) for separating a male–female *a cappella* duet in a CD-quality stereo audio recording [44]. This 16-bit PCM stereo recording sampled at $f_s = 44.1$kHz contains close harmonies with significant spectral overlap of the individual vocalists' voices as well as some reverberation effects.

The algorithm used in the experiments employed a block-based update whereby $L + 1$ individual updates of the form of the right-hand side of Equation (7.69) were summed across each block. By choosing $(L + 1)$ to be a power of two, we can implement all filtering and block averaging steps within the update using fast convolution procedures. The resulting implementation has computational elements that are similar to the block LMS algorithm in frequency-domain adaptive filtering [45].

We have chosen the output nonlinearity $f(y) = f_i(y)$ within the algorithm as

$$f(y) = \text{sgn}(y) = \begin{cases} 1 & \text{if } y \geq 0 \\ -1 & \text{if } y < 0 \,. \end{cases} \tag{7.79}$$

This choice is motivated by statistical studies of human speech [46]. These studies indicate that human speech has a nearly Laplacian amplitude PDF, which yields the nonlinearity in Equation (7.79) through the relationship below Equation (7.13). As for the step size matrix $\mathbf{M}(k)$ in the coefficient updates, we have chosen the diagonal entries of this matrix as

$$\mu_i(k) = \frac{\mu_0}{\beta + \sum_{j=L}^{2L} y_i(k-j) f(y_i(k-j))} \tag{7.80}$$

where μ_0 and β are fixed constants. Such choices make the resulting updates less sensitive to long-term changes in output signal amplitudes. The relevant parameter choices were $L = 4095$, $\mu_0 = 5/L$, and $\beta = 0.01$.

Because the impulse responses of the individual source-to-recording transfer functions of the two-channel recorded mixture are unavailable, it is challenging to determine the level of crosstalk in either the original mixtures or in the separated signals. Rather than employ a separation metric, we provide spectrograms of the individual channels. Figure 7.12a and b shows the spectrograms of the left and right channels, respectively, of the original recording over the interval $113 \leq t \leq 114.2$ sec. In these segments, the male singer is singing the syllables "I'm gon-na tell her now that" at different pitches, whereas the female singer is holding the "short-i" vowel sound of the word "him" at a single pitch. The female singer's voice clearly provides the dominant features in both spectrograms. Figure 7.13a and b is the spectrograms of the left and right channels, respectively, of the separation system's stereo output over the same time interval, in which the system has been adapted in a single pass over the previous 112 seconds of music. As can be seen, the male's voice is enhanced in the left output channel, whereas the female's voice is enhanced in the right output channel. Informal experiments with both trained and untrained listeners indicate that the individual singers' voices are easier to distinguish in each of the separation system's outputs.

One artifact of the processing method is a whitening of the output signals, such that the extracted signals have increased energy at high frequencies. While this artifact does not significantly affect the intelligibilities of the extracted outputs, it would have to be compensated for in a high-quality audio application. In situations where the source signals have easily characterized temporal features, this separation method can actually result in partial temporal deconvolution of the corresponding source signals. For example, experiments in separating a male voice–piano duet yielded an extracted piano signal in which the characteristic near-exponential envelope of the piano notes was shortened to a near-impulsive envelope. To avoid this problem, algorithms must be developed that do not impose specific temporal structure on the extracted output signals, as do all multichannel blind deconvolution algorithms. See Douglas [42] for a discussion of these issues.

7.6 Conclusions and Open Issues

This chapter has described the related problems of blind signal separation and blind deconvolution. Various formulations of each problem have been given, and each of these formulations yields several useful algorithms for practical implementation. In addition, we have described the spatio-temporal extensions of blind signal separation for convolutive mixtures and multichannel blind deconvolution. Examples illustrate the usefulness of several algorithms for BSS and blind deconvolution tasks.

While BSS and blind deconvolution are well studied topics, numerous issues remain largely unresolved in these fields. Some of the most important open issues are now discussed:

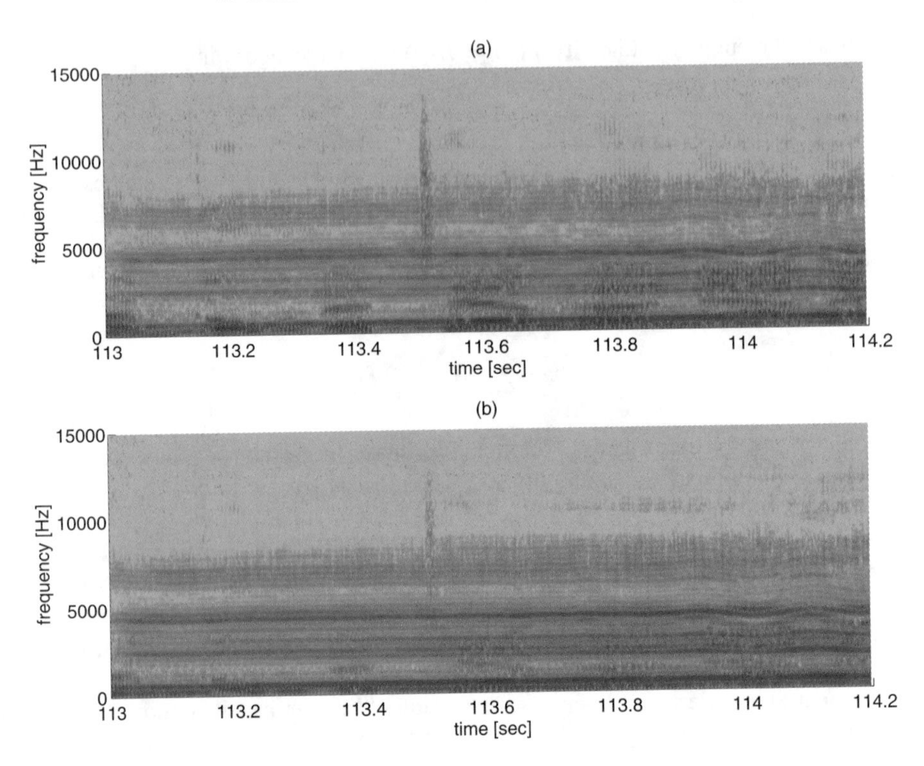

7.12 Spectrograms of the (a) left and (b) right channels of the original male–female *a cappella* duet audio recording.

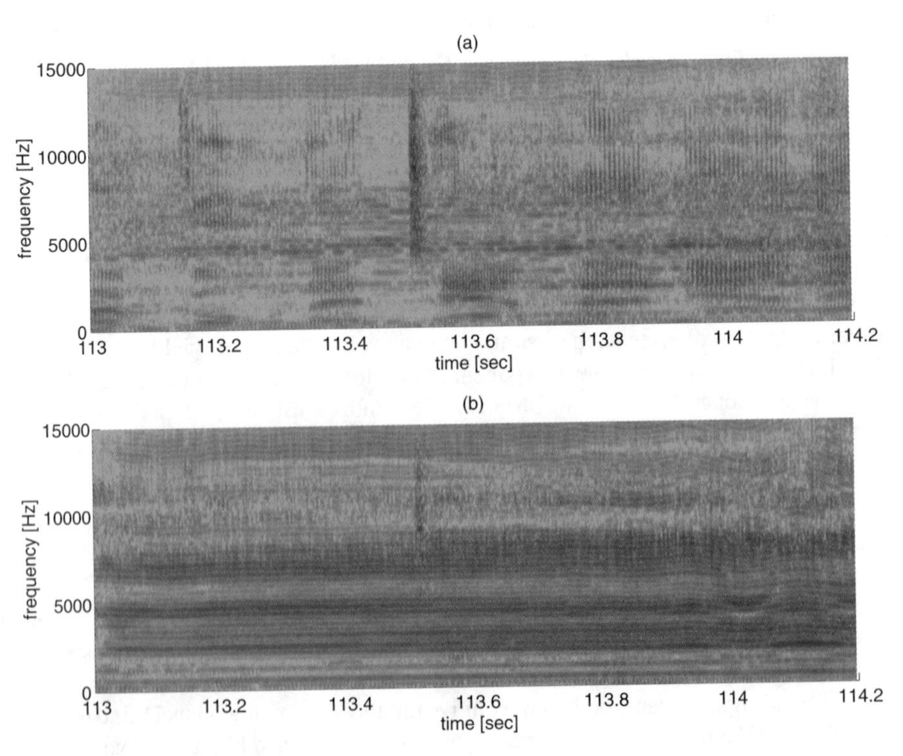

7.13 Spectrograms of the (a) left and (b) right output channels of the separation system as applied to the male–female *a cappella* duet audio recording.

Step size/data block size choices — Almost all BSS and blind deconvolution algorithms employ the received signals to train a set of system coefficients. For iterative training methods that employ an algorithm step size, one must choose the value of this step size in real-world applications. In algorithms that train on blocks of received data, such as the fastICA algorithm, the size of the data block must be selected. Both choices affect the degree of separation and/or deconvolution achieved. Theoretical analyses of the impacts of these choices on overall system behavior appear to be difficult to perform in all but the simplest situations. Currently, trial and error adjustment of these parameters appears to be the best way to design such systems.

Speed of convergence and tracking behavior — Iterative algorithms that employ non-quadratic blind criteria for training purposes often suffer from slow convergence properties. Such slow convergence properties hamper the use of these algorithms in some practical situations. In addition, slow convergence may prevent adequate tracking of unknown system conditions in situations where the unknown system is changing with time.

Generalized criteria for BSS and blind deconvolution — Many BSS and blind deconvolution methods are designed to separate only a certain class of signal types (such as spatially independent sources with a negative kurtosis). When some of the source signals in the signal mixtures do not fall into the appropriate signal class, a given algorithm usually fails to adequately separate any signals. It would be desirable to design separation/deconvolution criteria that separate/deconvolve source signals from a wider class, such as all spatially independent sources or all temporally independent sources.

"Separating" more signals than measurements — When the number of sources m is greater than the number of sensors n, it is impossible to design a linear separation system that extracts all source signals. The problem is one of dimensionality; that is, the combined system matrix $\mathbf{C}(k)$ can only be of rank $\min\{m, n\}$. It remains an open problem how to extract useful source estimates in such situations. Such problems have significant practical interest, as it is often the case that mixtures of a great many source signals are measured by only a few sensors in an array.

Using temporal information of the sources in convolutive BSS — Algorithms for separating convolutive mixtures of temporally dependent sources should not significantly modify the temporal structure of the source signals. It appears impossible, however, to know which temporal features are channel-dependent (i.e., multipath propagation) and which are signal-dependent (i.e., source content). Moreover, imposing a temporal structure to the extracted sources requires a temporal model of the source signals, which is generally unavailable.

Despite these challenges, the fields of BSS, blind deconvolution, multichannel blind deconvolution, and convolutive BSS are highly active, with many advances being developed by researchers in these fields. For those who are interested in developing advancements in the field, the references at the end of this chapter provide good starting points for future efforts.

References

[1] A.J. Paulraj and C.B. Papadias, Space-time processing for wireless communications, *IEEE Signal Processing Magazine,* vol. 14, no. 6, pp. 49–83, 1997.

[2] M.J. McKeown, S. Makeig, G.G. Brown, T.P. Jung, S.S. Kindermann, A.J. Bell, and T.J. Sejnowski, Analysis of fMRI data by blind separation into independent spatial components, *Human Brain Mapping,* vol. 6, pp. 160–188, 1998.

[3] K. Torkkola, Blind separation of delayed and convolved sources, in *Unsupervised Adaptive Filtering, Vol. I: Blind Signal Separation,* S. Haykin, Ed., (New York: John Wiley & Sons, 2000), pp. 321–375.
[4] S.U.H. Qureshi, Adaptive equalization, *Proceedings of the IEEE,* vol. 73, pp. 1349–1387, 1985.
[5] E.A. Robinson and S. Treitel, *Geophysical Signal Analysis,* (Englewood Cliffs, NJ: Prentice-Hall, 1980).
[6] P.A. Jansson, Ed., *Deconvolution of Images and Spectra,* 2nd. ed., (San Diego, CA: Academic Press, 1997).
[7] S. Bose and B. Friedlander, On the direct estimation of the Wiener beamformer using second and fourth-order cumulants, *Proceedings of the 31st Asilomar Conference on Signals, Systems, and Computing,* Pacific Grove, CA, vol. 1, pp. 370–374, 1997.
[8] S.C. Douglas, Combined subspace tracking, prewhitening, and contrast optimization for noisy blind signal separation, *Proceedings of the IEEE International Workshop Indep. Compon. Anal. Signal Sep.,* Helsinki, Finland, pp. 579–584, Jan. 2000.
[9] K. Matsuoka, M. Ohya, and M. Kawamoto, A neural net for blind separation of nonstationary signal sources, *Neural Networks,* vol. 8, no. 3, pp. 411–419, 1995.
[10] M.K. Tsatsanis and C. Kweon, Blind source separation of non-stationary sources using second-order statistics, *Proceedings of the 32th Asilomar Conference on Signals, Systems, and Computing,* Pacific Grove, CA, vol. 2, pp. 1574–1578, 1998.
[11] D.T. Pham and J.F. Cardoso, Blind separation of instantaneous mixtures of non stationary sources, *IEEE Transactions on Signal Processing,* in press.
[12] T.M. Cover and J.A. Thomas, *Elements of Information Theory,* (New York: John Wiley & Sons, 1991).
[13] A.J. Bell and T.J. Sejnowski, An information maximization approach to blind separation and blind deconvolution, *Neural Computation,* vol. 7, pp. 1129–1159, 1995.
[14] S. Amari, A. Cichocki, and H.H. Yang, A new learning algorithm for blind signal separation, *Advances in Neural Information Processing Systems 8,* (Cambridge, MA: MIT Press, 1996), pp. 757–763.
[15] J.F. Cardoso, Blind signal separation: statistical principles, *Proceedings of the IEEE,* vol. 86, pp. 2009–2025, 1998.
[16] S. Amari, T.P. Chen, and A. Cichocki, Stability analysis of learning algorithms for blind source separation, *Neural Networks,* vol. 10, no. 8, pp. 1345–1351, 1997.
[17] D.G. Luenberger, *Linear and Nonlinear Programming,* 2nd. ed., (Reading, MA: Addison-Wesley, 1984).
[18] S.I. Amari, Natural gradient works efficiently in learning, *Neural Computation,* vol. 10, pp. 251–276, 1998.
[19] S.C. Douglas and S.I. Amari, Natural gradient adaptation, in *Unsupervised Adaptive Filtering, vol. I: Blind Signal Separation,* S. Haykin, Ed., (New York: John Wiley & Sons, 2000), pp. 13–61.
[20] P. Comon, Independent component analysis: A new concept? *Signal Processing,* vol. 36, pp. 287–314, 1994.
[21] S.C. Douglas and A. Cichocki, Neural networks for blind decorrelation of signals, *IEEE Transactions on Signal Processing,* vol. 45, pp. 2829–2842, 1997.
[22] A. Hyvärinen and E. Oja, A fast fixed-point algorithm for independent component analysis, *Neural Computation,* vol. 9, no. 7, pp. 1483–1492, 1997.
[23] S.Y. Kung, Independent component analysis: extrema-correspondence properties for higher-order moment functions, in *Proceedings of the IEEE Workshop on Neural Networks Signal Processing,* Cambridge, UK, pp. 53–62, Aug. 1998.
[24] L. Molgedey and H.G. Schuster, Separation of a mixture of independent signals using time delayed correlations, *Physics Review Letters,* no. 72, no. 23, pp. 3634–3637, 1994.
[25] A. Belouchrani, K. Abed-Meraim, J.F. Cardoso, and E. Moulines, A blind source separation technique using second-order statistics, *IEEE Transactions on Signal Processing,* vol. 45, pp. 434–444, 1997.
[26] K.I. Diamantaras, Asymmetric PCA neural networks for adaptive blind source separation, *Proceedings of the IEEE Workshop on Neural Networks Signal Processing,* Cambridge, UK, pp. 103–112, Aug. 1998.
[27] S. Haykin, *Adaptive Filter Theory,* 3rd. ed., (Englewood Cliffs, NJ: Prentice-Hall, 1996.)
[28] S.C. Douglas and S. Haykin, Relationships between blind deconvolution and blind source separation, in *Unsupervised Adaptive Filtering, Vol. II: Blind Deconvolution,* S. Haykin, Ed., (New York: John Wiley & Sons, 2000), pp. 113–145.

[29] R.M. Gray, Toeplitz and circulant matrices: a review, Technical Rept. no. 6504–1, Information Systems Laboratory, Stanford University, Stanford, CA, April 1977.
[30] S.C. Douglas and S.Y. Kung, Gradient adaptive algorithms for contrast-based blind deconvolution, *Journal of VLSI Signal Processing Systems,* vol. 26, no. 1/2, pp. 47–60, 2000.
[31] S. Amari, S.C. Douglas, A. Cichocki, and H.H. Yang, Multichannel blind deconvolution and equalization using the natural gradient, *Proceedings of the IEEE Workshop on Signal Processing and Advances in Wireless Communication,* Paris, France, pp. 101–104, Apr. 1997.
[32] P.P. Vaidyanathan, *Multirate Systems and Filter Banks,* (Englewood Cliffs, NJ: Prentice-Hall, 1993).
[33] S.C. Douglas, S. Amari, and S.Y. Kung, Adaptive paraunitary filter banks for spatio-temporal principal and minor subspace analysis, *Proceedings of IEEE International Conference on Acoustics, Speech, and Signal Processing,* Phoenix, AZ, vol. 2, pp. 1089–1092, Mar. 1999.
[34] X. Sun and S.C. Douglas, Multichannel blind deconvolution of arbitrary signals: adaptive algorithms and stability analyses, *Proceedings of the 34th Asilomar Conference on Signals, Systems, and Computing,* Pacific Grove, CA, Oct. 2000.
[35] E. Weinstein, M. Feder, and A.V. Oppenheim, Multi-channel signal separation by decorrelation, *IEEE Transactions on Signal Processing,* vol. 1, pp. 405–413, 1993.
[36] S. Van Gerven and D. Van Compernolle, Signal separation by symmetric adaptive decorrelation: stability, convergence, and uniqueness, *IEEE Transactions on Signal Processing,* vol. 43, pp. 1602–1612, 1995.
[37] K.C. Yen and Y. Zhao, Adaptive co-channel speech separation and recognition, *IEEE Transactions on Speech Audio Processing,* vol. 7, pp. 138–151, 1999.
[38] L. Parra and C. Spence, Convolutive blind separation of non-stationary sources, *IEEE Transactions Speech Audio Processing,* vol. 8, pp. 320–327, 2000.
[39] R.H. Lambert, Multichannel blind deconvolution: FIR matrix algebra and separation of multipath mixtures, Ph.D. dissertation, University of Southern California, Los Angeles, 1996.
[40] R.H. Lambert and A.J. Bell, Blind separation of multiple speakers in a multipath environment, *Proceedings of the IEEE International Conference on Acoustics, Speech, and Signal Processing,* Munich, Germany, vol. 1, pp. 423–426, Apr. 1997.
[41] S. Amari, S.C. Douglas, A. Cichocki, and H.H. Yang, Novel online adaptive learning algorithms for blind deconvolution using the natural gradient approach, *Proceedings of the 11th IFAC Symposium on Systems Identification,* Kitakyushu City, Japan, vol. 3, pp. 1057–1062, July 1997.
[42] S.C. Douglas, Blind separation of acoustic signals, in *Microphone Arrays: Techniques and Applications,* M. Brandstein and D. Ward, Eds., (New York: Springer-Verlag, 2001).
[43] S. Jones, R. Meddis, S.C. Lim, and A.R. Temple, Toward a digital neuromorphic pitch extraction system, *IEEE Transactions on Neural Networks,* vol. 11, pp. 978–987, July 2000.
[44] The Bobs, Boy around the corner, from *Songs For Tomorrow Morning,* Rhino Records, 1988 [audio recording].
[45] J.J. Shynk, Frequency-domain and multirate adaptive filtering, *IEEE Signal Processing Magazine,* vol. 9, pp. 14–37, 1992.
[46] W.P. Davenport, Jr., A study of speech probability distributions, Tech. Rep. no. 148, MIT Research Laboratory of Electronics, Cambridge, MA, Aug. 1950.

8

Neural Networks and Principal Component Analysis

Konstantinos I. Diamantaras
Technological Education Institute of Thessaloniki

8.1 Introduction

Self-organization is one of the most important learning paradigms of neural systems. The ability to adapt to the environment without the provision of an external teacher is encountered in nature in most intelligent organisms. In this paradigm, the lack of teaching signals is compensated for by an inner purpose, i.e., some built-in criterion or objective function that the system seeks to optimize. Typically, the purpose is either (1) the extraction of significant features of the input data, or (2) the clustering of the data in neighborhoods based on similarity.

The discussion in this chapter is restricted to the class of feature-extracting unsupervised neural networks. We analyze the close relationship between the biologically motivated Hebbian self-organizing principle which governs neural assemblies and the classical principal component analysis (PCA) method used by statisticians for almost a century for multivariate data analysis and feature extraction. Both ends of the connection have appealing properties. On one end, Hebbian learning is based on the principles of simplicity and locality. Simplicity is, of course, intuitively appealing. Locality conforms with neurobiological evidence that does not favor action at great distance. According to this evidence, synapses are not likely to be modified based on electrical activity that happens far away from them. On the other end, PCA is also appealing because it is the optimal linear dimensionality reduction method. This has been known in the statistics community for a long time. The method first appeared in the works of Pearson [1] on linear regression and Hotelling [2] on psychometry. Donald Hebb also proposed his learning principle many decades ago [3]. The connection between the two, however, came much later in the works of Oja [4] and Karhunen [5]. Since then, the literature on PCA neural networks has multiplied. In addition to self-organized networks, other

0-8493-2359-2/01/$0.00+$1.50

models were also found to be related to PCA, such as linear auto-associative back-propagation networks. More recently, extensions to the classical PCA models were proposed to cope with nonlinear data dependencies. Classical PCA is based on the second-order statistics of the data and, in particular, on the eigenstructure of the data covariance matrix. Classical PCA neural models incorporate only cells with linear activation functions. Nonlinear PCA involves higher than second-order statistics, and it is implemented with neural models incorporating nonlinear units.

The chapter is organized as follows. Section 8.2 discusses the PCA method from a strictly statistical point of view. We offer the basic PCA theorem along with examples illustrating the related concepts. Section 8.3 introduces and analyzes the Hebbian learning principle from a pure neurobiological perspective. Section 8.4 studies the models and algorithms of PCA neural networks. We make the connection between PCA and Hebbian learning and we present the most prominent unsupervised neural models based on the Hebbian rule. Furthermore, we show that linear back-propagation models are related to PCA when operating in auto-associative mode. Finally, Section 8.5 discusses nonlinear PCA extensions and corresponding models.

8.2 Principal Component Analysis

Principal component analysis (PCA) is a classical linear feature extraction method. It is based on the analysis of the second order statistics of the data, and, in particular, the eigenvalue analysis of the covariance matrix. PCA is essentially equivalent to the Karhunen–Loève transform used in signal and image processing. The roots of PCA come from the work of Pearson [1] almost a century ago. Pearson proposed a linear regression method in n dimensions based on least squares optimization. However, the "father" of PCA is considered to be Hotelling, who proposed a new method for the variance analysis of multidimensional random variables [2].

The method is concerned with the analysis of multivariate observations. These observations can describe anything from stock prices to biometrical data of the turtle. The basic idea comes from the fact that, in many such measurements, the n observation variables $x_1, \ldots, x_n$ can be well fitted by an m-parametric surface where m is much smaller than n. This means that there are, in fact, m hidden degrees of freedom corresponding to some underlying parameters $y_1, \ldots, y_m$. We can say that n is the superficial dimensionality of $\mathbf{x}$, while m is its intrinsic dimensionality. The hidden parameters y_i are called factors or features, and $\mathbf{y} = [y_1, \ldots, y_m]^T$ is the feature vector.

To illustrate these concepts, we consider the following simplified scenario where the observation variables $x_1, \ldots, x_n$ can be written as perfect (noiseless) functions of m hidden uncorrelated factors $y_1, \ldots, y_m$.

$$
\begin{aligned}
x_1 &= f_1(y_1, \ldots, y_m) = f_1(\mathbf{y}) \\
&\vdots \\
x_n &= f_n(y_1, \ldots, y_m) = f_n(\mathbf{y}) .
\end{aligned}
\tag{8.1}
$$

In this scenario, the observation vector $\mathbf{x}$ lies in an m-parametric surface described by the vector function $\mathbf{f}(\mathbf{y}) = [f_1(\mathbf{y}), \ldots, f_n(\mathbf{y})]^T$. PCA treats the case where the functions $f_1(), \ldots, f_n()$, are linear:

$$
\begin{aligned}
x_1 &= \mathbf{f}_1^T \mathbf{y} \\
&\vdots \\
x_n &= \mathbf{f}_n^T \mathbf{y}
\end{aligned}
\tag{8.2}
$$

where we took the liberty of writing $\mathbf{f}_i^T \mathbf{y}$ instead of the function $f_i(\mathbf{y})$. More compactly, we can express the observation vector $\mathbf{x}$ as a linear function of the feature vector $\mathbf{y}$

$$\mathbf{x} = \mathbf{F}\mathbf{y} \tag{8.3}$$

where $\mathbf{F}$ is an $n \times m$ matrix ($m < n$). In this case, the surface described by the function $\mathbf{f}(\mathbf{y}) = \mathbf{F}\mathbf{y}$ is an m-dimensional hyperplane in $\mathbb{R}^n$. $\mathbf{F}$ is a "tall" matrix, i.e., it has more rows than columns. If $\mathbf{F}$ is known, then the features can be obtained from a linear operation on the data

$$\mathbf{y} = \mathbf{F}^{+}\mathbf{x} \tag{8.4}$$

where the superscript $^{+}$ denotes matrix pseudoinverse. PCA's task is to extract the hyperplane corresponding to $\mathbf{F}$ and the feature vector that lies on this hyperplane when $\mathbf{F}$ is unknown.

An interesting point to note is the close relationship among the observation variables x_i derived from Equation (8.3) and $m < n$. Consider any subset of m observation variables such as, for example, the subset $\{x_1, \ldots, x_m\}$. Let us partition

$$\mathbf{x} = \begin{bmatrix} x_1 \\ \vdots \\ x_m \\ \hline x_{m+1} \\ \vdots \\ x_n \end{bmatrix} = \begin{bmatrix} \mathbf{x}^{\mathrm{m}} \\ \hline \mathbf{x}^{\mathrm{n\text{-}m}} \end{bmatrix}, \qquad \mathbf{F} = \begin{bmatrix} \mathbf{f}_1^T \\ \vdots \\ \mathbf{f}_m^T \\ \hline \mathbf{f}_{m+1}^T \\ \vdots \\ \mathbf{f}_n^T \end{bmatrix} = \begin{bmatrix} \mathbf{F}_m \\ \hline \mathbf{F}_{n-m} \end{bmatrix}$$

and rewrite Equation (8.3) as

$$\begin{bmatrix} \mathbf{x}^{\mathrm{m}} \\ \mathbf{x}^{\mathrm{n\text{-}m}} \end{bmatrix} = \begin{bmatrix} \mathbf{F}_m \\ \mathbf{F}_{n-m} \end{bmatrix} \mathbf{y} .$$

Assuming that the $m \times m$ matrix $\mathbf{F}_m$ is invertible, we have $\mathbf{y} = \mathbf{F}_m^{-1}\mathbf{x}^{\mathrm{m}}$, and

$$\mathbf{x}^{\mathrm{n\text{-}m}} = \mathbf{F}_{n-m}\mathbf{F}_m^{-1}\mathbf{x}^{\mathrm{m}} . \tag{8.5}$$

So, the remaining $n - m$ variables, $x_{m+1}, \ldots, x_n$, are linear functions of the first m variables,

$$\begin{aligned} x_{m+1} &= \mathbf{g}_{m+1}^T \mathbf{x}^{\mathrm{m}} \\ &\vdots \\ x_n &= \mathbf{g}_n^T \mathbf{x}^{\mathrm{m}} \end{aligned} \tag{8.6}$$

$$\mathbf{G} = \left[\mathbf{g}_{m+1}, \ldots, \mathbf{g}_n\right]^T = \mathbf{F}_{n-m}\mathbf{F}_m^{-1} . \tag{8.7}$$

Moreover, if the covariance $E\{\mathbf{x}_m\mathbf{x}_m^T\}$ is positive definite, then there is a non-zero correlation between $\mathbf{x}_{n-m}$ and $\mathbf{x}_m$:

$$E\left\{\mathbf{x}_{n-m}\mathbf{x}_m^T\right\} = \mathbf{G}E\left\{\mathbf{x}_m\mathbf{x}_m^T\right\} \neq 0 \tag{8.8}$$

Equation (8.8) touches on a key characteristic of PCA: if there exists an m-dimensional hyperplane $\mathbf{x} = \mathbf{F}\mathbf{y}$ that describes the data, then the observation variables are correlated. Conversely, if there is complete correlation between a subset of the observation variables and the rest of the observation variables, then there must exist a hyperplane describing the data. In the extreme case where the variables $x_1, \ldots, x_n$ are totally uncorrelated, no relation such as Equation (8.5) can be derived for any $m < n$, and PCA will not be of much use.

In the following, we give a more rigorous treatment of PCA while simultaneously considering the most general case where the data do not lie exactly on some linear subspace of $\mathbb{R}^n$. Consider the random observation vector $\mathbf{x}$, with mean $E\{\mathbf{x}\} = 0$ and positive definite covariance matrix $\mathbf{R}_x = E\{\mathbf{x}\mathbf{x}^T\}$. According to our previous scenario, if the intrinsic dimensionality of $\mathbf{x}$ is m, then we may perfectly reconstruct the data $\mathbf{x}$ from the feature vector $\mathbf{y}$ using Equation (8.3) and the feature vector from the data using Equation (8.4). In a more realistic scenario, however, the reconstructed vector

$$\hat{\mathbf{x}} = \mathbf{F}\mathbf{y} \tag{8.9}$$

contains an error term $\mathbf{e}$

$$\mathbf{x} = \hat{\mathbf{x}} + \mathbf{e} \tag{8.10}$$

The feature vector $\mathbf{y} \in \mathbb{R}^m$ is a linear function of $\mathbf{x}$

$$\mathbf{y} = \mathbf{W}\mathbf{x} \tag{8.11}$$

where $\mathbf{W} \in \mathbb{R}^{m \times n}$ is a "wide" matrix with fewer rows than columns. Putting all this together, we obtain

$$\mathbf{x} = \mathbf{F}\mathbf{y} + \mathbf{e} = \mathbf{F}\mathbf{W}\mathbf{x} + \mathbf{e}\,.$$

In this general case, the goal of PCA is to minimize the reconstruction error

$$J_e = E\left\{\left\|\mathbf{x} - \hat{\mathbf{x}}\right\|^2\right\}$$

by appropriately selecting the linear feature and reconstruction operators $\mathbf{W}$ and $\mathbf{F}$.

The problem will be solved in two steps: (1) obtain the optimal $\mathbf{W}$ as a function of $\mathbf{F}$, expressing J_e as a function of $\mathbf{F}$ only, and (2) optimize J_e with respect to $\mathbf{F}$. To that end, we rewrite J_e using the matrix trace operator tr(), and we interchange expectation with trace since both are linear operations:

$$\begin{aligned} J_e &= E\left\{\mathrm{tr}\left[\left(\mathbf{x} - \hat{\mathbf{x}}\right)\left(\mathbf{x} - \hat{\mathbf{x}}\right)^T\right]\right\} \\ &= \mathrm{tr}\left\{E\mathbf{x}\mathbf{x}^T\right\} + \mathrm{tr}\left\{E\mathbf{F}\mathbf{W}\mathbf{x}\mathbf{x}^T\mathbf{W}^T\mathbf{F}^T\right\} - 2\,\mathrm{tr}\left\{E\mathbf{F}\mathbf{W}\mathbf{x}\mathbf{x}^T\right\} \\ &= \mathrm{tr}\,\mathbf{R}_x + \mathrm{tr}\left\{\mathbf{F}\mathbf{W}\mathbf{R}_x\mathbf{W}^T\mathbf{F}^T\right\} - 2\,\mathrm{tr}\left\{\mathbf{F}\mathbf{W}\mathbf{R}_x\right\}\,. \end{aligned} \tag{8.12}$$

In the first step, we consider $\mathbf{F}$ to be constant and we optimize J_e with respect to $\mathbf{W}$ by solving the Karush–Kühn–Tucker conditions:

$$\nabla_W J_e = 2\mathbf{F}^T\mathbf{F}\mathbf{W}\mathbf{R}_x - 2\mathbf{F}^T\mathbf{R}_x = 0\,. \tag{8.13}$$

In computing the derivative $\nabla_W J_e$ of J_e with respect to $\mathbf{W}$, we made use of the following facts:

- The trace operator has the property $\mathrm{tr}(\mathbf{AB}) = \mathrm{tr}(\mathbf{BA})$.
- The derivative of $\mathrm{tr}(\mathbf{A}\mathbf{B}^T)$ with respect to the matrix $\mathbf{B}$ is the matrix $\mathbf{A}$.

Now, Equation (8.13) easily leads to the desired relation between $\mathbf{W}$ and $\mathbf{F}$

$$\mathbf{F}^T\mathbf{F}\mathbf{W} = \mathbf{F}^T \tag{8.14}$$

$$\mathbf{W} = \left[\mathbf{F}^T\mathbf{F}\right]^{-1}\mathbf{F}^T = \mathbf{F}^+\,. \tag{8.15}$$

Consequently, the reconstruction error can be simplified into

$$J_e = \operatorname{tr} \mathbf{R}_x + \operatorname{tr}\left[\mathbf{F}\mathbf{F}^+\mathbf{R}_x \left\{\mathbf{F}^+\right\}^T \mathbf{F}^T\right] - 2\operatorname{tr}\left[\mathbf{F}\mathbf{F}^+\mathbf{R}_x\right] \tag{8.16}$$

thus completing step 1 above. In step 2, we define $\mathcal{L}$ to be the m-dimensional subspace spanned by the columns of $\mathbf{F}$. $\mathcal{L}$ is referred to as the feature subspace because it is spanned with the help of the feature vector $\mathbf{y}$. $\mathbf{F}$ being a "tall" matrix, it can be written as the product of an $n \times m$ matrix $\mathbf{U}$, whose columns form an orthonormal basis of $\mathcal{L}$, and an $m \times m$ invertible matrix $\mathbf{T}$

$$\mathbf{F} = \mathbf{U}\mathbf{T}, \qquad \mathbf{U}^T\mathbf{U} = \mathbf{I}\,.$$

Using the above notation, the pseudoinverse of $\mathbf{F}$ is simply $\mathbf{F}^+ = \mathbf{T}^{-1}\mathbf{U}^T$. Substituting into Equation (8.16), we express J_e as a function of $\mathbf{U}$:

$$\begin{aligned} J_e &= \operatorname{tr} \mathbf{R}_x + \operatorname{tr}\left\{\mathbf{U}\mathbf{U}^T\mathbf{R}_x\mathbf{U}\mathbf{U}^T\right\} - 2\operatorname{tr}\{\mathbf{U}\mathbf{U}^T\mathbf{R}_x\} \\ J_e &= \operatorname{tr} \mathbf{R}_x - \operatorname{tr}\left\{\mathbf{U}^T\mathbf{R}_x\mathbf{U}\right\}\,. \end{aligned} \tag{8.17}$$

A first observation is that the error J_e does not depend on the matrix $\mathbf{T}$; therefore, for every minimizer $\mathbf{U}$, there exists an infinite number of solutions $\mathbf{F}$. However, the subspace $\mathcal{L}$ spanned by the columns of $\mathbf{F}$ is the same as the one spanned by the columns of $\mathbf{U}$ since left multiplication by an invertible matrix does not affect the column span

$$\text{span}\, col(\mathbf{F}) = \text{span}\, col(\mathbf{U}\mathbf{T}) = \text{span}\, col(\mathbf{U})\,.$$

So, the optimal $\mathcal{L}$ is invariant for all minimizers $\mathbf{F}$. $\mathcal{L}$ is also known as the principal component subspace (PCS) of dimension m. The projection of the data $\mathbf{x}$ on the PCS $\mathcal{L}$ is the optimal linear reconstruction of $\mathbf{x}$ from m features.

A second observation is that the minimization of mean squared error J_e is equivalent to the maximization of the term

$$J_v = \operatorname{tr}\left\{\mathbf{U}^T\mathbf{R}_x\mathbf{U}\right\} \tag{8.18}$$

which appears in the right-hand side of Equation (8.17). On closer inspection, J_v is recognized to be the variance of the projection of $\mathbf{x}$ on the PCS. Indeed,

$$J_v = \operatorname{tr}\left\{E\mathbf{z}\mathbf{z}^T\right\} = \sum_{i=1}^{m} E z_i^2$$

where $\mathbf{z} = \mathbf{U}^T\mathbf{x}$ is the projection of $\mathbf{x}$ on $\mathcal{L}$ since the columns of $\mathbf{U}$ form an orthonormal basis of $\mathcal{L}$. It follows that the minimization of the mean squared reconstruction error J_e is equivalent to the maximization of the variance J_v of the projection of $\mathbf{x}$. Figure 8.1 illustrates the trade-off between projection error and projection variance. Step 2 of our analysis is completed by the following theorem.

THEOREM 8.1 *(PCA) Let the eigenvalues $\lambda_1, \lambda_2, \ldots, \lambda_n$ of the correlation matrix $\mathbf{R}_x$ be arranged in decreasing order, and the corresponding unit-length eigenvectors are $\mathbf{e}_1, \mathbf{e}_2, \ldots, \mathbf{e}_n$. Then the mean squared error J_e in Equation* (8.17) *is minimized (correspondingly, the variance J_v is maximized) for*

$$\mathbf{F} = \mathbf{U}\mathbf{T}$$

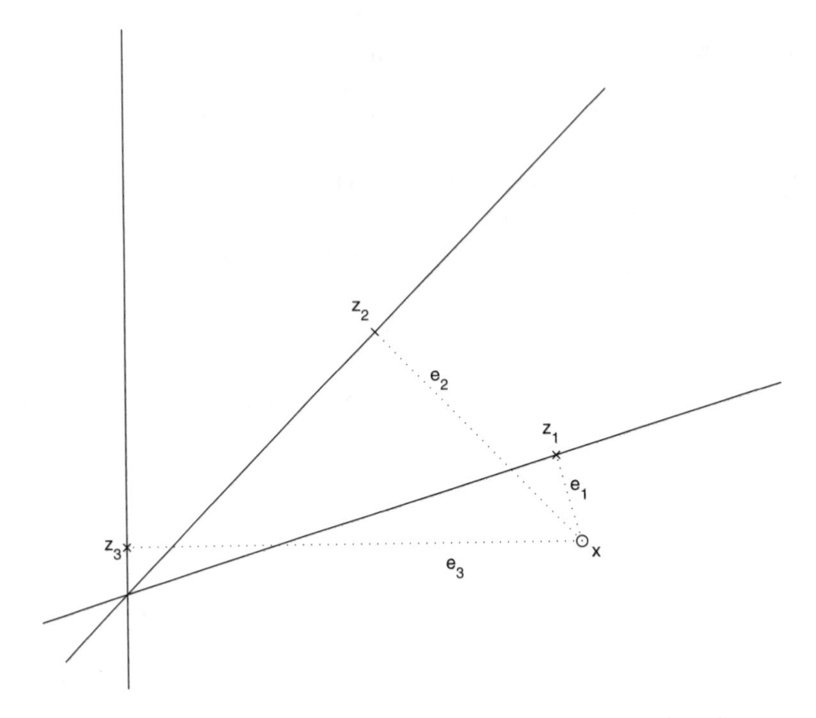

8.1 The antagonistic relationship between projection length and projection error. The points $\mathbf{z}_1$, $\mathbf{z}_2$, and $\mathbf{z}_3$ are projections of the point $\mathbf{x}$ on three different one-dimensional subspaces. Observe that the projection errors $\|\mathbf{e}_i\|$ increase as the projection lengths $\|\mathbf{z}_i\|$ decrease and vice versa.

where

$$\mathbf{U} = [\mathbf{e}_1, \mathbf{e}_2, \ldots, \mathbf{e}_m]^T$$

and $\mathbf{T}$ *is any* $m \times m$*, invertible matrix. The minimum squared error is*

$$\min J_e = \sum_{i=m+1}^{n} \lambda_i$$

while the maximum projection variance is

$$\max J_v = \sum_{i=1}^{m} \lambda_i \,.$$

Some nomenclature is in order here:

The eigenvectors $\mathbf{e}_1, \mathbf{e}_2, \ldots, \mathbf{e}_m$, are called principal eigenvectors.
The eigenvalues $\lambda_1, \ldots, \lambda_m$, are called principal eigenvalues.
The transformation

$$\mathbf{y} = \mathbf{U}\mathbf{x} \tag{8.19}$$

is called the Karhunen–Loève transform (KLT).
The features $y_1, y_2, \ldots, y_m$, which are the components of the transform vector $\mathbf{y}$, are called principal components (PCs).

It is straightforward to obtain the following properties for the PCs:

- The PCs have zero mean:

$$Ey_i = 0, \text{ for all } i$$

- Different PCs are uncorrelated with each other:

$$Ey_i y_j = 0, \quad i \neq j$$

- The variance of the ith PC is equal to the ith eigenvalue:

$$\text{var}(y_i) = Ey_i^2 = E\left(\mathbf{e}_i^T \mathbf{x}\right)^2 = \mathbf{e}_i^T \mathbf{R}_x \mathbf{e}_i = \lambda_i$$

- The components are hierarchically organized with respect to their variance. The first PC (y_1) has the largest variance, the second PC (y_2) has the second largest variance, and the last PC (y_m) has the smallest one:

$$\text{var}(y_1) > \text{var}(y_2) > \cdots > \text{var}(y_m) \ .$$

If, as it often happens in practice, the eigenvalues of $\mathbf{R}_x$ decay rapidly towards zero, then the basic corollary of Theorem 8.1 is that the random vector $\mathbf{x}$ can be well approximated (i.e., with small error J_e) using very few components y_i. In this light, PCA can be seen as an efficient, lossy data compression method, where n variables $x_1, \ldots, x_n$ can be represented by much fewer variables $y_1, \ldots, y_m$.

EXAMPLE 8.1:

Consider the extreme situation where the n-dimensional random vector $\mathbf{x} = [x_1, x_2, \ldots, x_n]^T$ always lies on some one-dimensional subspace $\mathcal{L}$ of $\mathbb{R}^n$. If we call $\mathbf{e}_1$ the unit length vector parallel to $\mathcal{L}$, then

$$\mathbf{x} = c_1 \mathbf{e}_1$$

where c_1 is a scalar random variable. In this case, the covariance matrix has rank 1 since $\mathbf{R}_x = E\{c_1^2\}\mathbf{e}_1\mathbf{e}_1^T$. All the eigenvalues of $\mathbf{R}_x$ except for the first one are zero, whereas the first eigenvalue can be shown to be equal to the variance of c_1, $\lambda_1 = E\{c_1^2\}$. Thus, the first principal component is the projection of $\mathbf{x}$ on $\mathcal{L}$ and is equal to c_1:

$$y_1 = \mathbf{e}_1^T \mathbf{x} = c_1 \ .$$

The first PC together with the constant vector $\mathbf{e}_1$ are enough to losslessly describe the random vector $\mathbf{x}$, since this vector can be reconstructed without error ($J_e = 0$) from the formula $\mathbf{x} = \hat{\mathbf{x}} = y_1\mathbf{e}_1$. Furthermore, although the apparent dimensionality of $\mathbf{x}$ is n, in reality there is only one degree of freedom (intrinsic dimensionality = 1). Figure 8.2 depicts many instantiations of such a random vector in two dimensions. As we can see in this figure, all the instantiations of this vector lie on the axis $\mathcal{L}$, and, therefore, the projection on this axis is a perfect reconstruction of the original point.

8.3 Hebb's Learning Rule

The important work of Donald Hebb published in the late 1940s marked the beginning of a new era in the development of the theory for neural self-organization based on local interactions between neurons. In his book, *The Organization of Behavior* [3], Hebb postulated that the development of

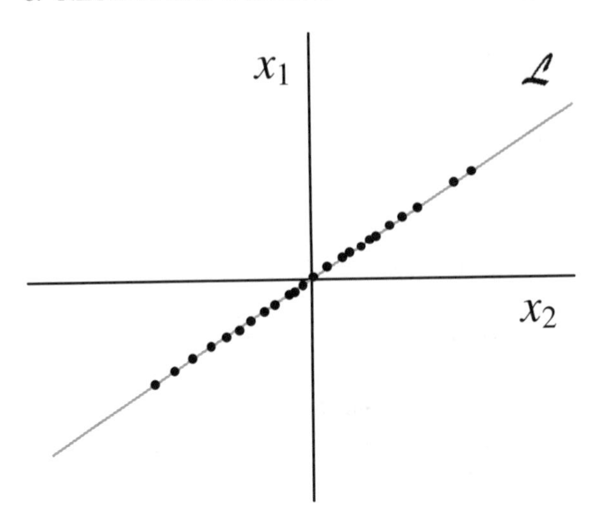

8.2 The axis $\mathcal{L}$ contains all the variance of the two-dimensional random vector $[x_1, x_2]$. Any instantiation of this vector can be losslessly described by its one-dimensional projection on $\mathcal{L}$.

neuronal synapses is governed by the correlation of electrical activity between the afferent axon and the efferent soma, i.e., between the two players involved in the synapse

> When an axon of cell A is near enough to excite cell B and repeatedly and persistently takes part in firing it, some growth process or metabolic change takes place in one or both cells such that A's efficiency, as one of the cells firing B, is increased.

This basic hypothesis is intuitively appealing since it does not assume action at great distance. It is much more plausible that local, rather than remote, electrical activity is responsible for synaptic development. Furthermore, it turns out that this hypothesis is well supported by experimental results. The Hebbian model has been used for the analysis of plasticity phenomena in various parts of the brain such as, for example, the long term potentiation in the hippocampus [6], the respiratory control by the central brain stem [7], the development of the visual cortex [8, 9], etc.

According to Hebb, the most likely way of increasing the efficiency of cell A in exciting cell B is through the growth of a synaptic knob between the axon of A and the soma of B. In this context, the word "growth" means either the creation of a new knob or the enlargement of an already existing one. In either case, any excitatory or inhibitory signal from cell A propagates more easily to cell B and, thus, it carries more "weight" in the final decision about the activation state of B ("firing" or "not firing"). This synaptic development process creates structural changes in the neural network and modifies the behavior of the neural assembly. Mathematically speaking, in a feed-forward neural network, this process implies modification of the input-output mapping function. In a dynamic (or recurrent) network, it may lead to the modification of the system steady states or the creation of new attractor points. Clearly, in either case, this process constitutes a learning method which does not use any supervising signals. The cell assembly self-organizes by modifying the synaptic weights of the network using the local neural activations and without reference to any external teachers or target values.

As with any unsupervised learning rule, an underlying mathematical principle is needed for guiding the Hebbian metabolic change into something meaningful and, perhaps, useful. Thus, the key question now is, "what principle guides Hebbian learning?" Unfortunately, Hebb's neurophysiological postulate described above does not involve any rigorous mathematical treatment. It is more like a general statement describing the philosophy behind self-organization of neural assemblies than a solid mathematical tool modeling this self-organizing process. Nevertheless, the Hebbian rule gives enough hints that allow a rather straightforward mathematical interpretation. Consider, for example, the two cells, A and B, and their synaptic weight w depicted in Figure 8.3. Let a be the activation

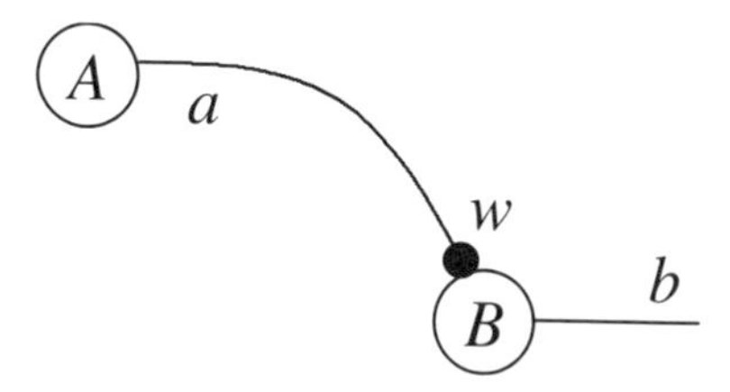

8.3 According to Hebb's rule, the synaptic weight w between neuron A and neuron B grows proportionally to the product of the activations of the two neurons.

of cell A, b the activation of cell B, and assume that these activations can take both positive and negative values. Clearly, if A assists the excitation of B, then b will tend to be positive (negative) whenever a is positive (negative). Therefore, according to the Hebbian philosophy, the synaptic weight between the two cells should increase when the two activations agree in their signs (they are either both positive or both negative), while it should decrease when the two neurons disagree in their signs (one is positive and the other is negative). It follows that this philosophy rewards positive correlation between the activations a and b and punishes negative correlation. Thus, a simple mathematical formulation of the Hebbian rule is that the synaptic weight w changes proportionally to the activation product $(a \cdot b)$:

$$w^{\text{new}} = w^{\text{old}} + \beta \cdot a \cdot b \tag{8.20}$$

where the parameter β is a small, positive, possibly time-varying number called learning rate.

Of course, the two other important characteristics of the Hebbian learning philosophy, namely locality and the lack supervision, are also present in Equation (8.20). Indeed, all the information used for the adaptation of w are the local activations a and b. Furthermore, Equation (8.20) expresses an unsupervised learning algorithm as no external target values are used.

The simple learning rule in Equation (8.20) is not immediately useful. However, it is quite interesting because of its relationship with principal component analysis. Using a simple normalization procedure and applying the algorithm in linear neurons, it turns into a principal component analyzer as shown by Oja [4] and Karhunen and Oja [5].

8.4 PCA and Linear Hebbian Models

The simplest Hebbian learning models — in terms of mathematical form — are those related to cells with linear activation functions. This section examines the relationship between such Hebbian models and principal component analysis. The importance of this relationship becomes apparent when we combine the biological origin of the Hebbian rule and the fact that any pattern recognition method relies on some kind of feature extracted from the raw data.

8.4.1 Unconstrained Hebbian Learning

Consider a neuron cell described by a linear activation function (see Figure 8.4). The output y of

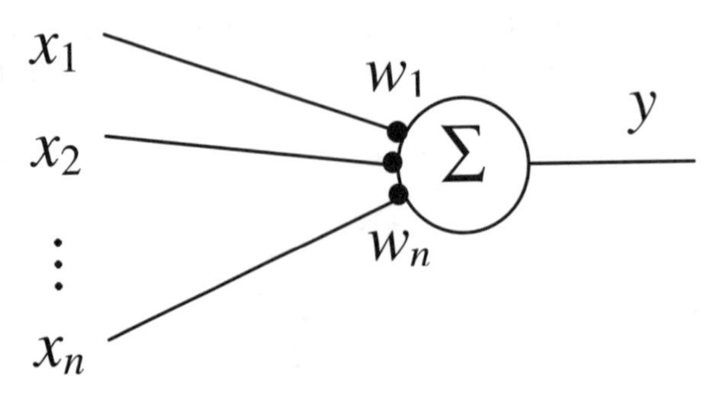

8.4 Model of a linear neuron.

such a cell is given by the relation

$$y = \sum_{i=1}^{n} w_i x_i = \mathbf{w}^T \mathbf{x} \tag{8.21}$$

where w_i is the synaptic weight corresponding to the input x_i, and we defined the synaptic weight vector $\mathbf{w} = [w_1 \dots w_n]^T$ and the input vector $\mathbf{x} = [x_1 \dots x_n]^T$. In the classical McCulloch–Pitts theory, neurons are typically modeled by nonlinear activation functions of the form $y = f(\mathbf{w}^T \mathbf{x})$, where the sigmoid function $f(u)$ tends to some finite values ($1/0$ or $1/-1$) as $u \to \pm\infty$. However, around $u = 0$, the function behaves in an approximately linear fashion and so nonlinear neurons can emulate linear ones in a small signal scenario, i.e., for small input values.

Let us now rewrite the simple Hebbian rule in Equation (8.20) using vector notation and introducing a time index k

$$\mathbf{w}(k+1) = \mathbf{w}(k) + \beta(k) y(k) \mathbf{x}(k) \ . \tag{8.22}$$

At first sight, Equation (8.23) is not interesting because it is unstable. It is straightforward to show that the norm of the weight vector is monotonically increasing

$$\begin{aligned} \|\mathbf{w}(k+1)\|^2 &= \left(\mathbf{w}(k)^T + \beta(k) y(k) \mathbf{x}(k)^T\right) (\mathbf{w}(k) + \beta(k) y(k) \mathbf{x}(k)) \\ &= \|\mathbf{w}(k)\|^2 + 2\beta(k) y(k)^2 + \beta(k)^2 y(k)^2 \|\mathbf{x}(k)\|^2 \\ &\geq \|\mathbf{w}(k)\|^2 \ . \end{aligned}$$

Suppose that the input signal $\mathbf{x} \in \mathbb{R}^n$ is a wide-sense-stationary process with zero mean $E\{\mathbf{x}(k)\} = 0$ and covariance matrix

$$\mathbf{R}_x = E\left\{\mathbf{x}(k)\mathbf{x}(k)^T\right\} \ .$$

Let $\lambda_1 > \dots > \lambda_n$ be the eigenvalues of $\mathbf{R}_x$ and $\mathbf{e}_1, \dots, \mathbf{e}_n$ be the corresponding eigenvectors. Substituting Equation (8.21) into Equation (8.22), we can write

$$\frac{1}{\beta(k)} \Delta \mathbf{w}(k) = \mathbf{x}(k)\mathbf{x}(k)^T \mathbf{w}(k) \tag{8.23}$$

where $\Delta \mathbf{w}(k) = \mathbf{w}(k+1) - \mathbf{w}(k)$.

According to the theory of stochastic recursive equations developed by Ljung [10] and Kushner and Clark [11], the difference equation (Equation (8.23)) can be approximated by an ordinary differential equation (ODE) treating $\mathbf{w}$ as deterministic and taking expectation with respect to $\mathbf{x}$:

$$\frac{d}{dt}\mathbf{w}(t) = E\left\{\mathbf{x}\mathbf{x}^T\right\} \mathbf{w}(t) = \mathbf{R}_x \mathbf{w}(t) \ . \tag{8.24}$$

The relation between the discrete time k in Equation (8.23) and the continuous time t in the ODE (Equation (8.24)) is described by the formula

$$t = t(k) = \sum_{m=0}^{k} \beta(m) . \tag{8.25}$$

A closer inspection of the associated ODE (Equation (8.24)) reveals that our learning rule is a principal component analyzer with unstable dynamics. We next show that the angle between $\mathbf{w}(t)$ and $\mathbf{e}_1$ asymptotically tends to zero, but at the same time, the norm $\|\mathbf{w}(t)\|$ tends to infinity. Let us expand $\mathbf{w}(t)$ into the orthonormal basis $\mathbf{e}_1, \ldots, \mathbf{e}_n$ of the eigenvectors of $\mathbf{R}_x$

$$\mathbf{w}(t) = \sum_{i=1}^{n} \alpha_i(t)\mathbf{e}_i . \tag{8.26}$$

We will show that $|\alpha_1(t)| \to \infty$, and $\alpha_i(t)/\alpha_1(t) \to 0$, $i = 2, 3, \ldots, n$, as $t \to \infty$. Substituting Equation (8.26) into Equation (8.24), we obtain

$$\sum_{i=1}^{n} \frac{d\alpha_i(t)}{dt}\mathbf{e}_i = \sum_{i=1}^{n} \alpha_i(t)\mathbf{R}_x\mathbf{e}_i$$

$$\frac{d\alpha_i(t)}{dt} = \lambda_i\alpha_i(t), \qquad i = 1, 2, \ldots, n \tag{8.27}$$

$$\alpha_i(t) = \alpha_i(0)e^{\lambda_i t}, \qquad i = 1, 2, \ldots, n . \tag{8.28}$$

All the eigenvalues λ_i are positive since $\mathbf{R}_x$ is positive definite. In addition, we have arranged them in decreasing order. Therefore, $\lambda_i > 0$ and $\lambda_1 > \lambda_i$, $i = 2, 3, \ldots, n$, so for $t \to \infty$ and assuming $\alpha_1(0) \neq 0$, Equation (8.28) yields

$$|\alpha_1(t)| \to \infty \tag{8.29}$$

$$\alpha_i(t)/\alpha_1(t) = \alpha_i(0)/\alpha_1(0)e^{(\lambda_i-\lambda_1)t} \tag{8.30}$$

$$\alpha_i(t)/\alpha_1(t) \to 0, \quad i \geq 2 . \tag{8.31}$$

It follows that the vector $\mathbf{w}(t)$ tends to become parallel to the first PC $\mathbf{e}_1$, since $\alpha_i/\alpha_1 \to 0$, for $i \geq 2$. At the same time, the length $\|\mathbf{w}(t)\|^2 = \Sigma_i\alpha_i(t)^2$ tends to infinity since $|\alpha_1| \to \infty$.

Alternatively, one can view Equation (8.24) as a gradient ascent rule

$$\frac{d\mathbf{w}}{dt} = \frac{\partial J}{\partial \mathbf{w}}$$

on the following energy function:

$$J = E\left\{\left(\mathbf{w}^T\mathbf{x}\right)^2\right\} = \mathbf{w}^T\mathbf{R}_x\mathbf{w} .$$

Define $\mathbf{u} = \mathbf{w}/\|\mathbf{w}\|$ to be the unit-length vector parallel to $\mathbf{w}$. The energy becomes

$$J = \|\mathbf{w}\|^2 E\left\{\left(\mathbf{u}^T\mathbf{x}\right)^2\right\}$$

J can be readily interpreted as the variance of the projected data on the subspace spanned by $\mathbf{w}$ and multiplied by the squared norm of $\mathbf{w}$. Clearly, if $\|\mathbf{w}\|$ is not constrained, the maximization of the energy leads to $J = \infty$ for $\|\mathbf{w}\| = \infty$. Under this new light, it is not surprising that the simple Hebbian rule, being a gradient ascent on J, diverges. However, the relation between PCA and the simple Hebbian rule is more important than divergence. As we will see, small modifications of the rule will lead to PCA without stability problems.

8.4.2 Constrained Hebbian Rules

Equation (8.23) already points to the close relationship between Hebbian learning and PCA. Instability is the only obstacle inhibiting Equation (8.23) from being a real principal component analyzer. This leads to the thought that a modified learning rule devoid of instability problems may lead to the extraction of the first PC. Such modifications will be discussed next.

8.4.2.1 The Normalized Hebbian Rule

One possible way of achieving stability is the division of $\mathbf{w}(k)$ by a scalar factor $\rho(k)$, such that the norm would be constrained between certain limits. This could lead to the desired result because the division $\mathbf{w}(k)/\rho(k)$ does not affect the ratio α_i/α_1.

The normalized Hebbian rule uses the factor $\rho(k) = \|\mathbf{w}(k)\|$ which keeps the norm constantly equal to one (hence the name "normalized" Hebbian rule):

$$\mathbf{v}(k) = \mathbf{w}(k) + \beta(k)y(k)\mathbf{x}(k) \tag{8.32}$$

$$\mathbf{w}(k+1) = \mathbf{v}(k)/\|\mathbf{v}(k)\| \,. \tag{8.33}$$

The normalized Hebbian rule does converge, asymptotically, to the first PC: $\mathbf{w}(t) \to \mathbf{w}(\infty) = \mathbf{e}_1$. However, a new problem emerges: the rule is no longer local because the norm $\|\mathbf{w}\|$ involves all the weights $w_1, \ldots, w_n$. In other words, the development of the synaptic weight $w_i(k)$ depends not only on the local values $y(k)$ and $x_i(k)$ but also on the values of all the other synaptic weights of the same cell.

8.4.2.2 Linearized Normalization (Oja's Single Unit Rule)

Fortunately, there is a rather elegant solution to the locality problem of the normalized Hebbian rule. In 1982, Oja [4] and Karhunen [5] proposed linearization of the normalization division in Equation (8.33). This is done by the linear approximation of the Taylor series expansion assuming small values of β:

$$\begin{aligned} \|\mathbf{v}(k)\|^{-1} &= \left[\mathbf{v}(k)^T\mathbf{v}(k)\right]^{-1/2} \\ &= \left[\|\mathbf{w}(k)\|^2 + 2\beta(k)y(k)\mathbf{w}(k)^T\mathbf{x}(k)\right]^{-1/2} \\ &= \left[1 + 2\beta(k)y(k)^2\right]^{-1/2} \\ &= 1 - \beta(k)y(k)^2 \,. \end{aligned} \tag{8.34}$$

Substituting into Equation (8.33), we get

$$\begin{aligned} \mathbf{w}(k+1) &= \mathbf{v}(k)\|\mathbf{v}(k)\|^{-1} \\ &= [\mathbf{w}(k) + \beta(k)y(k)\mathbf{x}(k)]\left[1 - \beta(k)y(k)^2\right] \end{aligned}$$

$$\mathbf{w}(k+1) = \mathbf{w}(k) + \beta(k)\left[y(k)\mathbf{x}(k) - \mathbf{w}(k)y(k)^2\right] \tag{8.35}$$

where we ignore all terms involving β^2 or higher order powers of β.

Equation (8.35) is known as Oja's rule. It is straightforward to show that Oja's rule is local. We simply inspect the adaptation equation for the ith weight

$$w_i(k+1) = w_i(k) + \beta(k)\left[y(k)x_i(k) - y(k)^2 w_i(k)\right] \tag{8.36}$$

and observe that it involves nothing but the local variables w_i, x_i, and y.

The following theorem shows that the rule also extracts the first PC and that the stable attractors have unit length.

THEOREM 8.2 *[4] Let the following assumptions hold:*

A1. *The sequence $\mathbf{x}(k)$ is zero-mean, wide-sense stationary, the eigenvalues of the covariance matrix $\mathbf{R}_x$ are positive, and the largest eigenvalue has multiplicity 1. In addition, we assume that the eigenvalues are arranged in decreasing order $\lambda_1 > \lambda_2 \geq \cdots \geq \lambda_n > 0$.*

A2. *The learning parameter $\beta(k)$ satisfies*

$$\lim_{k\to\infty} \beta(k) = 0 \tag{8.37}$$

$$\sum_{k=0}^{\infty} \beta(k) = \infty\,. \tag{8.38}$$

Let $\mathbf{e}_1, \ldots, \mathbf{e}_n$ denote a set of orthonormal eigenvectors of $\mathbf{R}_x$ corresponding to the eigenvalues $\lambda_1, \ldots, \lambda_n$, and let us consider the learning rule (Equation (8.35)) where the following condition holds: $\mathbf{e}_1^T \mathbf{w}(0) \neq 0$. Then, with probability 1, we have $\mathbf{w}(k) \to \pm\mathbf{e}_1$ as $k \to \infty$.

The complete proof of this theorem is given by Oja and Karhunen [12], Diamantaras [13], and Haykin [14]. Here we shall only briefly sketch the proof. Our aim is to illustrate its underlying ideas and expose the properties of the algorithm without getting lost in too many details. We use again the theory of stochastic recursive equations and associate the difference equation (Equation (8.35)) with the following deterministic ODE:

$$\frac{d}{dt}\mathbf{w}(t) = \mathbf{R}_x \mathbf{w}(t) - \left[\mathbf{w}(t)^T \mathbf{R}_x \mathbf{w}(t)\right] \mathbf{w}(t)\,. \tag{8.39}$$

We first observe that the equilibrium points of Equation (8.39) must satisfy

$$\mathbf{R}_x \mathbf{w} = \lambda \mathbf{w}$$

where $\lambda = \mathbf{w}^T \mathbf{R}_x \mathbf{w}$. It follows that the only possible equilibrium points are the eigenvectors of $\mathbf{R}_x$ and the zero vector.

As usual, we expand $\mathbf{w}(t)$ into the orthonormal basis $\mathbf{e}_1, \ldots, \mathbf{e}_n$,

$$\mathbf{w}(t) = \sum_{i=1}^{n} \alpha_i(t)\mathbf{e}_i$$

to obtain the following dynamics

$$\begin{aligned} \frac{d\alpha_i}{dt} &= \left(\lambda_i - \sigma^2\right)\alpha_i \\ \sigma^2 &= \sum_{i=1}^{n} \lambda_i \alpha_i^2\,. \end{aligned}$$

So,

$$\begin{aligned} \frac{d}{dt}\frac{\alpha_i}{\alpha_j} &= \frac{\alpha_i}{\alpha_j}\left[\frac{1}{\alpha_i}\frac{d\alpha_i}{dt} - \frac{1}{\alpha_j}\frac{d\alpha_j}{dt}\right] \\ &= \frac{\alpha_i}{\alpha_j}\left[\lambda_i - \lambda_j\right]\,. \end{aligned} \tag{8.40}$$

For all $i > 1$, we have $\lambda_i - \lambda_1 < 0$, and so $\lim_{t\to\infty} \alpha_i(t)/\alpha_1(t) = 0$. In addition, $\lim_{t\to\infty} \Sigma_i \alpha_i(t)^2 = 1$. It follows that

$$\lim_{t\to\infty} |\alpha_1(t)| = 1 ,$$

$$\lim_{t\to\infty} \alpha_i(t) = 0, \qquad i = 2, 3, \ldots, n$$

and, thus, the theorem holds.

Two points are worth noting here:

1. Convergence of the associated ODE is exponential as becomes evident from the dynamics of the ratio α_i/α_1. According to Equation (8.40), we have $\alpha_i(t)/\alpha_1(t) = \exp\{(\lambda_i - \lambda_1)t\}$ with $\lambda_i - \lambda_1 < 0$ for $i \geq 2$. The speed of convergence is illustrated by the example in Figure 8.5. In this experiment, we used 200 samples from a five-dimensional, zero-mean random sequence $\mathbf{x}(k)$ with principal eigenvalues $\lambda_1 = 2.5$, $\lambda_2 = 2.0$, $\lambda_3 = 1.6$, $\lambda_4 = 0.9$, and $\lambda_5 = 0.3$. The samples are recycled in 20 sweeps. From the evolution of the components $\alpha_2(k), \ldots, \alpha_5(k)$, it is evident that the convergence is exponential and that $\alpha_1(k)$ tends to a steady state equal to one.

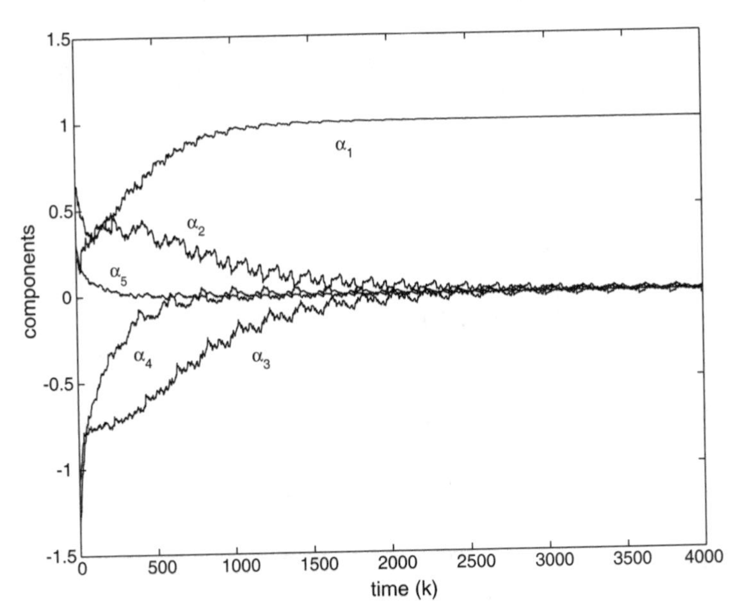

8.5 Typical experiment illustrating the dynamics of Oja's single unit rule.

2. Oja's rule (Equation (8.35)) differs from the simple Hebbian rule (Equation (8.22)) only in the term $-\beta(k)y(k)^2\mathbf{w}(k)$. This is the stabilizing term which also leads to a unit-length stable attractor. In fact, it can be shown that any term of the form $-\beta(k)\sigma(k)\mathbf{w}(k)$ stabilizes the simple Hebbian rule if $\sigma(k)$ is any positive definite function of $\mathbf{w}$. In this general case, however, the norm of the final convergence point may not be one [13].

8.4.2.3 The Generalized Hebbian Algorithm (GHA)

The generalized Hebbian algorithm (GHA) [15] is one of the first neural models that were proposed in the literature for extracting multiple PCs. There are two slightly different versions of the algorithm: the original GHA and the local GHA.

8.4.2.3.1 Original GHA

The original GHA rule is applicable to a linear neural network with one layer of m output units and one layer of $n > m$ input units (see Figure 8.6). The output y_i of the ith neuron is described by a linear equation

$$y_i = \mathbf{w}_i^T \mathbf{x} \tag{8.41}$$

where $\mathbf{x}$ is the input vector and $\mathbf{w}_i$ is the vector of synaptic weights for neuron i. The GHA learning rule is similar to Oja's rule. In fact, for neuron 1, it is exactly the same:

$$\Delta\mathbf{w}_1(k) = \beta(k) \left[y_1(k)\mathbf{x}(k) - y_1^2(k)\mathbf{w}_1(k) \right] . \tag{8.42}$$

For neurons 2, 3, ..., m, the rule is slightly different:

$$\Delta\mathbf{w}_i(k) = \beta(k) \left[y_i(k)\mathbf{x}(k) - y_i(k) \sum_{l=1}^{i} y_l(k)\mathbf{w}_l(k) \right] . \tag{8.43}$$

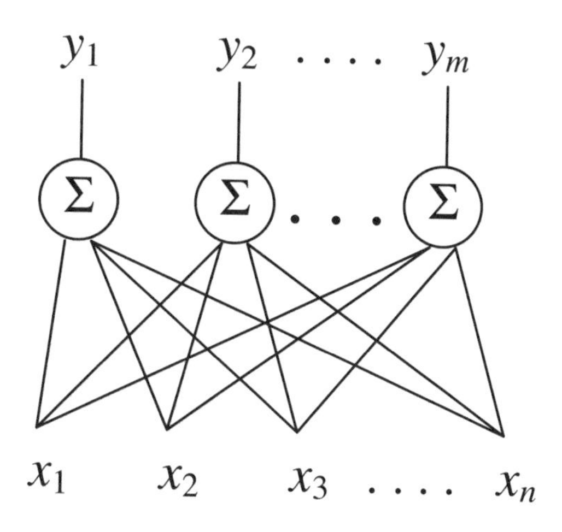

8.6 The network of the original generalized Hebbian algorithm comprises m linear neurons and n inputs ($n > m$).

The original GHA creates a hierarchical structure in the output neurons. The highest ranking neuron is neuron 1, whose output value y_1 and synaptic weight vector $\mathbf{w}_1$ affect the training of all the other neurons. At the same time, the training of neuron 1 is affected only by its own values y_1, $\mathbf{w}_1$, and not by the other neurons. Neuron 2, the second in the hierarchy, is affected only by y_1, y_2, $\mathbf{w}_1$, $\mathbf{w}_2$, and affects the training of neurons 3, ..., m. In general, neuron i uses the values $y_1, \ldots, y_i$, $\mathbf{w}_1, \ldots, \mathbf{w}_i$ of all the higher neurons in the hierarchy, and, at the same time, it affects the training of all the lower neurons, i.e., the neurons $i + 1, \ldots, m$, through the values y_i, $\mathbf{w}_i$.

It can be proven that the algorithm is uniformly, asymptotically stable, and at equilibrium we have

$$\mathbf{w}_i = \pm\mathbf{e}_i , \qquad i = 1, \ldots, m .$$

In other words, GHA is a principal component analyzer which extracts multiple PCs. The algorithm is clearly unsupervised and has partly Hebbian characteristics. For neuron 1, the rule is the same as Oja's rule, while for neurons 2, ..., m it only looks similar. However, for neurons 2 through m, the rule is obviously not local since every neuron $i \geq 2$ uses parameters from previous neurons.

8.4.2.3.2 Local GHA

The major criticism of original GHA is its lack of locality, an important ingredient of Hebbianity. Sanger himself [15] proposed an amendment through the local GHA, described as follows:

$$\Delta \mathbf{w}_i(k) = \beta(k) \left[y_i(k) \left(\mathbf{x}(k) - \sum_{l=1}^{i-1} y_l(k)\mathbf{w}_l(k) \right) - y_i(k)^2 \mathbf{w}_i(k) \right] . \tag{8.44}$$

If we define the vector,

$$\mathbf{x}^{(i)} = \mathbf{x} - \sum_{l<i} y_l \mathbf{w}_l \tag{8.45}$$

the algorithm takes the form of Oja's rule on $\mathbf{x}^{(i)}$:

$$\Delta \mathbf{w}_i(k) = \beta(k) \left[y_i(k)\mathbf{x}^{(i)}(k) - y_i(k)^2 \mathbf{w}_i(k) \right] \tag{8.46}$$

where

$$y_i = \mathbf{w}_i^T \mathbf{x}^{(i)} . \tag{8.47}$$

The difference between the output of the local algorithm (Equation (8.47)) and the output (Equation (8.41)) of the original algorithm is the basic difference between the two versions of GHA. This difference aside, Equation (8.44) is just a rearrangement of the terms in Equation (8.43).

The local GHA algorithm is based on the so called deflation transform [16] implemented in Equation (8.45). The deflation transform is the key for extracting components 2, 3, etc. For this reason, this transform is described in more detail in the next subsection.

8.4.2.3.3 The Deflation Transform

The orthonormal principal eigenvectors $\mathbf{e}_1, \ldots, \mathbf{e}_n$ of $\mathbf{R}_x$ have the following properties

$$\mathbf{e}_i^T \mathbf{e}_j = \begin{cases} 1 & \text{if } i = j \\ 0 & \text{if } i \neq j \end{cases}$$

$$\mathbf{e}_i^T \mathbf{R}_x \mathbf{e}_j = \begin{cases} \lambda_i & \text{if } i = j \\ 0 & \text{if } i \neq j . \end{cases}$$

Suppose that we are given some of these eigenvectors, for example, the set $\{\mathbf{e}_1, \ldots, \mathbf{e}_{m-1}\}$, $m < n$, and let $\mathcal{L}_{m-1}$ be the subspace spanned by them. The deflation transform is described by the following equation:

$$\mathbf{x}^{(m)} = \mathbf{x} - \sum_{l=1}^{m-1} \mathbf{e}_l \mathbf{e}_l^T \mathbf{x}$$

$$\mathbf{x}^{(m)} = \mathbf{P}_{m-1}\mathbf{x} \tag{8.48}$$

$$\mathbf{P}_{m-1} = \left[\mathbf{I} - \sum_{l=1}^{m-1} \mathbf{e}_l \mathbf{e}_l^T \right] \tag{8.49}$$

$\mathbf{x}^{(m)}$ is the projection of $\mathbf{x}$ on the subspace orthogonal to $\mathcal{L}_{m-1}$. The projector operator $\mathbf{P}_{m-1}$ corresponds to the orthogonal subspace. It has the following basic properties:

$$\mathbf{P}_{m-1} = \mathbf{P}_{m-1}^T$$

$$\mathbf{P}_{m-1}\mathbf{P}_{m-1} = \mathbf{P}_{m-1}$$

$$\mathbf{P}_{m-1}\mathbf{e}_i = \begin{cases} 0 & i = 1, \ldots, m-1 \\ \mathbf{e}_i & i = m, \ldots, n \, . \end{cases}$$

Simple mathematical manipulations show that the auto-correlation matrix of $\mathbf{x}^{(m)}$ can be written as:

$$\mathbf{R}_{x^{(m)}} = \mathbf{P}_{m-1}\mathbf{R}_x\mathbf{P}_{m-1} = \sum_{i=m}^{n} \lambda_i \mathbf{e}_i \mathbf{e}_i^T$$

therefore,

$$\mathbf{R}_{x^{(m)}}\mathbf{e}_i = E\{\mathbf{x}^{(m)}\mathbf{x}^{(m)T}\} = \begin{cases} 0 & i = 1, \ldots, m-1 \\ \lambda_i \mathbf{e}_i & i = m, \ldots, n \, . \end{cases}$$

Since $\mathbf{e}_1, \ldots, \mathbf{e}_n$ is an orthonormal basis of $\mathbb{R}^n$, it follows that $\mathbf{R}_{x^{(m)}}$ has one eigenvalue equal to zero with multiplicity $m - 1$, and the remaining $n - m + 1$ eigenvalues are $\lambda_m, \ldots, \lambda_n$.

What is the result of all this? First, the dimension of the subspace spanned by $\mathbf{R}_{x^{(m)}}$ (i.e., the rank of $\mathbf{R}_{x^{(m)}}$) is $n - m + 1$. Thus, deflation reduces the rank of the covariance matrix from n to $n - m + 1$. Figure 8.7 shows a geometrical interpretation of this rank reduction property. Second, but more important, is the fact that, now, the largest eigenvalue is λ_m and, therefore, the original mth PC becomes the new first PC. It follows that a principal component analyzer that extracts the first PC of the deflated data $\mathbf{x}^{(m)}$, such as Oja's algorithm, will extract the mth PC of $\mathbf{x}$.

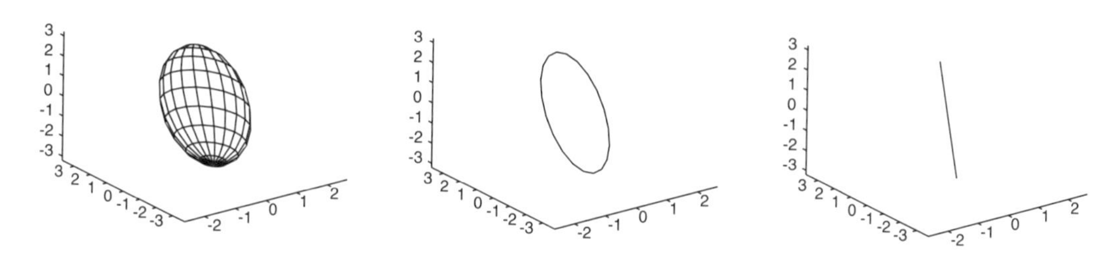

8.7 The locus of points $\mathbf{y} = \mathbf{R}\mathbf{x}$, $\|\mathbf{x}\| = 1$, for a 3×3 symmetric, prositive definite matrix $\mathbf{R}$ is a three-dimensional ellipsoid (left). The same locus for the deflated matrix $\mathbf{R}_1 = [\mathbf{I} - \mathbf{e}_3\mathbf{e}_3^T]\mathbf{R}[\mathbf{I} - \mathbf{e}_3\mathbf{e}_3^T]$ is a two-dimensional ellipse in three-dimensional space (middle). The locus for the twice deflated matrix $\mathbf{R}_2 = [\mathbf{I} - \mathbf{e}_2\mathbf{e}_2^T - \mathbf{e}_3\mathbf{e}_3^T]\mathbf{R}[\mathbf{I} - \mathbf{e}_2\mathbf{e}_2^T - \mathbf{e}_3\mathbf{e}_3^T]$ is a line in three-dimensional space (right).

The second observation is the basis of an inductive argument which shows that local GHA will extract as many PCs as needed. The proof starts with the fact that the first unit-length eigenvector $\mathbf{e}_1$ will be extracted by the first neuron, which is trained using Oja's algorithm. Then, the second neuron will extract the first principal eigenvector $\mathbf{e}_2$ of the deflated data $\mathbf{x}^{(2)} = \mathbf{P}_1\mathbf{x}$, which are created using $\mathbf{e}_1$. Consequently, the third neuron will extract $\mathbf{e}_3$ as it will be the first principal eigenvector of $\mathbf{x}^{(3)}$, which is created using $\mathbf{e}_1$ and $\mathbf{e}_2$, and so on. In general, if the first $m - 1$ neurons have extracted the first $m - 1$ orthonormal principal eigenvectors $\mathbf{e}_1, \ldots, \mathbf{e}_{m-1}$, the mth neuron will extract the $\mathbf{e}_m$ based on the analysis of $\mathbf{x}^{(m)}$. In practice, all the neurons may be trained in parallel, but convergence of the mth unit is not expected sooner than the convergence of the previous $m - 1$ units.

8.4.2.4 The APEX Learning Rule

The adaptive principal component extraction (APEX) rule was proposed by Kung and Diamantaras [13, 17]. The model extracts multiple PCs using lateral connections between the output neurons instead of using an explicit, off-line deflation transformation. The network architecture is shown in

Figure 8.8. It can be shown that deflation is implicitly accomplished by the lateral weights if they

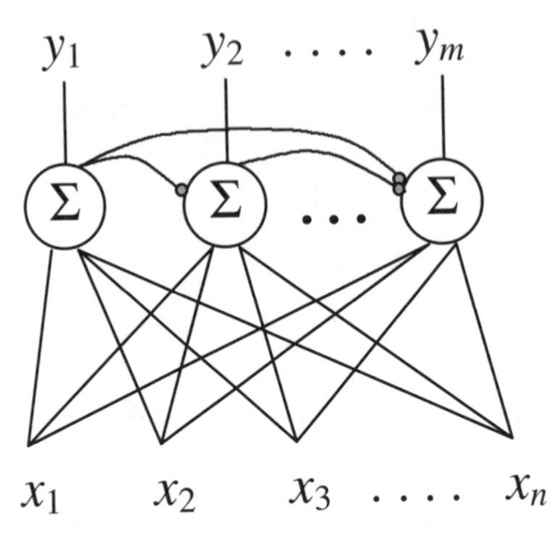

8.8 The architecture of the APEX network.

are trained using Oja's rule. The output y_i of the ith neuron is given by a linear relation involving the inputs $x_1, \ldots, x_n$ and the outputs $y_1, \ldots, y_{i-1}$ of neurons 1 through $i-1$. In particular, we have

$$y_i = \sum_{j=1}^{n} w_{ij} x_j - \sum_{j=1}^{i-1} c_{ij} y_j \tag{8.50}$$

$$\mathbf{y} = \mathbf{W}\mathbf{x} - \mathbf{C}\mathbf{y} \tag{8.51}$$

where $\mathbf{y} = [y_1, \ldots, y_m]^T$ is the output vector, $\mathbf{W} = [w_{ij}]$, $i = 1, \ldots, m$, $j = 1, \ldots, n$ is the matrix of the forward synaptic weights, and

$$\mathbf{C} = \begin{bmatrix} 0 & \cdots & \cdots & \cdots & 0 \\ c_{21} & 0 & \cdots & \cdots & 0 \\ \vdots & & \ddots & & \vdots \\ c_{m-1,1} & \cdots & c_{m-1,m-2} & 0 & 0 \\ c_{m,1} & \cdots & \cdots & c_{m,m-1} & 0 \end{bmatrix}$$

is the lower-triangular lateral weight matrix. Due to the special form of $\mathbf{C}$, there is no need for explicitly inverting it in order to compute the outputs in Equation (8.51), and the recursive relation Equation (8.50) can be used instead.

As with the GHA model, the APEX model maintains a hierarchical order for the output neurons since the ith output depends on the output of the previous $i-1$ neurons. In the input-output relationship (Equation (8.50)), the forward synaptic weights w_{ij} appear with a positive sign contrast to the lateral synaptic weights, which participate with a minus sign. The former work towards the positive correlation between input and output, while the latter work towards the orthogonalization (decorrelation) of the outputs. Often, w_{ij} are called Hebbian connections, and c_{ij} are called anti-Hebbian.

Both Hebbian and anti-Hebbian connections are trained using the same algorithm, i.e., single unit Oja's rule (compare the following rules with Equation (8.36)):

$$\Delta w_{ij}(k) = \beta(k)\left[y_i(k)x_j(k) - y_i(k)^2 w_{ij}(k)\right] \qquad i = 1, \ldots, m, \; j = 1, \ldots, n \tag{8.52}$$

$$\Delta c_{ij}(k) = \beta(k)\left[y_i(k)y_j(k) - y_i(k)^2 c_{ij}(k)\right] \qquad i = 1, \ldots, m, \; j < i\,. \tag{8.53}$$

A consequence of using Oja's rule for all synapses is the locality of the APEX algorithm. Indeed, Equation (8.52) for synapse w_{ij} connecting input j with output i uses only the local values x_j, y_i, and w_{ij}. Similarly, Equation (8.53) for the lateral connection c_{ij} between outputs i and j uses only the values y_i, y_j, and c_{ij}.

THEOREM 8.3 *[13] Let the following assumptions hold*

A1. *The sequence $\mathbf{x}(k)$ is wide sense stationary; its covariance matrix $\mathbf{R}_x$ is positive definite with eigenvalues arranged in decreasing order $\lambda_1 > \cdots > \lambda_m > \lambda_{m+1} \geq \lambda_{m+2} \geq \cdots \geq \lambda_n > 0$.*

A2. *The learning rate parameter $\beta(k)$ satisfies Equations (8.37) and (8.38).*

Consider the APEX learning equations, Equations (8.52) and (8.53), with initial condition $\mathbf{e}_i^T \mathbf{w}_i(0) \neq 0$ for $i = 1, \ldots, m$. Then, with probability 1, we have $\mathbf{w}_i(k) \to \pm\mathbf{e}_i$, $c_{ij}(k) \to 0$, $i = 1, \ldots, m$, $j = 1, \ldots, i-1$, as $k \to \infty$.

In the APEX model, the neurons are assumed to be trained in parallel. There is, however, a sequential variation of the algorithm, known as sequential APEX, in which the neurons are trained one at a time starting with neuron 1, continuing with neuron 2, etc. It turns out that the sequential model has a close relationship with the recursive least squares (RLS) algorithm [18] if the learning rate β is inversely proportional to the output variance weighted by some forgetting factor γ:

$$\beta(k) = \frac{1}{\sum_{i=1}^{k} \gamma^{k-i} y(i)^2} . \tag{8.54}$$

Recursively,

$$\beta(k) = \frac{\beta(k-1)}{\gamma + y(k)^2 \beta(k-1)} . \tag{8.55}$$

Since the RLS algorithm is deterministic, it is faster compared to stochastic methods where $\beta(k)$ tends to zero. Using the optimal learning rate (Equation (8.55)), APEX becomes faster than neural PCA models where the assumption of Equation (8.37) is used.

8.4.2.5 Other Hebbian PCA Learning Rules

This subsection briefly describes some important Hebbian models that extract either the PC eigenvectors or the PCS of the data. Most of these models use Oja's model as the starting point. There is a wide variety of PCA neural models in the literature [5, 12] [19]–[30].

8.4.2.5.1 Földiák's Model [31]

The network architecture proposed by Földiák [31] is shown in Figure 8.9. In this model, there is full connectivity between the output neurons, except for self-feedback connections. This destroys the hierarchy among the neurons which is present in both GHA and APEX models. Földiák's model is characterized by symmetry. The neurons have linear activation functions and the ith output is

$$y_i = \mathbf{w}_i^T \mathbf{x} - \sum_{j \neq i} c_{ij} y_j \tag{8.56}$$

$$\mathbf{y} = \mathbf{W}\mathbf{x} - \mathbf{C}\mathbf{y} . \tag{8.57}$$

Földiák's equation (Equation (8.57)) is similar to Equation (8.51) of the APEX model, except that $\mathbf{C}$ is a full matrix and, therefore, its inversion is required for the computation of the output vector $\mathbf{y}$:

$$\mathbf{y} = (\mathbf{I} + \mathbf{C})^{-1} \mathbf{W}\mathbf{x} \equiv \mathbf{F}\mathbf{x} .$$

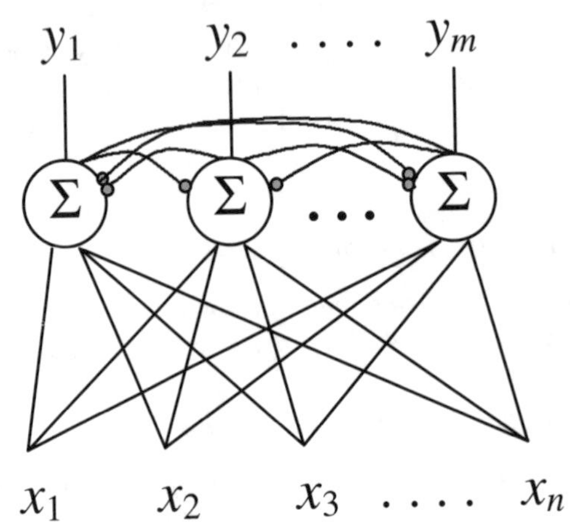

8.9 The network proposed by Földiák empoys full bidirectional connections between the output neurons.

Matrix inversion inhibits any locality aspirations of the algorithm. This problem aside, the learning rule is Hebbian both in relation to the forward weights w_{ij} and with respect to the lateral weights c_{ij}:

$$\Delta w_{ij}(k) = \beta(k)\left[y_i(k)x_j(k) - y_i(k)^2 w_{ij}(k)\right] \tag{8.58}$$

$$\Delta c_{ij}(k) = \beta(k)y_i(k)y_j(k), \qquad i \neq j\,. \tag{8.59}$$

A Földiák network with m output neurons learns the m-dimensional PCS of the input data. The lack of hierarchy does not allow for the extraction of the principal eigenvectors or the principal components themselves. Because of the network symmetry, there is no reason why, for instance, neuron 1 should converge to component 1, while neuron 2 should converge to component 2. Each neuron converges to a linear mixture of components. What can be shown, however, is that the components $m+1$ through n are absent in the steady states of the neurons. In other words, the rows of $\mathbf{F}$ span the same subspace spanned by $\mathbf{e}_1, \ldots, \mathbf{e}_m$, i.e., the m-dimensional PCS

$$\mathbf{F} = \mathbf{T}\left[\mathbf{e}_1, \ldots, \mathbf{e}_m\right]^T\,.$$

$\mathbf{T}$ is an unknown $m \times m$ matrix. Thus, the network outputs y_i are an unknown linear combination of the principal components 1 through m. This is not necessarily a drawback if we are not interested in the PCs themselves but rather in the projection of $\mathbf{x}$ on the PCS. The reconstruction of $\mathbf{x}$ from its projection is computed using the pseudoinverse of $\mathbf{F}$: $\hat{\mathbf{x}} = \mathbf{F}^+\mathbf{y}$.

8.4.2.5.2 The Subspace Rule [5, 32, 33]

This rule is an extension of Oja's single unit algorithm in multiple dimensions. Compare Equation (8.35) with the following describing the subspace rule:

$$\mathbf{y} = \mathbf{W}\mathbf{x} \tag{8.60}$$

$$\Delta\mathbf{W}(k) = \beta(k)\left[\mathbf{y}(k)\mathbf{x}(k)^T - \mathbf{y}(k)\mathbf{y}(k)^T\mathbf{W}(k)\right]\,. \tag{8.61}$$

Similar to Földiák's model, the subspace rule will not extract the principal eigenvectors themselves but some unknown linear combination which, however, spans the m-dimensional PCS: $\mathbf{W} = \mathbf{T}[\mathbf{e}_1, \ldots, \mathbf{e}_m]^T$.

8.4.2.5.3 The Model of Rubner [34]

The architecture of Rubner is the same as that of the APEX model (see Figure 8.8). The output function is also the same as the APEX model:

$$y_i = \sum_{j=1}^{n} w_{ij} x_j - \sum_{j=1}^{i-1} c_{ij} y_j \ .$$

The difference is in the learning rule, which is based on the normalized Hebbian algorithm and is, therefore, non-local:

$$\mathbf{v}_i(k) = \mathbf{w}_i(k) + \beta(k) y_i(k) \mathbf{x}(k) \tag{8.62}$$

$$\mathbf{w}_i(k+1) = \frac{1}{\|\mathbf{v}_i(k)\|} \mathbf{v}_i(k) \tag{8.63}$$

$$\Delta c_{ij}(k) = \beta(k) y_i(k) y_j(k), \qquad i > j \ . \tag{8.64}$$

Although there is no rigorous mathematical proof, the network does converge to the principal components: $\mathbf{w}_i \to \mathbf{e}_i$, $c_{ij} \to 0$, as $k \to \infty$.

8.4.2.6 Assessment of Hebbian PCA Models

An attempt to unify the major Hebbian PCA models was undertaken by Diamantaras and Kung [13]. It was found that they can be expressed as special cases of the following general formula:

$$\begin{aligned} \mathbf{y} &= \mathbf{W}\mathbf{x} - \mathbf{C}\mathbf{y} \\ \mathbf{W}(k+1) &= \mathbf{W}(k) + \beta(k)\left[\mathbf{y}(k)\mathbf{x}(k)^T - F(\mathbf{y}(k)\mathbf{y}(k)^T)\mathbf{W}(k)\right] \\ \mathbf{C}(k+1) &= \mathbf{C}(k) + \beta(k)\left[G(\mathbf{y}(k)\mathbf{y}(k)^T) - H(\mathbf{y}(k)\mathbf{y}(k)^T)\mathbf{C}(k)\right] \end{aligned}$$

or

$$\mathbf{C}(k) = 0$$

for some functions $F(\cdot)$, $G(\cdot)$, and $H(\cdot)$. Models with non-zero lateral weight matrix $\mathbf{C}$ are said to be in asymmetric mode if $\mathbf{C}$ is lower triangular (e.g., the APEX model) and in symmetric mode otherwise (e.g., Földiák's model). It turns out that asymmetric models have advantages over symmetric ones in terms of performance and biological plausibility [35]. Symmetric models require matrix inversion for the computation of $\mathbf{y} = (\mathbf{I}+\mathbf{C})^{-1}\mathbf{W}\mathbf{x}$. The use of standard finite methods, such as the Gauss–Seidel iteration, is biologically implausible. Infinite, iterative schemes can be used at the obvious expense in speed. To make things worse, if we truncate the matrix inversion series $(\mathbf{I}+\mathbf{C})^{-1} = \Sigma_{p=0}^{\infty}(-1)^p \mathbf{C}^p$ at some finite point, these algorithms become unstable. In asymmetric models, on the contrary, the inversion can be expressed in a finite series because $\mathbf{C}^p = 0$ for $p > m$. In fact, the outputs y_i can be computed using a finite recursive formula: $y_i = \mathbf{w}_i^T \mathbf{x} + \Sigma_{j=1}^{i-1} c_{ij} y_j$. Finally, for asymmetric models, the only asymptotic equilibria are the points

$$\mathbf{W} = [\pm\mathbf{e}_1, \ldots, \pm\mathbf{e}_m]^T \ , \qquad \mathbf{C} = 0$$

and all other equilibria are unstable.

Another interesting point is the comparison between neural PCA methods and standard batch approaches in which the covariance matrix is first estimated from the data and then eigenvalue analysis is performed on it. Both approaches have advantages and disadvantages depending on the problem setting, as explained next.

Classical eigenvalue decomposition methods are preferred when the covariance matrix $\mathbf{R}_x$ is known or when the data are finite and of small dimension. On the contrary, neural PCA methods are suitable for problems where the data keep coming continuously from some stochastic source.

Another case of advantage for neural methods is when the data have very large dimension, e.g., 1000. In that case, the covariance matrix is huge (e.g., 1000×1000) and the number of operations needed for a full classical eigenvalue decomposition becomes prohibitively large. On the other hand, neural models never compute the covariance matrix explicitly nor do they store it in memory. Thus, these models can be effectively used provided that only a few components are required. For further discussion on comparisons between PCA models and between neural models and batch methods, the interested reader is referred to Diamantaras and Kung [13].

8.4.2.7 Multilayer Perceptrons and PCA

Principal component analysis represents n-dimensional data using a smaller number of variables and reconstructs the original data from the representation variables. Consider a multilayer perceptron network like the one shown in Figure 8.10. It has the n input and n output units, but the hidden layer is an information bottleneck as it contains a smaller number of hidden units $m < n$. The network operates in auto-associative mode: the targets t_i are equal to the inputs x_i. The model squeezes the input information through m hidden units and is required to reconstruct the input at the output. It turns out that such a network structure is closely related with PCA if the model is trained on a least squares algorithm such as back-propagation (BP).

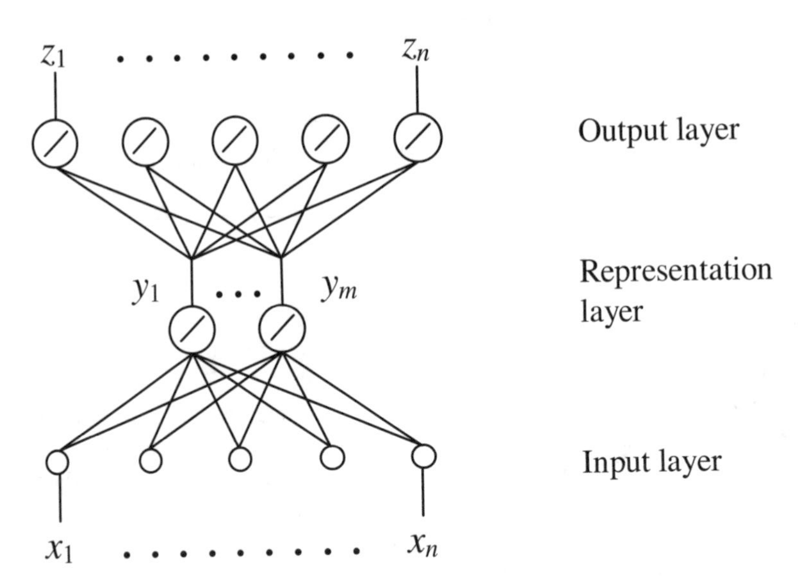

8.10 A multilayer perceptron network implements PCA if (a) the output layer comprises linear units, (b) the network operates in auto-associative mode, and (c) the hidden layer has fewer units than the input and output layers. After back-propagation training, the synaptic weight matrix spans the principal component subspace (PCS).

Let us use the following notations:

- $\mathbf{x} \in \mathbb{R}^n$ = the network input vector.
- $\mathbf{a} \in \mathbb{R}^p$ = the activation vector of the hidden layer.
- $\overline{\mathbf{W}}, \overline{\theta}$ = the matrix of synaptic weights and thresholds of the output layer.
- $\underline{\mathbf{W}}, \underline{\theta}$ = the matrix of synaptic weights and thresholds of the hidden layer.

The network output units have a linear activation function

$$\mathbf{y} = \overline{\mathbf{W}}\mathbf{a} + \overline{\theta} \,. \tag{8.65}$$

The hidden units, on the contrary, may have a nonlinear activation function f. The hidden layer activation vector is

$$\mathbf{a} = \mathbf{f}\left(\underline{\mathbf{W}}^T \mathbf{x} + \underline{\theta}\right) \tag{8.66}$$

where $\mathbf{f}(\mathbf{u}) = [f(u_1), \ldots, f(u_m)]^T$.

Given that the target vector is equal to the input vector, the network squared error is

$$J = \frac{1}{2N} \sum_{k=1}^{N} \|\mathbf{x}(k) - \mathbf{y}(k)\|^2 . \tag{8.67}$$

Bourlard and Kamp [36] showed that J is minimized for

$$\overline{\mathbf{W}} = \mathbf{U}_m \mathbf{T} \tag{8.68}$$

$$\underline{\mathbf{W}} = \frac{1}{b} \mathbf{U}_m \mathbf{T}^{-T} \tag{8.69}$$

$$\overline{\theta} = \langle \mathbf{x} \rangle - \overline{\mathbf{W}} \langle \mathbf{a} \rangle \tag{8.70}$$

$$\underline{\theta} = 0 . \tag{8.71}$$

The notations $\langle \mathbf{x} \rangle$ and $\langle \mathbf{a} \rangle$ correspond to the ensemble averages of the vectors $\mathbf{x}$, $\mathbf{a}$. The matrix $\mathbf{U}_m = [\mathbf{e}_1, \ldots, \mathbf{e}_m]^T$ contains the principal eigenvectors and spans the m-dimensional PCS. $\mathbf{T}$ is some square invertible matrix, and b is the slope of $f(u)$ at $u = 0$. According to Equations (8.68) and (8.69), both upper and lower layer weights $\overline{\mathbf{W}}$, $\underline{\mathbf{W}}$ involve the principal component eigenvectors, and their respective column-/row-spans are the m-dimensional PCS. If $b = 1$ and $f(u) = u$ is a linear function, then the MLP will implement the PCA transform:

$$\mathbf{y} = b \mathbf{U}_m \mathbf{U}_m^T \mathbf{x} .$$

The interesting point is that even if $f(u)$ is a nonlinear function, the weights are still related to the PCS.

The work of Bourlard and Kamp shows that Hebbian learning is not the sole connection between PCA and neural networks. PCA is a minimum mean-squared-error method, and so, back-propagation being another least-squares method, turns out to be related to it. Another important conclusion refers to the use of nonlinear units in the hidden layer. The result is the same if linear units are used. As a matter of fact, nonlinear units add local minima in the energy function and thus are preferably avoided. It is also possible to show that the same conclusions hold for networks with more than two networks provided that the second-to-last layer is a bottleneck [13]. It is noted that the transformation implemented by the hidden layer of the two-layer BP network does not involve the pure principal eigenvectors since an unknown invertible matrix $\mathbf{T}$ is involved. Thus, the activation values of the hidden units are not the exact signal PCs but some linear combination of them. What is extracted by the network is the mth dimensional PCS. In that sense, BP is similar to many Hebbian PCA techniques (see, for example, Földiák's rule, the subspace rule, etc).

8.4.3 Application: Image Compression

The use of PCA for data compression is related to the fact that the method produces the optimal linear transformation among those mapping n-dimensional data into m dimensions, where $m < n$. PCA optimality is in the least-mean-squared-error sense, meaning that the original n-dimensional data can be reconstructed from the m-dimensional transform data achieving the minimum possible MSE.

Let us look at a specific example that illustrates the idea of data compression with PCA. Consider an image like "Lenna" shown in Figure 8.11a. Every pixel is represented by an integer between 0 and 255 corresponding to the pixel luminance (0 = black, 255 = white). The image has a size of 256×256 pixels. We partition the image into a block of size 8×8, thus creating data vectors in the 64-dimensional space. Each block creates data by stacking the 64 pixels of the block on top of each other. The gray value of each pixel is treated as a random variable. In high-resolution, low-noise images such as "Lenna," most neighboring pixels have similar values unless they lie on different sides of an edge. Therefore, we expect to have high correlation between pixels and we know that high correlation is the case where PCA may yield the best results. Indeed, although the superficial dimensionality of the blocks is 64, the intrinsic dimensionality can be as low as 8 or 12 depending on the acceptable level of error (see Figure 8.11).

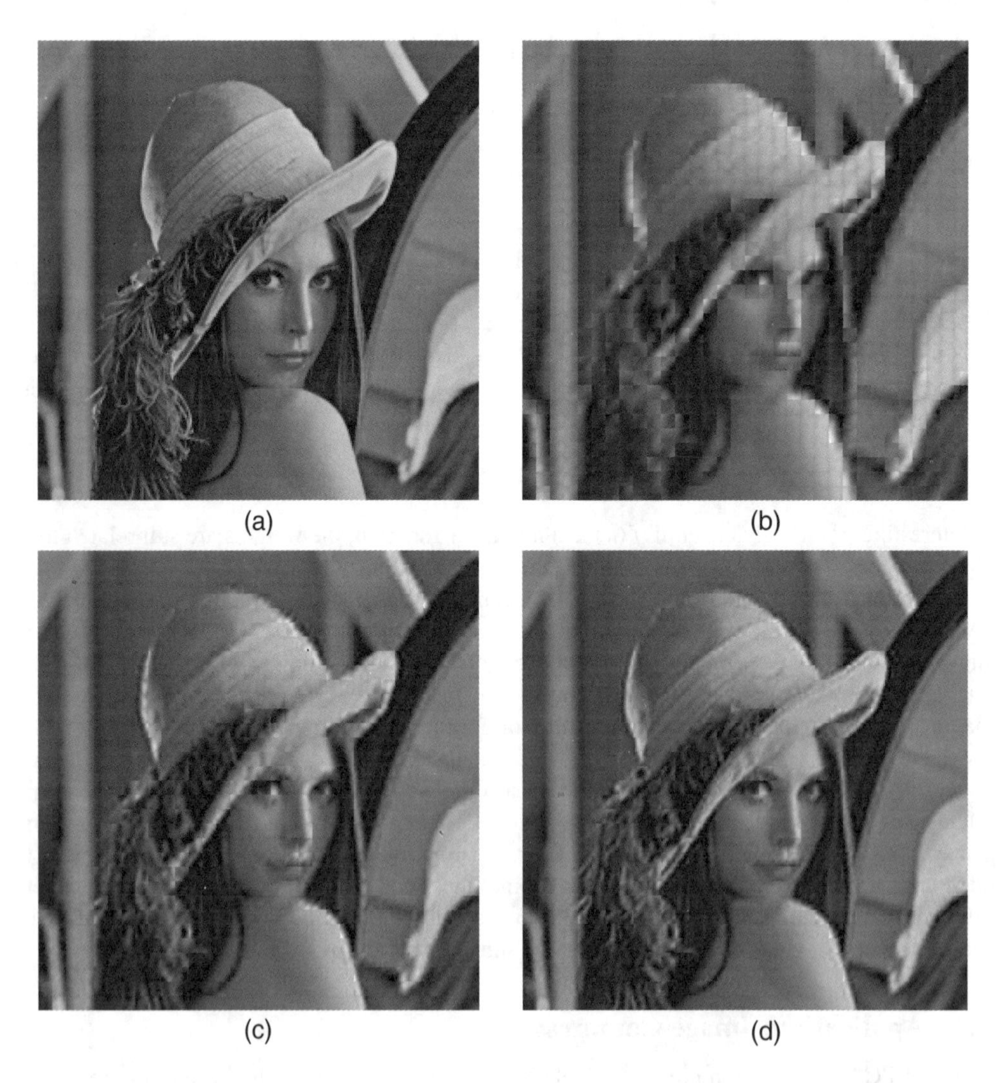

8.11 (a) The original "Lenna" image. Compressed "Lenna" using PCs obtained from the APEX model; (b) 4 PCs; (c) 8 PCs; and (d) 12 PCs.

8.4.4 PCA and Blind Source Separation

Consider n signals $x_1, \ldots, x_n$ resulting from the linear combination of an equal number of source signals $s_1, \ldots, s_n$,

$$\begin{bmatrix} x_1(k) \\ \vdots \\ x_n(k) \end{bmatrix} = \begin{bmatrix} h_{11} & \cdots & h_{1n} \\ \vdots & & \vdots \\ h_{n1} & \cdots & h_{nn} \end{bmatrix} \begin{bmatrix} s_1(k) \\ \vdots \\ s_n(k) \end{bmatrix} . \tag{8.72}$$

$$\mathbf{x}(k) = \mathbf{Hs}(k) . \tag{8.73}$$

The signals x_i are observed at the outputs of some receiving devices, e.g., microphones, antennas, etc. The sources s_i contain information that needs to be extracted at the receiver, but they are unknown. If the mixing matrix $\mathbf{H}$ is known, then the problem can be formulated as classical least squares optimization. If $\mathbf{H}$ is unknown, then the problem is called blind source separation (BSS). The term "blind" refers to fact that we are "blindly" looking for the sources without knowledge of the mixing parameters. In BSS, the solution is based on certain statistical properties of the sources, such as independence. BSS is a part of a large family of blind problems including blind deconvolution, blind system identification, and blind channel equalization.

Until recently, the only tool for blind problems was the analysis of higher order statistics (HOS). The use of second order statistics (SOS) was first noted by Tong et al. [37] in the 1990s. The problem studied in this classic paper was blind equalization. It was found that eigenvalue analysis of the oversampled observation covariance leads to blind recovery of the unknown filter coefficients. Nevertheless, second order methods do not really replace higher order methods since each approach is based on different assumptions. For example, second order methods assume that the sources are temporally colored, whereas higher order methods assume white sources. Another difference is that higher order methods do not apply on Gaussian signals, but second order methods do not have any such constraint.

Blind equalization is related to blind source separation, but it was not until 1997 that second order methods were proposed for BSS by Belouchrani et al. [38]. Here we shall offer a slightly different formulation which shows that BSS can be addressed with the help of PCA.

Before we proceed, note that the solution to the BSS problem posed above is not unique. This is because we can multiply source s_i by any non-zero scaling factor α and, at the same time, divide the ith column of $\mathbf{H}$ by α without affecting the observation sequence $\mathbf{x}$. Furthermore, we can change the order of the sources and similarly permute the columns of $\mathbf{H}$ and still obtain the same observation sequence $\mathbf{x}$. Thus, the scale and the order of the sources are unobservable.

Our assumptions are as follows:

A1. The observation vector sequence $\mathbf{x}(k)$ is spatially white:

$$\mathbf{R}_x(0) = E\left\{\mathbf{x}(k)\mathbf{x}(k)^T\right\} = \mathbf{I} . \tag{8.74}$$

If it is not white, it can always be whitened by a transformation of the form $\mathbf{x}'(k) \leftarrow \mathbf{R}_x(0)^{-1/2}\mathbf{x}(k)$.

A2. The sources are unit variance, pairwise uncorrelated, and each one is temporally colored:

$$E\left\{s_i(k)s_j(k)\right\} = \begin{cases} 0 & \text{if } i \neq j \\ r_i(0) = 1 & \text{if } i = j \end{cases} \tag{8.75}$$

$$E\left\{s_i(k)s_j(k-1)\right\} = \begin{cases} 0 & \text{if } i \neq j \\ r_i(1) \neq 0 & \text{if } i = j \end{cases} \tag{8.76}$$

$$\mathbf{R}_s(0) = E\left\{\mathbf{s}(k)\mathbf{s}(k)^T\right\} = \mathbf{I} \tag{8.77}$$

$$\mathbf{R}_s(1) \triangleq E\left\{\mathbf{s}(k)\mathbf{s}(k-1)^T\right\} = \operatorname{diag}\left[r_1(1), \ldots, r_n(1)\right] \neq 0\,. \tag{8.78}$$

The assumption that the sources are unit variance removes the part of the scaling ambiguity related to the magnitude of the scaling. There remains the sign ambiguity: if we change both the sign of s_i and the sign of the ith column of $\mathbf{H}$, then neither the observed sequence $\mathbf{x}$ nor the variance of s_i will change. It follows that if $\hat{\mathbf{H}}$ is a solution to the BSS problem, then so is $\hat{\mathbf{H}}\mathbf{P}$ for any a signed permutation matrix $\mathbf{P}$.

Consider the PCA of the signal:

$$\mathbf{y}(k) = \mathbf{x}(k) + \mathbf{x}(k-1)\,.$$

The covariance matrix of $\mathbf{y}$ is easily computed to be:

$$\begin{aligned} \mathbf{R}_y(0) &= E\left\{[\mathbf{x}(k) + \mathbf{x}(k-1)]\,[\mathbf{x}(k) + \mathbf{x}(k-1)]^T\right\} \\ &= 2\mathbf{R}_x(0) + \mathbf{R}_x(1) + \mathbf{R}_x(1)^T \\ &= 2\mathbf{I} + \mathbf{R}_x(1) + \mathbf{R}_x(1)^T \end{aligned}$$

where we define the lagged covariance,

$$\mathbf{R}_x(1) = E\left\{\mathbf{x}(k)\mathbf{x}(k-1)^T\right\} = \mathbf{H}\,\mathbf{R}_s(1)\,\mathbf{H}^T\,. \tag{8.79}$$

So,

$$\mathbf{R}_y(0) = \mathbf{H}\mathbf{D}\mathbf{H}^T\,. \tag{8.80}$$

Using assumption A2, the matrix

$$\mathbf{D} = 2\mathbf{I} + \mathbf{R}_s(1) + \mathbf{R}_s(1)^T \tag{8.81}$$

is diagonal. In addition, $\mathbf{H}$ is orthogonal since $\mathbf{H}\mathbf{H}^T = \mathbf{H}\mathbf{R}_s(0)\mathbf{H}^T = \mathbf{R}_x(0) = \mathbf{I}$. Hence, Equation (8.80) represents the eigenvalue decomposition of $\mathbf{R}_y(0)$. Moreover, the eigenvalues are given by the formula

$$d_i = 2 + 2E\left\{s_i(k)s_i(k-1)\right\} = 2\left(1 + r_i(1)\right)\,.$$

If $d_1, \ldots, d_n$ are distinct, then the eigen-decomposition is unique up to a permutation and sign of the eigenvectors.

We must stop for a moment and understand the consequences of this observation. First, it is obvious that the principal component analysis of $\mathbf{y}$ leads to an estimate of $\mathbf{H}$. If the columns of the matrix $\mathbf{U}$ are the n principal eigenvectors of $\mathbf{R}_y(0)$, then

$$\mathbf{U} = \mathbf{H}\mathbf{P}$$

where **P** is a signed permutation matrix. We can take this further and extract the source signals with arbitrary order and sign

$$\begin{aligned} \hat{\mathbf{s}}(k) &= \mathbf{U}^T \mathbf{x}(k) = \mathbf{P}^T \mathbf{s}(k) \\ \hat{s}_i(k) &= \pm s_{\pi(i)}(k) \, . \end{aligned}$$

Since the order and sign of the source signals are unobservable, this is the best estimate we can hope for. Figure 8.12 shows the block diagram of the overall BSS system using PCA.

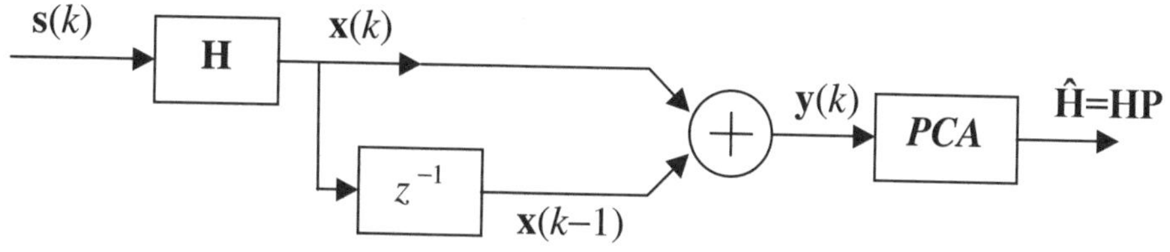

8.12 A model for blind source separation using PCA.

Second, our analysis holds for any signal $\mathbf{y}(k) = \mathbf{x}(k) + \mathbf{x}(k-l)$, where l is any non-zero time lag such that $\mathbf{R}_s(l) = E\{\mathbf{s}(k)\mathbf{s}(k-l)^T\} \neq 0$.

An adaptive solution of the BSS problem can be implemented using neural PCA models that can extract a complete set of principal eigenvectors. Such models include GHA, APEX, etc. Figure 8.13 shows the results of a blind separation experiment using the APEX model. The data were artificially created in two steps. First, we randomly generated $N = 3000$ samples of four pulse amplitude modulated (PAM) signals with 5 amplitude levels. Then, the signals were colored using the following FIR filters,

$$\begin{aligned} g_1 &= [0.8559,\ -0.8510,\ 0.8119,\ 0.7002,\ 0.7599,\ -1.7129,\ 1.5370,\ -1.6098,\ 1.1095,\ -1.1097] \\ g_2 &= [0.3855,\ 0.9652,\ 0.8183,\ 0.0370,\ -0.9260,\ -0.1119,\ -0.8030,\ -1.6650,\ -0.9014, \\ &\quad 0.5883] \\ g_3 &= [0.5542,\ -0.4152,\ 0.0618,\ 0.4574,\ 0.1990,\ 0.2576,\ 2.0807,\ -2.2772,\ 0.3390,\ 0.2899] \\ g_4 &= [0.6623,\ -0.5809,\ 0.8878,\ 0.1719,\ 0.8488,\ 0.9638,\ 1.3219,\ -0.0643,\ 1.3171,\ 0.2280] \end{aligned}$$

thus creating the sources s_1, s_2, s_3, and s_4. The mixing matrix

$$\mathbf{A} = \begin{bmatrix} -0.7283 & -0.5760 & 0.8701 & 0.8784 \\ -0.8719 & -0.6425 & 0.7825 & 0.9195 \\ -0.6235 & 0.8974 & -0.5981 & 0.5525 \\ -0.7057 & 0.6310 & -0.5692 & -0.6003 \end{bmatrix}$$

was used to derive the four observed signals x_1, x_2, x_3, and x_4, shown in Figure 8.13b. The vector sequence $\mathbf{x}(k)$ was spatially whitened,

$$\mathbf{x}'(k) = \mathbf{R}_x(0)^{-1/2}\mathbf{x}(k) = \mathbf{A}'\mathbf{s}(k)$$

and then the sources were blindly separated using the sequential APEX model on $\mathbf{y}(k) = \mathbf{x}'(k) + \mathbf{x}'(k-1)$. The steady-state forward weight matrix **W** attains the following unmixing performance:

$$\mathbf{W}\mathbf{A}' = \begin{bmatrix} 0.0142 & 1.0002 & -0.0171 & -0.0291 \\ -0.0381 & -0.0437 & 0.0163 & -1.0012 \\ -0.0800 & -0.0068 & -1.0002 & -0.0071 \\ 0.9988 & 0.0199 & -0.0385 & 0.0104 \end{bmatrix} .$$

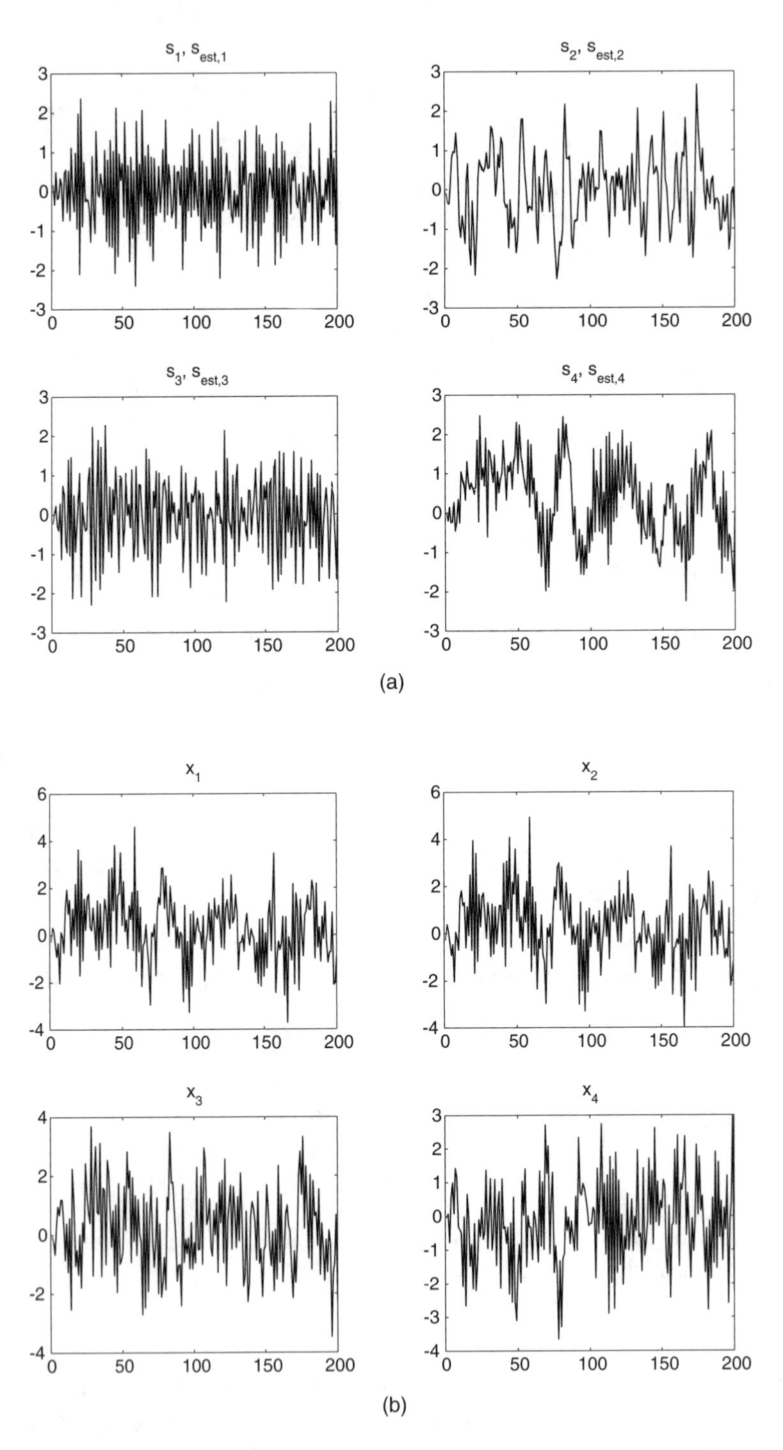

8.13 Blind separation of four sources, s_1, s_2, s_3, and s_4, using the APEX model. (a) A window of 200 samples of the sources, superimposed with the reconstructed signals. The error is so small that true and reconstructed signals can not be visually separated. (b) The same time window for the four observed mixtures.

The original and reconstructed sources are shown in Figure 8.13a. We have appropriately changed the signs and the order of the reconstructed sources in order to facilitate the comparison.

An alternative approach for second order neural BSS has been proposed [39, 40]. This approach is based on neural SVD analyzers known as asymmetric PCA models. One such model, the cross-coupled Hebbian rule [41], has been applied for the blind extraction of sources such as images or speech signals using a preselected time lag l. A discussion of asymmetric PCA models extends beyond the scope of this chapter.

8.5 Nonlinear PCA

There is more than one way to extend classical, linear PCA into the nonlinear domain. One approach is related to the functions $f_i()$ described in Section 8.2, and another approach is related to the neural PCA learning rules described in Section 8.4. The first approach leads to nonlinear multilayer perceptron architectures for the implementation of the representation and reconstruction functions. The second approach leads to nonlinear extensions of Hebbian learning rules. Both approaches have their own merits, deserve a closer look, and are discussed in the following sections.

8.5.1 Nonlinear PCA: A Functional Approach

Let us revisit the starting point of PCA analysis, namely the functions used for reconstructing the data,

$$\begin{aligned} x_1 &= f_1(y_1, \ldots, y_m) = f_1(\mathbf{y}) \\ &\vdots \\ x_n &= f_n(y_1, \ldots, y_m) = f_n(\mathbf{y}) \end{aligned}$$

as they appear in Equation (8.1). The PCA vector function $\mathbf{x} = \mathbf{f}(\mathbf{y})$ is linear and, therefore, it represents a linear m-dimensional manifold, i.e., a hyperplane, in the n-dimensional space. An obvious extension is to assume that $\mathbf{f}()$ is a nonlinear function representing an m-parametric nonlinear manifold in $\mathbb{R}^n$. The difference between linear and nonlinear manifolds can be easily visualized in $\mathbb{R}^2$ (see Figure 8.14).

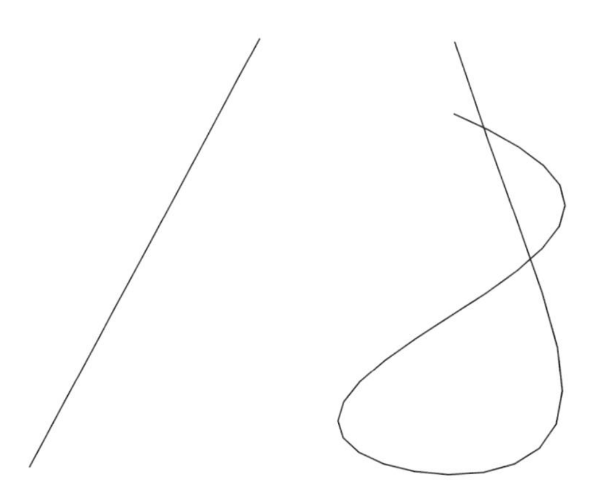

8.14 A linear mono-parametric manifold in R^2 is a straight line (left). A nonlinear mono-parametric manifold can be a curly shape (right).

In the same spirit, the representation function $\mathbf{y} = \mathbf{W}(\mathbf{x})$ is also nonlinear. The representation function expresses the feature vector $\mathbf{y}$ — now called the nonlinear principal component vector — as a function of the data $\mathbf{x}$. Obviously, nonlinear PCA, as described above, has a greater representation power than PCA, provided that the classes of functions $\mathcal{S}_f$, $\mathcal{S}_w$, where $\mathbf{f}()$ and $\mathbf{W}()$ belong, are supersets of the linear class L.

There are very few analytical results for nonlinear PCA. The second order statistics are no longer useful, and there are no analytical tools in nonlinear analysis as powerful as eigenvalue decomposition. However, if we know the representation function $\mathbf{W}()$, then the optimal reconstruction function is given by following theorem:

THEOREM 8.4 *[42] If the vectors $\mathbf{x} \in \mathbb{R}^n$ and $\mathbf{y} \in \mathbb{R}^m$ are jointly distributed, then the optimal estimate of $\mathbf{x}$ by a function of $\mathbf{y}$ is the conditional expectation $g(\mathbf{y}) = E\{\mathbf{x} \,|\, \mathbf{y}\}$:*

$$\min_{g(\mathbf{y})} E\left\{\|\mathbf{x} - g(\mathbf{y})\|^2\right\} = E\left\{\|\mathbf{x} - E\{\mathbf{x} \,|\, \mathbf{y}\}\|^2\right\} .$$

Applied to nonlinear PCA, Theorem 8.4 implies that, given $\mathbf{W}()$, the optimal reconstruction function $\mathbf{f}()$ is [13]:

$$\mathbf{f}(\mathbf{y}) = E\{\mathbf{x} \,|\, \mathbf{y} = \mathbf{W}(\mathbf{x})\} = \int_{\mathbf{x} \in \mathbf{W}^{-1}(\mathbf{y})} \mathbf{x}\, dP(\mathbf{x}) \tag{8.82}$$

where $\mathbf{W}^{-1}(\mathbf{y}) \equiv \{\mathbf{x} : \mathbf{W}(\mathbf{x}) = \mathbf{y}\}$ and $P(\mathbf{x})$ is the cumulative probability distribution function of $\mathbf{x}$. If $\mathbf{W}()$ is not given, the optimizing pair of functions $[\mathbf{f}(), \mathbf{W}()]$ may not be unique. However, the following two objects are unique and characterize $\mathbf{x}$ for a specific dimension m and classes $\mathcal{S}_f$, $\mathcal{S}_w$:

1. the contour set $\mathcal{I} = \{\mathbf{W}^{-1}(\mathbf{y}) : \text{ all } \mathbf{y}\}$
2. the optimal m-parametric surface $\mathcal{C}$ generated by $\mathbf{f}$. We call $\mathcal{C}$ the m-parametric nonlinear principal component surface (NPCS) of $\mathbf{x}$.

EXAMPLE 8.2:

Consider the representation of two-dimensional data by a single nonlinear component y. Let the reconstruction function $\mathbf{f}(y)$ belong to the class $\mathcal{S}_f$ of 2-D ellipses, i.e.,

$$\begin{aligned} \hat{x}_1 &= f_1(y) = a_1 \cos(y) + b_1 \sin(y) + c_1 \\ \hat{x}_2 &= f_2(y) = a_2 \cos(y) + b_2 \sin(y) + c_2 . \end{aligned}$$

Let the data be scattered around a specific ellipse:

$$\begin{aligned} x_1 &= 2\cos(y) + 0.5 \sin(y) + e_1 \\ x_2 &= \cos(y) - \sin(y) - 1 + e_2 \end{aligned}$$

as in Figure 8.15. The terms e_1 and e_2 are small additive noises. The one-parametric NPCS C is the ellipse shown in the figure. It fits the data with $MSE = 0.0128$. For the sake of comparison, we also show the corresponding linear one-dimensional PCS (straight line). Obviously, the linear PCS is not a good fit for the data ($MSE = 0.6414$).

8.5.1.1 Kramer's Neural Model

Kramer's nonlinear PCA neural network [43] is a multilayer perceptron with a special structure. The model has five layers: the input and output layers have the same number of units n; the first and

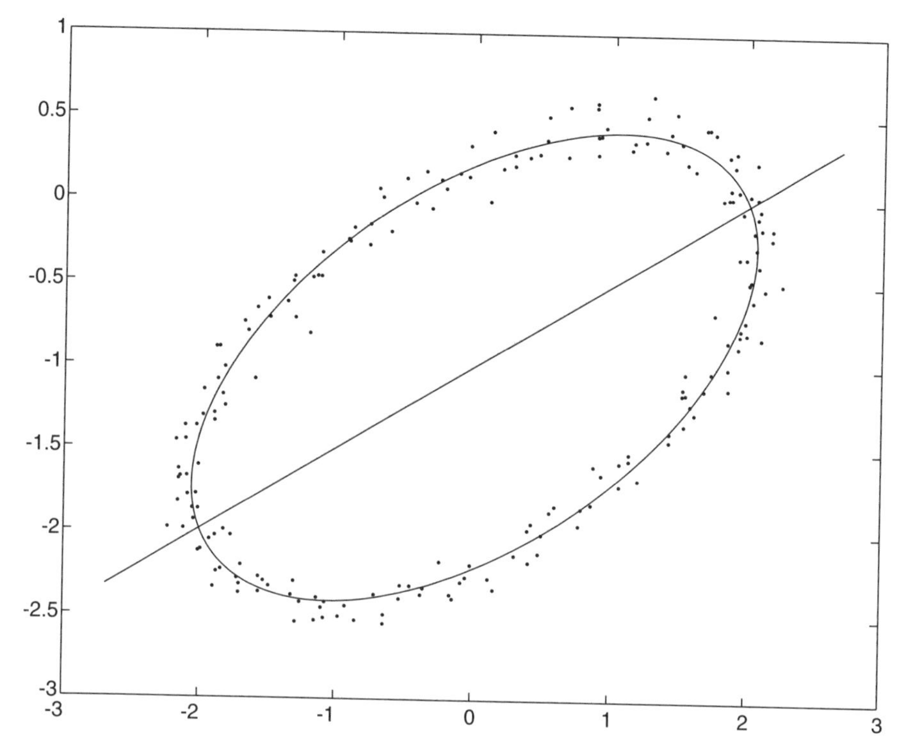

8.15 Nonlinear vs. linear PCS. For these data, the nonlinear PCS (ellipse) is a much better fit than the linear PCS (straight line).

third layers are nonlinear, and the second and fourth are linear. Layers 1 and 3 have enough units to represent the functions $\mathbf{f}()$ and $\mathbf{W}()$ with acceptable accuracy. Layer 2 contains m units, i.e., as many as the nonlinear PCs. The activations of the neurons in Layer 2 are the nonlinear PCs of the input data.

The architecture of the network is the cascade of two modules: the representation subnetwork (layers 0–2) and the reconstruction subnetwork (layers 3–4). These two modules have the same structure: they have two layers of neurons (excluding the input layer), where the first layer is wide and nonlinear and the second layer is narrow and linear. It is known [44, 45] that the functions of the form,

$$\phi(\mathbf{x}) = \sum_{i=1}^{N} \alpha_i\, f\left(\sum_{j=1}^{n} \beta_{ij} x_j + \gamma_i\right) + \delta \tag{8.83}$$

where $f()$ is the sigmoid function, are universal approximators. This means that $\phi(\mathbf{x})$ can approximate any continuous bounded function $g(\mathbf{x})$ on the n-dimensional unit hypercube $I_n = [0, 1]^n$ with arbitrary accuracy provided that N can be arbitrarily large. In other words, for any given error threshold ε, there exists an integer N and real numbers α_i, β_{ij}, γ_i, and δ such that $|g(\mathbf{x}) - \phi(\mathbf{x})| < \varepsilon$, for all $\mathbf{x} \in I_n$.

This result applies directly to neural networks with structures like those of the representation and reconstruction subnetworks in Figure 8.16. Equation (8.83) expresses the input-output relationship of a two layer network with a nonlinear first layer and a linear second layer. The second layer weights/thresholds are equal to α_i, δ, and the first layer weights/thresholds are equal to β_{ij}, γ_i. Thus, the representation and reconstruction subnetworks in Kramer's net are universal approximators. Provided that enough units are present in layers 1 and 3, the total network can represent any continuous representation or reconstruction function on I_n. The network can represent very complex continuous nonlinear PCA; therefore, it is useful for problems where the data relationships are not adequately described by linear relations.

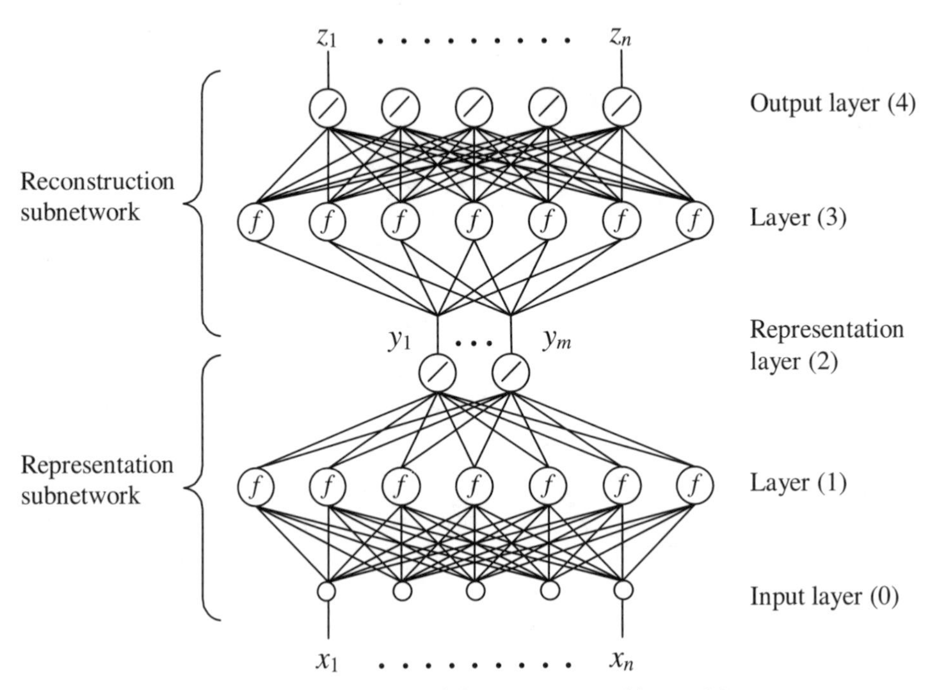

8.16 Kramer's nonlinear PCA neural network is a multilayer perceptron with a special structure.

8.5.2 Application: Ischemia Detection

The high representation power of the nonlinear PCA features has been used in the classification of ischemic episodes using patient ECG signals [46]. Ischemia is related to the shape of a specific part of the cardiac beat known as the ST segment. The analysis of the ST segment is far from trivial for many reasons, including inaccurate determination of the ST segment boundaries, drifting signal baseline, signal artefacts due to a patient's movements or sensor noise, patient-dependent ischemic signatures, and appropriate feature selection from the ST segment data. Careful preprocessing of the ECG signal can remove the baseline drift and help estimate the starting and ending points of the ST segment. Once the ST segment is extracted, it is sampled and calibrated by subtracting the average ST segment of the specific patient. The resulting vector forms the raw data for a nonlinear classification algorithm. The idea is that normal raw data have different nonlinear features than abnormal (ischemic) data. The idea is put to the test using a Kramer nonlinear PCA network. The network is trained using only normal (healthy) data and is tested on both normal and abnormal data. The nonlinear features are the activation vector of the second layer of the network. The distribution of the normal features is modeled using an RBF neural network. Classification into the abnormal category happens when the activation vector of the second layer lies in a low probability area of the normal PDF, as modeled above.

The results reported by Stamkopoulos et al. [46] are based on data from the European ST-T ECG signal database. Using only two nonlinear components and a threshold allowing 80% correct classification on the normal beats, the authors report classification results for the abnormal beats ranging between 60 and 100%, with an average rate at 75%. This performance is far better than the other ischemic beat detection algorithms proposed in the literature [47]–[50].

8.5.3 Nonlinear PCA: A Hebbian Approach

Another approach for defining nonlinear PCA is the extension of linear Hebbian PCA models to nonlinear ones. This is accomplished with the introduction of a nonlinear function $g()$ in the learning algorithm. Two basic questions need to be answered here: (1) how is this done? and (2) what is the motivation behind it? The "how-to" question relates to numerical stability issues. One needs to find a proper way to introduce g so that the modified algorithm remains stable. The "why" question is more important because it relates to the meaning of the stability points of the new algorithm(s). At first sight, the nonlinear extension of Hebbian rules may seem like a mathematical exercise motivated more by curiosity than by application. It turns out, however, that the problem has more depth as it leads to the blind separation of independent sources from their linear mixtures.

Consider, for example, the nonlinear PCA subspace rule introduced by Oja et al. [51] as an extension to the linear PCA subspace rule (see Equation (8.61)):

$$\Delta\mathbf{W}(k) = \beta(k)[\mathbf{x}(k) - \mathbf{W}(k)\mathbf{g}(\mathbf{y}(k))]\mathbf{g}(\mathbf{y}(k))^T . \tag{8.84}$$

Let us again consider the BSS problem

$$\mathbf{x}(k) = \mathbf{H}\mathbf{s}(k) \tag{8.85}$$

where the sources $s_1(k), \ldots, s_n(k)$ are zero-mean, unit-variance, statistically independent variables:

$$\mathbf{R}_s = E\left\{\mathbf{s}(k)\mathbf{s}(k)^T\right\} = \mathbf{I} . \tag{8.86}$$

The problem is identical to the BSS problem discussed in Section 8.4.4 except for the assumptions on the sources. As before, without affecting generality, we may assume that the vector $\mathbf{x}(k)$ is spatially white: $E\{\mathbf{x}(k)\mathbf{x}(k)^T\} = \mathbf{I}$. The next theorem shows that Equation (8.84) extracts the unknown matrix $\mathbf{H}$ and, consequently, the hidden independent sources s_i.

THEOREM 8.5 *[52, 53] Assume the following:*

1. *The random vector* $\mathbf{s}$ *has symmetrical density with* $E\{\mathbf{s}\} = 0$.
2. *The elements* $s_1, \ldots, s_n$ *of* $\mathbf{s}$ *are statistically mutually independent and have the same density* $P_s(s)$.
3. *The function* $g()$ *is odd and at least twice differentiable everywhere.*
4. *The following conditions are satisfied by* $g()$ *and* $P_s()$:

$$E\left\{s^2 g'(\alpha s)\right\} - 2\alpha E\left\{g(\alpha s)g'(\alpha s)s\right\} - E\left\{g(\alpha s)^2\right\} < 0$$

where $g'()$ *denotes the derivative of* $g()$ *and* α *is a scalar such that*

$$E\{sg(\alpha s)\} = \alpha E\left\{g(\alpha s)^2\right\} .$$

5. *The following holds true:*

$$E\left\{s^2\right\} E\left\{g'(\alpha s)\right\} - E\left\{g(\alpha s)^2\right\} < 0 .$$

Then the matrix,

$$\mathbf{D} = \alpha \mathbf{P} \mathbf{H}^T$$

where **P** *is an arbitrary* $n \times n$ *permutation matrix, is an asymptotically stable stationary point of Equation* (8.84).

The theorem implies that, at equilibrium, the outputs y_i will be scaled versions of the independent sources s_i with a possible change in order:

$$\mathbf{y}(k) = \mathbf{W}\mathbf{x}(k) = \alpha \mathbf{P}\mathbf{s}(k) \quad (8.87)$$

$$y_i(k) = \alpha s_{\pi(i)}(k) \,. \quad (8.88)$$

We say that the algorithm performs the analysis of the signal $\mathbf{x}(k)$ into independent components. The term independent component analysis (ICA) first appeared in the works of Jutten and Herault [54] and Comon et al. [55]. The analogy between PCA and ICA is summarized below:

- It is possible to obtain ICA neural models by nonlinear extensions of Hebbian PCA models.
- PCA extracts uncorrelated components of the signal, whereas ICA extracts independent components.
- PCA is based on second order statistics, whereas ICA is based on higher-than-second order statistics (higher order statistics, or HOS).
- The neural models implementing PCA involve linear units, whereas ICA neural models involve nonlinear functions.

Many different nonlinear functions $g()$ can be applied in Equation (8.84) as long as they satisfy the conditions set in Theorem 8.5. A simple nonlinear function is $g(z) = z^3$. Some mathematical manipulations based on the theorem conditions lead to the conclusion that, for $g(z) = z^3$, the algorithm is asymptotically stable if

$$E\left\{s^4\right\} - 3\left(E\left\{s^2\right\}\right)^2 > 0 \,.$$

The expression $k(s) = E\{s^4\} - 3(E\{s^2\})^2$ is the fourth order cumulant of the variable s also known as the kurtosis of s. Other nonlinear functions, such as $g(z) = \tanh(z)$, are stable under negative kurtosis conditions.

Higher-than-second order cumulants (and especially the kurtosis) play a central role in the blind recovery of independent signals from linear mixtures and also in the blind deconvolution of non-Gaussian signals [56]. The subjects of ICA, blind source separation (BSS), and blind deconvolution (BD) in conjunction with neural models are very wide and extend beyond the scope of this chapter. A large variety of neural models for ICA have been proposed in the literature [52]–[54], [57]–[61]. The reader interested in delving into the theory of ICA should refer to the books of Lee [62], Girolami [63], Haykin [64, 65], and Cichocki and Unbehauen [66].

8.5.4 Application: Blind Image Separation

We mixed three negative kurtotic images, $s1$, $s2$, $s3$, to produce three confused images, $x1$, $x2$, $x3$, as shown in Figure 8.17. The mixing matrix **A** was randomly chosen:

$$\mathbf{A} = \begin{bmatrix} -0.7224 & 0.9609 & -0.7029 \\ -0.8077 & -0.8691 & -0.9677 \\ 0.8960 & -0.5881 & 0.9585 \end{bmatrix} .$$

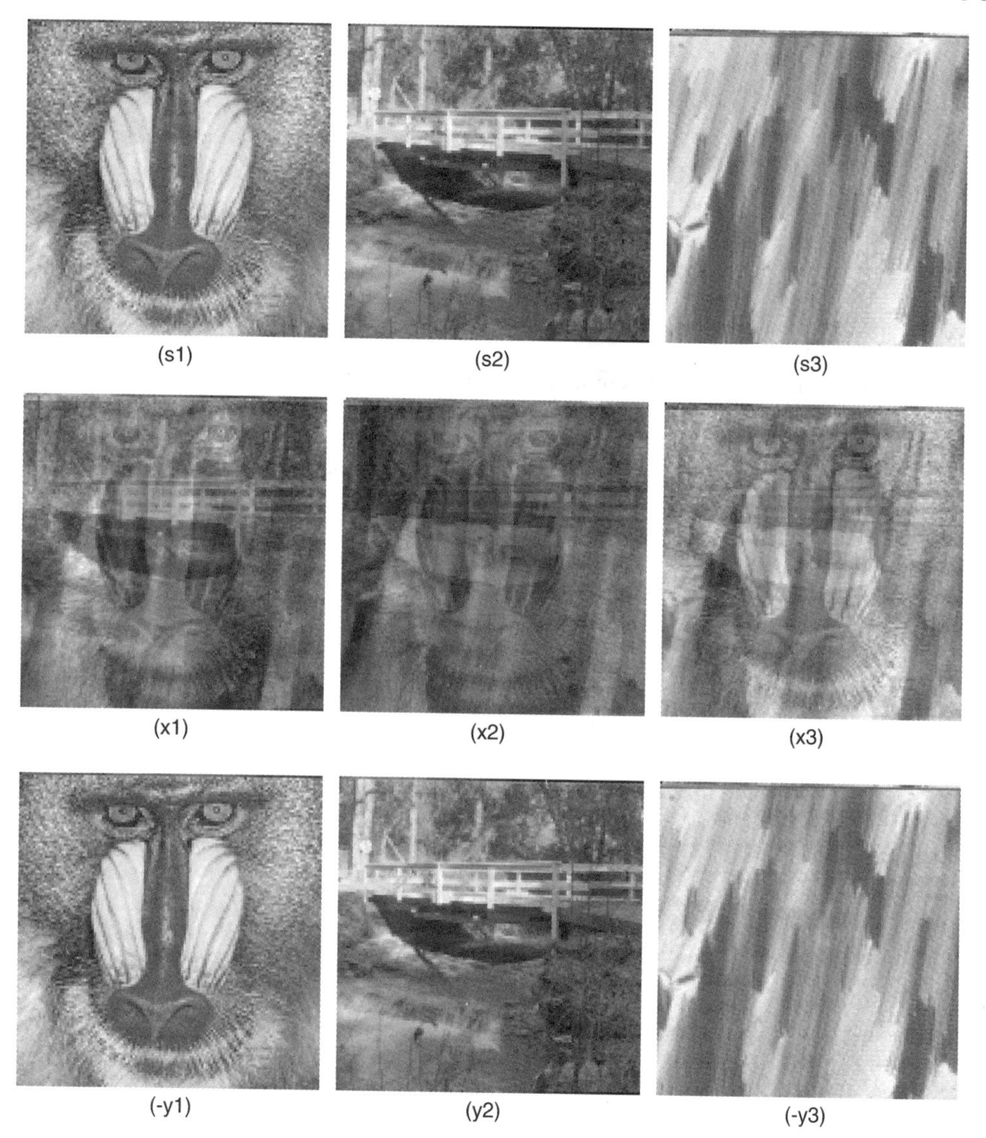

8.17 The source images, S1, S2, and S3, (top row) are mixed into the confused images, X1, X2, and X3 (middle row). The nonlinear PCA rule performs almost perfect unmixing of the sources into the images Y1, Y2, and Y3 (bottom row).

All images were transformed into one-dimensional signals by stacking the image columns on top of each other. We then created a three-dimensional vector signal $\mathbf{x}(k) = [x1(k)\, x2(k)\, x3(k)]^T$, where k is the pixel position (if the image has size $N \times N$, then $k = 1, \ldots, N^2$).

The nonlinear PCA rule Equation (8.84) with $g(z) = \tanh(z)$ was applied to the spatially whitened vector $\mathbf{x}(k)$. The algorithm converged very fast. After only six sweeps over the data, the following unmixing operator was obtained:

$$\mathbf{W}^T\mathbf{A} = \begin{bmatrix} -1.1942 & -0.0383 & 0.0663 \\ -0.0426 & 1.2142 & -0.0597 \\ -0.0389 & -0.0801 & -1.3220 \end{bmatrix}$$

so

$$\mathbf{y} = \mathbf{W}^T \mathbf{x} = \mathbf{W}^T \mathbf{A} \mathbf{s} .$$

Since the unmixing operator is very close to a permutation matrix (except for the signs), the images have been successfully separated. Figure 8.17 verifies that the unmixing result is almost perfect.

References

[1] Pearson, K., On lines and planes of closest fit to systems of points in space. *Philos. Mag.*, ser. 6, 2:559–572, 1901.

[2] Hotelling, H., Analysis of complex of statistical variables into principal components. *J. Educ. Psych.*, 24:498–520, 1933.

[3] Hebb, D.O., *The Organization of Behavior.* John Wiley & Sons, Inc., New York, 1949.

[4] Oja, E., A simplified neuron model as a principal component analyzer. *J. Math. Biology,* 15:267–273, 1982.

[5] Karhunen, J. and Oja, E., New methods for stochastic approximation of truncated Karhunen–Loeve expansions. In *Proc. 6th Int. Conf. on Pattern Recognition.* Springer-Verlag, New York, 1982, 550–553.

[6] Otsu, Y., Kimura, F., and Tsumoto, T., Hebbian induction of LTP in visual cortex: perforated patch-clamp study in cultured neurons. *J. Neurophysiol.*, 74:2437–2443, 1995.

[7] Poon, C.S., Self-Tuning optimal regulation of respiratory motor output by Hebbian covariance learning. *Neural Networks,* 9(8):1367–1383, 1996.

[8] Hubel, D.H., *Eye, Brain, and Vision.* Scientific American Library, 1988.

[9] Fregnác, Y., Schultz, D., and Thorp, S., A cellular analog of visual cortical plasticity. *Nature,* 333:367–370, 1988.

[10] Ljung, L., Analysis of recursive stochastic algortihms. *IEEE Trans. Automat. Contr.,* AC-22(4):551–575, 1977.

[11] Kushner, H.J. and Clark, D.S., *Stochastic Approximation Methods for Constrained and Unconstrained Systems.* Springer-Verlag, New York, 1978.

[12] Oja, E. and Karhunen, J., On stochastic approximation of the eigenvectors and eigenvalues of the expectation of a random matrix. *J. Math. Anal. and Appl.*, 106:69–84, 1985.

[13] Diamantaras, K.I. and Kung, S.Y., *Principal Component Neural Networks: Theory and Applications.* Wiley Interscience, New York, 1996.

[14] Haykin, S., Editor. *Blind Deconvolution.* Prentice-Hall, Englewood Cliffs, NJ, 1994.

[15] Sanger, T. D., Optimal unsupervised learning in a single-layer linear feedforward neural network. *Neural Networks,* 2(6):459–473, 1989.

[16] Golub, G.H. and Van Loan, C.F., *Matrix Computations,* 2nd edition. Johns Hopkins University Press, Baltimore, MD, 1989.

[17] Kung, S.Y. and Diamantaras, K.I., A neural network learning algorithm for adaptive principal component extraction (APEX). In *Proc. IEEE Int. Conf. Acoustics, Speech Signal Process.,* Albuquerque, April 1990, 861–864.

[18] Ljung, L. and Söderström, T., *Theory and Practice of Recursive Identification.* MIT Press, Cambridge, MA, 1983.

[19] Chauvin, Y., Principal component analysis by gradient descent on a constrained linear Hebbian cell. In *Proc. Int. Joint Conf. Neural Networks (IJCNN).* Washington, DC, 1989, 373–380.

[20] Cichocki, A. and Unbehauen, R., Neural networks for computing eigenvalues and eigenvectors. *Biol. Cybern.,* 68:155–164, 1992.

[21] Krasulina, T.P., Method of stochastic approximation in the determination of the largest eigenvalue of the mathematical expectation of random matrices. *Automation Remote Control,* 215–221, February 1970.

[22] Leen, T., Dynamics of learning in linear feature-discovery networks. *Network,* 2:85–105, 1991.

[23] Lenz, R. and Österberg, M., A parallel learning filter system that learns the KL-expansion from examples. In B.H. Juang, S.Y. Kung, and C.A. Kamm, Editors, *Neural Networks for Signal Processing.* IEEE, New York, 1991, 121–130.

[24] Luo, F.L., Unbehauen, R., and Li, Y.D., A principal component analysis algorithm with invariant norm. *Neurocomputing,* 8(2):213–221, 1995.

[25] Oja, E., Principal components, minor components, and linear networks. *Neural Networks,* 5(6):927–935, 1992.

[26] Owsley, N.L., Adaptive data orthogonalization. In *Proc. IEEE Int. Conf. Acoustics, Speech Signal Proc.,* Tulsa, OK, April 1978, 109–112.

[27] Palmieri, F., A self-organizing neural network for multidimensional approximation. In *Proc. Int. Joint Conf. Neural Networks (IJCNN),* volume 4. Baltimore, June 1992, 802–807.

[28] Russo, L.E., An outer product neural net for extracting principal components from a time series. In B.H. Juang, S.Y. Kung, and C.A. Kamm, Editors, *Neural Networks for Signal Processing.* IEEE, New York, 1991, 161–170.

[29] Smith, S.T., Dynamical systems that perform the singular value decomposition. *Syst. Control Lett.,* 16:319–327, 1991.

[30] White, R.H., Competitive Hebbian learning: algorithm and demonstrations. *Neural Networks,* 5(2):261–275, 1992.

[31] Földiák, P., Adaptive network for optimal linear feature extraction. In *Int. Joint Conf. Neural Networks,* volume 1. Washington DC, 1989, 401–406.

[32] Baldi, P., Linear learning: landscapes and algorithms. In D.S. Touretzky, Editor, *Advances in Neural Information Processing Systems I,* (Denver 1988), Morgan Kaufmann, San Mateo, CA, 1989.

[33] Oja, E., Neural networks, principal components, and subspaces. *Int. J. Neural Syst.,* 1(1):61–68, 1989.

[34] Rubner, J. and Tavan, P., A self-organizing network for principal-components analysis. *Europhysics Lett.,* 10(7):693–698, 1989.

[35] Hornik, K. and Kuan, C.M., Convergence analysis of local feature extraction algorithms. *Neural Networks,* 5:229–240, 1992.

[36] Bourlard, H. and Kamp, Y., Auto-Association by multilayer perceptrons and singular value decomposition. *Biol. Cybern.,* 59:291–294, 1988.

[37] Tong, L., Xu, G., and Kailath, T., Blind identification and equalization based on second-order statistics: a time domain approach. *IEEE Trans. Inf. Theory,* 40(2):340–349, 1994.

[38] Belouchrani, A., Abed-Meraim, K., Cardoso, J.F., and Moulines, E., A blind source separation technique using second-order statistics. *IEEE Trans. Signal Proc.,* 45(2):434–444, 1997.

[39] Diamantaras, K.I., Asymmetric PCA neural networks for adaptive blind source separation. In *Proc. IEEE Workshop Neural Networks Signal Proc. (NNSP'98).* Cambridge, UK, August 1998, 103–112.

[40] Diamantaras, K.I., Second order Hebbian neural networks and blind source separation. In *Proc. EUSIPCO'98 (Eur. Signal Process. Conf.).* Rhodes, Greece, September 1998, 1317–1320.

[41] Diamantaras, K.I. and Kung, S.Y., Multilayer neural networks for reduced rank approximation. *IEEE Trans. Neural Networks,* 5(5):684–697, 1994.

[42] Anderson, B.D.O. and Moore, J.B., Editors. *Optimal Filtering,* Prentice-Hall, Englewood Cliffs, NJ, 1979.

[43] Kramer, M.A., Nonlinear principal component analysis using autoassociative neural networks. *J. Am. Institute Chem. Eng. (AIChE),* 37(2):233–243, 1991.

[44] Cybenko, G., Approximation by superpositions of a sigmoidal function. *Math. Control Signals Syst.,* 2:303–314, 1989.

[45] Hornik, K., Strinchcombe, M., and White, H., Multilayer feedforward networks are universal approximators. *Neural Networks,* 2(5):359–366, 1989.

[46] Stamkopoulos, T., Diamantaras, K.I., Maglaveras, N., and Strintzis, M.G., ECG Analysis using nonlinear PCA neural networks for ischemia detection. *IEEE Trans. Signal Process.,* 46(11):3058–3067, 1998.

[47] Maglaveras, N., Stamkopoulos, T., Pappas, C., and Strintzis, M.G., Use of neural networks in detection of ischemic episodes from ECG leads. In J. Vlontzos, J.N. Hwang, and E. Wilson, Editors, *Neural Networks for Signal Processing IV.* IEEE Press, New York, 1994, 518–524.

[48] Silipo, R., Laguna, P., Marchesi, C., and Mark, R.G., ST-T segment change recognition using artificial neural networks and principal component analysis. In *Computers in Cardiology.* IEEE Computer Society Press, New York, 1995, 213–216.

[49] Jager, F., Mark, R.G., Moody, G.B., and Divjak, S., Analysis of transient ST segment changes during ambulatory monitoring using the Karhunen–Loeve transform. In *Computers in Cardiology.* IEEE Computer Society Press, New York, 1992, 691–694.

[50] Jager, F., Moody, G.B., Taddei, A., and Mark, R.G., Performance measures for algorithms to detect transient ischemic ST segment changes. In *Computers in Cardiology.* IEEE Computer Society Press, New York, 1991, 369–372.

[51] Oja, E., Ogawa, H., and Wangviwattana, J., Learning in nonlinear constrained Hebbian networks. In T. Kohonen et al., Editor, *Artificial Neural Networks.* Amsterdam: North Holland, 1991, 385–390.

[52] Oja, E., The nonlinear PCA learning rule and signal separation — mathematical analysis. Technical Report TR. A26, Lab of Computer and Information Science, Helsinki University of Technology, Espoo, Finland, August 1995.

[53] Karhunen, J., Oja, E., Wang, L., Vigario, R., and Joutsensalo, J., A class of neural networks for independent component analysis. *IEEE Trans. Neural Networks,* 8(3):486–504, 1997.

[54] Jutten, C. and Herault, J., Blind separation of sources, part I: an adaptive algorithm based on neuromimetic architecture. *Signal Process.,* 24(1):1–10, 1991.

[55] Comon, P., Jutten, C., and Herault, J., Blind separation of sources, part II: problems statement. *Signal Process.,* 24:11–20, 1991.

[56] Gadzow, J.A., Blind deconvolution via cumulant extrema. *IEEE Signal Process. Mag.,* 13(3):24–42, 1996.

[57] Bell, A.J. and Sejnowski, T.J., An information-maximization approach to blind separation and blind deconvolution. *Neural Computation,* 7(6):1129–1159, 1995.

[58] Cardoso, J.F. and Laheld, B.H., Equivariant adaptive source separation. *IEEE Trans. Signal Process.,* 44(12):3017–3030, 1996.

[59] Cichocki, A., Amari, S., Adachi, M., and Kasprzak, W., Self adaptive neural networks for blind separation of sources. In *Proc. Int. Symp. Circuits Syst., (ISCAS-96).* Atlanta, GA, 1996, 157–161.

[60] Girolami, M. and Fyfe, C., An extended exploratory projection pursuit network with linear and nonlinear anti-Hebbian lateral connections applied to the cocktail party problem. *Neural Networks,* 10(9):1607–1618, 1997.

[61] Hyvärinen, A. and Oja, E., A fast fixed-point algorithm for independent component analysis. *Neural Computation,* 9(7):1483–1492, 1997.

[62] Lee, T.W., *Independent Component Analysis — Theory and Applications.* Kluwer Academic Publishers, 1998.

[63] Girolami, M., *Self-Organising Neural Networks: Independent Component Analysis and Blind Source Separation.* Springer-Verlag, New York, 1998.

[64] Haykin, S., *Unsupervised Adaptive Filtering, Vol 1, Blind Source Separation.* John Wiley & Sons, New York, 2000.

[65] Haykin, S., *Unsupervised Adaptive Filtering, Vol 2, Blind Deconvolution.* John Wiley & Sons, New York, 2000.

[66] Cichocki, A. and Unbehauen, R., Robust estimation of principal components by using neural network learning algorithms. *IEEE Electron. Lett.,* 29(21):1869–1870, 1993.

9

Applications of Artificial Neural Networks to Time Series Prediction

Yuansong Liao
Oregon Graduate Institute of Science and Technology

John Moody
Oregon Graduate Institute of Science and Technology

Lizhong Wu
HNC Software, Inc.

This chapter provides a technical overview of neural network approaches to time series prediction problems and discusses challenges associated with time series prediction and neural network solutions. Some of the important issues related to neural network time series modeling include incorporating temporal information, selecting input variables, and balancing model bias/variance trade-off. Three techniques — sensitivity based input selection and pruning, constructing committee prediction models using input feature grouping, and smoothing regularizer for recurrent neural networks — and their application to an economic time series prediction problem are presented in detail. This case study demonstrates how to tackle a time series prediction problem in the neural network paradigm.

9.1 Introduction

A time series is a set of observations obtained sequentially in time. Observations in a time series can be spaced in a physical time scale (e.g., hourly, daily), a business time scale (e.g., transaction

0-8493-2359-2/01/$0.00+$1.50

tick), or other user-defined time scales (e.g., θ-time[1]). If a time series can be forecasted exactly, it is said to be deterministic. Usually, practical time series are stochastic processes because of the existence of observation noises whose characteristics can change over time. In consequence, the future observation of a time series is only partially determined by past observations and has a probability distribution conditioned by its past observations and other prior knowledge. The goal of time series prediction is to model the underlying mechanism that generates the time series so that the value of the series for a short to intermediate term into the future can be predicted.

Artificial neural networks are statistical modeling tools that have a wide range of applications, including time series prediction. Examples include power load forecasting [48], medical risk prediction [47, 76], economic and financial forecasting [27, 37, 52, 53, 55, 57, 85], and chaotic time series prediction [50, 67, 79]. In most cases, neural network prediction models demonstrate better performance than other approaches. For example, Moody, Levin, and Rehfuss [53] convincingly demonstrated the superiority of neural network forecasting techniques in predicting some indicators of the U.S. economy; Hutchinson, Lo, and Poggio [37] showed that their neural network based pricing model outperforms the Black–Scholes model in delta-hedging daily call option prices on S&P futures; and Giles, Lawrence, and Tsoi [27] found significant predictability in daily foreign exchange rates using their neural network models. Furthermore, almost all top systems in several recent time series prediction competitions (as listed in the Appendix at the end of this chapter) are neural network based. In conclusion, artificial neural networks are considered one of the best and most promising techniques for time series predictions.

This chapter is organized as follows. Section 9.2 gives a general overview of time series prediction problems and traditional approaches to time series prediction. Section 9.3 introduces neural network modeling for time series prediction and discusses challenges of time series predictions and neural network solutions. Some references are provided for the interested reader. Section 9.4 provides a case study on an economic time series forecasting problem and demonstrates how to apply advanced neural network techniques to real-world time series prediction tasks. Section 9.5 summarizes the chapter.

9.2 Time Series Prediction

Time series can be linear or nonlinear and stationary or nonstationary. Let $s(t)$ be a time series. If the join probability distribution of $\{s(t_1), s(t_2), \ldots, s(t_n)\}$ is the same as the join probability distribution of $\{s(t_1 + \tau), s(t_2 + \tau), \ldots, s(t_n + \tau)\}$ for all $t_1, \ldots, t_n$, and τ, the time series $s(t)$ is said to be strictly stationary. In practice, it is difficult to obtain all moments of the join distribution. A time series is usually called stationary when its mean is time-independent and its auto-covariance depends only on the time lag. Time series often exhibit nonstationarity. There are four major situations that give rise to nonstationary time series: transients, trends, discontinuities, and multiple equilibria. Some nonstationary time series can be reduced to stationary series by proper transformation, such as differencing. In other time series, time-varying adaptive models need to be used for modeling. A practical approach to modeling nonstationary series is using the combination of rolling training window and nonadaptive models, where models are retrained using new data once in a while to capture the changes of the underlying dynamics. How frequently the retraining is needed depends on the speed of the changes of the underlying dynamics.

[1] θ-time was introduced by Dacorogna et al. [17] in order to remove the seasonal pattern of intraday volatility in foreign exchange price change series.

The time series analysis can be performed in either the time domain (e.g., autocorrelation) or the frequency domain (e.g., spectral analysis). There are two basic approaches for forecasting time series: the univariate approach, where forecasts of a time series are based on a model fitted only to the past observations of the series, and the multivariate or cause-and-effect approach, where forecasts of a time series depend, at least partly, on some other series that are believed to cause the behavior of the forecasted series.

9.2.1 Time Series Prediction

Time series prediction can be defined as follows:[2] given p previous observations of the signal $s(t)$, $\mathbf{X} = (s(t-1), \ldots, s(t-p))^T$, find a function $g(\cdot)$ which minimizes the prediction residual

$$D = \int \int \| s - g(\mathbf{X}) \|^2 P(\mathbf{X}, s) dX ds \tag{9.1}$$

where $P(\mathbf{X}, s)$ is the density function of the joint probability of $\mathbf{X}$ and s. The theoretical solution of Equation (9.1) is the posterior mean estimator:

$$g(\mathbf{X}) = \int s P_{s|\mathbf{X}}(\mathbf{X}, s) ds \tag{9.2}$$

where $P_{s|\mathbf{X}}(\mathbf{X}, s)$ is the density function of the conditional probability of s given $\mathbf{X}$.

Equations (9.1) and (9.2) describe the general time series prediction problem and its theoretically optimal solution.

9.2.2 Traditional Approaches to Time Series Prediction

Traditional time series techniques [7, 11, 20, 21, 29, 31, 46] usually assume that a signal is stationary and can be described by a set of linear equations. Popular models include AR (autoregressive), ARX (AR with external input series), VAR (vector autoregression [45]), ARMA (autoregressive moving average), ARMAX (ARMA with external input series), ARIMA (autoregressive integrated moving average), ARIMAX (ARIMA with external input series), and ARFIMA (autoregressive fractionally integrated moving average [19, 26, 70]).[3] Advantages of linear time series models are that: (1) they have been studied for a long time and can be understood in great detail, and (2) they are straightforward to implement. However, because of the limitation of linearity, they cannot be applied to many more complicated problems. Instead, nonlinear models, such as TAR (threshold autoregressive model) [64, 65, 72, 73] and state-space models [3], are used for nonlinear time series modeling. For these techniques, model types and complexities need to be predefined. Some of these models work very well for specific problems, for example, TAR for Sunspots series prediction [74]. However, for most time series, *a priori* models are unknown and it is difficult to obtain a good guess due to the large number of variables involved, the high level of noise, and the limited amount of training data.

---

[2]For simplicity, Equations (9.1) and (9.2) present a univariate case, but it is straightforward to extend it to a multivariate case.

[3]In many empirical time series, particularly in finance, economics, and hydrology, the dependence between distant observations, though small, is by no means negligible. ARFIMA is one of the models developed to deal with such time series.

9.3 Neural Network Techniques for Time Series Prediction

Neural networks with hidden units are universal approximators, which means that, in theory, they are capable of learning an arbitrarily accurate approximation to any unknown function, provided that they increase in complexity at a rate approximately proportional to the size of the training data. Neural networks can be applied to time series modeling without assuming *a priori* function forms of models. A variety of neural network techniques have been proposed, investigated, and successfully applied to time series prediction.

9.3.1 Feedforward, Time Delay, and Recurrent Neural Networks

9.3.1.1 Multilayer Feedforward Neural Networks

One of the challenges of applying static neural network models to time series prediction is to incorporate the temporal relationship between observations at different time steps into the model. The simplest way to include temporal information into a multilayer feedforward network is by using different time-lagged input variables. For example, for a target series $s(t)$, series $\{s(t-1), s(t-2), \ldots, s(t-\tau)\}$ can be used as input variables. Selecting proper time lags and an informative set of input variables is critical to the solution of any time series prediction problems. Davey et al. [18] suggested that the embedding theorem and the false nearest neighbor method can provide useful heuristics for selecting proper time lags. Later in this chapter, we will present the sensitivity-based input feature selection method for choosing an informative set of input variables. Since choosing suitable time lags is a difficult problem, another practical approach is to first select as many lagged input variables as possible, then apply principle component analysis to the input space and transform input variables into new variables in the principle component space, which usually has a much lower dimensionality than the original space. Transformed variables are then used to train neural networks.

9.3.1.2 Time Delay Neural Network

The time delay neural network (TDNN) and its functional equivalent, finite impulse response (FIR) filter network or unfold-in-time static approach, can also be used for time series prediction [78, 80]. TDNNs are feedforward networks. They do not have feedback connections between units. TDNNs provide simple forms of dynamics by buffering lagged input variables at the input layer and/or lagged hidden unit outputs at the hidden layer. The FIR filter network [2] is a feedforward network whose static connection weights between units are replaced by an FIR linear filter that can be modeled with tapped delay lines. After applying the unfold-in-time technique to a TDNN or an FIR filter network, which removes all time delays by expanding the network into a large equivalent static structure, we can use the standard back-propagation algorithm for training. An alternative is to use the temporal back-propagation learning [80]. Another variation on TDNNs is the Gamma filter network [66], where the tapped delay line is replaced by a set of cascaded filters.

9.3.1.3 Recurrent Neural Network

Recurrent neural networks (RNNs) have feedback connections. They address the temporal relationship of inputs by maintaining internal states that have memory. RNNs have proven to be effective in learning time-dependent signals that have short term structure. For signals with long term dependencies, RNNs are less successful, since during training, the error gets "diluted" when passed back through the layers many times [5]. Due to their dynamic nature, RNNs have found great use in time series prediction [14, 15, 24, 27, 60, 84, 87]. Real time recurrent learning and back-propagation through time are two popular training algorithms for RNNs. Training RNNs tends to be difficult because of the feedback connections. The comparative study done by Horne and Giles [36] shows that RNNs do better than TDNNs in the tasks of finite state machine induction and nonlinear system identification, even though the performance differences are not significant. Two other comparative studies [15, 30] on feedforward and recurrent neural networks in time series prediction show that feedforward networks consistently outperform recurrent networks for their time series prediction tasks.

Many challenges, such as lack of prior knowledge, high noise level, nonlinearity, and nonstationarity, are associated with time series modeling. The success of applying neural networks to time series predictions comes from proper input variable selection and effectively balancing model complexity (bias/variance trade-off [25]). Controlling model complexity can be difficult due to the following three key facts:

- Unlike linear systems, general theoretical analysis for nonlinear neural networks is usually intractable, especially for models with dynamic connections.
- The error surface of nonlinear neural networks has multiple local minima. Neural networks are "unstable" with respect to choices of training and validation data, initial weights, architectures, and training parameters. The mapping functions of neural networks trained with different setups may vary greatly, especially for networks with embedded feedback connections and other time factors.
- Training data are usually limited and noisy.

Many model selection and pruning techniques have been developed for controlling the bias/variance trade-off for a given problem. These include, among others, sequential network construction [8, 55], optimal brain damage [16], optimal brain surgeon [32], principle component pruning [41], FARM (Frobenius approximation reduction method) [38], and skeletonization [58]. The rest of this chapter describes three other techniques for variable selection and controlling neural network model complexity, as well as their applications to an economic time series prediction problem.

9.3.2 Sensitivity Analysis Based Input Variable Selection

Input variable selection is one of the most important stages of a modeling process. The number of input variables used during learning affects the quantity of training data needed for learning. Redundant, irrelevant, or misleading features make the training data less comprehensible. Both data collection and the learning process can be expensive and time consuming. There are two types of feature selection procedures:

- the model-independent (filtered) approach, where statistical merits of input variables, for example, joint mutual information of input variables and target variables, are directly evaluated using data
- the model-dependent (wrapper) approach, which evaluates input features together with learning algorithms. That is, a learning algorithm is applied to the data, and the subset of input features that gives the best result for the algorithm is used for modeling.

Sensitivity-based input variable selection techniques are model-dependent algorithms that prune unnecessary or harmful input variables from a trained network. The following sections describe four average sensitivity measures that are calculated based on the entire data set, as well as two sensitivity measures for individual data exemplars [42]. These measures can be used to guide input feature selection and the pruning of hidden layer units. The sensitivities for individual exemplars can provide insight into which inputs are important for specific predictions.

9.3.2.1 Average Sensitivity Measures

One of the sensitivity measures, delta error [55], is defined in terms of the increase of the average square error when replacing a variable x with its mean $\overline{x}$. The sensitivity S_i of the ith variable is:

$$S_i = \frac{1}{N}\sum_{n=1}^{N} S_i^{(n)}$$

$$S_i^{(n)} = \mathrm{SE}\,(\overline{x_i}, \mathbf{W}) - \mathrm{SE}\left(x_i^{(n)}, \mathbf{W}\right)$$

where SE denotes the square error, which is a function of network weights and data exemplars, and $S_i^{(n)}$ is the delta error measure of the nth data exemplar. If S_i is large, the network error will be largely changed by replacing the ith input variable with its mean. If S_i is small, other measures are needed to decide whether the ith input variable is useful. Three additional sensitivity measures are computed based on perturbating an input or a hidden variable and monitoring network output variations:

1. **Average Gradient (AG):** $S_i = \frac{1}{N}\sum_{n=1}^{N}\frac{\partial f^{(n)}}{\partial x_i}$

2. **Average Absolute Gradient (AAG):** $S_i = \frac{1}{N}\sum_{n=1}^{N}\left|\frac{\partial f^{(n)}}{\partial x_i}\right|$

3. **RMS Gradient (RMSG):** $S_i = \sqrt{\frac{1}{N}\sum_{n=1}^{N}\left[\frac{\partial f^{(n)}}{\partial x_i}\right]^2}$

where $f^{(n)} = f(x_1^{(n)}, \ldots, x_i^{(n)}, \ldots, x_d^{(n)})$ is the network output given the nth input data pattern.

These three sensitivity measures considered together offer useful information. If $S_i^{\mathbf{AG}}$ is positive and large, then, on average, the change of the direction of the network output f is the same as that of the ith input variable. If $S_i^{\mathbf{AG}}$ is negative and large, on average, the change of the direction of f is opposite to that of the ith input variable. If $S_i^{\mathbf{AAG}}$ is large, the output f is sensitive to the ith input variable. If $S_i^{\mathbf{AAG}}$ is small, f is not sensitive to the ith input variable. If $S_i^{\mathbf{RMSG}}$ is very different from $S_i^{\mathbf{AAG}}$, the ith input series could be very noisy and have a lot of outliers.

9.3.2.2 Sensitivities for Individual Exemplars

When we apply a data exemplar to a trained neural network, the network outputs a result. Sensitivity analysis performed for an individual exemplar provides information about which input features play an important role in producing the current network output. It helps to interpret how the network is making a prediction. Two types of sensitivity measures for individual exemplars are calculated. These measures are defined as

1. **Delta Output (DO):** $S_i = \Delta f_i = f\left(x_1^{(n)}, \ldots, x_i^{(n)}, \ldots, x_d^{(n)}\right) - f\left(x_1^{(n)}, \ldots, \overline{x_i}, \ldots, x_d^{(n)}\right)$

2. **Output Gradient (OG):** $S_i = \frac{\partial f^{(n)}}{\partial x_i}$.

where $f^{(n)} = f(x_1^{(n)}, \ldots, x_i^{(n)}, \ldots, x_d^{(n)})$.

For a given data exemplar, if $S_i^{\mathbf{DO}}$ or $S_i^{\mathbf{OG}}$ is large, then the ith variable plays an important role in the current network output, and slightly changing the value of the variable may cause a large change in the network output. Figure 9.1 gives an example of visualization of the individual exemplar sensitivity analysis. Black and gray represent negative and positive, respectively. The size of a rectangle represents the magnitude of a sensitivity value. The indices of data exemplars change along the horizontal direction, and the indices of input variables change along the vertical direction.

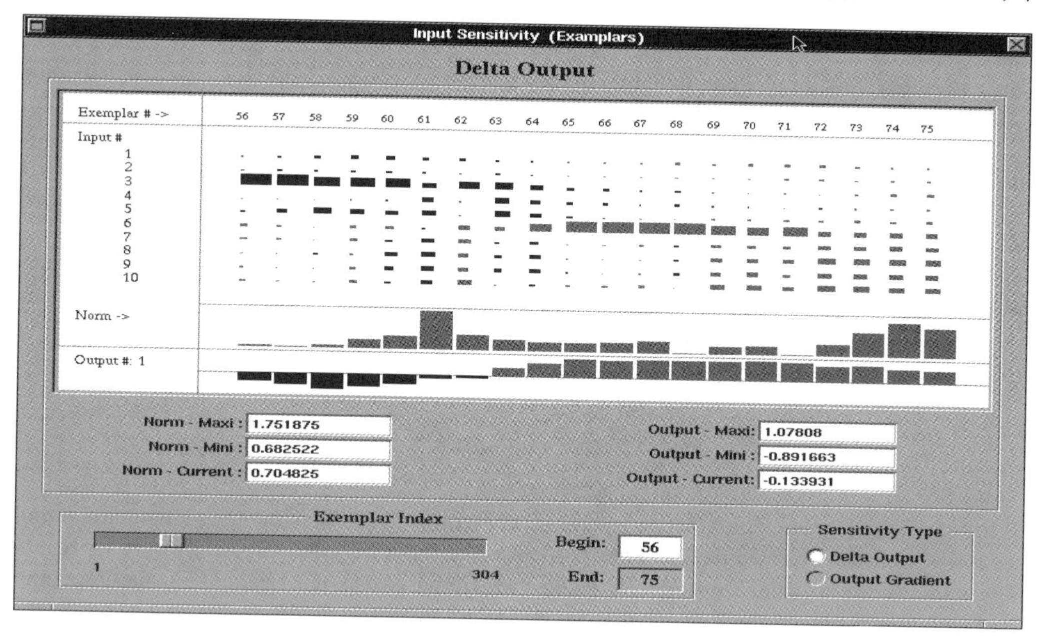

9.1 Sensitivity analysis results for individual exemplars. Black and gray represent negative and positive, respectively. The size of a rectangle represents the magnitude of a value. The indices of exemplars change along the horizontal direction. The indices of input variables change along the vertical direction.

Using this visualization, we can observe which input variables play important roles on the current network output or which input variables, when we change them, can largely increase or decrease errors. For time series prediction, we can also observe how the roles of different input series change over time. For example, in Figure 9.1, for exemplars with indices from 56 to 60, the third input series has large negative sensitivity measures. Starting with the 65th exemplar, the 6th input series starts to play an important role, and this lasts until the 71st exemplar.

9.3.3 Committees of Predictors

One way to deal with instability and noise during neural network modeling is to train a set of neural networks that have different initial weights, training parameters, or architectures, then choose the network that performs the best on a validation data set. An alternative approach is to use committees.

A committee consists of a set of member models. The committee approach has been used to reduce model variance and improve generalization performance. Researchers of economics have studied and used committees for economic time series prediction for a long time and generally find that they outperform their member estimators and that unweighted averages tend to outperform weighted averages for a variety of weighting methods [13].

If member neural network models of a committee use the same input variables and architecture, the committee formed by these members is called a homogeneous committee. Because a lot of time series prediction problems only have a limited amount of data, and data are usually noisy, bagging [9] or double-bagging [44] techniques, where member models of a committee are trained and validated using different bootstrap replicas of the original data set, are effective approaches for constructing committees for these problems.

For committees to achieve substantial generalization performance improvement over single models, committee members need to satisfy two criteria — have reasonable individual performance and make decisions as independently as possible. The input feature grouping technique we proposed [43] aims to generate members that provide a good balance between the two criteria. The idea is to give each member estimator of a committee a rich but distinct feature set, in the hope that each member will generalize independently with reduced error correlations.

The input grouping method first groups features using a hierarchical clustering algorithm based on a relevance measure in such a way that features between different groups are less related to one another and features within a group are more related to one another. Then, the feature set for each committee member is formed by selecting a feature from each group.

The mutual information $I(x_i; x_j)$ between two input variables x_i and x_j is used as the relevance measure to group inputs. The mutual information $I(x_i; x_j)$, defined in Equation (9.3), measures the reduction of uncertainty by introducing another random variable. It reflects the dependence between the two random variables.

$$I\left(x_i; x_j\right) = H\left(x_i\right) - H\left(x_i|x_j\right) = \sum_{x_i, x_j} p\left(x_i, y_i\right) \log \frac{p(x_i, x_j)}{p(x_i)p(x_j)} . \tag{9.3}$$

If features x_i and x_j are highly dependent, $I(x_i; x_j)$ will be large. Because the mutual information measures arbitrary dependencies between random variables, it has been effectively used for feature selections in complex prediction tasks [4], where methods based on linear relations like the correlation are likely to make mistakes. The fact that the mutual information is independent of the coordinates chosen permits a robust estimation.

Because members of committees designed by the input grouping technique observe different combinations of input variables, they will have fewer error correlations between each other. The feature sets of individual members will contain less redundant information because highly correlated variables will not be used for the same model. Also, the feature sets of members contain almost complete information because every set includes features from all information groups. Section 9.4.2 describes a case study using this technique.

9.3.4 Regularizer for Recurrent Learning

Overfitting modeling solutions are generally characterized by mappings which have relatively high curvature and structure. Regularization is an effective technique to encourage smoother network mappings. Other techniques to prevent overfitting include early stopping of training, which has an effect similar to weight decay [69], and using prior knowledge in the form of hints [1, 75]. Well established regularization techniques include ridge regression [34, 35], and, more generally, spline smoothing functions or Tikhonov stabilizers that penalize the mth-order squared derivatives of the function being fit [22, 33, 71, 77]. These methods were extended to radial basis function networks [28, 62, 63], and several heuristic approaches, such as quadratic weight decay [61], weight elimination [12, 68, 83], soft weight sharing [59], and curvature-driven smoothing [6, 40, 54], were also developed for sigmoidal neural networks. All these regularizers are designed for feedforward neural networks.

Wu and Moody [86] derived a smoothing regularizer for general dynamic models by requiring robustness in prediction performance to perturbations on training data. The regularizer can be viewed as a generalization of the first order Tikhonov stabilizer to dynamic models. A two-layer network with recurrent connections can be described by equations:

$$\begin{aligned} Y(t) &= f\left(WY(t-\tau) + VX(t)\right) \\ \hat{Z}(t) &= UY(t) \end{aligned} \tag{9.4}$$

where $X(t)$, $Y(t)$, and $\hat{Z}(t)$ are, respectively, the network input vector, the hidden output vector, and the network output vector; U, V, and W are the output, input, and recurrent connection weights, respectively; $f(\cdot)$ is the nonlinear transfer function of hidden units; and τ is the time delay in the feedback connections of the hidden layer. The training criterion that includes the regularizer is defined as:

$$D = \frac{1}{N}\sum_{t=1}^{N}\left\|Z(t) - \hat{Z}(\Phi, I(t))\right\|^2 + \lambda {\rho_\tau}^2(\Phi) \quad (9.5)$$

where $\Phi = \{U, V, W\}$ is the network parameter set, $Z(t)$ is the target, $I(t) = \{X(s)|s = 1, 2, \ldots, t\}$ represents the current and all historical input information, N is the size of the training data, ${\rho_\tau}^2(\Phi)$ is the regularizer, and λ is the regularization parameter. The closed-form expression of the regularizer for time-lagged recurrent networks is

$$\rho_\tau(\Phi) = \frac{\gamma||U||||V||}{1-\gamma||W||}\left[1 - e^{\frac{\gamma||W||-1}{\tau}}\right] \quad (9.6)$$

where $||\cdot||$ is the Euclidean matrix norm and γ is a factor that depends on the maximal value of the first derivatives of the internal unit activations $f(\cdot)$. Simplifications of the regularizer can be obtained for simultaneous recurrent nets ($\tau \mapsto 0$), two-layer feedforward nets, and one-layer linear nets. Section 9.4.3 describes a case study using this technique.

9.4 A Case Study

9.4.1 Task, Data, and Performance Measure

The task is to predict the one-month rate of change of the U.S. Index of Industrial Production (IP), one of the key measures of economic activity. It is computed and published monthly. Figure 9.2 plots monthly IP data from 1967 to 1993.

Nine macroeconomic time series, as listed in Table 9.1, are used for forecasting IP. Macroeconomic forecasting is a difficult task because data are usually limited, and these series are intrinsically very noisy and nonstationary. The nine series are preprocessed before they are applied to the forecasting

TABLE 9.1 Input Data Series

Series	Description
IP	Index of Industrial Production
SP	Standard & Poor's 500
DL	Index of Leading Indicators
M2	Money Supply
CP	Consumer Price Index
CB	Moody's AAA Bond Yield
HS	Housing Starts
TB3	Three-month Treasury Bill Yield
Tr	Yield Curve Slope: (10-Year Bond Composite)–(3-Month Treasury Bill)

Data are taken from the Citibase database [53].

models. The representation is the first difference on one-month time scales of the logged series. For example, the notation IP.L.D1 represents IP.L.D1 $\equiv$ ln(IP(t)) – ln(IP(t-1)). The target series is IP.L.FD1, which is defined as IP.L.FD1 $\equiv$ ln(IP(t+1)) – ln(IP(t)). Data from January 1950 to December 1979 are used to train models, and data from January 1980 to December 1989 are used for testing.

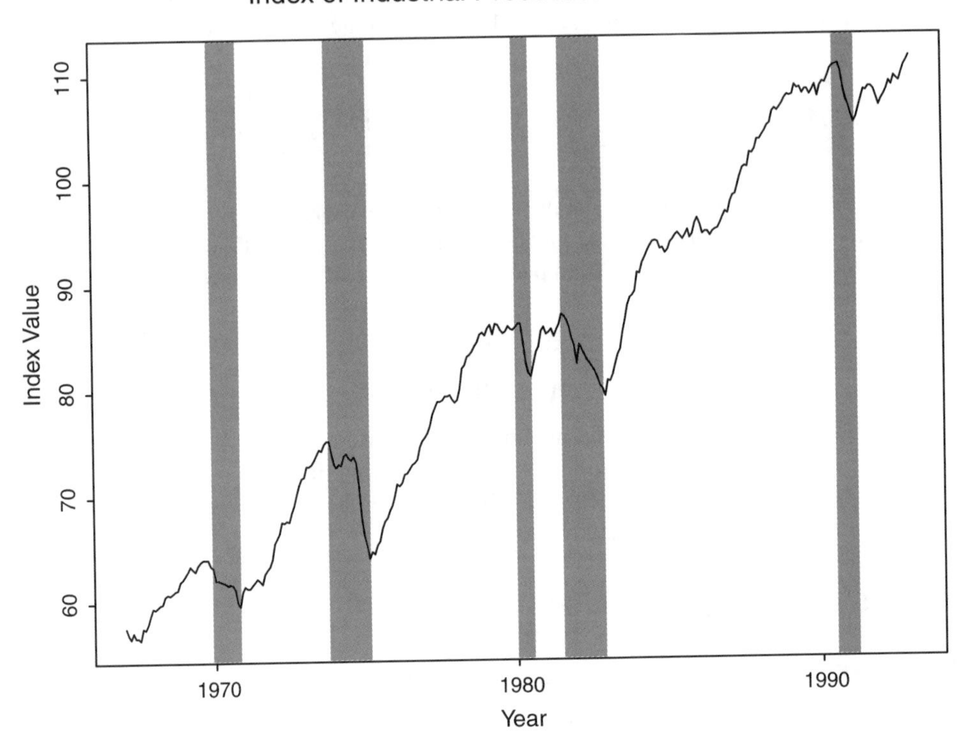

9.2 U.S. Index of Industrial Production (IP) for the period 1967 to 1993. Shaded regions denote official recessions, while unshaded regions denote official expansions. The boundaries for recessions and expansions are determined by the National Bureau of Economic Research based on several macroeconomic series. As is evident for IP, business cycles are irregular in magnitude, duration, and structure, making prediction of IP an interesting challenge [53].

The performance measure is the normalized prediction error, which is defined as

$$D_Q = \frac{\sum_{t \in Q}[S(t) - \hat{S(t)}]^2}{\sum_{t \in Q}[S(t) - \bar{S}]^2} \tag{9.7}$$

where $S(t)$ is the target series, Q represents the test data set, and $\bar{S}$ is the mean of $S(t)$ over the training data set. This measure evaluates prediction accuracy by comparing model predicted value $\hat{S}(t)$ to the trivial predictor $\bar{S}$.

9.4.2 Applying the Input Feature Grouping Committee Technique

In this experiment, the input feature grouping technique is used to construct heterogeneous committees for IP prediction. During the input feature grouping procedure, measures of mutual information between all pairs of input variables are computed first. A histogram-based method is used to calculate these estimates. Then, a hierarchical clustering algorithm is applied to these values to group inputs. Hierarchical clustering proceeds by a series of successive fusions of the nine input variables into groups. At any particular stage, the process fuses variables or groups of variables which are closest, based on their mutual information estimates. The distance between two groups is defined as the average of the distances between all pairs of individuals in the two groups. The result is represented by a tree in Figure 9.3, which illustrates the fusions made at every successive level.

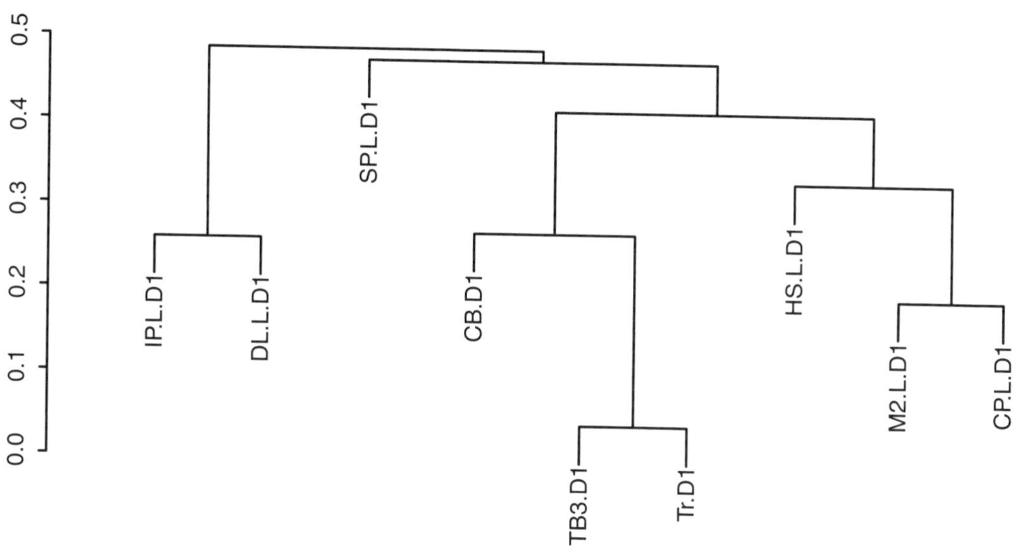

9.3 Variable grouping based on mutual information. Y label is the distance.

From the clustering tree, it is clear that we can break the input variables into four groups: (IP.L.D1 and DL.L.D1) measure recent economic changes, (SP.L.D1) reflects recent stock market momentum, (CB.D1, TB3.D1, and Tr.D1) give interest rate information, and (M2.L.D1, CP.L.D1, and HS.L.D1) provide inflation information. The grouping algorithm meaningfully clusters the nine input series.

Eighteen different subsets of features can be generated from the four groups by selecting one feature from each group. Each subset is given to a committee member. For example, the subsets (IP.L.D1, SP.L.D1, CB.D1, and M2.L.D1) and (DL.L.D1, SP.L.D1, TB3.D1, and M2.L.D1) are used as feature sets for two different committee members. A committee has, in total, 18 members. Each member is a neural network model.

We compare the input grouping method with three other committee member generating methods: baseline, random selection, and bootstrapping. The baseline method is to train a committee member using all the input variables. Members are only different in their initial weights. The bootstrapping method also trains a member using all the input features, but each member has different bootstrap replicates of the original training data as its training and validation sets. The random selection method constructs a feature set for a member by randomly picking a subset from the available features. For comparison with the grouping method, each committee generated by these three methods also has 18 members.

Twenty runs are performed for each of the four methods in order to get reliable performance measures. Figure 9.4 shows the boxplots of normalized MSE for the four methods. The grouping method gives the best result, and the performance improvement is significant compared to other methods. The grouping method outperforms the random selection method by meaningfully grouping input features. The committees constructed using the input feature grouping method have much less performance variance compared to those constructed using the random picking method. It is interesting to note that the heterogeneous committee methods, grouping and random selection, perform better than homogeneous methods for this data set. One of the reasons for this is that giving different members different input sets increases model independence between members. Another reason may be that the problem becomes easier to model because of smaller feature sets.

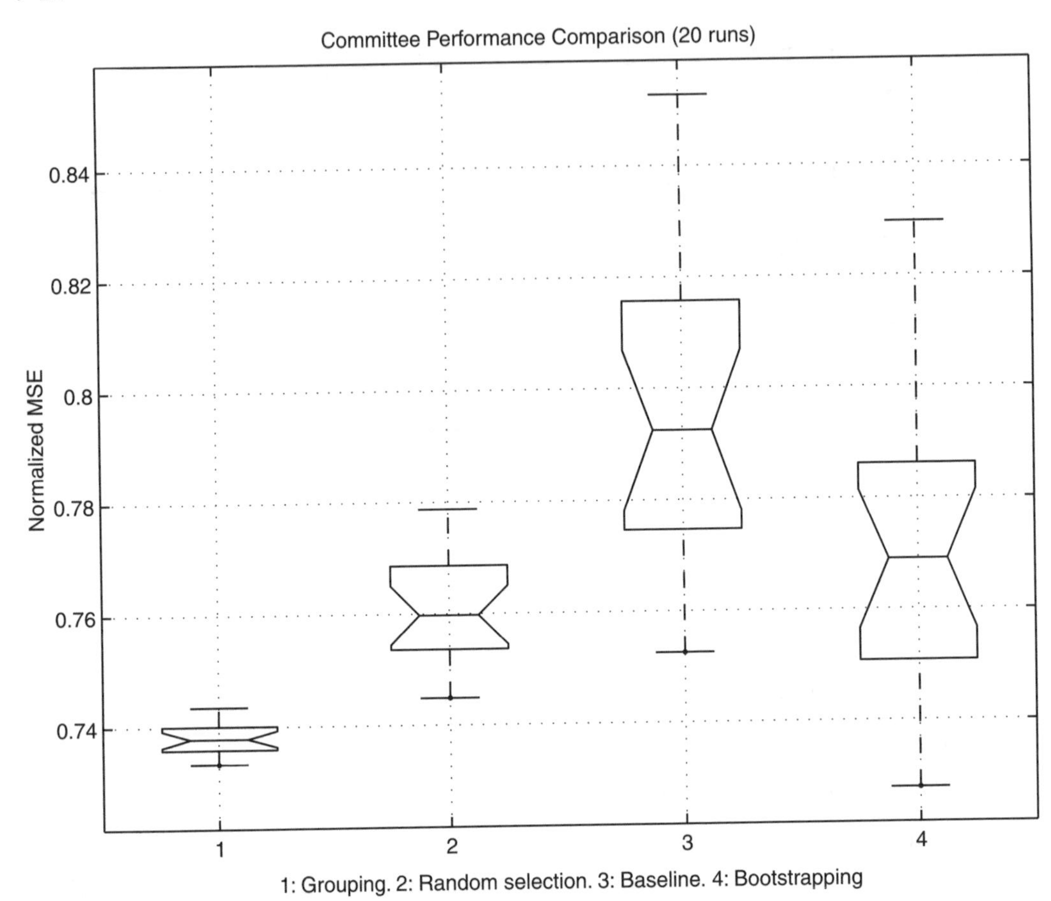

9.4 Comparison among four different committee member generating methods. The proposed grouping method gives the best result, and the performance improvement is significant compared to the other three methods.

9.4.3 Applying the Regularized Recurrent Learning Technique

In this study, a recurrent neural network model, which has nine input units and a time-delayed length (τ) that equals one in the recurrent connections, is used for the IP prediction task. The training data are divided into four nonoverlapping subsets. The subset that has 70% of the original data is used for training. The other three subsets, each with 10% of the original data, are used for early stopping, selecting the regularization parameter and the number of hidden units, respectively. Ten random training and validation partitions are used. For each training and validation partition, 3 networks with different initial weight parameters are trained, so a total of 30 networks are trained.

Table 9.2 lists the results of the test data set. It compares the out-of-sample performance of networks trained with our smoothing regularizer to those networks trained with the standard weight decay regularizer. The results are summarized based on the performance of all 30 networks. The last column gives the performance of the committee, which is the equal weight average of the predictions of all 30 networks. The median, minimal, and maximal prediction errors of the 30 predictors are also listed. In terms of the mean of errors, the smoothing regularizer outperforms the standard weight decay regularizer with 95% confidence (in t-distribution hypothesis). The smoothing regularizer performs better than the weight decay in the median, minima, and maxima comparisons as well.

Figure 9.5 plots the changes of prediction errors with the regularization parameter. As shown, the prediction error on the training data set increases when the regularization parameter increases,

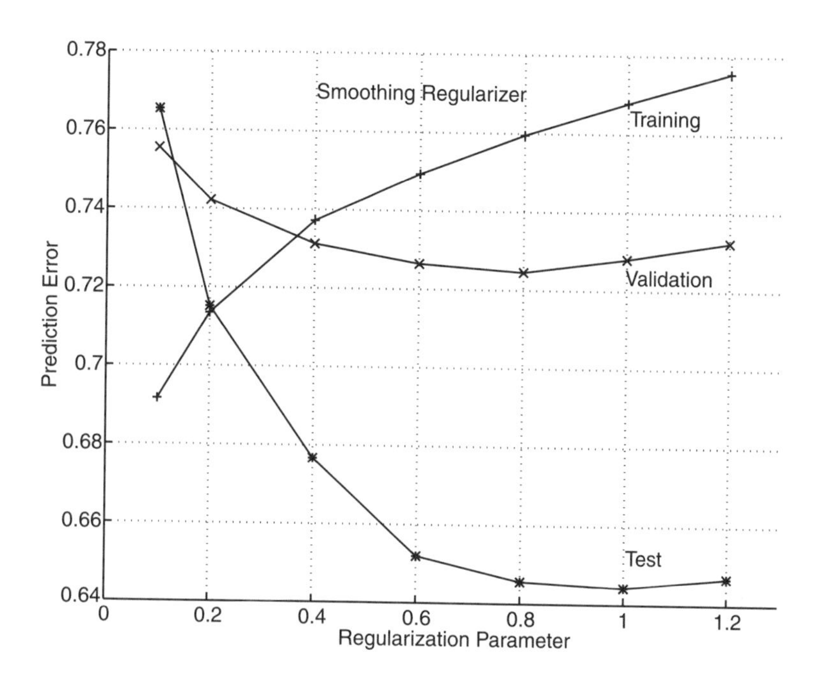

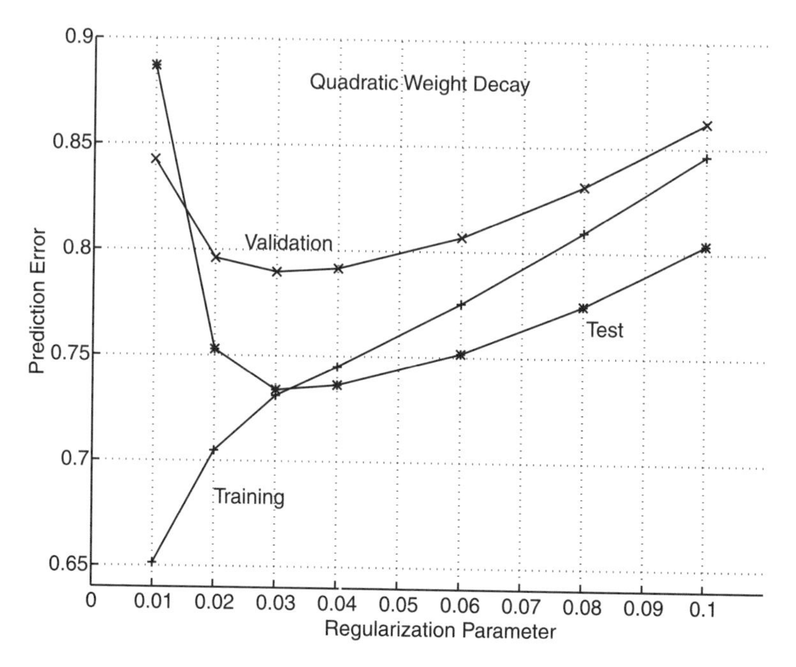

9.5 Regularization parameter vs. normalized prediction errors for the task of predicting the rate of changes of the U.S. Index of Industrial Production. The plots are for a recurrent neural network trained with the smoothing regularizer (upper panel) and an RNN trained with the standard weight decay regularizer (lower panel).

TABLE 9.2 Normalized Prediction Errors for the One-Month Rate of Changes of the U.S. Index of Industrial Production (Jan. 1980–Dec. 1989).

Regularizer	Mean ± Std	Median	Max	Min	Committee
Smoothing	0.646 ± 0.008	0.647	0.657	0.632	0.639
Weight Decay	0.734 ± 0.018	0.737	0.767	0.704	0.734

Results are summarized based on the performance of 30 networks.

and the prediction errors on the validation and test data sets first decrease and then increase when the regularization parameter increases. The optimal regularization parameter that gives the smallest validation error is 0.8 for the smoothing regularizer and 0.03 for the standard weight decay regularizer. For both the smoothing regularizer and the weight decay regularizer, the regularization parameters should be larger than zero in order to achieve optimal prediction performance. This suggests that it is necessary to use both regularization and early stopping during training.

9.5 Conclusion

In theory, neural networks are capable of modeling any time series without assuming *a priori* function forms and degrees of nonlinearity about a series. Challenges to time series prediction include nonlinearity, nonstationarity, noise, and limit quantity of data. When applying neural networks to time series modeling, important issues include incorporating temporal information, proper input variable selections, and balancing bias/variance trade-off of a model. Many neural network techniques are proposed and successfully applied to real-world time series problems. This chapter only addresses some of them. Other important issues include prediction risk [51], generalization error estimates [39], Bayesian methods [48], nonstationary time series modeling [82], and incorporation of prior knowledge [1]. A large number of empirical simulations have demonstrated that no technique alone is sufficient, but a combination of selected models and techniques could yield superior results.

Appendix

A.1 Benchmark Data Sets for Time Series Prediction Modeling

Benchmark data sets (which can easily be found and downloaded from the Internet) for testing neural network models for time series prediction include:

- Sunspots series [56, 59, 65, 74, 83]
- Boston housing data [56]
- Mackey–Glass series [23, 49]

A.2 Time Series Prediction Competitions

Several competitions have been organized for evaluating and benchmarking new and existing techniques in time series prediction. These include:

- Santa Fe Institute Time Series Prediction and Analysis Competition [81]
- The Great Energy Shootout: a building energy forecasting competition organized by the American Society of Heating and Refrigeration and Air Conditioning Engineers [48]
- The First International Nonlinear Financial Forecasting Competition sponsored by Finance & Technology Publishing [10]

Acknowledgments

Yuansong Liao's work was supported by NSF ECS-9626406.

References

[1] Y.S. Abu-Mostafa. Hints. *Neural Computation,* 7(4):639–671, 1995.

[2] A.D. Back, E. Wan, S. Lawrence, and A.C. Tsoi. A unifying view of some training algorithms for multilayer perceptrons with FIR filter synapses. In J. Vlontzos, J. Hwang, and E. Wilson, Editors, *Neural Networks for Signal Processing 4,* pages 146–154. IEEE Press, New York, 1995.

[3] Y. Bar-Shalom and X. Li. *Estimation and Tracking: Principles, Techniques and Software.* Artech House, Norwood, MA, 1993.

[4] R. Battiti. Using mutual information for selecting features in supervised neural net learning. *IEEE Transactions on Neural Networks,* 5(4), 537–550, 1994.

[5] Y. Bengio, P. Frasconi, and P. Simard. The problem of learning long-term dependencies in recurrent networks. In *International Conference on Neural Networks,* San Francisco, 1993.

[6] C.M. Bishop. Curvature-driven smoothing: a learning algorithm for feedforward networks. *IEEE Transactions on Neural Networks,* 4(5):882–884, 1993.

[7] G.E.P. Box and F.M. Jenkins. *Time Series Analysis: Forecasting and Control.* Holder-Day, San Francisco, 1976.

[8] L. Breiman. Heuristics of instability in model selection. Technical report, Department of Statistics, University of California at Berkeley, 1994.

[9] L. Breiman. Bagging predictors. *Machine Learning,* 24(2):123–40, 1996.

[10] R.B. Caldwell. *Nonlinear Financial Forecasting, Proceedings of the First INFFC.* Finance & Technology Publishing, Haymarket, VA, 1997.

[11] C. Chatfield. *The Analysis of Time Series.* Chapman & Hall, London, 1989.

[12] Y. Chauvin. Dynamic behavior of constrained back-propagation networks. In D.S. Touretzky, Editor, *Advances in Neural Information Processing Systems 2,* pages 642–649. Morgan Kaufmann Publishers, San Mateo, CA, 1990.

[13] R. Clemen. Combining forecast: a review and annotated bibliography. *International Journal on Forecasting,* 5:559–583, 1989.

[14] J. Conner, R. Douglas Martin, and L. Atlas. Recurrent neural networks and robust time series prediction. *IEEE Transactions on Neural Networks,* 5:240–254, 1994.

[15] M. Crucianu, R. Bone, and J.P.A. de Beauville. Model comparison for monthly forecasts of the CAC 40. In *International Conference on Neural Information Processing,* Kitakyushu, Japan, 1998.

[16] Y. Le Cun, J.S. Denker, and S.A. Solla. Optimal brain damage. In D.S. Touretzky, Editor, *Advances in Neural Information Processing Systems 2,* pages 598–605, Morgan Kaufmann Publishers, San Mateo, CA, 1990.

[17] M.M. Dacorogna, U.A. Muller, R.J. Nagler, R.B. Oslen, and O.V. Pictet. A geographical model for the daily and weekly seasonal volatility in the FX market. *Journal of International Money and Finance,* 12(4):413–438, 1993.

[18] N. Davey, S.P. Hunt, and R.J. Frank. Time series prediction and neural networks. In W. Duch, Editor, *5th International Conference on Engineering Applications of Neural Networks (EANN'99),* 1999.

[19] F.X. Diebold and G.D. Rudebusch. Long memory and persistence in aggregate output. *Journal of Monetary Economics,* 24:189–209, 1989.

[20] N.R. Draper and H. Smith. *Applied Regression Analysis.* John Wiley & Sons, New York, 1981.

[21] W. Enders. *Applied Econometric Time Series.* John Wiley & Sons, New York, 1994.

[22] R.L. Eubank. *Spline Smoothing and Nonparametric Regression.* Marcel Dekker, Inc., New York, 1988.

[23] J.D. Farmer. Chaotic attractors of an infinite-dimentional dynamical system. *Physica D,* 4:366–383, 1982.

[24] F. Fessant, S. Bengio, and D. Collobert. On the prediction of solar activity using different neural network models. *Annales Geophysicae,* 14:20–26, 1995.

[25] S. Geman, E. Bienenstock, and R. Doursat. Neural networks and the bias/variance dilemma. *Neural Computation,* 4(1):1–58, 1992.

[26] J. Geweke and S. Porter-Hudak. The estimation and application of long memory time series models. *Journal of Time Series Analysis,* 4:221–238, 1983.

[27] C. Lee Giles, S. Lawrence, and A.C. Tsoi. Rule inference for financial prediction using recurrent neural networks. In *Proceedings of IEEE/IAFE Conference on Computational Intelligence for Financial Engineering (CIFEr),* pages 253–259. IEEE, Piscataway, NJ, 1997.

[28] F. Girosi, M. Jones, and T. Poggio. Regularization theory and neural networks architectures. *Neural Computation,* 7:219–269, 1995.

[29] W. Greene. *Econometric Analysis.* Prentice-Hall, Englewood Cliffs, NJ, 1999.

[30] M. Hallas and G. Dorffner. A comparative study on feedforward and recurrent neural networks in time series prediction using gradient descent learning. In R. Trappl, Editor, *Cybernetics and Systems '98: Proceedings of 14th European Meeting on Cybernetics and Systems Research, Austrian Society for Cybernetic Studies,* pages 644–647, Vienna, 1998.

[31] J. Hamilton. *Time Series Analysis.* Princeton University Press, Princeton, NJ, 1994.

[32] B. Hassibi, D.G. Stork, and G. Wolf. Optimal brain surgeon and general network pruning. In *Proceedings of the 1993 IEEE International Conference on Neural Networks,* San Francisco, 1993.

[33] T.J. Hastie and R.J. Tibshirani. *Generalized Additive Models,* volume 43 of *Monographs on Statistics and Applied Probability.* Chapman & Hall, London, 1990.

[34] A.E. Hoerl and R.W. Kennard. Ridge regression: applications to nonorthogonal problems. *Technometrics,* 12:69–82, 1970.

[35] A.E. Hoerl and R.W. Kennard. Ridge regression: biased estimation for nonorthogonal problems. *Technometrics,* 12:55–67, 1970.

[36] B.G. Horne and C.L. Giles. An experimental comparison of recurrent neural networks. In G. Tesauro, D. Touretzky, and T. Leen, Editors, *Advances in Neural Information Processing Systems,* page 697. MIT Press, Cambridge, MA, 1995.

[37] J. Hutchinson, A. Lo, and T. Poggio. A nonparametric approach to pricing and hedging derivative securities via learning networks. Technical Report A.I. No. 1471, MIT, AI Lab., April 1994.

[38] S.Y. Kung and Y.H. Hu. A frobenius approximation reduction method (FARM) for determining optimal number of hidden units. In *Proceedings of International Conference on Neural Networks,* pages 163–168, Seattle, WA, 1991.

[39] J. Larson. A generalization error estimate for nonlinear systems. In S.Y. Kung, F. Fallside, J.A. Sorensen, and C.A. Kamm, Editors, *Neural Networks for Signal Processing II,* pages 29–38. IEEE, Piscataway, NJ, 1992.

[40] T.K. Leen. From data distributions to regularization in invariant learning. *Neural Computation,* 5:974–981, 1995.

[41] A.U. Levin, T.K. Leen, and J.E. Moody. Fast pruning using principal components. In J. Cowan, G. Tesauro, and J. Alspector, Editors, *Advances in Neural Information Processing Systems 6.* Morgan Kaufmann Publishers, San Mateo, CA, 1994.

[42] Y. Liao and J. Moody. A neural network visualization and sensitivity analysis toolkit. In S. Amari, L. Xu, L. Chan, I. King, and K. Leung, Editors, *Proceedings of the International Conference on Neural Information Processing,* pages 1069–1074. Springer-Verlag Singapore Pte. Ltd., Hong Kong, 1996.

[43] Y. Liao and J. Moody. Constructing heterogeneous committees using input feature grouping: application to economic forecasting. In S.A. Solla, T.K. Leen, and K.R. Muller, Editors, *Advances in Neural Information Processing Systems 12.* MIT Press, Cambridge, MA, 2000.

[44] Y. Liao and J.E. Moody. Double bagging. Oregon Graduate Institute Technical Report, 1996.

[45] R.B. Litterman. Forecasting with Bayesian vector autoregressions — five years of experience. *Journal of Business & Economics,* 4(1):25–37, 1986.

[46] L. Ljung. *System Identification: Theory for the User.* Prentice-Hall, Englewood Cliffs, NJ, 1987.

[47] D.R. Lovell, M.J.J. Scott, M. Niranjan, R.W. Prager, K.J. Dalton, and R. Derom. On the use of expected attainable discrimination for feature selection in large scale medical risk prediction problems. Technical Report CUED/F-INFENG/TR299, Cambridge University Engineering Department, August 1997.

[48] D.J.C. MacKay. Bayesian non-linear modelling for the 1993 energy prediction competition. In G. Heidbreder, Editor, *Maximum Entropy and Bayesian Methods, Santa Barbara 1993,* pages 221–234. Kluwer, Dordrecht, 1996.

[49] M.C. Mackey and L. Glass. Oscillation and chaos in physiological control systems. *Science,* 197:287–289, 1977.

[50] J. Moody. Fast learning in multi-resolution hierarchies. In D.S. Touretzky, Editor, *Advances in Neural Information Processing Systems 2,* Morgan Kaufmann Publishers, San Mateo, CA, 1989.

[51] J. Moody. Prediction risk and neural network architecture selection. In V. Cherkassky, J.H. Friedman, and H. Wechsler, Editors, *From Statistics to Neural Networks: Theory and Pattern Recognition Applications.* Springer-Verlag, New York, 1994.

[52] J. Moody. Economic forecasting: challenges and neural network solutions. In *Proceedings of the International Symposium on Artificial Neural Networks,* Hsinchu, Taiwan, 1995.

[53] J. Moody, U. Levin, and S. Rehfuss. Predicting the U.S. index of industrial production. In *Proceedings of the 1993 Parallel Applications in Statistics and Economics Conference, Zeist. The Netherlands.* Special issue of *Neural Network World,* 3(6):791–794, 1993.

[54] J. Moody and T. Rögnvaldsson. Smoothing regularizers for projective basis function networks. In M.C. Mozer, M.I. Jordan, and T. Petsche, Editors, *Advances in Neural Information Processing Systems 9.* MIT Press, Cambridge, MA, 1997.

[55] J. Moody and J. Utans. Architecture selection strategies for neural networks: Application to corporate bond rating prediction. In A.N. Refenes, Editor, *Neural Networks in the Capital Markets.* John Wiley & Sons, New York, 1994.

[56] J.E. Moody and N. Yarvin. Networks with learned unit response functions. In J.E. Moody, S.J. Hanson, and R.P. Lippmann, Editors, *Advances in Neural Information Processing Systems 4,* pages 1048–55. Morgan Kaufmann Publishers, San Mateo, CA, 1992.

[57] M.C. Mozer. Neural net architectures for temporal sequence processing. In A. Weigend and N. Gershenfeld, Editors, *Predicting the Future and Understanding the past, SFI Studies in the Science of Complexity, Proc. Vol. XVII.* Addison-Wesley, Reading, MA, 1993.

[58] M.C. Mozer and P. Smolensky. Skeletonization: a technique for triming the fat from a network via relevance assessment. In D.S. Touretzky, Editor, *Advances in Neural Information Processing Systems 2,* pages 107–115. Morgan Kaufmann Publishers, San Mateo, CA, 1989.

[59] S.J. Nowlan and G.E. Hinton. Simplifying neural networks by soft weight-sharing. *Neural Computation,* 4(4):473–493, 1992.

[60] V. Petridis and A. Kehagias. A recurrent network implementation of time series classification. *Neural Computation,* 8:357–372, 1996.

[61] D.C. Plaut, S.J. Nowlan, and G.E. Hinton. Experiments on learning by back propagation. Technical Report CMU-CS-86-126, Carnegie–Mellon University, 1986.

[62] T. Poggio and F. Girosi. Networks for approximation and learning. *IEEE Proceedings,* 78(9), 1481–1497, 1990.

[63] M.J.D. Powell. Radial basis functions for multivariable interpolation: a review. In J.C. Mason and M.G. Cox, Editors, *Algorithms for Approximation.* Clarendon Press, Oxford, UK, 1987.

[64] M.B. Priestley. *Spectral Analysis and Time Series.* Academic Press, London, 1981.

[65] M.B. Priestley. *Non-Linear and Non-Stationary Time Series Analysis.* Academic Press, London, 1988.

[66] J.C. Principe, B. de Vries, and P. Oliveira. The Gamma filter — a new class of adaptive IIR filters with restricted feedback. *IEEE Transactions on Signal Processing,* 41:649–656, 1993.

[67] R. Rosipal, M. Koska, and I. Farkas. Prediction of chaotic time-series with a resource-allocating RBF network. *Neural Processing Letters,* 7:1–13, 1998.

[68] R. Scalettar and A. Zee. Emergence of grandmother memory in feed forward networks: learning with noise and forgetfulness. In D. Waltz and J.A. Feldman, Editors, *Connectionist Models and Their Implications: Readings from Cognitive Science.* Ablex Publishing Corp., New Jersey, 1988.

[69] J. Sjöberg and L. Ljung. Overtraining, regularization and searching for minimum in neural nets. In *Preprint 4th IFAC Symposium on Adaptive Systems in Control and Signal Processing,* Grenoble, France, pages 669–674, 1992.

[70] F. Sowell. Modelling long-run behavior with the fractional ARIMA model. *Journal of Monetary Economics,* 29:277–302, 1992.

[71] A.N. Tikhonov and V.I.A. Arsenin. *Solutions of Ill-Posed Problems.* Winston, New York (distributed solely by Halsted Press), 1977.

[72] H. Tong. *Threshold Models in Non-Linear Time Series Analysis.* Springer-Verlag, New York, 1983.

[73] H. Tong. *Non-Linear Time Series: A Dynamical System Approach.* Oxford University Press, Oxford, UK, 1990.

[74] H. Tong and K.S. Lim. Threshold autoregression, limit cycles, and cyclical data. *Journal Royal Statistical Society B,* 42:245–253, 1980.

[75] V. Tresp, J. Hollatz, and S. Ahmad. Network structuring and training using rule-based knowledge. In S.J. Hanson, J.D. Cowan, and C.L. Giles, Editors, *Advances in Neural Information Processing Systems 4,* pages 871–878. Morgan Kaufmann Publishers, San Mateo, CA, 1993.

[76] V. Tresp, J. Moody, and W. Delong. Prediction and control of the glucose metabolism of a diabetic. *NIPS Post-Conference Workshop: Neural Network Applications in Medicine,* Vail, CO, 1994.

[77] G. Wahba. *Spline Models for Observational Data.* CBMS-NSF Regional Conference Series in Applied Mathematics, Philadelphia, PA, 1990.

[78] A. Waibel, T. Hanazawa, G. Hinton, K. Shikano, and K. Lang. Phoneme recognition using time-delay neural networks. Technical Report TR-1-0006, ATR Interpreting Telephony Research Laboratories, 1987.

[79] E. Wan. Autoregressive neural network prediction: learning chaotic time series and attractors. In *Proceeding of the Summer Workshop on Neural Network Computing for the Electric Power Industry,* Stanford, CA, 1992.

[80] E. Wan. Finite impulse response neural networks with applications in time series prediction. Ph.D. thesis, Stanford University, 1993.

[81] A. Weigend and N. Gershenfeld. *Predicting the Future and Understanding the Past, SFI Studies in the Science of Complexity, Proc. Vol. XVII.* Addison-Wesley, Reading, MA, 1993.

[82] A.S. Weigend, M. Mangeas, and A.N. Srivastava. Nonlinear gated experts for time series: discovering regimes and avoiding overfitting. *International Journal of Neural Systems,* 6:373–399, 1995.

[83] A.S. Weigend, D.E. Rumelhart, and B.A. Huberman. Back-propagation, weight-elimination and time series prediction. In T.J. Sejnowski, G.E. Hinton, and D.S. Touretzky, Editors, *Proceedings of the Connectionist Models Summer School,* pages 105–116. Morgan Kaufmann Publishers, San Mateo, CA, 1990.

[84] A.S. Weigend, D.E. Rumelhart, and B.A. Huberman. Generalization by weight-elimination applied to currency exchange rate prediction. In *International Joint Conference on Neural Networks,* pages 837–841, IEEE, Seattle, WA, 1991.

[85] P.J. Werbos and J. Titus. An empirical test of new forecasting methods derived from a theory of intelligence: the prediction of conflict in Latin America. *IEEE Transactions Systems, Man & Cybernetics,* SMC-8(9):657–666, 1978.

[86] L. Wu and J. Moody. A smoothing regularizer for feedforward and recurrent neural networks. *Neural Computation,* 8(3):463–491, 1996.

[87] L. Wu, M. Niranjan, and F. Fallside. Fully vector-quantized neural network-based code-excited nonlinear predictive speech coding. *IEEE Transactions on Speech and Audio Processing,* 2(1):482–489, 1994.

10

Applications of Artificial Neural Networks (ANNs) to Speech Processing

Shigeru Katagiri
NTT Communication Science Laboratories

10.1 Introduction

A speech signal is the most fundamental human communication medium filled with various types of information, such as linguistic information, the speaker's identity, and emotional information. To use this medium effectively, speech processing technologies have been vigorously investigated in recent decades.

In most conventional cases, speech processing technologies employ classical disciplines such as probability theories, the Bayes decision theory [11, 14], vector quantization (VQ) [18], and spectrum analysis [51]. For example, speech recognition systems usually use a typical probabilistic framework for modeling dynamic (variable-durational) signals, i.e., a hidden Markov model (HMM). VQ was the core algorithm for most examples of speech coding systems, and auto-regressive (AR) modeling, a fundamental algorithm for estimating short-time spectra of time-series signals in a parametric form, mostly occupied a standard position of algorithmic selection for representing salient acoustic features of speech signals.

In the 1980s, due to the re-advent of the system concept of the artificial neural network (ANN) [21, 37, 38, 49, 55], there was a big boom of new research on ANN-based speech processing [47]. Since then, supported by advantages of the ANN such as a nonlinear modeling capability, high

0-8493-2359-2/01/$0.00+$1.50

discriminative capability, and adaptation capability, ANN-based speech processing technologies have been extensively investigated.

The period from the 1980s until today can be divided into two types of contrasting days: the high-tide days of the 1980s, in which ANN-based speech technologies were booming dramatically, and the low-tide days of the latter half of the 1990s, in which people rapidly came (at least seemingly) to lose research interest in ANN-based approaches. From this view, it might be plausible to say that ANN research is coming to an end. In reality, however, many important research issues remain, and the value of ANN research is still large. Actually, it should be noted that the importance of ANN research is increasing rather than decreasing. It can probably be said that ANN research has shifted in these past two decades from an early phase to a mature phase.

Indeed, the 1980s were a very productive research period for ANN-based speech processing technologies, even though research was still young at that point. A quick recall of those days may remind one of many valuable development examples, such as the time-delay neural network (TDNN) [62], the shift-tolerant learning vector quantization (STLVQ) [44], and the multi-state time-delay neural network (MSTDNN) [19, 20]. These results were actually useful for improving the performance of traditional speech processing technologies. However, the most important result during this period was the classification of the principal frameworks/criteria needed to study ANNs for speech processing applications; they were made mathematically sound. For example, it was shown that most ANN systems can be categorized according to four rather classic system design criteria and that further research should be executed along the guidelines of these criteria. The criteria are (1) network structure (measurement), (2) design (training) objective, (3) optimization, and (4) robustness to unknown samples (generalization) [11, 31]. Indeed, based on past results, enthusiastic research is currently being conducted, with a focus on advanced and difficult issues of speech-related ANN technologies.

The results of the first research period were published in many different places [32, 47]. To avoid duplication, this chapter focuses on four emerging and ongoing topics, most of which are related to speech recognition: (1) the generalized probabilistic descent (GPD) method, (2) recurrent neural networks (RNNs), (3) the support vector machine (SVM), and (4) signal separation technologies. Actually, speech recognition has always been a central stream of recent ANN applications to speech processing.

GPD [31] is a family of discriminative training algorithms for general pattern recognizers and was originally developed in the context of ANN design, especially LVQ [34, 35]. The range of GPD usage is not limited to ANNs or to speech, but research on GPD can directly contribute to an understanding of ANN-based speech recognizer design.

The heart of the RNN concept is the network structure of data recurrency. This recurrent structure is clearly suited towards modeling the temporal structure of speech signals, and the RNN is considered to possess high potential for alleviating limitations of the current standards, i.e., HMM and AR modeling [53].

SVM, the third focus of this chapter, is a novel pattern recognition concept that utilizes the nonlinear projections of input vector patterns to a higher dimensional (i.e., easier to classify) pattern space [61]. Similar to GPD, the concept has high generality, and it is not limited to ANN-based speech recognition. However, a close relation has been shown between SVMs and ANNs, and it is therefore clearly worthwhile to investigate this new theoretical paradigm in the chapter.

The final topic of this chapter is signal separation. Acoustic signals coexist in a mixed form, and humans can separate a target signal from all the other signals and recognize the target signal [10, 12]. Compared to this human ability, the function of current speech recognizers is seriously limited. Such recognizers usually assume that an input speech signal is spoken close to a system's input microphone so that they can simplify the problem, i.e., the separation and recognition of the target speech signal, to only the recognition of an *a priori* segmented speech signal.

There are two types of approaches to signal separation: (1) blind signal separation (BSS) [2, 26] and (2) model-based signal separation (MSS) [64]. Specifically, BSS is often formalized in an ANN framework, and it is rapidly comprising a new ANN-based research sub-area.

This chapter is organized as follows. Section 10.2 summarizes the fundamentals of speech signal processing and the background of ANN application to speech recognition. GPD is introduced in Section 10.3. Section 10.4 is dedicated to the RNN. Sections 10.5 and 10.6 are dedicated to SVMs and signal separation, respectively. Finally, Section 10.7 consists of concluding remarks.

10.2 Preparations

10.2.1 Fundamentals of Speech Recognition

10.2.1.1 Variety of Problem Formalizations

Based on the flexibility of human speech communication styles, speech recognition can be formalized in various ways. Typical formalization cases are summarized in Table 10.1. Generally, isolated-word recognition is easier than its counterpart, connected-word recognition. Read-speech recognition, in which text can basically be expected to satisfy grammatical rules, is easier than the recognition of spontaneous speech, which often includes out-of-grammar utterances. Speaker-dependent recognition is easier than speaker-independent recognition, which must cope with the speaker-oriented variety of acoustical and phonological characteristics. Closed-vocabulary recognition is more tractable than open-vocabulary recognition, which is basically based on keyword spotting techniques, even if the size of the closed set is large. Most of today's speech recognizers assume an input is spoken close to a microphone. This assumption is effective to avoid acoustic interferences, such as reverberations and background noise. Compared to this, distant-talk recognition is more difficult, but it basically enables one to communicate with a recognizer in a natural human-to-human conversational style.

TABLE 10.1 Variety of Speech Recognition Formalizations

Isolated-word recognition	–	Connected-word recognition
Read-speech recognition	–	Spontaneous-speech recognition
Speaker-dependent recognition	–	Speaker-independent recognition
Closed-vocabulary recognition	–	Open-vocabulary recognition
Close-talk recognition	–	Distant-talk recognition

Different problem settings should be tackled by different recognizers. To achieve the best matching between problems and systems, recognizers have been developed on a case-by-case basis, enabling them to satisfy the conditions required by individual formalization cases.

10.2.1.2 Nature of Speech Signals

A speech wave is a one-dimensional signal with a temporal structure. As can easily be experienced, a speech sound varies in length based on changes in the speaking speed (rate), although its linguistic information does not change. In addition, the temporal warping (extension and shrinking) range of speech is, in general, large for vowel classes and small for consonant classes. That is, the temporal structure of a speech sound is non-uniform or, in other words, nonlinearly time-warped.

Obviously, it is not appropriate to model a nonlinearly warping, dynamic (various-length) speech signal as a single static (fixed-length or fixed-dimensional) pattern. The desirable way of modeling such a speech signal should reflect the temporal structure that is specific to speech. One widely used solution is to model the observed speech as a dynamic sequence of short-time spectra. In this scheme, the short-time spectra are usually modeled using a static vector format called an acoustic feature vector.

As illustrated in Figure 10.1, a speech signal can be considered an output of a vocal track filter that is excited by either a noise source or a pulse train. A noise-driven output corresponds to an unvoiced

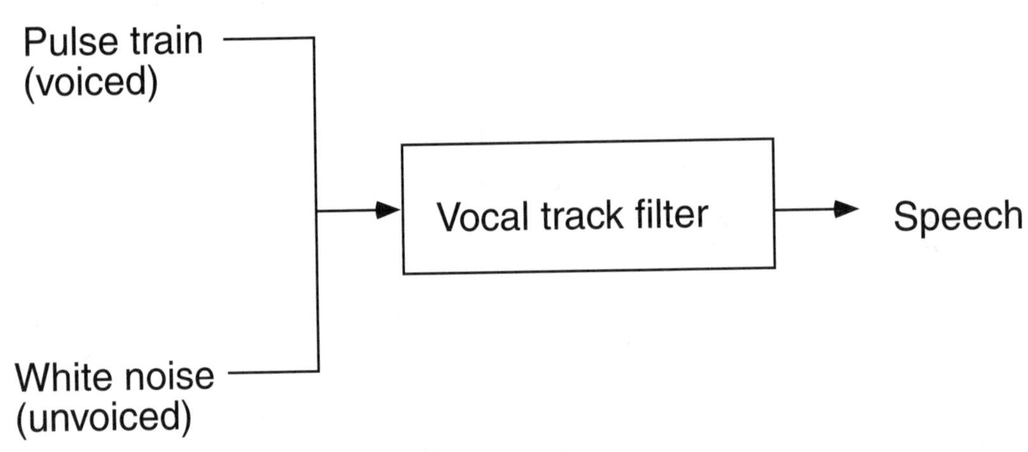

10.1 Schematic diagram of a speech production process.

phoneme sound, such as /p/ or /s/, and a pulse-driven output corresponds to a voiced phoneme, such as a vowel or nasal. Generally, the characteristics of the vocal tract shape represent phonemic information, and they principally form feature patterns used for speech recognition. According to the distinction between a vocal tract filter and the source signals, the phonemic information based on the vocal tract appears in a smoothed envelope shape of a short-time spectrum, and the source information appears in a minute structure of the spectrum. For speech recognition, therefore, an acoustic feature vector is computed so that it appropriately represents the spectral envelope information.

Readers are referred to textbooks such as Denes and Pinson [10] and Fant [12] for further information about the human speech communication process and the nature of speech signals.

10.2.1.3 Feature Representation for Speech Recognition

The spectral envelope defined in the frequency domain is rather redundant in terms of the phonemic information. For computational efficiency, it is usually expressed by some parametric form. A typical example of a parametric expression includes a bank-of-filter power spectrum estimation, homomorphic transform, and AR modeling. The bank-of-filter method is a straight model of the human auditory peripheral. The homomorphic transform is a signal-processing oriented method that expresses the spectral envelope as a small set of cepstrum coefficients. The AR modeling is a mathematical standard for linearly modeling time series signals, and it also has a unique relationship with the human speech production mechanism. Accordingly, in most cases of speech recognition, a speech wave is represented as a sequence of parametric-form acoustic feature vectors. Details of the feature representation methods are found in textbooks such as Markel and Gray [41] and Rabiner and Juang [51].

10.2.1.4 Modular Recognition Process

Regardless of the selection of problem settings, recognizer standards have long been a modular system that consists of a front-end feature extraction module (feature extractor) and a post-end classification module (classifier). A typical structure of a modular speech recognizer is illustrated in Figure 10.2. The feature extractor first converts an input speech wave to some acoustic feature

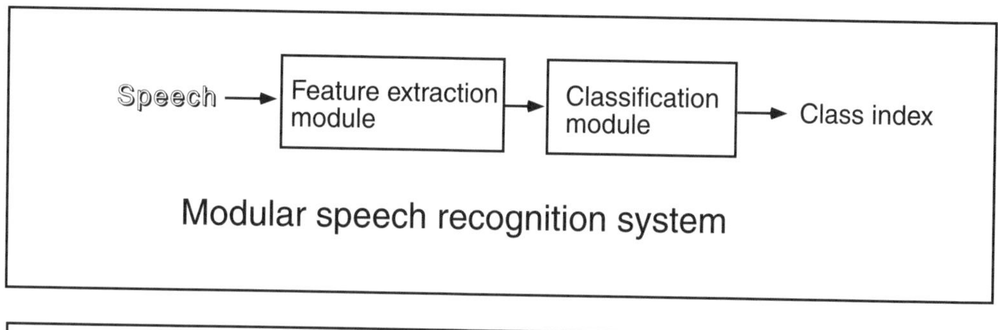

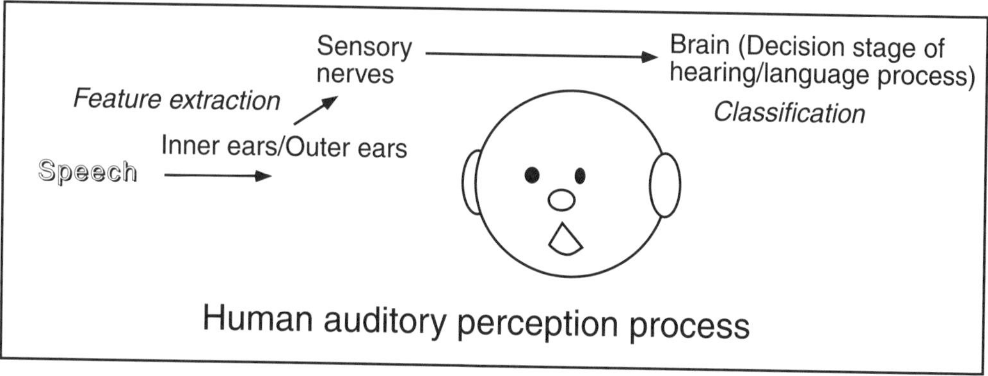

10.2 A typical structure of a modular speech recognizer. The conceptual correspondence between the modular recognizer and the human perception process is additionally illustrated.

pattern (see Section 10.2.1.3), and then the classifier decodes the pattern to a linguistic class such as a word sequence.

The modular structure of a recognizer can be considered to model the human mechanism of speech perception. The feature extractor roughly corresponds to the human auditory peripheral, such as the outer/inner ears, and the classifier simulates the decision stage of the human hearing/language process. The conceptual correspondence between the modular recognizer and the human perception mechanism is also depicted in Figure 10.2.

An acoustic feature pattern computed at the feature extractor is generally in the form of a parametric-form acoustic feature vector sequence, as cited above. An acoustic feature pattern is fed to the classifier as input. Accordingly, the class separability of the acoustic feature pattern space dominates the achievable performance of classifying the pattern. In this light, the design of feature extraction functions such as the bank-of-filter is of great importance. However, conventional approaches to such designs are often heuristic and empirical.

Traditionally, the classifier was embodied in the template/reference matching paradigm. Here, an input feature pattern produced at the feature extractor is compared to template patterns, the template pattern closest (in some preset distance measure) to the input pattern is selected, and the linguistic class to which the closest template belongs is emitted as a classification result. To cope with the dynamic nature of speech signals, the dynamic time-warping (DTW) scheme was specifically employed in the distance computation.

Distance measures such as the Euclidean distance and the Mahalanobis distance have a close link to the probability measure. Nowadays, template matching recognizers using DTW-distance computation are being replaced by a probability-based system framework that consists of HMM acoustic models and probabilistic language models such as the N-gram. In this present scheme, the *a posteriori* probability that an input feature pattern belongs to its corresponding linguistic class is measured for every possible class, and the most likely class is selected as a classification result.

Similar to most cases of pattern recognizer design, a central discipline of designing probabilistic models is the maximum likelihood (ML) method. However, for the HMM that inevitably contains unobservable components, i.e., states, an advanced version of the ML method called the expectation–maximization (EM) method is employed [11, 14, 51].

Readers are referred to textbooks such as Huang et al. [23], Lee et al. [39], and Rabiner and Juang [51] for more detailed information about recent speech recognition technologies.

10.2.2 Early Stage ANN Applications to Speech Recognition

Conventional speech recognizers based on HMMs have been shown to be useful under some limited conditions, e.g., the case of speaker-dependent, large-vocabulary recognition of short connected word sequences and the case of speaker-independent, small-vocabulary recognition of isolated words. Actually, these systems are now forming a new industrial opportunity using speech processing technologies [15, 46]. However, it has also been pointed out that these systems are unable to perform satisfactorily in more user-friendly task settings that enable people to speak to systems in the same manner as human-to-human speech communications.

The most serious reason for this dissatisfaction has been the limited classification accuracy of conventional systems. To alleviate this problem, early research interests focused on a promising alternative to the conventional system framework, i.e., the ANN, with an emphasis on its high discriminative capability. Most ANN-based speech recognizers, such as the TDNN and ANN/HMM hybrids, have been developed in this context. Several examples of such ANN-based recognizers are summarized in Table 10.2.

TABLE 10.2 Typical Examples of ANN-Based Speech Recognizers

- Time delay neural network (TDNN) [62]
- Multi-state TDNN [19, 20]
- Learning vector quantization (LVQ) network [34, 35]
- Shift-tolerant LVQ network [44]
- HMM-based time warping/ANN hybrid [16, 22, 28]
- ANN-based probability estimator/HMM hybrid [47]

In the earliest applications, the ANN was used to increase the recognition accuracy of short speech segments such as phonemes. The TDNN [62] and STLVQ [44] were typical examples of this type of ANN application. A time delay structure, or, in other words, a shift-tolerant structure, was incorporated into network architectures, aiming at normalizing the temporal variations of short segments. The effect of these ANN-based recognizers in phoneme recognition was remarkable. However, they were not sufficient for recognizing longer and more realistic speech segments, such as words and sentences, because the time delay structure was a simple normalization mechanism for comparatively short (and stationary) speech segments, which usually correspond to single phonemes at most. ANN-based recognizers could not handle the non-negligible dynamics of long segments such as words. Then, in the next advanced stage, ANN-based recognizers such as the TDNN were used in a hybrid form with DTW and HMMs, which have a state architecture suited to modeling the non-stationary characteristics of long speech segments [47].

Accordingly, the ANN has successfully contributed towards improving the recognition accuracy of preceding conventional systems in many experimental tasks. However, the scope of such ANN application has been limited to the simple recognition of speech signals that are extracted *a priori*. Obviously, many unsolved technical issues still remain, and ANN-based research challenges, such as some of the topics introduced in later sections, need to be conducted with vigor.

10.3 Generalized Probabilistic Descent Method

10.3.1 Formalization

10.3.1.1 Preparations

For description purposes, let us consider the following M class speech pattern recognition task defined in Equation (10.1).

$$C(X) = C_i \qquad \text{iff } i = \arg\max_j g_j(X; \Psi) \tag{10.1}$$

where X is a speech signal, Ψ is a trainable (designable) parameter set of our recognizer, $C(\,)$ is a recognition operation executed by the recognizer, and $g_j(X; \Psi)$ is a discriminant function that indicates the possibility with which X belongs to C_j. Following the descriptions in Section 10.2, we assume the recognizer to be a modular system that consists of a feature extractor and a classifier; the designable parameter sets of the feature extractor and the classifier are defined as Φ and Λ, respectively. Naturally, here we define our design goal as finding a status of Ψ $(= \Phi \cup \Lambda)$ that corresponds to the minimum misrecognition count condition.

Based on the definition of the recognizer, we assume that the recognition operation is composed of feature extraction and classification. Clearly, however, the recognition/misrecognition count (result) can be considered the same as the classification/misclassification count (result), which has been widely used in pattern recognition theory. For clarity of presentation, we use the terms recognition and misrecognition in the following sections.

10.3.1.2 Functional Form Embodiment of the Entire Process

The heart of the GPD formalization is to directly embed the overall process of recognizing an input pattern in a tractable functional form. In principle, there are many ways of defining tractable forms. In the spirit of mathematical and computational convenience, GPD assumes a functional form to be at least first-order differentiable with respect to the recognizer parameters [24, 27].

Based on an observation of the decision procedure in Equation (10.1), GPD first defines a misrecognition measure that emulates the procedure in a tractable smooth functional form. It should be noted here that the term misrecognition measure was originally introduced as misclassification measure, due to historical reasons of GPD development [24, 31]. Among many possibilities, the following is a typical definition of the misrecognition measure for a design sample X $(\in C_k)$:

$$d_k(X; \Psi) = -g_k(X; \Psi) + \left[\frac{1}{M-1} \sum_{j, j \neq k} \{g_j(X; \Psi)\}^{\mu} \right]^{1/\mu} \tag{10.2}$$

where μ is a positive constant. Clearly, $d_k(\,) > 0$ indicates a misrecognition and $d_k(\,) < 0$ indicates a correct recognition. That is, the recognition decision result of Equation (10.1) is expressed by a simple scalar value. In addition, we find that controlling μ enables the simulation of various decision rules. In particular, when μ approaches ∞, Equation (10.2) resembles Equation (10.1).

The next step of the GPD formalization is to introduce a mechanism for evaluating recognition results, similar to the standard discriminant function approaches to pattern recognizer design. That is, these approaches introduce an objective function for every design sample such as X, and specifically define the function as a smooth, monotonically increasing function of the misrecognition measure:

$$\ell_k(X; \Psi) = l\,(d_k(X; \Psi)) \tag{10.3}$$

where $l(\cdot)$ is a scalar function that determines the characteristics of the objective function. Similar to the misrecognition measure case, there are many possibilities for defining the objective. Among them, the GPD method usually uses the following smooth sigmoidal function:

$$\ell_k(X, \Psi) = l(d_k(X; \Psi)) = \frac{1}{1 + e^{-(\alpha d_k(X;\Psi)+\beta)}} \quad (\alpha > 0) \tag{10.4}$$

where α and β are constants. Note that the objective of Equation (10.4) is a smoothed version of the error count objective:

$$\ell_k(X, \Psi) = \begin{cases} 0 & (C(X) = k) \\ 1 & (\text{others}) \,. \end{cases} \tag{10.5}$$

The intuition here is that our design should aim to minimize the smooth loss of Equation (10.3) over design samples. Actually, this point is rigorously formalized in a fundamental theoretical basis of pattern recognition, i.e., the Bayes decision theory, by introducing the concept of expected loss. By using the individual loss functions, such as Equation (10.4), the expected loss is defined over all of the possible design samples, as follows:

$$L(\Psi) = \sum_k \int_\Omega p\,(X, C_k)\,\ell_k(X; \Psi) 1\,(X \in C_k)\,dX \tag{10.6}$$

where Ω is the entire sample space of the patterns Xs; it is assumed that $dp(X, C_k) = p(X, C_k)dX$ and that $1(\cdot)$ is an indicator function. Then, our design goal becomes the minimization of $L(\Psi)$ with respect to Ψ.

10.3.1.3 Optimization Based on the Probabilistic Descent Theorem

A standard approach to the minimization of the smooth functions is the use of gradient descent methods, such as the steepest descent method. In the GPD formalism, the probabilistic descent method, which is a stochastic approximation version of gradient descent methods, is employed for the minimization, with a focus on its adaptation mechanism. The essence of the probabilistic descent method is summarized in the following theorem [1].

10.3.1.3.1 Probabilistic Descent Theorem

Assume that a given design sample X belongs to C_k. If the recognizer parameter adjustment $\delta\Psi(X, C_k, \Psi)$ is specified by

$$\delta\Psi(X, C_k, \Psi) = -\epsilon \mathbf{U} \nabla \ell_k(X; \Psi) \tag{10.7}$$

where $\mathbf{U}$ is a positive-definite matrix and ϵ is a small positive real number, which is called a learning weight, then

$$E[\delta L(\Psi)] \leq 0 \tag{10.8}$$

Furthermore, if an infinite sequence of randomly selected samples $X(t)$ is used for the design ($X(t)$ is a design pattern sample given at time index t in the design stage) and the adjustment rule of Equation (10.7) is utilized with a corresponding learning weight sequence $\epsilon(t)$, which satisfies

$$\sum_{t=1}^{\infty} \epsilon(t) \rightarrow \infty \text{ and } \sum_{t=1}^{\infty} \epsilon(t)^2 < \infty \tag{10.9}$$

then the parameter sequence $\Psi(t)$ (i.e., the state of Ψ at t) according to

$$\Psi(t+1) = \Psi(t) + \delta\Psi\left(X, C_k, \Psi(t)\right) \tag{10.10}$$

converges with a probability of one, at least to Ψ^*, which results in a local minimum of $L(\Psi)$.

The above theorem obviously assumes an ideal but unrealistic design environment, where infinite design samples are available and an infinite training repetition is acceptable. In a realistic situation, where only a finite run of training over finite design samples is available, the state of Ψ that can be achieved by probabilistic descent training is, at most, a local optimum over a set of design samples. However, based on the directness of the formalization that embeds the recognition process in an optimizable functional form, the high utility of GPD has been clearly demonstrated in various speech recognition tasks [31].

10.3.1.4 Global Optimization Scope

We have assumed that our recognizer is a modular system that consists of a front-end feature extractor and a post-end classifier. However, the error minimization (optimization) of GPD is triggered at the classifier, and it seems that there is a gap between the two modules in terms of optimization computation. Indeed, in most conventional cases, the feature extractor has been designed heuristically or empirically, while the classifier has been trained with some mathematical optimization methods such as the ML method.

In contrast, GPD optimizes the entire recognizer with a single objective, i.e., the recognition error count loss, such as Equation (10.4). The mechanism underlying this global optimization is a simple extension of the chain rule of calculus that is used for optimization through loss, a misrecognition measure, and a discriminant function. Let us assume an output of the feature extractor to be $f(X; \Phi)$. Then,

$$g_j(X; \Psi) = g_j(f(X; \Phi); \Lambda)\ . \tag{10.11}$$

Clearly, the adjustment that is computed for the error minimization at the level of $g_j(\cdot; \Lambda)$ is easily propagated to the level of $f(X; \Phi)$, leading to a global optimization of the entire system.

10.3.2 Minimum Recognition Error Learning

In the case of using Equation (10.1) as a recognition decision rule, an ultimate goal of recognizer design is to find the parameter set that achieves the minimum recognition error condition. The relationship between this ultimate goal and the GPD design operation is summarized as follows.

Let us assume that (1) a probability measure $p(X)$ is provided in a known functional form for a pattern sample X, and (2) a parameter set determining the functional form is $\dot{\Psi}$. Then, considering the discriminant function

$$g_j(X; \dot{\Psi}) = p_{\dot{\Psi}}\left(C_j \mid X\right) \tag{10.12}$$

and the misrecognition measure of Equation (10.2), we can rewrite the expected loss, defined by using the smooth recognition error count loss Equation (10.4), as follows:

$$\begin{aligned} L(\dot{\Psi}) &= \sum_k \int_\Omega p\,(X, C_k)\,\ell_k(X; \dot{\Psi}) 1\,(X \in C_k)\,dX \\ &\simeq \sum_k \int_\Omega p\,(X, C_k)\,1\,(X \in C_k) \\ &\quad 1\left(p_{\dot{\Psi}}\,(C_k \mid X) \neq \max_j p_{\dot{\Psi}}\left(C_j \mid X\right)\right) dX \end{aligned} \tag{10.13}$$

Controlling the smoothness of functions such as the L_p norm used in Equation (10.2) and the sigmoidal function used in Equation (10.4), we can arbitrarily make $L(\dot{\Psi})$ closer to the last equation in Equation (10.13). Note that here we use $\dot{\Psi}$. Based on this fact, the status of $\dot{\Psi}$ that corresponds to the minimum of $L(\dot{\Psi})$ in Equation (10.13) (which is achieved by adjusting $\dot{\Psi}$) is clearly equal to the $\dot{\Psi}^*$ that corresponds to a true probability, or, in other words, achieves the maximum *a posteriori* probability condition. In short, it turns out that the minimum condition of $L(\dot{\Psi})$ can become arbitrarily close to the ideal minimum recognition error probability

$$\mathcal{E} = \sum_k \int_{\Omega_k} p_{\dot{\Psi}^*}\,(X, C_k)\,1\,(X \in C_k)\,dX \tag{10.14}$$

where Ω_k is a partial space of Ω that causes a recognition error according to the maximum *a posteriori* probability rule, i.e.,

$$\Omega_k = \left\{X \in \Omega \mid p_{\dot{\Psi}^*}\,(C_k \mid X) \neq \max_j p_{\dot{\Psi}^*}\left(C_j \mid X\right)\right\} \tag{10.15}$$

The above analysis of the minimum error condition is important from the mathematical viewpoint of showing the rationality of the GPD formalization. In reality, however, the parameter set $\dot{\Psi}$ is rarely known, and, accordingly, achieving the minimum recognition error probability condition through GPD-based design is usually impossible. The value of the analysis seems to be small; yet, the practical role of the analysis on the minimum recognition error learning continues to be large. It actually provides a mathematically sound background to practical attempts at recognizer design. The practical utility of GPD-based design has been successfully demonstrated in many experimental evaluations [31].

10.3.3 Links with Others

Our discussion of GPD has considered the entire process of recognition. However, in traditional cases, general mathematical discussions have been conducted only for the classification process, because the issue of feature extraction is essentially data-oriented, and discussing it from a general standpoint is often difficult. When limiting the formalization scope of GPD to the classification stage, we find that there are important links between GPD and many conventional classifier design approaches.

According to the technical issues described in the introduction, there are several possible ways to consider the links between GPD and other design methods.

We focus first on the selection of the objective function. In the case of using the classification (recognition) error count loss, it has been shown that a GPD training method for (multi-template) distance-based classifiers is similar to the discriminative versions of LVQ [27]. (It should be noted, however, that the LVQ methods were defined as heuristic rules [27, 35].)

Based on the theory of the minimum recognition error learning, GPD usually uses the smooth error count loss. In principle, however, it can also use other types of loss functions, such as the mutual information loss and the squared error loss, which have been widely used in speech recognition. Relationships between the minimization of the smooth error count loss and that of other loss functions have been analyzed, and it has been clarified that the minimization of the smooth error count loss is the most direct to the ideal minimum recognition error probability condition [31].

One may note that global optimization based on the chain rule of calculus is principally the same as the error back-propagation algorithm, which is an historic ANN-related idea [29, 30]. Indeed, there is an obvious similarity in the computation mechanisms of these two ideas. However, it should be remembered that GPD formalization emulates the recognition decision process in a functional form, while the standard error back-propagation is a simple embodiment of the chain rule for a hierarchical network structure or an embedded structure of functions.

10.3.4 GPD Families

For historical reasons relating to GPD development, and also based on the variety of task settings, GPD has been embodied in various different design methods. The following subsections introduce four exemplary topics of such embodiments.

10.3.4.1 Segmental GPD

Section 10.3.1.4 introduced the global optimization scope of GPD encompassing different modules of a recognizer. Under the classic (and standard) understanding that a dynamic (variable-length) pattern is a sequence of static (fixed-length) vectors and the design procedure for a whole dynamic pattern is a combination (in any form) of design procedures, each for an individual static vector, we can easily see that the GPD's formalization already embodies another type of global optimization scope. That is, GPD is a design method that optimizes the recognizer at hand with the global scope of minimizing the misrecognition of dynamic samples instead of their component vectors.

Segmental GPD was developed in the context of the classic understanding cited above, with special attention paid to the globalism extended over the time-axis of dynamic samples [6, 25]. Important here is that segmental GPD provides a powerful tool for a wide range of speech recognition tasks, such as connected-word recognition and conversational speech recognition; i.e., it discriminatively optimizes recognizers so that they can directly pursue the minimum error status in the recognition of preset speech units.

The effects of segmental GPD have been demonstrated in several common speech recognition tasks such as the TI digit [7]. In addition, the same design concept employed in segmental GPD has been tested in several similar formalizations, demonstrating the high utility of the design concept of segmental GPD [45, 52].

10.3.4.2 GPD for Open-Vocabulary Recognition

Generally, it is not easy to prepare a lexicon or language model set that completely covers all possible vocabularies. Even humans sometimes happen to meet unknown words in their daily speech communications, and they try to acquire the meanings of such new words through queries and other knowledge sources. A practical engineering solution to this difficulty in communications is the technology of open-vocabulary speech recognition. In this paradigm, a recognizer aims to correctly spot (extract) and recognize only keywords crucial for understanding the input speech.

Keyword spotting (for some particular words) is usually formalized by using keyword model λ and its corresponding threshold h. A spotting decision is fundamentally made at every time index over an input speech pattern X. Then, a discriminant function $g_t(X, S_t; \lambda)$ is defined as a function that measures the probability for observing a selected speech segment S_t of input utterance X, and the spotting decision rule is formulated as, "If the discriminant function meets

$$g_t(X, S_t; \lambda) > h \tag{10.16}$$

then the spotter judges at t that a keyword exists in segment S_t; no keyword is spotted otherwise."

A typical embodiment of GPD for the keyword spotting framework is minimum spotting error (MSPE) learning [36]. A goal of MSPE learning is to minimize spotting errors by adjusting both the keyword model λ and its corresponding threshold h. Note that the GPD's concept of global optimization is utilized in a twofold adjustment for the keyword model and the threshold.

Following the GPD formalization concept, the MSPE formalism aims to embed the above cited spotting decision process into an optimizable functional form and provide a concrete algorithm of optimization so that one can consequently reduce spotting errors. The spotting decision process is then emulated as spotting measure $d_t(X; \Lambda)$, which is defined as

$$d_t(X; \Lambda) = -h + \ln \left\{ \frac{1}{|I_t|} \sum_{\varsigma \in I_t} \exp\left(\xi g_\varsigma\left(X, S_\varsigma; \lambda\right)\right) \right\}^{1/\xi} \tag{10.17}$$

where I_t is a short segment, which is set for increasing the reliability and stability of the decision, around the time position t, $|I_t|$ is the size of I_t (the number of acoustic feature vectors in I_t), and ξ is a positive constant. A positive value for $d_t(X; \Lambda)$ implies that at least one keyword exists in I_t, and a negative value implies that no keyword exists in I_t. Importantly, this type of decision can produce, in principle, two types of decision errors: false detections (the spotter decides that S_t does not include a keyword when S_t actually does include a keyword) and false alarms (the spotter decides that S_t includes a keyword when S_t does not include a keyword). Decision results are evaluated by using a loss function defined by using two types of smoothed $0-1$ functions, $\acute{\ell}(\,)$ and $\hat{\ell}(\,)$, as [36]:

$$\ell_t(X; \Lambda) = \begin{cases} \acute{\ell}\left(d_t(X; \Lambda)\right) & \text{(if } I_t \text{ includes a training keyword)} \\ \gamma \hat{\ell}\left(d_t(X; \Lambda)\right) & \text{(if } I_t \text{ includes no training keyword)}\,. \end{cases} \tag{10.18}$$

Here, $\acute{\ell}(\,)$ and $\hat{\ell}(\,)$ are defined by using a sigmoidal function, such as Equation (10.4), and $\ell_t(\,)$ approximates (1) unity for one false detection, (2) γ for one false alarm, and (3) zero (0) for a correct spotting, where γ is a parameter controlling the characteristics of the spotting decision. Refer to Komori and Katagiri [36] for detailed definitions of $\acute{\ell}(\,)$ and $\hat{\ell}(\,)$.

The training procedure of MSPE is obtained by applying the adjustment rule [Equation (10.7)] of the probabilistic descent theorem to the above-defined functions, i.e., the loss, the spotting measure, and the discriminant function.

The mechanism of keyword spotting is similar to a hypothesis testing procedure based on Neyman–Pearson testing and the likelihood ratio test (LRT). The design concept of GPD has also been applied to the design of an LRT-based keyword spotting system in Rose et al. [54]. The resulting training procedure is similar to that in Komori and Katagiri [36].

10.3.4.3 GPD for Speaker Recognition

There are two types of speaker recognition tasks: (1) speaker identification, which is the process of identifying an unknown speaker from a known population, and (2) speaker verification, which is the process of verifying the identity of a claimed speaker from a known population. Given a test utterance X, the discriminant function $g_k(X; \Lambda)$ is defined as a function that measures the likelihood of observing X being generated by speaker k, where Λ is a set of trainable recognizer parameters.

Then, the decision operation of speaker identification is formalized as

$$\hat{k} = \arg\max_{k} g_k(X; \Lambda) \tag{10.19}$$

with $\hat{k}$ being the identified speaker, attaining the most likely score among all competing speakers.

In contrast, the decision operation of speaker verification is formalized as: "If the discriminant function meets

$$g_k(X; \Lambda) > h_k \tag{10.20}$$

then the recognizer accepts the claimed speaker's identity k; the recognizer rejects it otherwise."

Note that the formalization for speaker identification is equivalent to that for speech recognition and that the formalization for speaker verification is essentially the same as that for keyword spotting. Accordingly, GPD can be easily applied to the design of either a speaker identification system or a speaker verification system [40]. The derivation of GPD-based training is fundamentally the same as that for speech recognition. Refer to Liu et al. [40] for details on the implementation and experimental results.

To see other GPD applications to the task of speaker recognition, readers are referred to some of the recent literature on that topic [13, 43, 58, 59].

10.3.4.4 Discriminative Feature Extraction

Fundamentally, the global optimization scope of GPD can be applied to any module of the recognizer at hand. Focusing on a cascade architecture consisting of a feature extractor and a classifier, it is embodied as a discriminative feature extractor (DFE) that enables one to optimize the front-end feature extractor under a single design objective that is directly used for optimizing the post-end classifier [30]. The procedure of adjusting the system's trainable parameters is the same as that described in Section 10.3.1.3, and, in particular, the adjustment for the front-end feature extractor is made using the chain rule of differential calculus, which enables one to back-propagate the derivative of the objective function over the modules.

DFE can be applied to any reasonable system structure. In particular, Biem et al. [3, 4] tested DFE on an ANN-based feature extractor that is expected to discover features salient for recognition from cepstrum-based acoustic feature vectors. Note that cepstrum-based acoustic feature vectors have conventionally been computed using a heuristic and empirical lifter, and, accordingly, they are not guaranteed to be optimal for the recognition tasks at hand. Biem et al.'s [3, 4] expectation of DFE, therefore, is for the DFE training to lead to a more accurate recognition through the achievement of the optimal design for both the lifter feature extractor and the post-end classifier.

Focusing on the general perspective that feature extraction can be viewed as a process that forms a metric for measuring the class membership of an input pattern, DFE has also been embodied as a discriminative metric design method [63]. A key point in this embodiment was to introduce different metrics, one for each class, and optimize all of the metrics under a single minimization criterion using the classification error objective.

10.4 Recurrent Networks

10.4.1 Overview

Basically, a time-series signal has temporal correlations between its samples (or segments), each extracted at a different time position. This fact is a primary reason for the great success of using AR models, or, in other words, linear predictive coding, in a wide range of attempts at modeling time-series signals such as speech signals.

There are two main approaches to modeling the temporal information of speech signals: (1) memorizing the information spatially, and (2) modeling the information in a data-recurrent structure. The former case includes most methods of representing speech signals, such as the use of feature vector sequence patterns as reference patterns and the use of state models. The dynamics of signals are directly represented and memorized in the form of vector sequences or state sequences. The structure of the HMM is a typical example of a state model. The latter approach has been studied by using recurrent neural networks. In this case, in contrast to the direct memorization of the dynamics, the dynamics of signals are modeled, in some compressed parametric form, with network weights. The intuition and expectation do exist that recurrent network-based modeling leads to the discovery of essential components of information on the dynamics through the training (design) of a limited number of network weights. It should be noted that time delay (shift-tolerant) structures, e.g., those used in the TDNN and STLVQ, can be considered hybrids of spatial memorization and recurrent structure modeling.

Clearly, direct, spatial memorization is the most straightforward approach to the use of information on the dynamics, and its utility has been shown in many examples of speech recognizer design. However, the rather simple mechanism of this direct memorization sometimes results in a shortage of salient information and also in an excess storage of unnecessary (often noisy for classification decisions) information. Therefore, recurrent networks have been investigated, with the aim of extracting salient information for the task at hand effectively and efficiently.

There are various types of recurrent networks. Among them, this chapter introduces the following two cases: (1) unidirectional recurrent networks, and (2) bidirectional recurrent networks.

10.4.2 Unidirectional Network

Based on the causality of natural signals, temporal information goes, in principle, from the past to the future. A natural selection for modeling such information, therefore, has a unidirectional structure, illustrated in Figure 10.3. In that figure, the input speech signal is assumed to be converted *a priori* to a sequence of acoustic feature vectors, $\mathbf{u}(t)$ $(t = 1, \ldots, T)$, where T is the length of the acoustic feature vector sequence. Then, the input vector $\mathbf{u}(t)$ is presented to the network along with the state vector $\mathbf{x}(t)$, and these two vectors produce the output vector $\mathbf{y}(t)$ and the next state vector $\mathbf{x}(t+1)$. One design goal here is to determine two weight matrices, $\mathbf{W}$ and $\mathbf{V}$, so that $\mathbf{y}(t)$ can satisfy a preset design objective.

Among the many design methods for optimizing matrices, the back-propagation through time method has often been employed [66]. This method expands the network in time or, in other words, considers a recurrent net for all time indices as a single very large network with an input and output at each time index and shared weights over all time indices.

A network expansion scheme is illustrated in Figure 10.4. The training procedure is twofold: (1) forward-propagating the input vectors and the state vectors to get the final output vector at $T-1$ by using the initial (or adjusted) weight matrices, and (2) back-propagating the weight-update information calculated at the output position inversely in time.

Robinson [53] used the unidirectional recurrent network introduced above as a likelihood estimator, with some minor change in the output signal level, for an HMM-based speech recognizer.

10.4.3 Bidirectional Network

In addition to temporal correlation in the forward direction, which was described in the previous subsection, time series signals often possess backward correlation. In particular, it is an obvious observation that a speech signal possesses correlation in the backward direction. The speech signal is an output of an articulation system that is controlled by a speech production plan, which prepares future utterances and, accordingly, has influence on the future state (shape) of the articulators. In

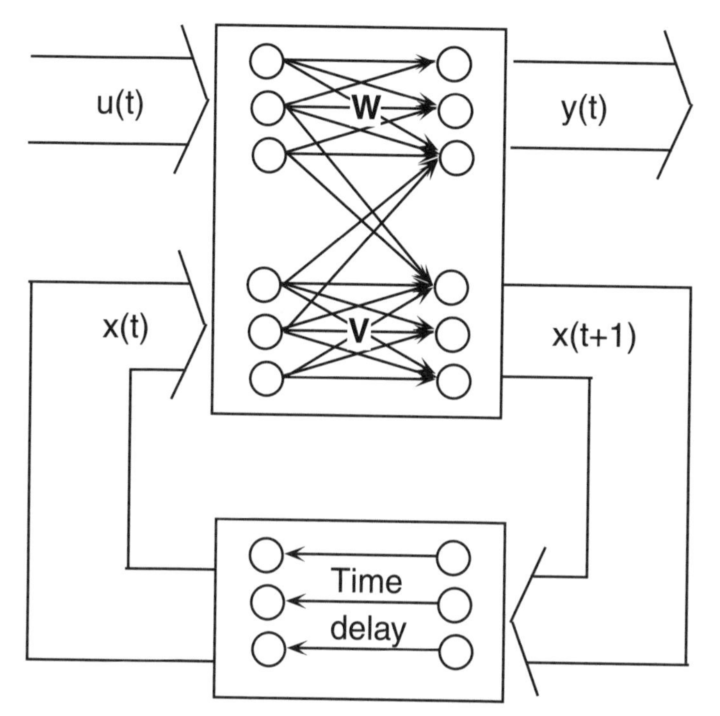

10.3 A typical structure of a unidirectional network [53].

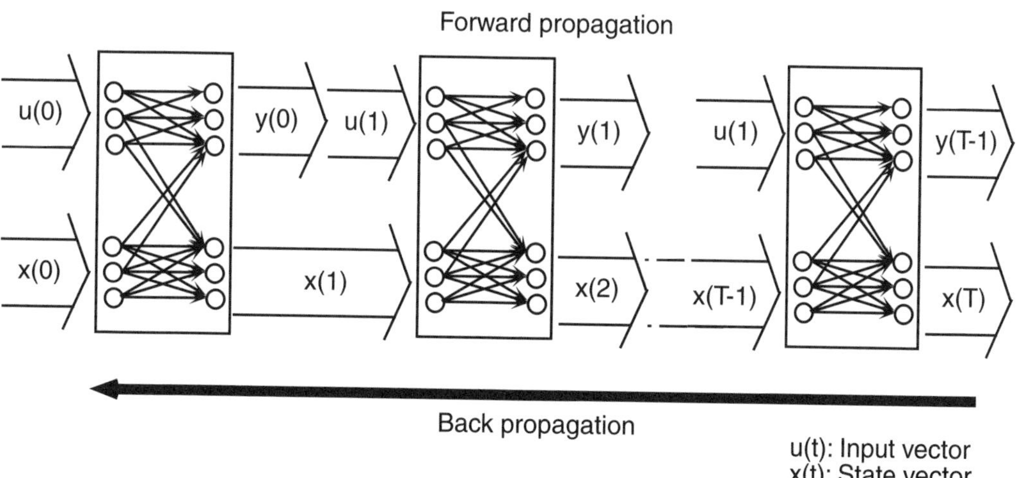

10.4 A schematic explanation of the back-propagation-through-time training method [53]).

conventional speech recognition approaches, this type of information is directly incorporated in the spatial memorization of signals.

Obviously, the unidirectional recurrent structure is not suited for representing backward information as well as forward information. A possible solution to this problem is a bidirectional recurrent network.

A sample structure of a bidirectional network is illustrated in Figure 10.5 [57]. A key idea in the structure is to split the state neurons into two parts: one part responsible for the forward time direction

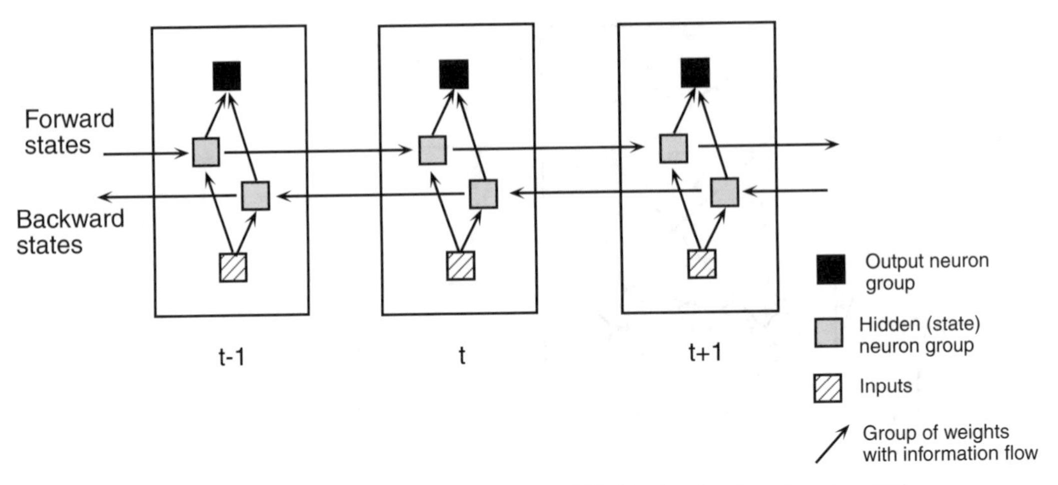

10.5 A sample structure of a bidirectional network shown unfolded in time for three time steps [57].

(forward states) and one part responsible for the backward time direction (backward states). Note that outputs from forward states are not connected to inputs of backward states and vice versa; in other words, the two networks run separately. It turns out, therefore, that in principle, the bidirectional recurrent network can be designed in the same way as the unidirectional recurrent network, e.g., by applying the back-propagation through time method to both networks.

Schuster and Paliwal [56, 57] tested the bidirectional network in phoneme recognition tasks and demonstrated its fundamental utility.

10.5 Support Vector Machines

10.5.1 Fundamentals

Generally, classification in a high-dimensional vector space is easier than in a low-dimensional vector space. In principle, even if sample (vector) distributions of different classes overlap in a low-dimensional sample space, they can be observed with less overlap in a high-dimensional space. Focusing on this general nature of sample observation, the SVM was developed as a new theoretical paradigm of pattern recognition [8, 61].

Consider a classification problem of linearly separable samples, $\{\mathbf{x}_1, \ldots, \mathbf{x}_m, \ldots, \mathbf{x}_M\}$, where $\mathbf{x}_m \in \mathcal{R}^n$. Each sample is associated with its corresponding class indicator; i.e., $(\mathbf{x}_1, y_1), \ldots, (\mathbf{x}_m, y_m), \ldots, (\mathbf{x}_M, y_M)$, where y_ms are class indicators ($y_m \in \{-1, 1\}$). Then, the hyperplane $(\mathbf{w} \cdot \mathbf{x}) + b$ completely separates these linearly separable samples if and only if

$$\begin{cases} (\mathbf{w} \cdot \mathbf{x}_i) + b \geq 1 & (\text{if } y_i = 1) \\ (\mathbf{w} \cdot \mathbf{x}_i) + b \leq -1 & (\text{if } y_i = -1) \end{cases} \tag{10.21}$$

where b is a constant. One goal of the classifier design is to determine the weight vector $\mathbf{w}$ (and, accordingly, its corresponding hyperplane) that satisfies Equation (10.21). Clearly, an optimal status of the weight vector can be the status with the largest distance between the hyperplane and its closest samples. Through a rewrite of the equations, the problem of finding the optimal weight vector becomes the problem of minimizing

$$\sum_i \alpha_i - \frac{1}{2} \sum_{i,j} \alpha_i \alpha_j y_i y_j \mathbf{x}_i \cdot \mathbf{x}_j \tag{10.22}$$

subject to

$$\alpha_i \geq 0 \qquad \sum_i \alpha_i y_i = 0 \tag{10.23}$$

where α_i are Lagrange multipliers and each design sample $\mathbf{x}_i$ has one Lagrange multiplier α_i. Here, the training sample whose corresponding multiplier is non-zero is a support vector that dominates the optimal hyperplane. This hyperplane is then achieved with a standard quadratic programming procedure.

In reality, however, samples of different classes are observed to overlap and are nonlinearly non-separable. Moreover, most realistic classification tasks are of the multiple class type. Therefore, the procedure for finding the optimal hyperplane, introduced above, is usually softened in terms of separability requirements. A nonlinear mapping from the original sample vector space to a high-dimensional pattern space is also incorporated, based on the expectation that classification in a high-dimensional space is generally easier than in a low-dimensional space. To cope with the multi-class settings, SVM-based classifiers designed for two-class settings are usually used in some combinatorial form.

The nonlinear mapping bridges the two paradigms, SVMs and ANNs. The final design formations, Equations (10.22) and (10.23), are only dot product computations, and their corresponding computations in a nonlinearly mapped high-dimensional space can be efficiently operated by using kernel functions such as polynominal kernel functions and Gaussian radial-basis functions, both of which are widely used in ANN systems.

10.5.2 Application Examples

Applications of the SVM to speech recognition are still in a preliminary stage, although the theoretical advantage involved is widely recognized. These circumstances may arise from the fact that the SVM is essentially a concept for static (fixed-length) vector patterns and is not suited for dynamic (variable-length) speech patterns. This subsection introduces two recent application examples [8, 50] which are not that mature but suggest a new promising technological direction using SVMs.

10.5.2.1 SVM-Based Phoneme Detection

In most cases of recent speech recognition, speech signals have been represented by common acoustic features, such as AR coefficients, cepstral coefficients, and bank-of-filter coefficients, regardless of phoneme class differences. On the other hand, phonetics has long suggested that each phoneme class should be characterized by its particular types of features, i.e., distinctive features. As an alternative to the current HMM-based speech recognition with generally high costs, an approach using distinctive features can be expected to be useful for developing simple and small-sized recognizers and also for achieving high flexibility in classification decisions, which is needed in conversational speech recognition and open-vocabulary speech recognition.

The detection operation is basically the same as the spotting described in Section 10.3.4, and it is essentially a two-class operation which outputs "detected" or "not detected." The use of SVMs is, therefore, straightforward. Niyogi et al. [50] investigated the feasibility of SVMs in a task of stop consonant detection, which is a typical example of the phoneme detection task described above. An SVM-based recognizer that works as a stop consonant detector at every time position over an input speech signal was designed by using three-dimensional vectors with components based on phonetic distinctive features. Experimental results demonstrated the superiority of a SVM-based recognizer to a conventional HMM-based recognizer using 39-dimensional cepstrum-based features. The results also showed that the nonlinearity in the mapping with radial-basis kernel functions is effective for increasing the detection accuracy.

10.5.2.2 SVM-Based Phoneme Classification

In the early stages of ANN application to speech recognition, several attempts were made to apply ANNs to static patterns converted from original dynamic speech patterns [16, 22, 28]. Clarkson and Moreno [8] represented phoneme segments as static feature vectors whose components were formant frequency values measured at the central positions of phonemes or average cepstral coefficients calculated over preset subsegments of phonemes, and SVM-based classification was evaluated over these static vector patterns.

The classification tasks used by Clarkson and Moreno [8] were of the multi-class type. Therefore, two combinatorial formations were tested: (1) the "one vs. one" formation and (2) the "one vs. all" formation. In the one vs. one formation, an SVM-based subclassifier was designed for every pair of two different classes. A test sample was preclassified by all of the designed subclassifiers and was then finally classified with a voting scheme over the subclassifiers. In the one vs. all formation, an SVM-based subclassifier was designed for every pair of a target class and remaining classes. A test sample was preclassified by all of the subclassifiers and its class label was then finally set to the class having the largest distance from the separating hyperplane.

For comparison, a conventional Gaussian mixture classifier was also designed for the same static data. Experiments demonstrated the superiority of the SVM-based classifier to the Gaussian mixture classifier and the superiority of the one vs. one formation to its counterpart. They also suggested the importance of the selection of nonlinear mapping kernel functions.

10.6 Signal Separation

10.6.1 Overview

There are three major approaches to speech signal separation: (1) an approach based on microphone-array technology [48], (2) an approach based on blind signal separation [2, 9, 26], and (3) an approach based on model-based separation [33, 42, 64]. The first approach, i.e., acoustic-technology-based, is the most traditional and orthodox, and is already used in real-world recognizers. However, although it works sufficiently under some limited conditions, it cannot emulate the high flexibility and capability of humans in separating a target speech signal with a reasonably small-size implementation. The second approach is based on the information theory, and it presently represents a main research trend in the field of signal separation. The third approach attempts to emulate the human hearing process to some extent by assuming the importance of model-based (top-down or *a priori*) knowledge about target signals. Compared to the second approach, blind signal separation, this model-based approach is still at the beginning stages of research. Nonetheless, the validity and prospects of this approach are supported by many psychological findings [5].

This chapter focuses on two recent trends, i.e., blind separation and model-based separation. From the standpoint of speech recognition, the techniques of these two separation approaches have not yet been fully developed. They also do not necessarily have a direct link to ANN technologies. Only a few links can be observed in the structural similarities between the ANN and the problem formalism of signal separation. However, studying these technical topics is clearly worthwhile because mathematics and ultimate research goals, i.e., the development of speech recognition technologies that successfully emulate humans, are common to both the ANN and signal separation.

10.6.2 Blind Separation

In the blind signal separation paradigm, a problem is generally formalized using a kind of network structure that has M inputs and N outputs. Figure 10.6 depicts a two-input and two-output case of a formalization. In that figure, there are four possible signal channels, and they are represented

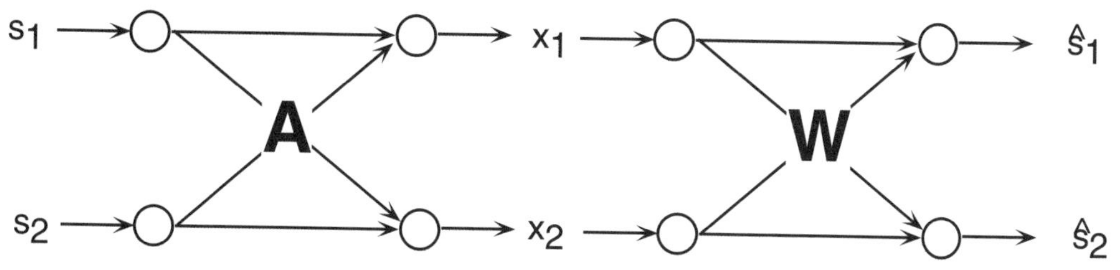

10.6 A schematic explanation of the formalization of two-input and two-output signal separation.

by a 2 × 2 mixing matrix **A**. The relation between the original source signals, s_1 and s_2, and the observations, x_1 and x_2, are represented as

$$\begin{pmatrix} x_1 \\ x_2 \end{pmatrix} = \mathbf{A} \begin{pmatrix} s_1 \\ s_2 \end{pmatrix} . \tag{10.24}$$

One goal is to then estimate the inverse matrix of **A**, i.e., **W**, which is defined as

$$\begin{pmatrix} \hat{s}_1 \\ \hat{s}_2 \end{pmatrix} = \mathbf{W} \begin{pmatrix} x_1 \\ x_2 \end{pmatrix} \tag{10.25}$$

where $\hat{s}_1$ and $\hat{s}_2$ are the estimates of s_1 and s_2, respectively.

Three major approaches to the estimation of the inverse matrix have been investigated: (1) signal decorrelation [65], (2) independent component analysis (ICA) [26], and (3) information-maximization-based separation [2]. The first, signal decorrelation, is mainly based on the correlation information between the estimated source signals. ICA additionally uses the independence between the estimates, which is prescribed by the estimates' higher-order statistics. The third approach is derived from the ICA-based approach with an additional nonlinear transform of the estimated source signals.

The following introduces a speech recognition example using the blind signal separation of Taniguchi et al. [60], where information-maximization-based separation is employed.

A basic strategy underlying the information-maximization-based approach is to estimate **W** such that its estimation, $\hat{\mathbf{W}}$, minimizes the mutual information $I(\hat{s}_1, \hat{s}_2)$ between the estimated source signals, based on the fact that when **W** is correctly estimated, $I(\hat{s}_1, \hat{s}_2)$ should be minimum due to the independence between the estimates:

$$\hat{\mathbf{W}} = \arg\min_{\mathbf{W}} I\left(\hat{s}_1, \hat{s}_2\right) . \tag{10.26}$$

Here, from the relationship between the mutual information and the entropy functions, i.e.,

$$I\left(\hat{s}_1, \hat{s}_2\right) = H\left(\hat{s}_1\right) + H\left(\hat{s}_2\right) - H\left(\hat{s}_1, \hat{s}_2\right) \tag{10.27}$$

it turns out that the estimation problem is equivalent to the maximization of $H(\hat{s}_1, \hat{s}_2)$ if $H(\hat{s}_1)$ and $H(\hat{s}_2)$ can be assumed to remain the same values, respectively. However, the entropy, such as $H(\hat{s}_1)$, usually increases as the signal's variance increases. Therefore, to meet the assumption of an unchangeable entropy, the value ranges of the signals are bounded to some fixed values using a nonlinear function $g(\cdot)$ such as a sigmoidal function (which is widely used in ANN systems).

$$y_i = g\left(\hat{s}_i\right) \qquad (i = 1, 2) . \tag{10.28}$$

The problem is then further reformed as

$$\begin{aligned} H\left(\hat{s}_1, \hat{s}_2\right) &= E\left[-\ln \frac{f_{x_1,x_2}\left(x_1, x_2\right)}{|J|}\right] \\ &= E[\ln |J|] - E\left[\ln f_{x_1,x_2}\left(x_1, x_2\right)\right] \end{aligned} \tag{10.29}$$

where $|J|$ is the Jacobian of the mapping from (x_1, x_2) to (y_1, y_2), and $f_{x_1,x_2}(x_1, x_2)$ is the joint distribution of x_1 and x_2. Here, because the second term of Equation (10.29) is independent from **W**, the final design target is to find the state of **W** that maximizes the first term of Equation (10.29), i.e., $E[\ln|J|]$, resulting in the following adjustment procedure for the estimation:

$$\mathbf{W}^{(i)} = \mathbf{W}^{(i-1)} + \epsilon\Delta\mathbf{W} \tag{10.30}$$

$$\Delta\mathbf{W} = E\left[\frac{\partial}{\partial\mathbf{W}}\ln|J|\right]. \tag{10.31}$$

In Taniguchi et al. [60], experimental evaluations were done by applying the information-maximization-based blind separation described above to a DTW speech recognizer and an HMM speech recognizer, for a task of recognizing 68 phonetically similar Japanese city names. Results demonstrated the utility of the separation method in both types of recognizers.

10.6.3 Model-Based Separation

An underlying concept of model-based signal separation is to use some *a priori* or top-down knowledge about signals to be separated and recognized, as humans do in their hearing procedures. Using such knowledge will generally increase the accuracy and robustness in both the separation and recognition processes. The following subsection introduces two recent embodiments of the model-based separation discussed by Gautama and Van Hulle [17] and Watanabe et al. [64].

10.6.3.1 Separation Using Codebook Projection

Figure 10.7 illustrates, for a case of two source signals, a diagram of a separation procedure that uses complex Fourier spectrum representations of input signals and an ANN-trained model codebook [17]. The signals in this scheme are all represented in complex short-time Fourier trans-

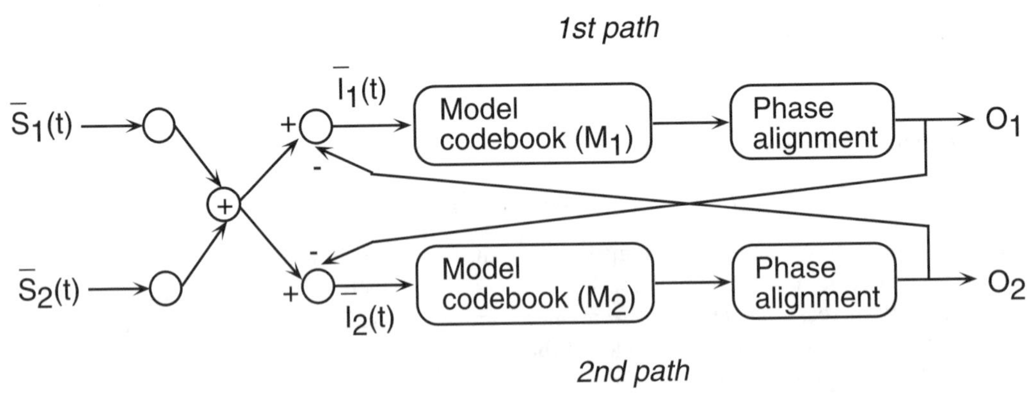

10.7 A schematic diagram of signal separation using codebook projection [17].

forms. An overlapped signal $\bar{C}(t)$ is a linear combination of two independent source signals, $\bar{S}_1(t)$ and $\bar{S}_2(t)$, at some time index t. The compound signal goes to both paths, each corresponding to one source. In the ith path ($i = 1, 2$ in the figure), the estimated spectrum of the other source is subtracted from $\bar{C}(t)$, and the subtraction result $\bar{I}_i(t)$ is quantized by the model M_i. The quantization is basically done based on the projection of $\bar{I}_i(t)$ onto the winning code model (vector), which produces the maximum dot product with $\bar{I}_i(t)$. Then, the quantized signal is converted to a source signal estimate $\bar{O}_i$ with the phase alignment ϕ. The expectation here is that repeating the subtraction of the interference and the model projection leads to a convergence towards accurate estimates of the original source signals.

Gautama and Van Hulle [17] used ANN-based algorithms, such as a self-organizing feature map, to train the model codebook, and the method was evaluated in a task of separating the sound signals of two instruments.

10.6.3.2 Separation Using a Speech Production Model

Another attempt at model-based separation is found in Watanabe et al. [64]. A basic scheme of this separation is illustrated in Figure 10.8. An observed signal is assumed to be a linear sum of

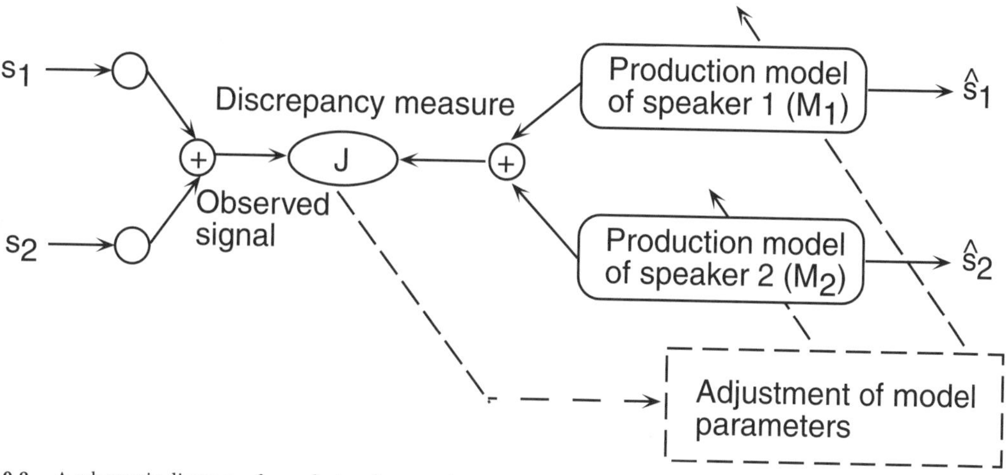

10.8 A schematic diagram of speech signal separation using a speech production model [64].

multiple speakers' utterances:

$$s(t) = s_1(t) + s_2(t) + \cdots + s_I(t) \tag{10.32}$$

where I is the number of speakers. One design goal here is to reconstruct the component signal sources $\{s_i(t)\}_{i=1}^{I}$ from the observed signal $s(t)$. Motivated by the idea of speech segregation based on the motor theory in human speech perception, a speech production model is incorporated as top-down knowledge in the process. As shown in the figure, one speech production model is prepared for each speaker, and the model parameters are estimated so that the summation of the signals synthesized by these models can approximate the observed overlapped speech accurately. Each synthesized signal is then expected to be a reasonable estimate of its corresponding speaker's original speech signal when the adjustment of the model parameters converges to some approximation quality. Of note in this method is that the speech production model used as *a priori* knowledge can produce speech recognition results in parallel with the separation: a speech production model, such as one based on AR modeling, can easily associate its parametric state to some phonetic category, and such phonetic information can be used as a recognition output.

Watanabe et al. [64] employed a simple speech production model using an autoregressive-model based vocal tract model and Klatt's vocal cord wave model for the separation/recognition of two speakers' utterances. The experiments were still in a preliminary stage, but they demonstrated the prospects of the unique approach.

10.7 Concluding Remarks

This chapter has summarized recent research on ANN applications to speech processing, specifically focusing on several example topics in speech recognition. The main topics introduced in the chapter include a general discriminative design method for pattern recognition, i.e., the generalized probabilistic descent method (GPD), a recurrent neural network (RNN) characterized by its data recurrency structure, a novel theoretical paradigm of pattern recognition, i.e., the support vector machine (SVM), and recent signal separation technologies that are mainly based on the statistics or mathematical modeling of the data at hand. These topics are all new and are in ongoing stages of research.

The title of this chapter may cause the reader to naturally expect to see many examples of ANN applications to a wide range of speech processing technologies such as speech recognition, speech synthesis, speech coding, and speech enhancement. In reality, however, most of the applications mentioned in this chapter were investigated in the speech recognition area, even in the high-tide stage of research through the middle of the 1990s. Today, when new technological paradigms such as the SVM and BSS are rapidly booming, applications to speech processing are not necessarily so active. There are several possible reasons for this situation; probably the most serious is that recent research still adheres to simple and old-fashioned approaches in the belief that, if a lot of data are available, a good system can and will be achieved — that is, anything is possible with a large amount of data. The fact that most current speech recognizers are being developed by applying the classic maximum likelihood method to a huge amount of design samples probably supports this observation. However, current technologies for computing acoustic feature vectors and the probabilistic modeling framework based on HMMs are obviously insufficient for handling more realistic tasks such as distant talk recognition, where systems have to perform signal separation accurately, and for developing more accurate and more efficient systems. Rather than having a large amount of design samples, novel frameworks are needed for modeling speech data and the tasks at hand. The topics introduced in this chapter have not yet formed a new trend of technology, but, hopefully, they will be useful for the reader to envision desired directions of future research.

References

[1] S. Amari; A theory of adaptive pattern classifiers, *IEEE Trans. EC,* vol. EC-16, pp. 299–307 (1967).

[2] A.J. Bell and T.J. Sejnowski; An information-maximization approach to blind separation and blind deconvolution, *Neural Comput.,* vol. 7, pp. 1129–1159 (1995).

[3] A. Biem, S. Katagiri, and B.H. Juang; Discriminative feature extraction for speech recognition, in *Neural Networks for Signal Processing III,* IEEE, pp. 392–401 (1993).

[4] A. Biem, S. Katagiri, and B.H. Juang; Pattern recognition using discriminative feature extraction, *IEEE Trans. SP,* vol. 45, pp. 500–504 (1997).

[5] A. de Cheveigne; Concurrent vowel identification. III. A neural model of harmonic interference cancellation, *J. Acoust. Soc. Am.,* vol. 101, no. 5, pp. 2857–2865 (1997).

[6] W. Chou, B.H. Juang, and C.H. Lee; Segmental GPD training of HMM based speech recognition, *Proc. IEEE ICASSP92,* vol. 1, pp. 473–476 (1992).

[7] W. Chou, C.H. Lee, and B.H. Juang; Minimum error rate training of inter-word context dependent acoustic model units in speech recognition, *Proc. ICSLP94,* pp. 439–442 (1994).

[8] P. Clarkson and P. Moreno; On the use of support vector machines for phonetic classification, *Proc. ICASSP99,* paper no. 2104 (1999).

[9] P. Common, C. Jutten, and J. Herault; Blind separation of sources, part II: Problems statement, *Signal Processing,* vol. 24, pp. 11–20 (1991).

[10] P.B. Denes and E.N. Pinson; *The Speech Chain: The Physics and Biology of Spoken Language,* New York: W.H. Freeman and Company (1993).

[11] R. Duda and P. Hart; *Pattern Classification and Scene Analysis,* New York: John Wiley & Sons (1973).

[12] G. Fant; *Speech Sounds and Features,* Cambridge, MA: MIT Press, (1973).

[13] K.R. Farrell, R.J. Mammone, and K.T. Assaleh; Speaker recognition using neural networks and conventional classifiers, *IEEE Trans. SAP,* vol. 2, no. 1, Part II, pp. 194–205 (1994).

[14] K. Fukunaga; *Introduction to Statistical Pattern Recognition,* New York: John Wiley & Sons (1972).

[15] S. Furui; Speech recognition technology in the ubiquitous/wearable computing environment, *Proc. ICASSP2000,* vol. 6, pp. 3735–3738 (2000).

[16] Y.Q. Gao, T.Y. Huang, and D.W. Chen; HMM-based warping in neural networks, *Proc. ICASSP90,* vol. 1, pp. 501–504 (1990).

[17] T. Gautama and M.M. Van Hulle; Separation of acoustic signals using self-organizing neural networks, in *Neural Networks for Signal Processing IX,* IEEE, pp. 324–332 (1999).

[18] R. Gray; Vector quantization, *IEEE ASSP Magazine,* pp. 4–29 (1984).

[19] P. Haffner, M. Franzini, and A. Waibel; Integrating time alignment and neural networks for high performance continuous speech recognition, *Proc. ICASSP91,* pp. 105–108 (1991).

[20] P. Haffner; A new probabilistic framework for connectionist time alignment, *Proc. ICSLP94,* pp. 1559–1562 (1994).

[21] S. Haykin; *Neural Networks: A Comprehensive Foundation,* New York: McMillan (1994).

[22] D. Howell; The multilayer perceptron as a discriminating post processor for hidden Markov networks, in *Proc. 7th FASE Symp.,* pp. 1389–1396 (1988).

[23] X. Huang, Y. Ariki, and M. Jack; *Hidden Markov Models for Speech Recognition,* Edinburgh, UK: Edinburgh University Press (1990).

[24] B.H. Juang and S. Katagiri; Discriminative learning for minimum error classification, *IEEE Trans. SP.,* vol. 40, no. 12, pp. 3043–3054 (1992).

[25] B.H. Juang, W. Chou, and C.H. Lee; Minimum classification error rate methods for speech recognition, *IEEE Trans. SAP,* vol. 5, pp. 257–265 (1997).

[26] C. Jutten and J. Herault; Blind separation of sources, part I: An adaptive algorithm based on neuromimetic architecture, *Signal Processing,* vol. 24, pp. 1–10 (1991).

[27] S. Katagiri, C.H. Lee, and B.H. Juang; New discriminative training algorithms based on the generalized probabilistic descent method, in *Neural Networks for Signal Processing,* IEEE, pp. 299–308 (1991).

[28] S. Katagiri and C.H. Lee; A new hybrid algorithm for speech recognition based on HMM segmentation and learning vector quantization, *IEEE Trans. SAP,* vol. 1, pp. 421–430 (1993).

[29] S. Katagiri; A unified approach to pattern recognition, *Proc. ISANN94,* pp. 561–570 (1994).

[30] S. Katagiri, B.H. Juang, and A. Biem; Discriminative feature extraction, in *Artificial Neural Networks for Speech and Vision,* (R. Mammon, Ed.), London, UK: Chapman & Hall, (1994), pp. 278–293.

[31] S. Katagiri, B.H. Juang, and C.H. Lee; Pattern recognition using a family of design algorithms based upon the generalized probabilistic descent method, *Proc. IEEE,* vol. 86, no. 11, pp. 2345–2373 (1998).

[32] S. Katagiri (Ed.); *Handbook of Neural Networks for Speech Processing,* Boston, MA: Artech House, 2000.

[33] H. Kawahara, I. Masuda-Katsuse, and A. de Cheveigne, Restructuring speech representations using a pitch-adaptive time-frequency smoothing and an instantaneous-frequency-based F0 extraction: possible role of a repetitive structure in sounds, *Speech Communication,* vol. 27, pp. 187–207 (1999).

[34] T. Kohonen, G. Barna, and R. Chrisley; Statistical pattern recognition with neural networks: benchmarking studies, *Proc. of ICNN,* vol. 1, pp. I-61–I-68 (1988).

[35] T. Kohonen; *Self-Organizing Feature Maps,* New York: Springer-Verlag (1995).

[36] T. Komori and S. Katagiri; A minimum error approach to spotting-based pattern recognition, *IEICE Trans. Inform. Syst.,* vol. E78-D, no. 8, pp. 1032–1043 (1995).

[37] B. Kosko (Ed.); *Neural Networks for Signal Processing,* Englewood Cliffs, NJ: Prentice-Hall (1992).

[38] S.Y. Kung; *Digital Neural Networks,* Englewood Cliffs, NJ: Prentice-Hall (1993).

[39] C.H. Lee, F.K. Soong, and K.K. Paliwal (Eds.); *Automatic Speech and Speaker Recognition,* Norwell, MA: Kluwer (1996).

[40] C.S. Liu, C.H. Lee, W. Chou, B.H. Juang, and A. Rosenberg; A study on minimum error discriminative training for speaker recognition, *J. Acoustical Soc. Amer.,* vol. 97, no. 1, pp. 637–648 (1995).

[41] J.D. Markel and A.H. Gray, Jr.; *Linear Prediction of Speech,* New York: Springer-Verlag (1976).

[42] I. Masuda-Katsuse and H. Kawahara; Dynamic sound stream formation based on continuity of spectral change, *Speech Communication,* vol. 27, pp. 235–259 (1999).

[43] T. Matsui and S. Furui; A study of speaker adaptation based on minimum classification error training, *Proc. Eurospeech 95,* pp. 81–84 (1995).

[44] E. McDermott and S. Katagiri; LVQ-based shift-tolerant phoneme recognition, *IEEE Trans. SP,* vol. 39, pp. 1398–1411 (1991).

[45] E. McDermott and S. Katagiri; Prototype-based MCE/GPD training for various speech units, *Comput. Speech Language,* vol. 8, pp. 351–368 (1994).

[46] E. McDermott, A. Biem, S. Tenpaku, and S. Katagiri; Discriminative training for large vocabulary telephone-based name recognition, *Proc. ICASSP2000,* vol. 6, pp. 3739–3442 (2000).

[47] N. Morgan and H. Bourlard; Continuous speech recognition — an introduction to the hybrid HMM/connectionist approach, *IEEE Signal Processing Mag.,* vol. 12, no. 3, pp. 25–42 (1995).

[48] S. Nakamura and K. Shikano; Room acoustics and reverberation: impact on hands-free recognition, *Proc. Eurospeech97,* vol. 5, pp. 2419–2422 (1997).

[49] N. Nilsson; *The Mathematical Foundations of Learning Machine,* San Mateo, CA: Morgan Kaufmann (1990).

[50] P. Niyogi, C. Burges, and P. Ramesh; Distinctive feature detection using support vector machines, *Proc. ICASSP99,* paper no. 1995 (1999).

[51] L. Rabiner and B.H. Juang; *Fundamentals of Speech Recognition,* Englewood Cliffs, NJ: Prentice-Hall (1993).

[52] D. Rainton and S. Sagayama; Minimum error classification training of HMMs: implementation details and experimental results, *J. Acoustical Soc. Japan (E),* vol. 13, no. 6, pp. 379–387 (1992).

[53] A.J. Robinson; An application of recurrent nets to phone probability estimation, *IEEE Trans. NN,* vol. 5, no. 2, pp. 298–305 (1994).

[54] R.C. Rose, B.H. Juang, and C.H. Lee; A training procedure for verifying string hypothesis in continuous speech recognition, *Proc. ICASSP95,* pp. 281–284 (1995).

[55] D.E. Rumelhart, G.E. Hinton, and R.J. Williams; Learning internal representations by error propagation, in *Parallel Distributed Processing: Explorations in the Microstructure of Cognition,* (D.E. Rumelhart et al., Eds.), Cambridge, MA: MIT Press (1986).

[56] M. Schuster; Learning out of time series with an extended recurrent neural network, in *Neural Networks for Signal Processing VI,* IEEE, pp. 170–179 (1996).

[57] M. Schuster and K.K. Paliwal; Bidirectional recurrent neural networks, *IEEE Trans. SP,* vol. 45, no. 11, pp. 2673–2681 (1997).

[58] A. Setlur and T. Jacobs; Results of a speaker verification service trial using HMM models, *Proc. Eurospeech 95,* pp. 639–642 (1995).

[59] M. Sugiyama and K. Kurinami; Minimal classification error optimization for a speaker mapping neural network, in *Neural Networks for Signal Processing II,* IEEE, pp. 233–242 (1992).

[60] T. Taniguchi, S. Kajita, K. Takeda, and F. Itakura; Applying blind signal separation to the recognition of overlapped speech, *Proc. Eurospeech 97,* pp. 1103–1106 (1997).

[61] V.N. Vapnik; *The Nature of Statistical Learning Theory,* New York: Springer-Verlag (1995).

[62] A. Waibel, T. Hanazawa, G. Hinton, K. Shikano, and K. Lang; Phoneme recognition using time-delay neural networks, *IEEE Trans. ASSP,* vol. 37, pp. 328–339 (1989).

[63] H. Watanabe, T. Yamaguchi, and S. Katagiri; Discriminative metric design for robust pattern recognition, *IEEE Trans. SP,* vol. 45, pp. 2655–2662 (1997).

[64] H. Watanabe, S. Fujita, and S. Katagiri; Separation of an overlapped signal using speech production models, in *Neural Networks for Signal Processing IX,* IEEE, pp. 293–302 (1999).

[65] E. Weinstein, M. Feder, and A.V. Oppenheim; Multi-channel signal separation by decorrelation, *IEEE Trans. SAP,* vol. 1, pp. 405–413 (1993).

[66] P.J. Werbos; Backpropagation through time: what it does and how to do it, *Proc. IEEE,* vol. 78, pp. 1550–1560 (1990).

11

Learning and Adaptive Characterization of Visual Contents in Image Retrieval Systems

Paisarn Muneesawang
The University of Sydney

Hau-San Wong
The University of Sydney

Jose Lay
The University of Sydney

Ling Guan
The University of Sydney

Accurate characterization of visual information is an important requirement for constructing an effective content-based image retrieval (CBIR) system. Conventional nonadaptive image models adopted in simple CBIR systems do not usually perform this task adequately. A more effective method is to adopt a machine learning approach where the system directly learns the image interpretation criteria from the users. As a result, we adopt neural network techniques to perform this characterization. More specifically, we have adopted a radial basis function (RBF) network for implementing an adaptive metric in image retrieval which progressively models the notion of image similarity through continual relevance feedback from users and a modular neural network for characterizing edge information in the front-end feature extraction module of the CBIR system. Experimental results have shown that the proposed methods outperform conventional techniques in terms of both accuracy and robustness.

11.1 Introduction

Multimedia data, which include digital images, video, audio, graphics, and text data, appear in diverse application domains such as the entertainment industry, education, medical imaging, and geographic information systems. While the individual needs for each of these domains may be different, they

0-8493-2359-2/01/$0.00+$1.50

all require the access and manipulation of large quantities of heterogeneous data. In view of this, there have been a lot of research efforts on how to improve the accuracy and efficiency of retrieving these data. In particular, content-based image retrieval (CBIR) has received a great deal of attention in the literature [1]–[8]. Research in this area includes the characterization of image contents using low-level features and the integration of these features to form a high-level semantic description for search and retrieval [1, 2]. In addition to these, one particularly important issue is how to apply adaptive mechanisms to tailor the search process to the needs of individual users, which is the main focus of this chapter.

Image content in a CBIR system is usually expressed in the form of a set of features which characterizes the color, texture, and shape information [6, 8] of individual images. These features are usually concatenated into a single feature vector for the purpose of matching the query image against the corresponding pre-extracted feature vectors in the database. The set of images with associated feature vectors closest to the query feature vector under a predefined metric (e.g., the Euclidean distance) is then displayed as the retrieved images. The operation of a simple CBIR system is illustrated in Figure 11.1a.

This chapter proposes the adoption of neural network techniques for implementing the relevance feedback module and the feature extraction module in the figure. The motivation for adopting this computational structure for performing these two operations is described below.

11.1.1 Relevance Feedback Module

In simple CBIR systems, the Euclidean distance measure between feature vectors is usually adopted in the matching stage to characterize the difference between images. However, this does not take into account the possible different variances of the individual vector components, which may arise due to their different physical origins. For example, heterogeneous feature types describing the color, texture, and shape of image components are usually combined by simply concatenating their associated attribute values into a single vector. A possible solution to this problem is to adopt a weighted Euclidean measure where different weights are assigned to the individual components in the vector. We can further generalize the measure by incorporating limited adaptivity in the form of a relevance feedback scheme [5, 9, 10], where the weights are modified according to the user's preference.

Originally, the relevance feedback technique was used in modern information retrieval (IR) by Salton and McGill [11]. In IR, each document in a collection is represented as a set of terms. These are concatenated into a vector and referred to as the term vector model. MARS (multimedia analysis and retrieval system) is one of the systems for extending the previous relevance feedback techniques to content-based image retrieval [5, 9, 10, 12, 13, 14]. In this system, an image is represented using a set of low-level features including color, texture, and shape. The numerical values of the various features are concatenated into a vector, and relevance feedback techniques can be applied based on these vectors. Gevers and Smeulders present PicToSeek [6], a retrieval system that exploits weighting techniques in IR for estimating the weight parameters of image features. Alternatively, retrieval systems proposed by Peng et al. [4] and Cox et al. [7] implement relevance feedback using a supervised learning process instead of query modification.

The methods described so far have proven somewhat successful in content-based image retrieval. The drawback of most methods, however, is the limited degree of adaptivity offered. In addition, the restriction of the distance measure to a quadratic form may not be adequate for modeling perceptual difference as seen from the user's point of view.

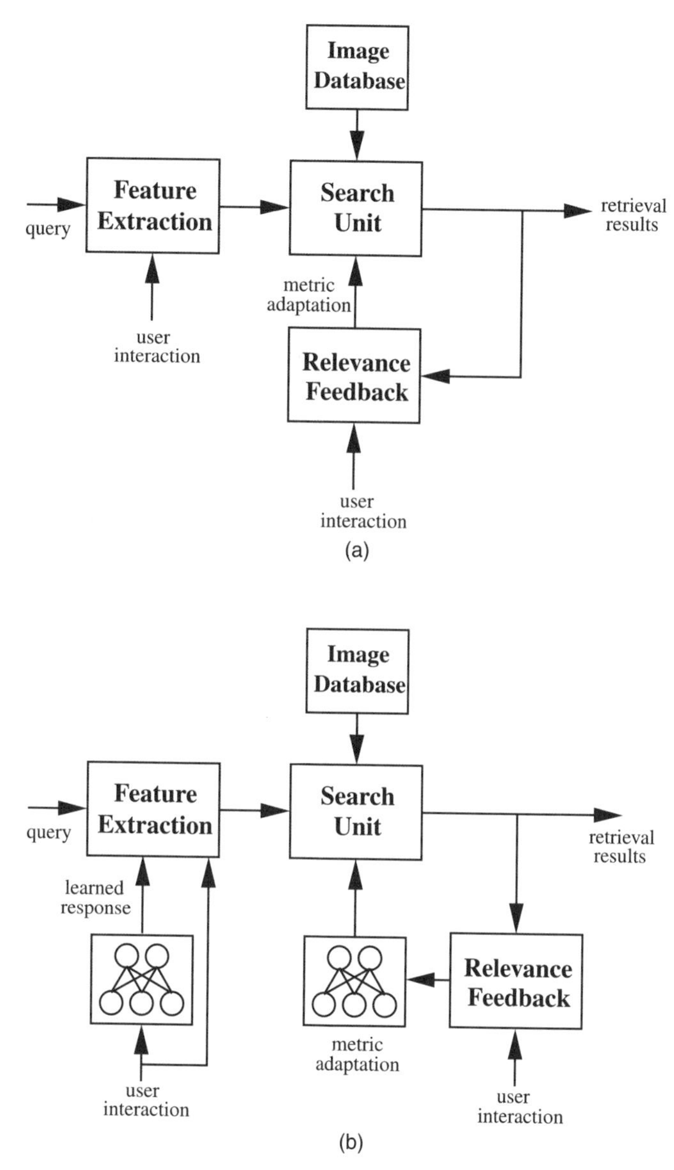

11.1 (a) Simple CBIR system (b) CBIR system with neural network processing.

11.1.2 Feature Extraction Module

The features extracted in the front-end module are usually in the form of color, texture, and shape, which describe complementary aspects of an image. In particular, the latter two feature categories, in turn, require the accurate characterization of edges in the image. An important issue here is how to establish a mechanism to distinguish the valid edge points from the non-edge points, which is compatible with the human user's point of view. In conventional edge detection approaches [15]–[17], a threshold on the edge magnitudes is usually chosen empirically by the user to produce a binary edge map. More advanced approaches such as the Canny edge detector [16] and the Shen–Castan edge detector [17] employ multiple thresholds and an edge tracing operation to take into account the nonstationary nature of the detection process. In general, the required threshold level will be highly dependent on the specific contents of the image and the additive noise level, and a threshold level chosen for a particular image is usually not applicable to other images, or even to the same image at a different noise level. This will, in turn, lead to the erroneous determination of texture and shape parameters. In current CBIR systems, an interface is usually provided where the user can interactively specify values of parameters for optimal retrieval results. However, this has to be performed separately for each query for the following reasons: the image models are usually not robust enough such that reselection of the parameters is required for different types of images, and the feature extraction module does not usually possess learning capability such that it cannot infer the user's current preference from previous inputs.

11.1.3 Adoption of Neural Network Techniques

In view of these problems, we propose the adoption of neural network techniques [18, 19] to perform the preceding two operations. A neural network is a specific computational structure where a set of nodes or neurons performs a predefined simple mathematical operation. These nodes are connected with each other through network weights which specify the strength of the connection. These network weights are adjustable through a learning process which enables the network to perform a variety of computational tasks.

We can see, therefore, the relevance of neural network techniques to these two operations in CBIR. To incorporate learning capabilities into the system, we replace the relevance feedback module with a specialized radial basis function (RBF) network [19, 20] for learning the user's notion of similarity between images. More specifically, in each interactive retrieval session, the user is asked to select, from the set of retrieved images, those which are most similar to the query image. The feature vectors extracted from the selected images are then used as training examples to determine the centers and widths of the different RBFs in the network. In other words, instead of relying on any preconceived notions of similarity through the enforcement of a fixed metric for comparison, the concept is adaptively redefined in accordance with different user's preferences and different types of images. Compared to the previous quadratic measure and the limited adaptivity allowed by its weighted form, the current approach offers an expanded parameter set, in the form of the RBF centers and widths, which allows a more accurate modeling of the notion of similarity from the user's point of view.

Similarly, for the front-end feature extraction module, we can implement an adaptive feature model in the form of a neural network, with the network weights representing the various parameters of the model. In this way, a human user can select what he/she regards as salient features on the query image. The selected pixels and their associated neighborhoods can then be incorporated directly as training examples for the network. It is then possible for the trained network to anticipate the preference of future users with regard to preferred feature selection. In this chapter, we investigate the adoption of neural network techniques to the task of the characterization of edges, which is usually considered one of the most significant features in images and is essential for the further extraction of texture and shape information for the purpose of retrieval.

As a result, we generalize the simple CBIR system of Figure 11.1a to include neural network processing, as shown in Figure. 11.1b. In this figure, the relevance feedback module and the feature extraction module are implemented in the form of specialized neural networks. In these highly user-oriented modules, the learning capability associated with the networks and their ability for general function approximation offer increased flexibility in the modeling of the user's visual response. The next section introduces our implementation of the relevance feedback module in the form of an RBF network, and our adoption of neural network for the purpose of feature extraction is described in Section 11.3.

11.2 Interactive CBIR Using RBF-Based Relevance Feedback

This section describes a specialized radial basis function (RBF) network [19, 20] for the implementation of the relevance feedback module in the CBIR system, as shown in Figure 11.1b. Specifically, the network allows the progressive modeling of the notion of image similarity through the adjustment of its associated RBF centers and widths. The image matching process is initiated when the user supplies a query image and the system retrieves the images in the data base which are closest to the query image. The user then selects, from the displayed images, those most similar to the current query image, which are then considered as examples of relevant images in this session, while the rest are regarded as counter examples. The feature vectors extracted from these images are then incorporated as training data for the RBF network to modify the centers and widths. The re-estimated RBF model is then used to evaluate the perceptual similarity in a new search; this process is repeated until the user is satisfied with the retrieval results.

11.2.1 RBF Network Architecture

Radial basis function (RBF) neural networks provide an excellent nonlinear approximation capability [19, 20]. As a result, we exploit this property to design a system of locally tuned processing units to approximate the target nonlinear function. A Gaussian-shaped RBF is chosen for this work. In our work, we associate a one-dimensional Gaussian RBF with each component of the feature vector, as follows:

$$S(\mathbf{z}, \mathbf{x}) = \sum_{i=1}^{P} G_i\,(x_i - z_i) = \sum_{i=1}^{P} \exp\left(-\frac{(x_i - z_i)^2}{2\sigma_i^2}\right) \tag{11.1}$$

where $\sigma_i, i = 1, \ldots P$ are the tuning parameters in the form of RBF widths, $\mathbf{x} = [x_1, \ldots, x_i, \ldots, x_P]^T$ is the feature vector associated with an image in the database, and $\mathbf{z} = [z_1, \ldots, z_i, \ldots, z_P]^T$ is the adjustable query position or the center of the RBF function. Each RBF unit implements an exponential function which constructs a local approximation to a nonlinear input–output mapping. The magnitude of $S(\mathbf{z}, \mathbf{x})$ represents the similarity between the input vector $\mathbf{x}$ and the query $\mathbf{z}$, where the highest similarity is attained when $\mathbf{x} = \mathbf{z}$.

Each RBF function is characterized by a set of tuning parameters $\sigma_i, i = 1, \ldots P$. In particular, these tuning parameters can reflect the relevance of individual features. If a feature is highly relevant, the value of σ_i should be small to allow higher sensitivity to any change of the difference $d_i \equiv |x_i - z_i|$. In contrast, a high value of σ_i is assigned to the nonrelevant features so that the corresponding vector component can be disregarded when determining the similarity, since the magnitude of $G_i(\cdot)$ is approximately equal to unity regardless of the difference d_i. The choice of σ_i according to this criterion will be discussed in the next section.

11.2.2 Training and Searching Algorithm

We propose a learning technique which enables the RBF network to progressively model the notion of image similarity for effective searching. This is implemented as an iterative search procedure which uses the information provided by the user to update the parameters of the RBF model. The process is summarized in the following subsections.

11.2.2.1 Initial Searching

A search unit uses the feature vector associated with the initial query to retrieve similar images from the database. In this first iteration, the similarity is measured by the Euclidean distance:

$$d(\mathbf{z}, \mathbf{x}) = \sqrt{\sum_{i=1}^{P} (z_i - x_i)^2} . \tag{11.2}$$

The distance values are then stored in ascending order, and the images corresponding to the N_R smallest distance values are displayed. It can be seen (Figure 11.5a) that some of the N_R best-matched images are not visually similar to the query.

11.2.2.2 Selection of Relevant Images by User

In this step, the N_R retrieved images are classified into a set of relevant images and a set of nonrelevant images. Formally, for each feature vector associated with one of the N_R images, the user supplies the training pattern $(\mathbf{x}_n, y_n), n = 1, \ldots, N_R$, where $y_n = 0$ indicates a nonrelevant image and $y_n = 1$ indicates a relevant image. These are then used as the training data in the next step.

11.2.2.3 Relevance Estimation

To estimate the relevance of individual features, the image feature vectors associated with the set of relevant images are used to form an $M \times P$ feature matrix $\mathbf{R}$:

$$\begin{aligned} \mathbf{R} &= \left[\mathbf{x}'_1, \ldots, \mathbf{x}'_m, \ldots, \mathbf{x}'_M\right]^T \\ &= \left[x'_{mi}\right] \; m = 1, \ldots, M, \; i = 1, \ldots, P \end{aligned} \tag{11.3}$$

where $\mathbf{x}'_m = [x'_{m1}, \ldots, x'_{mi}, \ldots, x'_{mP}]^T$ corresponds to one of the images marked as relevant, x'_{mi} is the ith component of the feature vector $\mathbf{x}'_m$, P is the total number of features, and M is the number of relevant images. According to our previous discussion, the tuning parameters σ_i should reflect the relevance of individual features. It has been proposed [4, 21] that, given a particular numerical value z_i for a component of the query vector, the length of the interval that completely encloses z_i and a predetermined number L of the set of values x'_{mi} in the relevant set that falls into its vicinity are a good indication of the relevancy of the feature. In other words, the relevancy of the ith feature is related to the density of x'_{mi} around z_i, which is inversely proportional to the length of the interval. A large density usually indicates high relevancy for a particular feature, while a low density implies that the corresponding feature is not critical to the similarity characterization. Setting $L = M$, the set of tuning parameters is thus estimated as follows:

$$\sigma_i = \eta \max_m \left|x'_{mi} - z_i\right| . \tag{11.4}$$

The additional factor η is for ensuring a reasonably large output $S(\mathbf{z}, \mathbf{x})$ for the exponential RBF unit, which indicates the degree of similarity, even for the member x'_{mi} furthest from z_i.

As a result, if the ith feature is highly relevant, Equation (11.4) gives a small value of σ_i to allow higher sensitivity to any change of the difference. In contrast, a high value of σ_i is assigned to the nonrelevant features so that the corresponding vector component can be disregarded when determining the similarity.

11.2.2.4 Weighted Searching

The tuning parameters σ_i obtained in the previous step are used for characterizing the Gaussian function in Equation (11.1). The estimated function $S(\mathbf{z}, \mathbf{x})$ is then used to determine the image similarity in a new search process, where the magnitude of the function $S(\mathbf{z}, \mathbf{x})$ is stored in descending order and a new set of best-matched images is obtained. The above iterative process is repeated by going back to the previous steps until convergence is achieved.

11.2.3 Query Modification

In the retrieval process, the user may have difficulty specifying a query that represents important aspects of the desired image or class of images. This suggests that the first iteration should be conducted as a trial search. After this initial iteration, the retrieved images should provide more choices of desired images to the user. Those initially retrieved images should then be evaluated according to relevance, and a modified query constructed with the objective of retrieving more relevant images in the next search operation. This is the idea of query modification, which is described in this section.

Consider the matrix $\mathbf{R}$ representing the feature vectors of relevant images in the training set. The entries in the ith column of the matrix indicate the possible values that the ith feature component will take on for a sample set of relevant images. Hence, a suitable statistical measure of values in this sequence should provide a good representation of the ith feature component. In particular, the mean value of this sequence $\overline{x}'_i = \Sigma_{m=1}^{M} x'_{mi}/M$ is a good statistical measure since this is the value which minimizes the average distance $\Sigma_{m=1}^{M}(x'_{mi} - \overline{x}'_i)^2/M$. As a result, after the first iteration, a suitable candidate for the modified query is the mean of the set of row vectors in $\mathbf{R}$. We refer to this approach as RBF1, which is formally defined as follows:

RBF1: Based on the selected relevant images in the previous iteration, the new query $\hat{\mathbf{z}}$ is chosen as

$$\hat{\mathbf{z}} = \frac{1}{M} \sum_{m=1}^{M} \mathbf{x}'_m \tag{11.5}$$

where $\mathbf{x}'_m$ is the feature vector from the mth row of matrix $\mathbf{R}$ in Equation (11.3). In other words, the modified query $\hat{\mathbf{z}}$ is the centroid of the relevant feature vectors. Since the relevant image group indicates the user's preference, the modified query obtained by Equation (11.5) will give a reasonable representation of the desired image.

11.2.3.1 Unfavorable Relevance Feedback Situation

Formally, we can refer to the complete relevant image set in the database as X_R. During relevance feedback, the set of images $X_{R'} \subset X_R$ chosen by the user can be considered an approximation of the actual set X_R. A problem that arises when using the subset $X_{R'}$ instead of X_R is that the corresponding modified query will not perform well unless the subset is a good representation of the actual relevant set for the given query. As an example, consider the situation depicted in Figure 11.2, where the original query is intended for retrieving images located inside the dashed line. There are three relevant images in the retrieved image set in the first iteration, and, hence, the modified query constructed by Equation (11.5) will lie in the center of this relevant image set (open triangle in Figure 11.2). When the modified query is used for retrieval, a great number of nonrelevant images located near the modified query will then be retrieved. This is undesirable since the modified query is located far away from a set of relevant images not previously retrieved. Instead, the ideal query indicated in Figure 11.2 will be more suitable.

One possible way to overcome this problem is to increase the size of the training set such that it is a better approximation of X_R. However, this technique may not be suitable in practice where the size of the training set is limited. Instead, we propose including the feature vectors associated with the nonrelevant images as part of the training set. More specifically, the presence of these feature

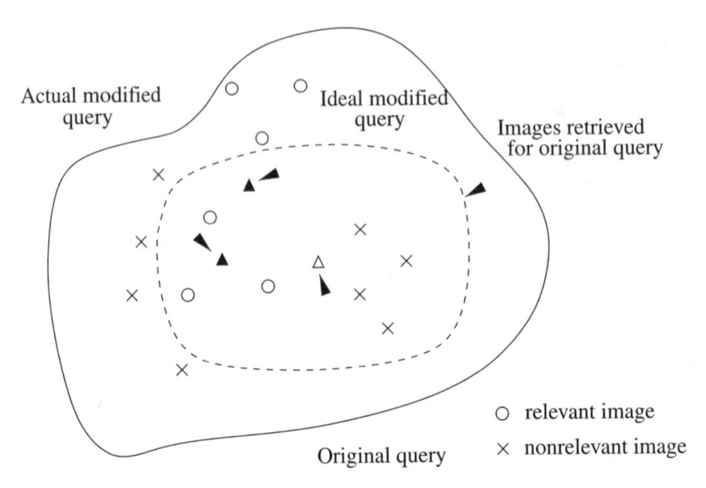

11.2 Suboptimal query selection.

vectors in the training set allows the current query to move away from those regions populated by nonrelevant images as well as moving towards the relevant regions.

Let **N** be the matrix containing the feature vectors of nonrelevant images in the training set:

$$\begin{aligned} \mathbf{N} &= \left[\mathbf{x}''_1, \ldots, \mathbf{x}''_q, \ldots, \mathbf{x}''_Q\right]^T \\ &= \left[x''_{qi}\right] \; q = 1, \ldots, Q, \; , i = 1, \ldots, P \end{aligned} \tag{11.6}$$

where $\mathbf{x}''_q = [x''_{q1}, \ldots, x''_{qi}, \ldots, x''_{qP}]^T$ is the feature vector of the nonrelevant images, and Q is the number of nonrelevant images in the training set. Note that the matrix **N** can be generated in a way similar to the matrix **R**. Given this set of nonrelevant feature vectors, we propose an alternative query update approach, which we refer to as RBF2.

RBF2: Based on the selected relevant and nonrelevant images in the previous iteration, the new query is chosen as

$$\hat{\mathbf{z}} = \mathbf{z}' + \alpha_R\left(\overline{\mathbf{x}}' - \mathbf{z}'\right) - \alpha_N\left(\overline{\mathbf{x}}'' - \mathbf{z}'\right) \tag{11.7}$$

$$\overline{\mathbf{x}}' = \frac{1}{M}\sum_{m=1}^{M}\mathbf{x}'_m \tag{11.8}$$

$$\overline{\mathbf{x}}'' = \frac{1}{Q}\sum_{q=1}^{Q}\mathbf{x}''_q \tag{11.9}$$

where $\mathbf{z}'$ is the previous query, and α_R, α_N are suitable positive constants.

Equation (11.7) can be illustrated using the one-dimensional example in Figure 11.3. Let the centers of the relevant image set and nonrelevant image set in the training data be R and N, respectively. As shown in Figure 11.3, the effect of the second term on the right-hand side of Equation (11.7) is to allow the new query to move towards R. On the other hand, if $N = N_1 < z'$ such that the third term is negative, the current query will move to the right, i.e., the position of z' will shift away from N_1 to $\hat{z}_1$. On the other hand, when $N = N_2 > z'$, the third term is positive, and, hence, z' will move to the left to $\hat{z}_2$, i.e., shifting away from N_2.

In practice, one finds that the relevant image set is more important in determining the modified query. The reason for this is that the set of relevant images is usually tightly clustered due to the similarities between its member images and, thus, specifies the modified query in a more unambiguous

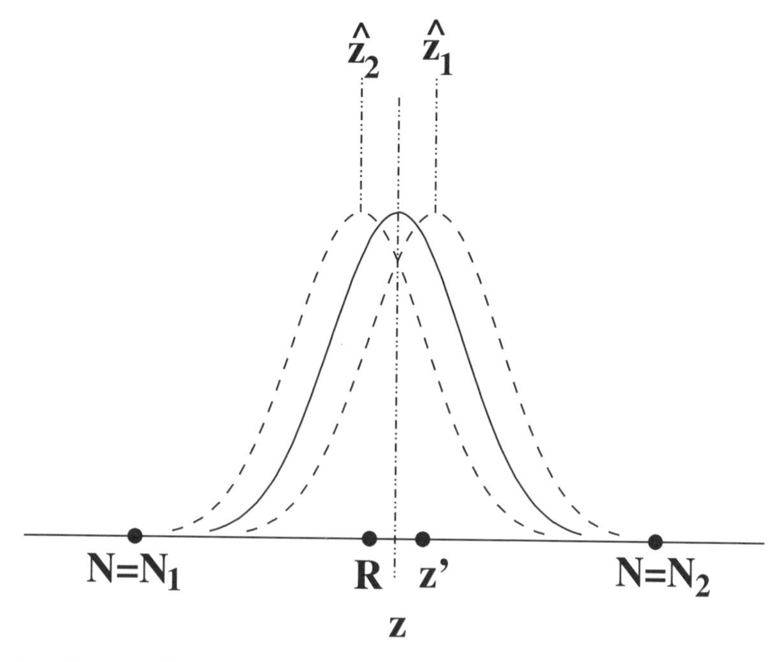

11.3 Illustration of query modification.

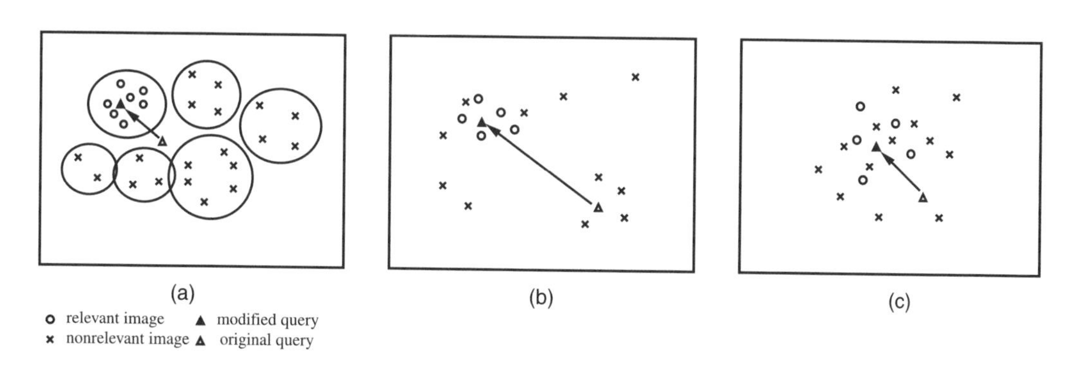

11.4 Query modification in the feature space: (a) ideal configuration; (b) favorable configuration; (c) unfavorable configuration.

way. This is illustrated in Figure 11.4a. On the other hand, the set of nonrelevant images is much more heterogeneous, and, therefore, the centroid of this nonrelevant image set may be located almost anywhere in the feature space, as shown in the figure. As a result, we have chosen $\alpha_R \gg \alpha_N$ in Equation (11.7) to allow a more definite movement toward the set of relevant images while permitting slight movement away from the nonrelevant regions.

The current approach works well when the sets of relevant and nonrelevant images are well separated, as in Figure 11.4a. In practice, the set of nonrelevant images usually covers a wider region of the space, as shown in Figure 11.4b and c. The effectiveness of the current approach will thus depend on the exact distribution of the nonrelevant images in the space. Figure 11.4b illustrates a particular distribution which is favorable to the current approach, while the case illustrated in Figure 11.4c may compromise its performance.

The complete algorithm can be summarized as follows:

1. For a given query $\mathbf{z}$, retrieve the N_R most similar images using the Euclidean distance measure.
2. Construct the training set $(\mathbf{x}_n, y_n), n = 1, \ldots, N_R$ from the relevant and nonrelevant images selected by the user.
3. Modify the query and estimate tuning parameters using $(\mathbf{x}_n, y_n)$:
   a. Construct **R** and **N** from Equations (11.3) and (11.6).
   b. Compute the modified query $\hat{\mathbf{z}}$ from Equations (11.5) or (11.7).
   c. Compute $\sigma_i, i = 1, \ldots, P$ from Equation (11.4) using $\hat{\mathbf{z}}$ and **R**.
4. Substitute the estimated parameters $\hat{\mathbf{z}}$ and σ_i into Equation (11.1) and use the resulting function $S(\mathbf{z}, \mathbf{x})$ to determine the similarity in the next iteration.
5. Store the magnitude of $S(\mathbf{z}, \mathbf{x})$ in descending order and obtain the set of new best-matched images.
6. Stop if convergence is achieved; otherwise go back to step 2.

11.2.4 Experimental Results

In the experiments reported in this section, we test the proposed approach using two image databases. The first is a standard texture database which has been used for testing a number of CBIR systems [4, 9, 10, 14]. The second database contains JPEG color images covering a wide range of real-life pictures.

The following experiments are designed for performance comparison between two methods: the interactive and the noninteractive CBIR methods:

1. **Method 1** — **RBF1:** Radial basis function method based on Equation (11.5) for query modification, and **RBF2:** Radial basis function method based on Equation (11.7) for query modification
2. **Method 2** — Simple CBIR using a noninteractive retrieval method, which corresponds to the first iteration of interactive search

11.2.4.1 The Database

The original test images were obtained from MIT Media Lab at ftp://whitechapel.media.mit.edu /pub/VisTex/ [4, 10]. There are 167 texture images which are manually classified into 79 classes, each of which is 512 × 512 pixels in size. Each of these images is then divided into 16 nonoverlapping images, each of which is 128 × 128 pixels in size. As a result, there are a total of 2672 images in the database. The number of images in each class varies from 16 to 80. The images in the same class are considered to be similar to one another.

Each texture image in this database is described by a 48-dimensional feature vector which is constructed as follows: we first apply Gabor wavelet transform to the image, where the set of basis functions consists of Gabor wavelets spanning four scales and six orientations. The mean and standard deviation of the transform coefficients are then used to form the feature vectors.

11.2.4.2 Summary of Comparison

A total of 79 images, one from each class, were selected as the query images. For each query, the top N_R images were retrieved to provide necessary relevance feedback, where $N_R = 16$ if the class size is equal to 16, and $N_R = 30$ if the class size is greater than 30. The performance is measured using the average retrieval precision of the 79 query images, which is defined as in Peng et al. [4]:

$$\text{precision} = \frac{\text{relevant images}}{\text{retrieved images}} \times 100\% .$$

The average retrieval precision of the 79 query images and the CPU time required are summarized in Tables 11.1 and 11.2, respectively. In the tables, i denotes the number of iterations.

TABLE 11.1 Average Retrieval Precision for MIT Database

Method	$i = 0$	$i = 1$	$i = 2$	$i = 3$	$i = 4$
Noninteractive CBIR	48.41	—	—	—	—
RBF1	48.41	78.26	83.31	83.31	83.90
RBF2	48.41	76.70	81.37	84.68	85.47

TABLE 11.2 Average CPU Time (on a Pentium III 550E) for a Single Query

Method	Processing Time (sec/iteration)
Noninteractive CBIR	0.110 sec
RBF1	0.237 sec
RBF2	0.257 sec

Does not include the time for displaying the images.

The following observations are made from the results:

1. The use of relevance feedback techniques results in significant improvement of the retrieval performance over the simple noninteractive CBIR technique.
2. For the two interactive methods, the greatest improvement is achieved in the first iteration, while the later iterations provide only miner improvements. Thus, good retrieval results can be achieved within a few iterations.
3. At the fourth iteration, RBF2 slightly outperforms RBF1. This is due to the inclusion of both the relevant image group and the nonrelevant image group in modifying the query, while RBF1 uses only the relevant image group for the query modification.
4. Although the interactive approach requires a longer CPU time than the noninteractive one, its response time of less than 0.3 seconds is still acceptable considering the associated improvements.

Figure 11.5 shows an example of a retrieval session. Figure 11.5a shows the retrieval result without relevance feedback and Figure 11.5b shows the result after relevance feedback. The improvement given by the proposed method is apparent.

11.2.5 Application to Compressed Domain Image Retrieval

In this experiment, we apply the proposed interactive approach to a compressed domain image retrieval system. Specifically, the matching process is directly performed on the DCT domain to avoid the costly operation of decompression. The image database consists of 4700 real-life images which cover a broad range of categories. Due to its excellent energy compaction property, DCT is widely used in JPEG and many other popular image and video compression standards. When a typical 8×8 block of data undergoes DCT transformation, most of the significant coefficients

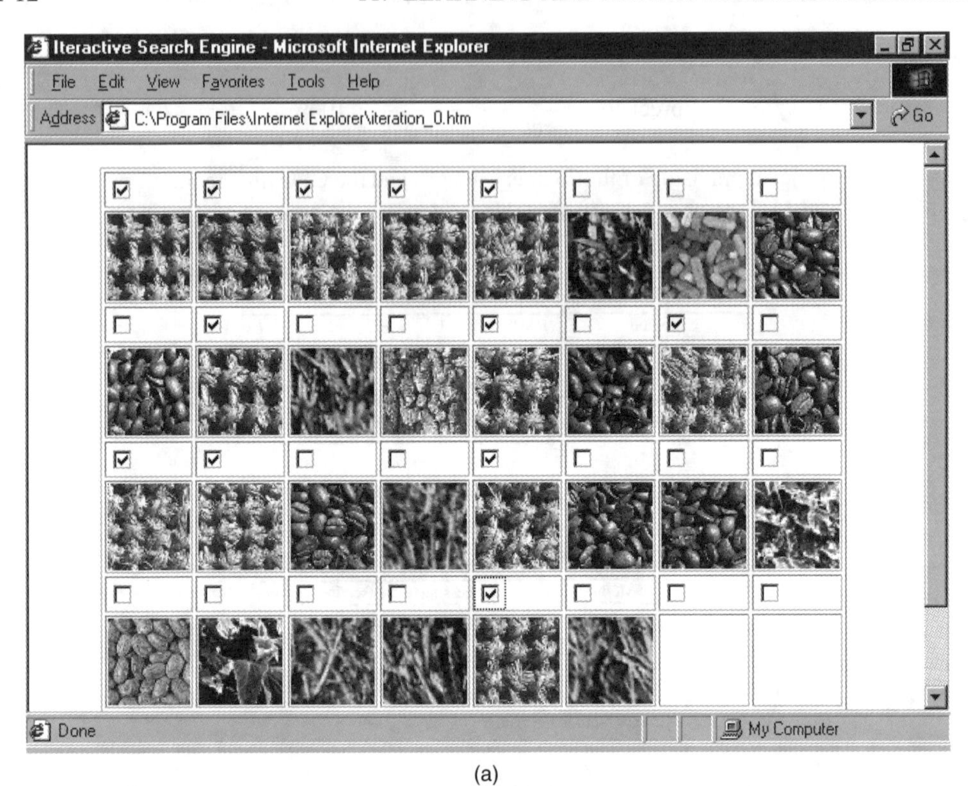

(a)

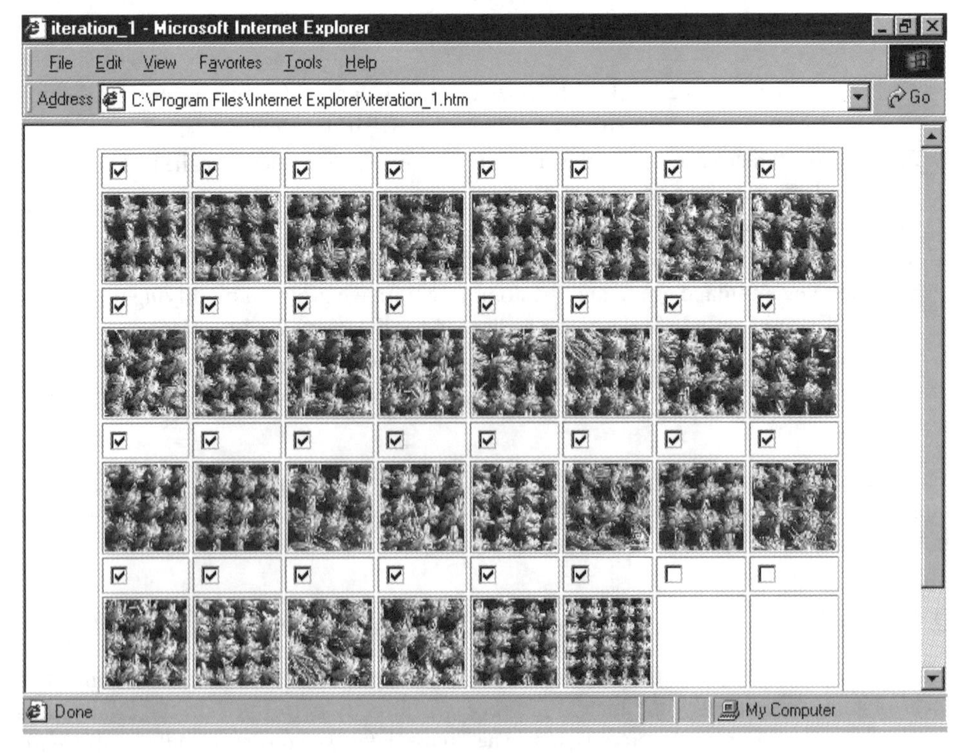

(b)

11.5 Retrieval results (query image is on the top left corner): (a) no relevance feedback (retrieval precision = 0.4); (b) relevance feedback (retrieval precision = 1.0).

are concentrated in the upper-left region of the transformed block, thus allowing the storage and transmission of a small number of coefficients.

In our system, each image in the database is described by the energy histogram of the DCT coefficients. An energy histogram of a DCT coefficient is obtained by counting the number of times a particular coefficient value appears in the 8×8 block. Formally, the value of the histogram in the mth bin can be written as:

$$h_c[m] = \sum_{u=0}^{7} \sum_{v=0}^{7} I(Q(F[u, v]) = m) \tag{11.10}$$

where $Q(F[u, v])$ denotes the value of the coefficient at the u, v locations, and m is the index of the current histogram bin. The function $I(\cdot)$ equals 1 if the argument is true, and it equals 0 otherwise.

For a chrominance DCT block, the DC coefficient is proportional to the average of the chrominance values in the block. As a result, the histogram of DC coefficients can be used as an approximation of the color histogram of the original image. On the other hand, a histogram of the AC coefficients can be used to characterize the frequency composition of the image. Studies have shown that the combination of DC and lower frequency AC coefficients is effective for measuring similarity in image retrieval applications [22]. In this work, the nine DCT coefficients in the upper left corner of the block are partitioned into three sets as follows (Figure 11.6):

$$\begin{aligned} F1D &= \{DC\} \\ F1A &= \{AC_{10}, AC_{11}, AC_{01}\} \\ F2A &= \{AC_{20}, AC_{21}, AC_{22}, AC_{12}, AC_{21}\} . \end{aligned}$$

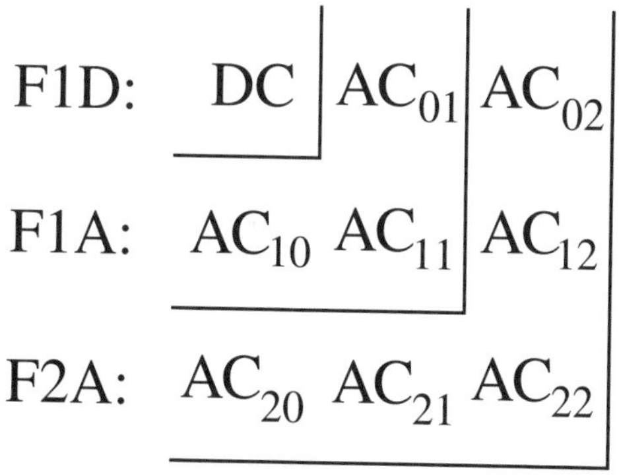

F1D: DC | AC_{01} | AC_{02}

F1A: AC_{10} AC_{11} | AC_{12}

F2A: AC_{20} AC_{21} AC_{22}

11.6 The four coefficient groups in the DCT domain.

For this experiment, the energy histogram features are based on the coefficients in two of these collections:

$$F = F1D \cup F1A = \{DC, AC_{01}, AC_{10}, AC_{11}\} .$$

Separate energy histograms are constructed for the DC and AC coefficients of each of the color channels, and 30 bins are used for each histogram.

After generating the feature database, the interactive search engine is applied to it. Typical retrieval sessions are shown in Figures 11.7 and 11.8. Figure 11.7a shows the 20 best-matched images before applying any feedback, with the query image displayed at the top left corner. It is observed that some retrieved images are similar to the query image in terms of color composition. At this iteration, five similar images are marked as relevant. Based on this information, the system dynamically readjusts

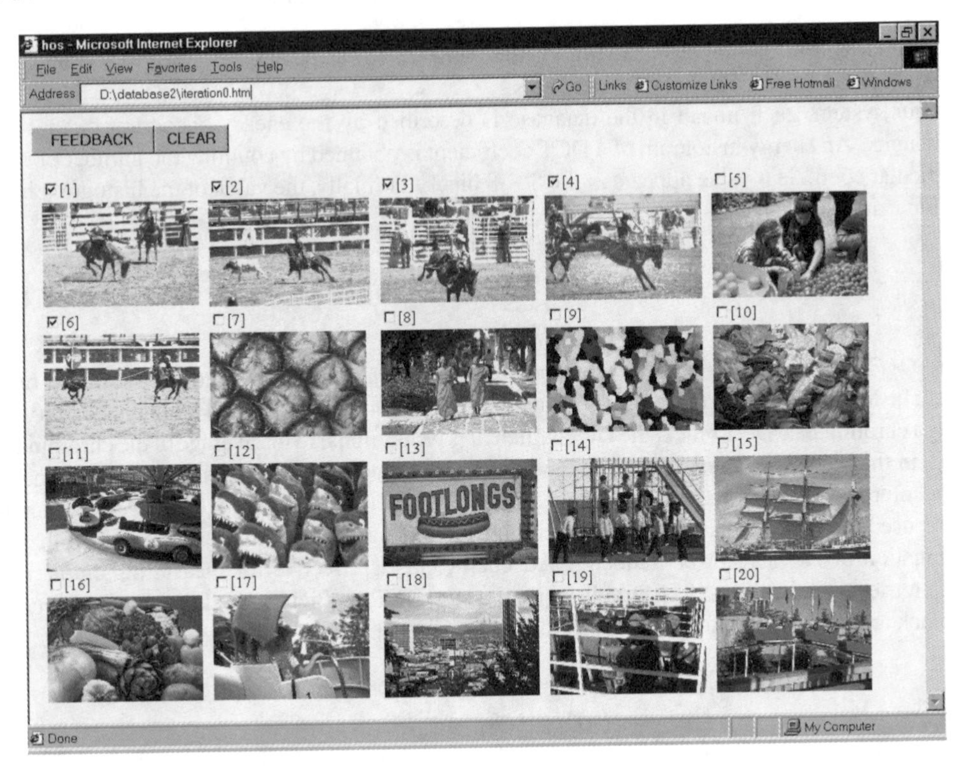

(a)

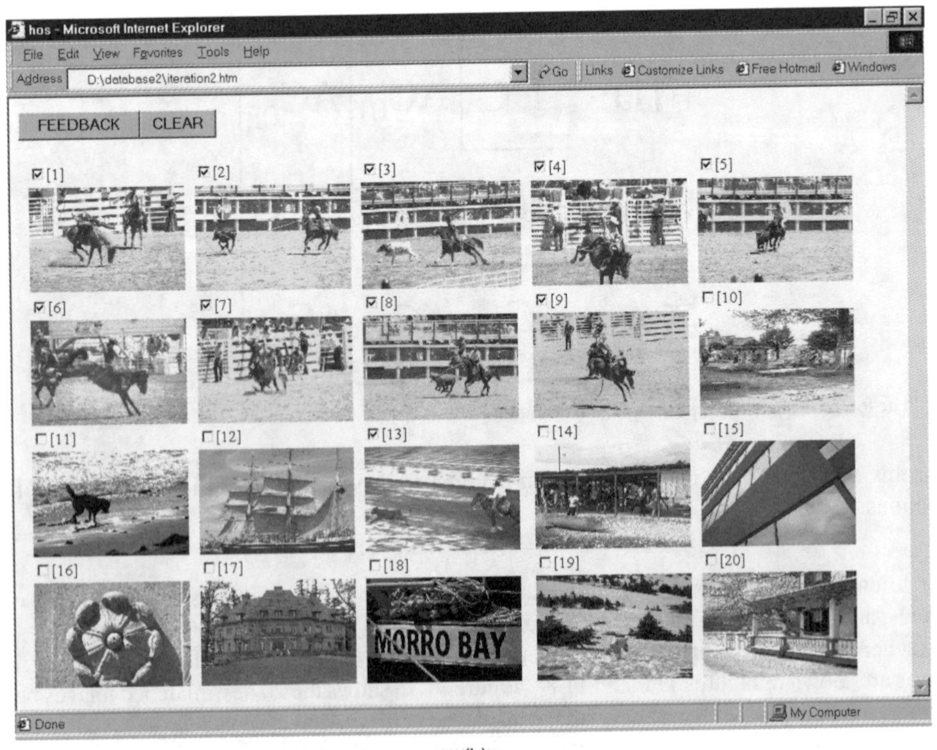

(b)

11.7 Retrieval results: (a) no relevance feedback; (b) relevance feedback.

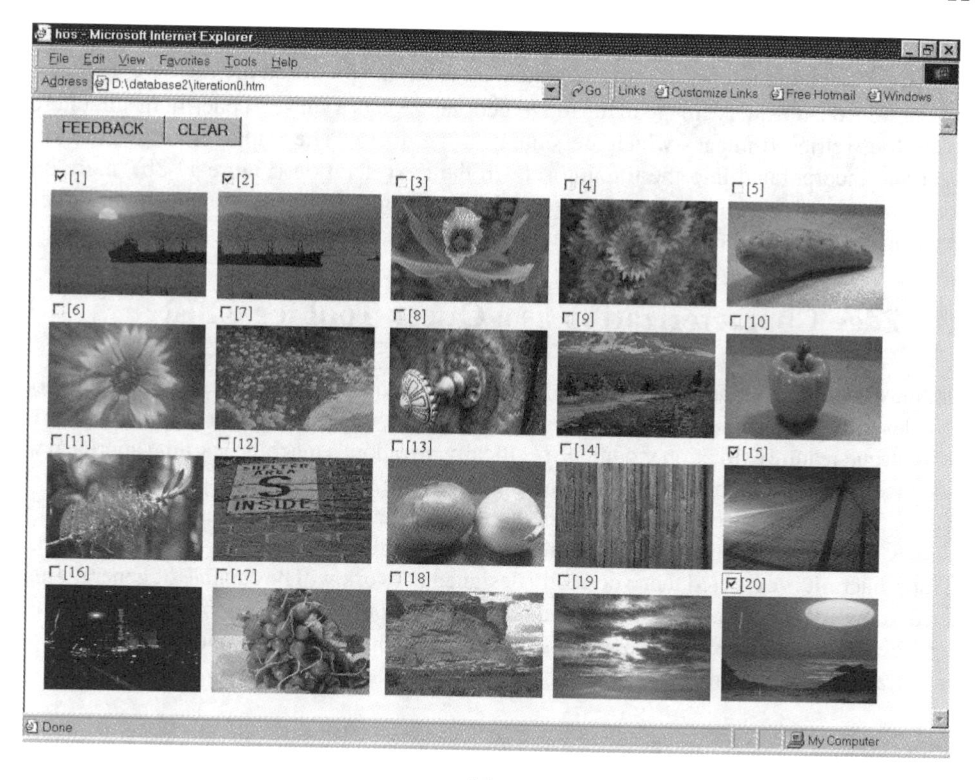

(a)

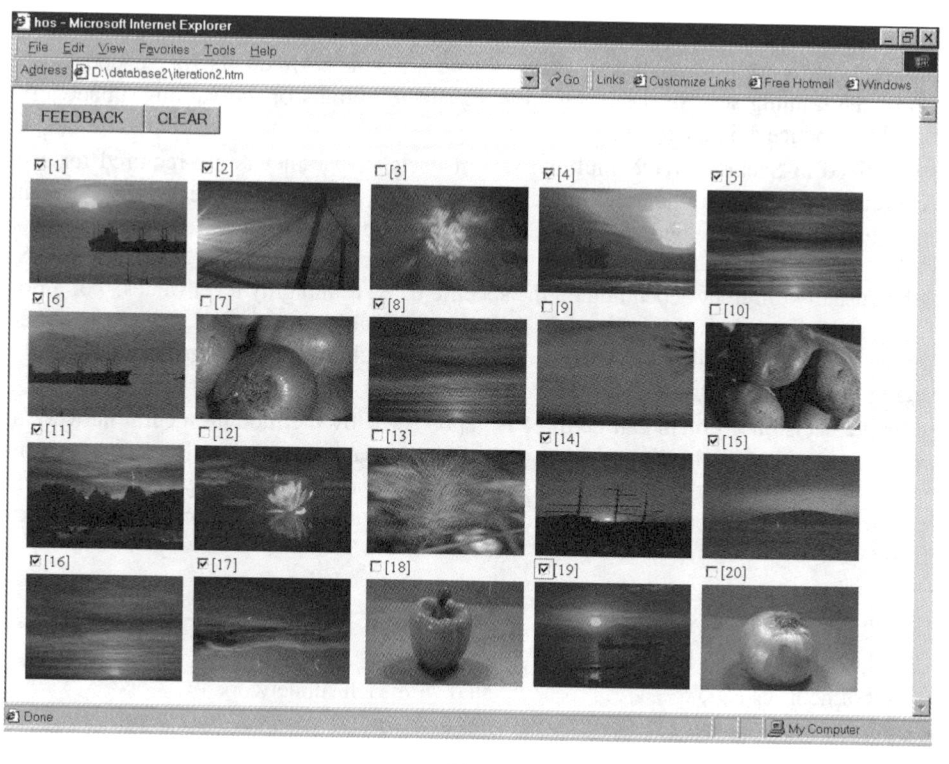

(b)

11.8 Retrieval results: (a) no relevance feedback; (b) relevance feedback.

the weight parameters of the RBF model to capture the notion of image similarity. Figure 11.7b shows the considerably improved retrieval results by using the proposed interactive approach.

In Figure 11.8a, the query image in the top left corner depicts a sunset scene. In the first iteration, there are four retrieved images which are similar to the query. These images are then marked as relevant and incorporated into the training set. In the next iteration (Figure 11.8b), more images depicting sunset and related images showing a red sky are returned. In addition, it was observed that good retrieval results can be achieved within one or two iterations.

11.3 Edge Characterization as a Query Tool for CBIR

In addition to our previous adoption of neural network techniques for the relevance feedback module, we now describe a specialized modular neural network for the characterization of salient image edges in the front-end feature extraction module. Specifically, we adopt a machine learning approach where user-defined edges are incorporated as training inputs for neural networks specially configured as edge detectors. In other words, we allow the network to automatically acquire the notion of what constitutes important edge features as defined by users through this human–computer interaction (HCI) approach. It is expected that a correctly designed network will be capable of generalizing this acquired knowledge to identify important edges in images not included in the training set, and we also require that the approach be robust enough to allow identification of similar sets of edge pixels under different noise conditions.

11.3.1 Network Architecture

In this work, the edge detector is modeled using a modular neural network architecture [23]–[29], which is composed of a hierarchical structure where clusters of neurons representing different classes of training patterns form separate subnetworks. As a result, each subnetwork encodes different aspects of the training set. In the recognition stage, the outputs of the various subnetworks are combined to produce a final decision.

As described in Section 11.1.2, multiple sets of decision parameters are required for accurate edge characterization due to the nonstationary nature of the problem. In other words, different sets of parameters should be applied depending on the local context instead of adopting a single set of parameters across the whole image. For example, the subjective visibility of an edge with a certain strength is usually different depending on the specific background gray level values. For a brightly lit background, even relatively weak edges which are invisible in dark backgrounds may become discernible. As a result, different threshold values corresponding to the background gray level value are usually required.

The above decision problem can be directly represented by the modular neural network architecture if we associate each subnetwork with a different background gray-level and each unit in the subnetwork with different edge prototypes under the corresponding gray-level value. The architecture of the feature detection network is shown in Figure 11.9 and consists of the following structures:

- input transformation stage
- a set of subnetworks $V_r, r = 1, \ldots, R$
- a set of neurons $U_{rs}, s = 1, \ldots, S$ associated with each subnetwork V_r
- a dynamic neuron U_d

The functions of the various structures are described next and summarized in Table 11.3.

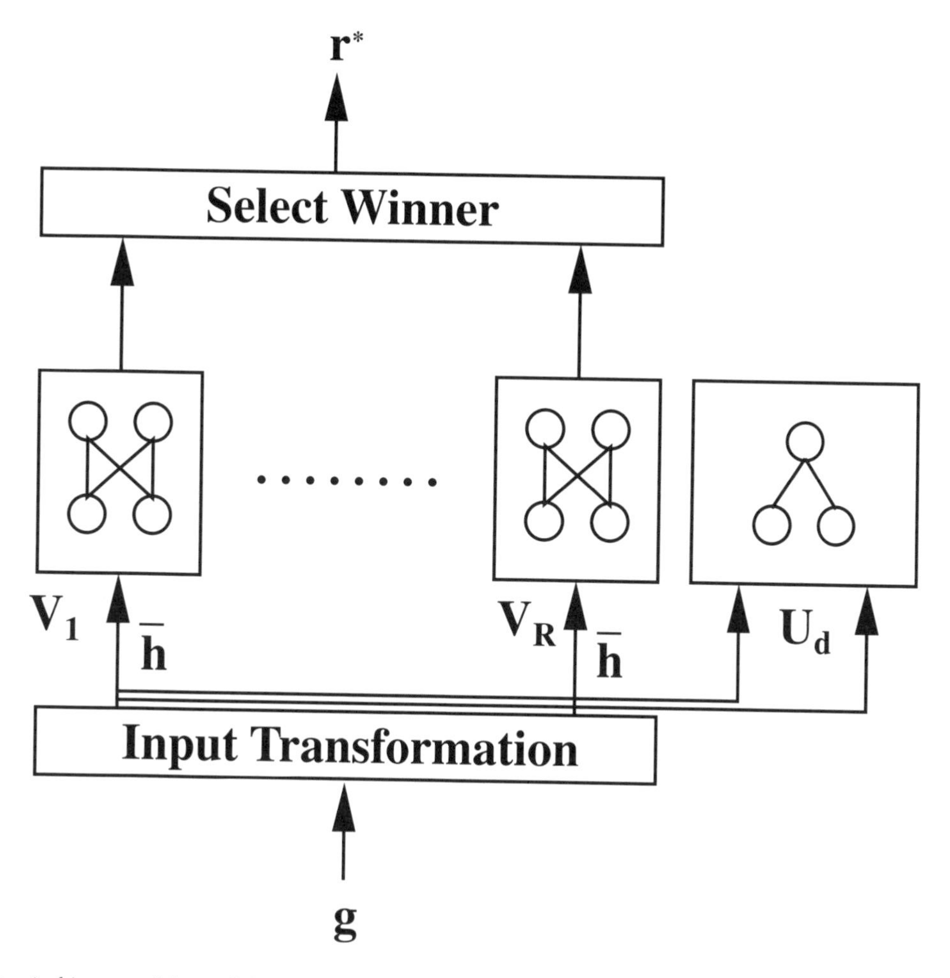

11.9 Architecture of the modular neural network for edge characterization.

TABLE 11.3 Functions of Different Structures in the Modular Neural Network

Structure	Function
Input transformation	Summarize information in $N \times N$ edge blocks
Subnetworks V_r	Characterize average gray level value of edge blocks
Neurons U_{rs}	Represent different edge types under each average gray value
Dynamic neuron U_d	Incremental parameter adaptation in edge tracing

11.3.1.1 Input Transformation

The query image is first partitioned into $N \times N$ windows and the associated gray-level values in the window are represented as a vector $\mathbf{g} = [g_1 \ldots g_{N^2}]^T \in \mathbf{R}^{N^2}$. The mean of the components is then defined as

$$\bar{g} = \frac{1}{N^2} \sum_{i=1}^{N^2} g_i \,. \tag{11.11}$$

From this initial representation, we further summarize the gray-level information in terms of a two-dimensional vector $\mathbf{h} = [h_1 \;\; h_2]^T \in \mathbf{R}^2$, which characterizes the two dominant gray-level values within the window, and the mean of the components $\overline{h}$. The components of this vector are defined as follows:

$$h_1 = \frac{\sum_{i=1}^{N^2} I(g_i < \overline{g}) g_i}{\sum_{i=1}^{N^2} I(g_i < \overline{g})} \tag{11.12}$$

$$h_2 = \frac{\sum_{i=1}^{N^2} I(g_i \geq \overline{g}) g_i}{\sum_{i=1}^{N^2} I(g_i \geq \overline{g})} \tag{11.13}$$

$$\overline{h} = \frac{h_1 + h_2}{2} \tag{11.14}$$

where the function $I(\cdot)$ equals 1 if the argument is true and equals 0 otherwise.

11.3.1.2 Functions of Subnetworks

We associate each subnetwork $V_r, r = 1, \ldots, R$ with a prototype background gray-level value p_r and assign all those windows with their background gray-level values close to p_r to the subnetwork V_r, in order that adaptive processing with respect to different illumination levels is allowed. Specifically, a particular window is assigned to the subnetwork V_{r^*} if the following conditions are satisfied:

N1. $p_{r^*} \in [h_1, h_2]$
N2. $|\overline{h} - p_{r^*}| < |\overline{h} - p_r| \quad r = 1, \ldots, R, r \neq r^*$

where $[h_1, h_2]$ is the closed interval with h_1, h_2 as its endpoints (to be distinguished from the two-dimensional vector $[h_1 \;\; h_2]^T$). In this way, all members in a single cluster exhibit similar levels of background gray-level values.

11.3.1.3 Functions of Neurons under Each Subnetwork

Each subnetwork V_r contains S neurons $U_{rs}, s = 1, \ldots, S$, with each neuron encoding the different edge prototypes under gray-level value p_r. Each neuron is associated with a weight vector $\mathbf{w}_{rs} = [w_{rs,1} \;\; w_{rs,2}]^T \in \mathbf{R}^2$, which serves as a prototype for the vector $\mathbf{h}$. A window with associated vector $\mathbf{h}$ is assigned to neuron $U_{r^*s^*}$ if the following condition is satisfied:

$$\|\mathbf{h} - \mathbf{w}_{r^*s^*}\| < \|\mathbf{h} - \mathbf{w}_{r^*s}\| \quad s = 1, \ldots, S, s \neq s^* . \tag{11.15}$$

In this work, we have incorporated two neurons into each subnetwork which, respectively, encode the prototype for weak edges and strong edges. In other words, we have set $S = 2$ in the above equation. Designating one of the weight vectors $\mathbf{w}_{r^*s}, s = 1, 2$ as the weak edge prototype $\mathbf{w}_{r^*}^l$ and the other one as the strong edge prototype $\mathbf{w}_{r^*}^u$, they are selected according to the following criteria:

- $\mathbf{w}_{r^*}^l = \mathbf{w}_{r^*s'}$, where $s' = \arg\min_s (w_{r^*s,2} - w_{r^*s,1})$
- $\mathbf{w}_{r^*}^u = \mathbf{w}_{r^*s''}$, where $s'' = \arg\max_s (w_{r^*s,2} - w_{r^*s,1})$

The difference of the components in the weak edge prototype vector, $(w_{r^*,2}^l - w_{r^*,1}^l)$ thus represents a learned threshold parameter for specifying the lower limit of visibility for edges and is useful for identifying potential starting points in the image for edge tracing. The structure of the subnetwork is illustrated in Figure 11.10.

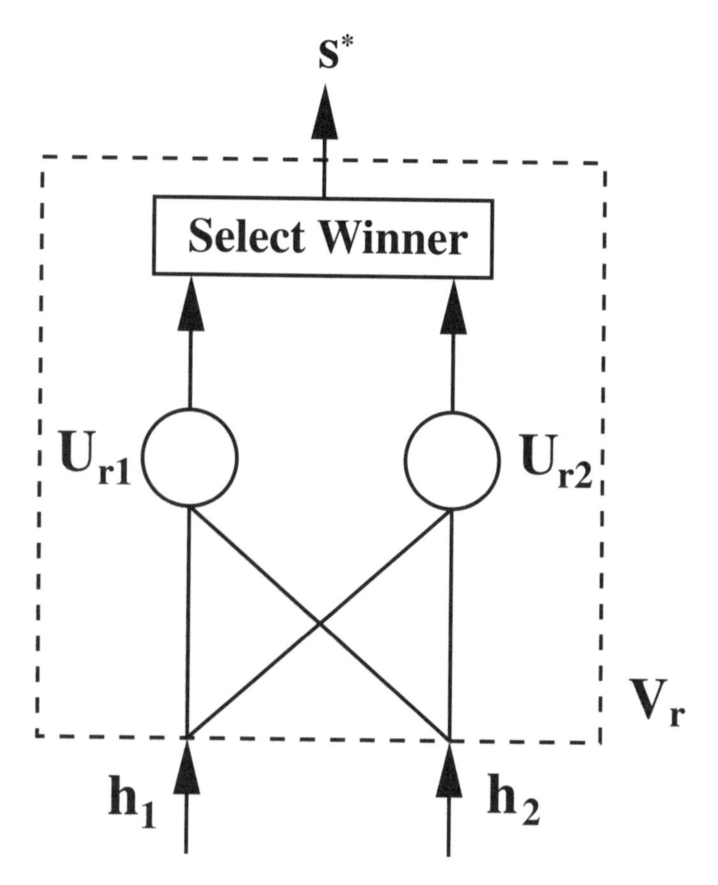

11.10 Structure of subnetwork.

11.3.1.4 Functions of the Dynamic Neuron

Independent of the neuron clusters V_r and U_{rs}, we associated a dynamic tracking neuron U_d with the network. The purpose of this neuron is to accommodate the nonstationary characteristics of an edge as it is being traced out in the recognition step. Similar to the neurons U_{rs} in each subnetwork V_r, the dynamic neuron is associated with a dynamic weight vector $\mathbf{w}_d = [w_{d,1} \;\; w_{d,2}]^T \in \mathbf{R}^2$ and a scalar parameter p_d which is similar in function to the scalar prototype p_r of each subnetwork. The structure of the dynamic tracking neuron is shown in Figure 11.11. The weight vector $\mathbf{w}_d$ and illumination level indicator p_d of this neuron are dynamically varied during the recognition step to trace out all those secondary edge points connected to the primary edge points (primary and secondary edge points are defined in Sections 11.3.3.1 and 11.3.3.2, respectively).

11.3.1.5 Edge Configurations

Apart from acquiring the gray-level difference values associated with user-specified features, it is also important for the network to learn the specific pixel configurations which are characteristic of these features. To formally express this requirement, we suppose that a certain vector $\mathbf{h}$ is assigned to neuron $U_{r^*s^*}$ with weight vector $\mathbf{w}_{r^*s^*}$. We then define the function $\mathcal{F} : \mathbf{R}^{N^2} \times \mathbf{R}^2 \longrightarrow \mathbf{B}^N$, where $\mathbf{B} = \{0, 1\}$, which maps the real vector $\mathbf{g} \in \mathbf{R}^{N^2}$ representing the gray-level values of the current window to a binary vector $\mathbf{c} = \mathcal{F}(\mathbf{g}, \mathbf{w}_{r^*s^*}) = [f(g_1, \mathbf{w}_{r^*s^*}) \;\; \ldots \;\; f(g_N, \mathbf{w}_{r^*s^*})]^T \in \mathbf{B}^{N^2}$,

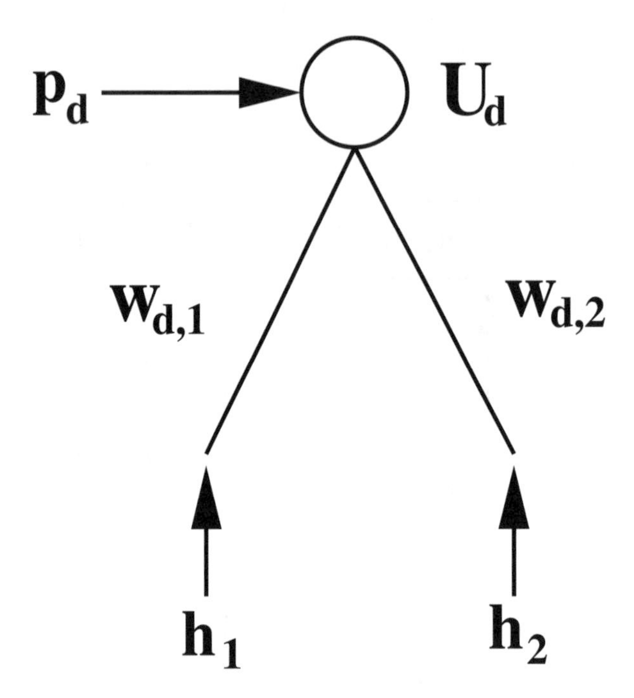

11.11 Structure of dynamic neuron.

in terms of the component mapping $f : \mathbf{R} \times \mathbf{R}^2 \longrightarrow \mathbf{B}$ as follows:

$$f\left(g_i, \mathbf{w}_{r^*s^*}\right) = \begin{cases} 0 & \text{if } \left|g_i - w_{r^*s^*,1}\right| < \left|g_i - w_{r^*s^*,2}\right| \\ 1 & \text{if } \left|g_i - w_{r^*s^*,1}\right| \geq \left|g_i - w_{r^*s^*,2}\right| \end{cases} . \tag{11.16}$$

The binary vector **c** assumes a special form for valid edge configurations. Some of the possible valid edge configurations are shown in Figure 11.12. During the network training phase, the network

1	0	0
1	0	0
1	0	0

1	1	1
0	0	0
0	0	0

0	0	0
1	0	0
1	1	0

11.12 Valid edge configurations.

applies the mapping to form a collection of the user-specified valid edge configuration patterns in an edge configuration set C, which forms part of the overall network. During the recognition phase, apart from ascertaining that the current pixel under consideration satisfies the previous edge strength requirement, we further require that the edge configuration requirement be satisfied at the same time.

11.3.2 Network Training Stage

The training of the network proceeds in three stages: in the first stage, the background gray-level prototypes $p_r, r = 1, \ldots, R$ are determined for each subnetwork V_r by competitive learning [19, 30].

In the second stage, the weight vectors $\mathbf{w}_{rs}$ associated with each subnetwork are determined, again using competitive learning, from the corresponding training pixels assigned to the subnetwork. In the third stage, the corresponding binary edge configuration pattern $\mathbf{c}$ of each training pixel is extracted as a function of the winning weight vector $\mathbf{w}_{r^*s^*}$ and inserted into the edge configuration set C (see Figure 11.13).

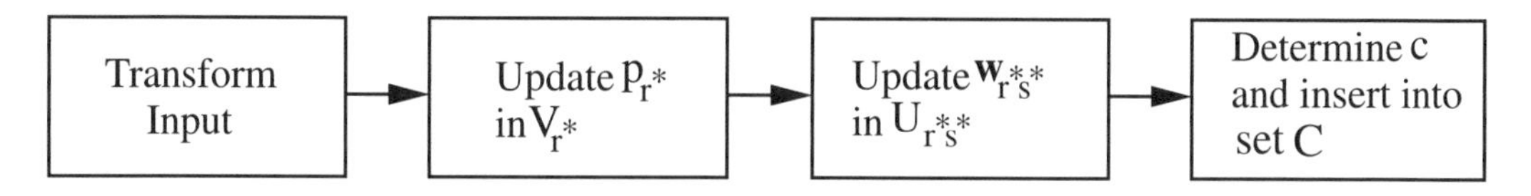

11.13 Stages in network training.

11.3.2.1 Determination of Background Gray-Level Prototypes

Assuming that the current training pixels with associated parameter $\overline{h}$ are assigned to subnetwork V_{r^*}, we update the value of the corresponding prototype p_{r^*} using the following equation:

$$p_{r^*}(t+1) = p_{r^*}(t) + \alpha(t)\left(\overline{h} - p_{r^*}(t)\right) . \tag{11.17}$$

The learning stepsize $\alpha(t)$ is successively decreased according to the following linear schedule [31]:

$$\alpha(t+1) = \alpha(0)\left(1 - \frac{t}{t_f}\right) \tag{11.18}$$

where t_f is the total number of iterations and should be large enough to ensure convergence of the prototype values p_r, $r = 1, \ldots R$. The suitable value of t_f can be determined by performing a number of independent training runs using a particular t_f and observing whether the final values for p_r are similar among the different trials.

11.3.2.2 Determination of Edge Prototypes

In the second stage, assuming that the current training pixel with associated feature vector $\mathbf{h}$ is assigned to neuron $U_{r^*s^*}$ of subnetwork V_{r^*}, we update the corresponding weight vector $\mathbf{w}_{r^*s^*}$ using the following equation:

$$\mathbf{w}_{r^*s^*}(t+1) = \mathbf{w}_{r^*s^*}(t) + \alpha(t)\left(\mathbf{h} - \mathbf{w}_{r^*s^*}(t)\right) . \tag{11.19}$$

11.3.2.3 Determination of Valid Edge Configurations

In the third stage, we once again assign all the training pixels to their corresponding neurons within the subnetworks. Assuming that the current training pixel belongs to neuron $U_{r^*s^*}$ within subnetwork V_{r^*}, we can transform the associated gray-level vector $\mathbf{g}$ of the training pixels into a binary edge configuration vector $\mathbf{c}$ according to Equation (11.16):

$$\mathbf{c} = \mathcal{F}\left(\mathbf{g}, \mathbf{w}_{r^*s^*}\right) . \tag{11.20}$$

This user-specified valid edge configuration is then inserted into the edge configuration set C.

11.3.3 Recognition Stage

In the recognition stage, the network is required to locate pixels in a test image which share similar edge properties with the training pixels as expressed through the acquired feature prototypes. The recognition phase proceeds in two stages: in the first stage, we locate all these primary edge pixels in the test image which share a high degree of similarity with the training pixels. In the second stage, starting from the primary edge pixels, we recursively locate all the secondary edge pixels connected to them which satisfy a relaxed conformance criterion. The purpose of this second stage is to allow the validation of comparatively nonprominent edge points through their connection to primary edge pixels.

11.3.3.1 Detection of Primary Edge Points

In this first stage, we regard those pixels with associated parameters $\overline{h}, h_1, h_2$ as primary edge points if the following requirements are fulfilled:

P1. satisfaction of conditions N1 and N2 in Section 11.3.1.2 for some r^*

P2. $h_2 - h_1 \geq w^l_{r^*,2} - w^l_{r^*,1}$, where $w^l_{r^*,1}$ and $w^l_{r^*,2}$ are the components of the weak edge prototype $\mathbf{w}^l_{r^*}$ associated with subnetwork V_{r^*}

P3. $\mathbf{c} = \mathcal{F}(\mathbf{g}, \mathbf{w}_{r^*s^*}) \in C$, where the weight vector $\mathbf{w}_{r^*s^*}$ is associated with the selected neuron $U_{r^*s^*}$

Condition P1 above specifies that the background gray-level value of the current training pixel should be reasonably close to one of the prototype levels. Condition P2 ensures that the magnitude of gray-level variations characterized by the difference $h_2 - h_1$ is greater than that specified by the weak edge prototype of the assigned subnetwork. Condition P3 ensures that the binary edge configuration of the current training pixel is included in the edge configuration set C.

11.3.3.2 Detection of Secondary Edge Points

At this stage, the dynamic tracking neuron U_d is used to trace the secondary edge pixels connected to the previously detected primary edge pixel. The weight vector $\mathbf{w}_d$ and gray-level prototype p_d of the tracking neuron are initialized using the associated parameters $\mathbf{h}^p$ and $\overline{h}^p$ of the initial primary edge pixel. Their values are continually updated as the edge is being traced out to account for the variation of the gray-level values along the edge.

After initialization, the pixels connected to the primary edge pixel are recursively located and designated as secondary edge pixels. They, in turn, are validated by the following conditions

S1. $p_d \in [h^s_1, h^s_2]$

S2. $\mathbf{c}^s = \mathcal{F}(\mathbf{g}, \mathbf{w}_d) \in C$

where h^s_1, h^s_2, and $\mathbf{c}^s$ describe the edge configuration of the current secondary pixel. Condition S2 above is similar to condition P3 for primary edge pixel detection. Condition S1 is a modified form of condition N1 (Section 11.3.1.2) where p_{r^*} is replaced by p_d. There are no conditions corresponding to P2 for primary edge pixel detection to allow the possibility of weak secondary edge pixels.

For each validated secondary edge pixel, the local illumination level indicator p_d is updated using the mean value $\overline{h}^s = (h^s_1 + h^s_2)/2$ of the current pixel:

$$p_d(t+1) = p_d(t) + \alpha(0)\left(\overline{h}^s - p_d(t)\right) . \tag{11.21}$$

In addition, if condition P2 for primary edge pixel detection is satisfied by the current secondary pixel, which implies that its edge strength is comparable with that of a primary edge pixel, the dynamic weight vector $\mathbf{w}_d$ is updated as follows:

$$\mathbf{w}_d(t+1) = \mathbf{w}_d(t) + \alpha(t)\left(\mathbf{h}^s - \mathbf{w}_d(t)\right) \tag{11.22}$$

where $\mathbf{h}^s$ is defined as the vector $[h^s_1 \ h^s_2]^T$ in the equation.

The conditions for primary and secondary edge detection are summarized in Table 11.4.

TABLE 11.4 Conditions for Primary and Secondary Edge Validation

Primary Edge Points	Secondary Edge Points
• $p_{r*} \in [h_1, h_2]$	• $p_d \in [h_1^s, h_2^s]$
• $\lvert \bar{h} - p_{r*} \rvert < \lvert \bar{h} - p_r \rvert,\ r \neq r^*$	• $\mathbf{c}^s = \mathcal{F}(\mathbf{g}, \mathbf{w}_d) \in C$
• $h_2 - h_1 \geq w^l_{r*,2} - w^l_{r*,1}$	
• $\mathbf{c} = \mathcal{F}\left(\mathbf{g}, \mathbf{w}_{r*,s*}\right) \in C$	

11.3.4 Experimental Results

For training, various edge examples from different images are selected, as shown in Figure 11.14. We first applied the trained network to images in the training set to test its performance in generalizing the initial sparse tracings to other edge-like features. The detected edges for an image depicting an eagle are shown in Figure 11.15a. We can see that the network is able to locate all the important edges in the image.

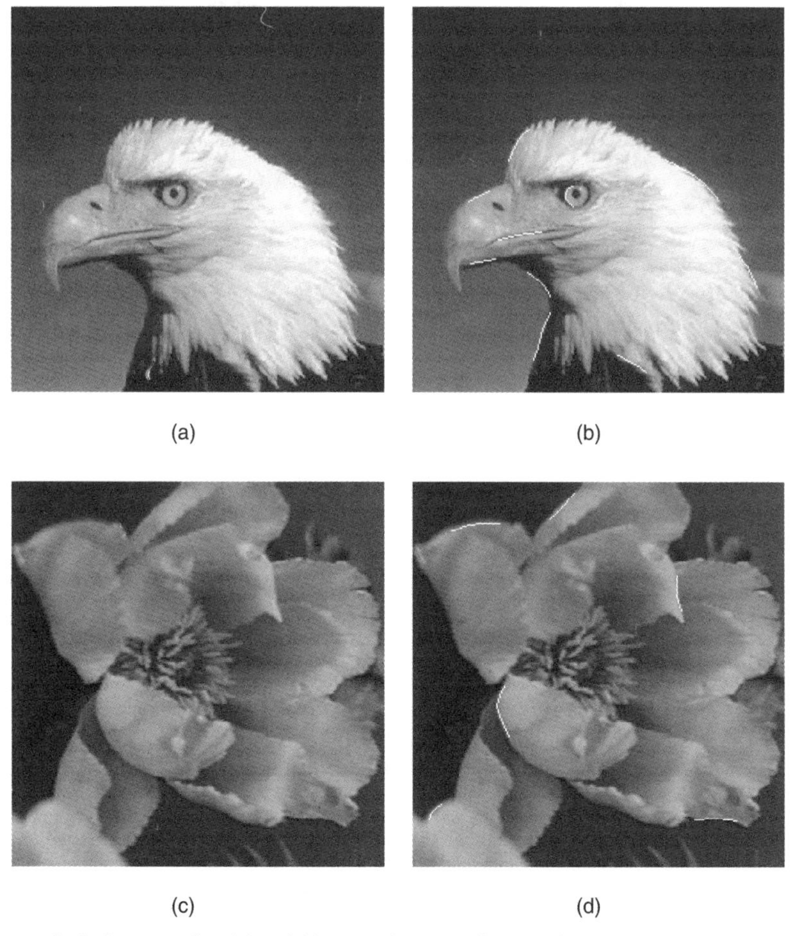

11.14 User-supplied edge examples: (a) and (c) original images; (b) and (d) examples of edges selected by users.

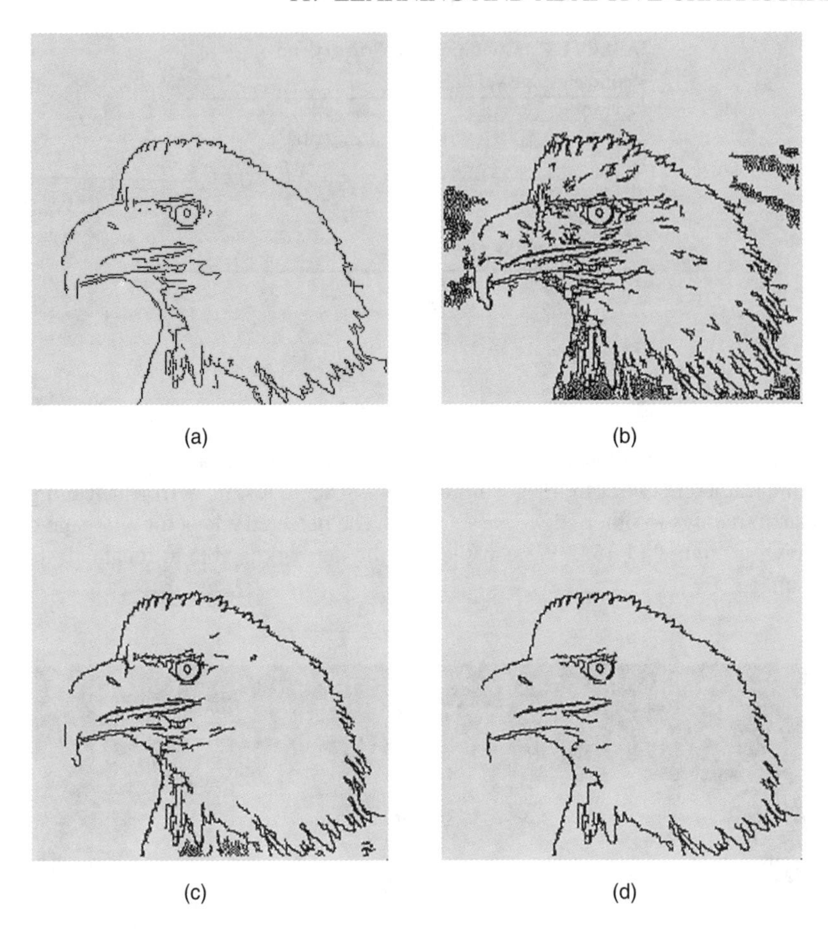

11.15 Edge detection results: (a) neural network detection result; (b) and (c) results using Shen–Castan edge detector: (b) $a_1 = 10, a_2 = 15$; (c) $a_1 = 20, a_2 = 25$; (d) $a_1 = 30, a_2 = 35$.

We also compared the performance of the neural network edge detector with that of the Shen–Castan edge detector [17], a modified form of the Canny edge detector [16] widely used as a comparison standard in edge detection research, in Figure 11.15b–d. The associated parameters of the Shen–Castan edge detector include the hysteresis thresholds a_1 and a_2. A large number of combinations of these two threshold values are possible, and each may result in a very different edge map. Figure 11.15 compares the neural network feature detector result with the Shen–Castan edge detector under various settings of a_1 and a_2. The lower hysteresis threshold ranges from $a_1 = 10$ to $a_1 = 30$ in Figure 11.15b–d, with $a_2 = a_1 + 5$ in each case. We can observe that the corresponding edge map is sensitive to the choice of a_1 and a_2; lower values of a_1 and a_2 will reveal more details but at the same time cause more false positive detections (Figure 11.15b), while higher threshold values lead to missed features (Figure 11.15d). With a proper choice of parameters, we can obtain an adequate representation of the underlying image features, as in Figure 11.15c with $a_1 = 20$ and $a_2 = 25$. If we compare this edge map with the result of the neural network edge detector in Figure 11.15a, we can observe that the neural network detection result is comparable to that obtained under near-optimal settings of the parameters for a conventional edge detector, and, most importantly, the current approach acquires the appropriate parameter settings directly through the user-specified features without extensive trial and error.

We further apply the trained network to other images not in the training set as shown in Figure 11.16. We can observe that the detection results are very satisfactory, considering that the network is trained

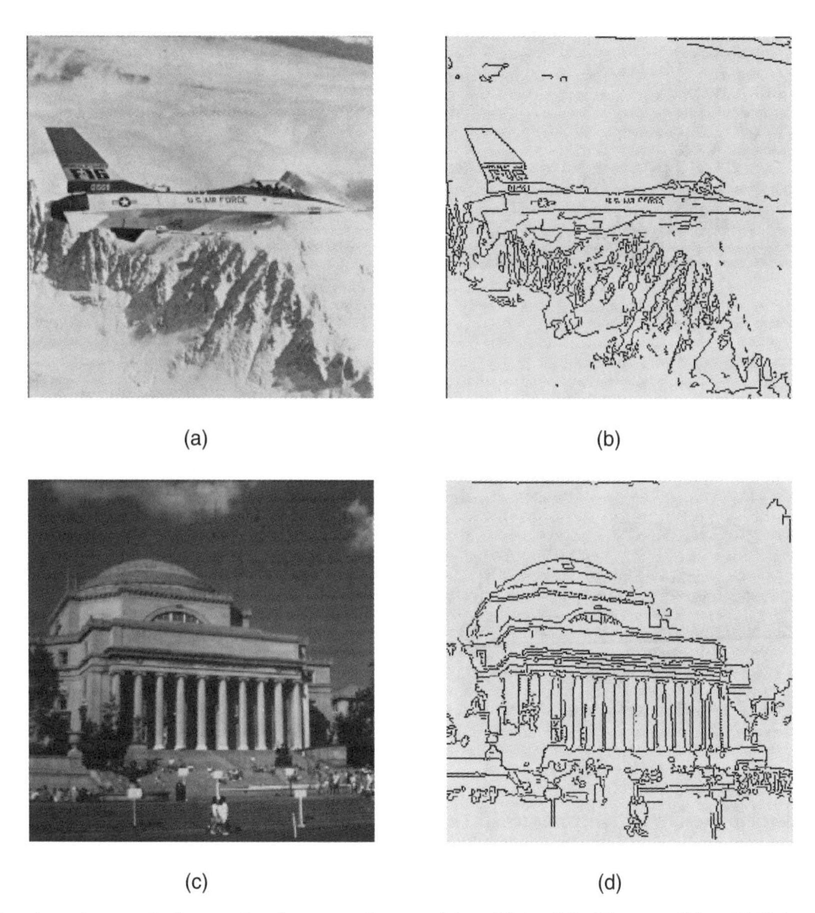

11.16 Edge detection results for previously unseen images: (a) and (c) original images; (b) and (d) detected edges.

only on the eagle and flower images, thus showing the effectiveness of the current architecture in characterizing edges.

We also tested the robustness of the current approach by applying the network to noisy images. In Figure 11.17a, Gaussian noise with standard deviation $\sigma_n = 10$ is added to the eagle image. We have applied the same neural network as in the previous noiseless case to this image without any retraining and alteration of architecture. The result is shown in Figure 11.17b. We can observe that, although some false detections are noticeable, the overall effect is not serious and the result is reasonably similar to the noiseless case. On the other hand, for the Shen–Castan edge detector, if we choose the previous optimal threshold of $a_1 = 20$ and $a_2 = 25$ (Figure 11.17c), the effect of noise is clearly noticeable, and the thresholds have to be readjusted to $a_1 = 25$ and $a_2 = 30$ to compensate for its effect (Figure 11.17d).

We also show the results of applying the same network to the noisy version of the other images in Figure 11.18. We can again notice that the effect of noise contamination is not serious, and we can still regard the edge maps as valid caricatures of the images.

From the results, we can conclude that the hierarchical network architecture can effectively represent the essential characteristics of user-specified edge features through a learning process. Another

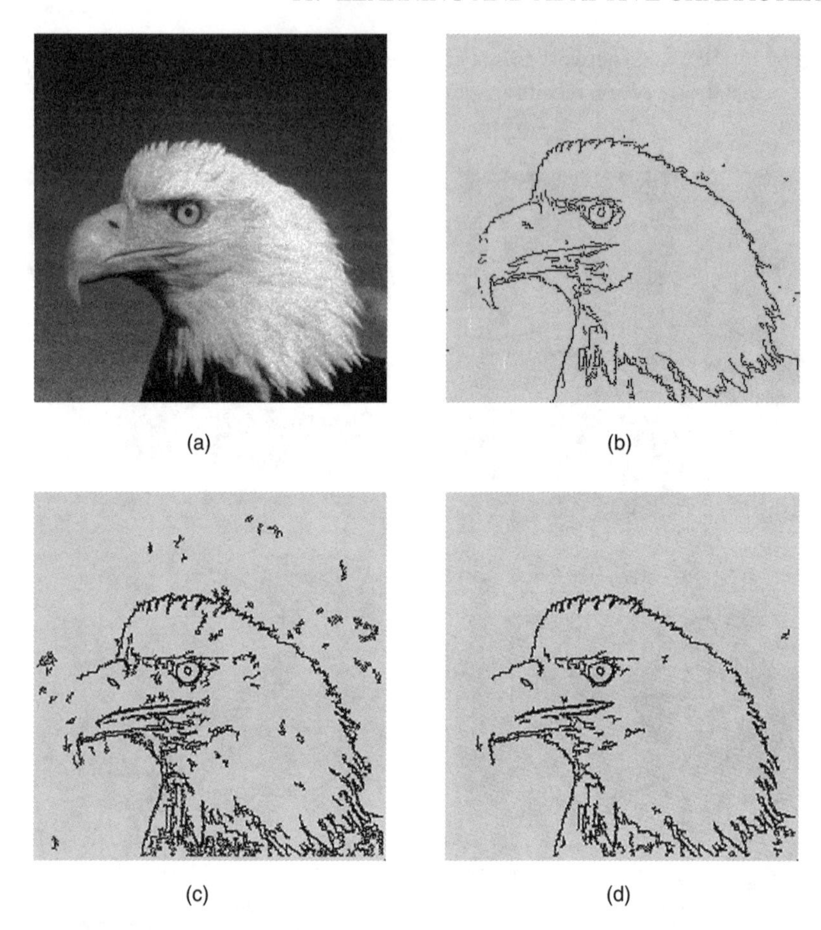

11.17 Edge detection results for noisy images: (a) noisy eagle image; (b) neural network detection result; (c) and (d) results using Shen–Castan edge detector: (c) $a_1 = 20, a_2 = 25$; (d) $a_1 = 25, a_2 = 30$.

important characteristic of this approach is that, unlike previous attempts of edge detection using neural network where both positive and negative training examples are required, the current algorithm requires only a small number of positive training examples in the form of sparse sketches. In other words, for image retrieval applications using edge features, the user is required to provide sketches on only a small subset of the images for training. In addition, it was shown that no retraining of the network and no alteration of architecture are required for applying the network to noisy images. This is particularly important when the quality of the supplied query image from the user is uncertain, in which case the current approach will still allow a reasonable characterization of the edges of the query image for feature matching without additional retraining.

11.4 Conclusion

This chapter has introduced different neural network techniques for the characterization of visual information in CBIR systems. In particular, we adopt an RBF network for characterizing the behavior of users in an interactive retrieval session where relevance feedback is applied. Specifically, the network implements an adaptive metric which progressively models the notion of image similarity from the users' viewpoints through their continual feedback. Compared with previous image matching approaches adopting either a fixed Euclidean metric or its weighted form, which provides limited

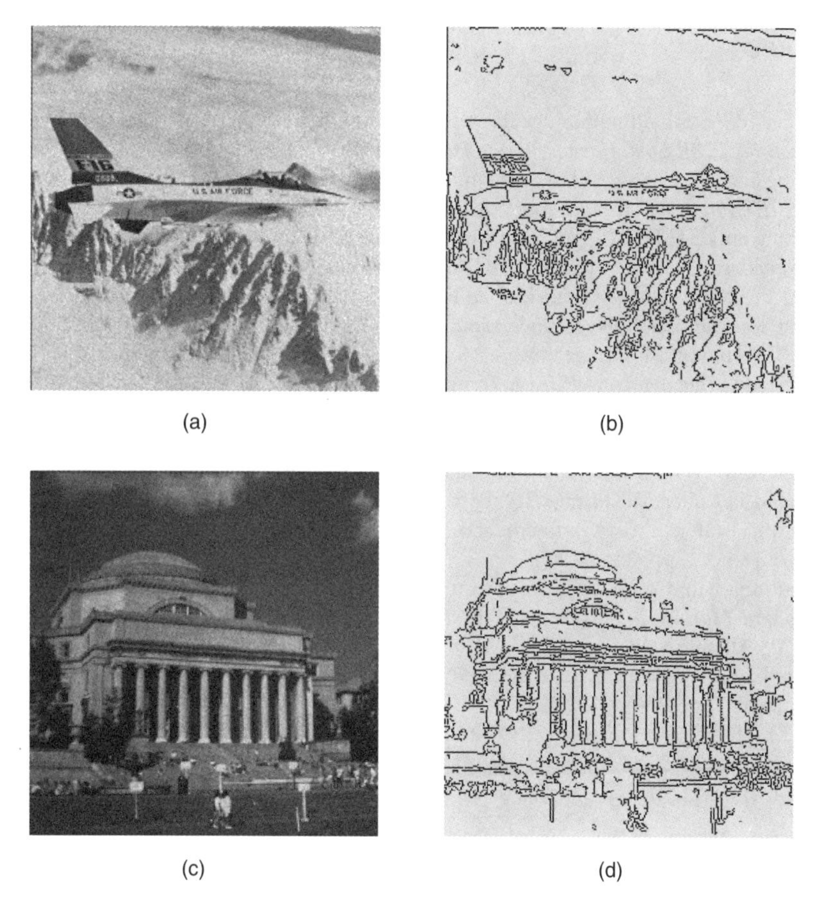

11.18 Edge detection results for previously unseen noisy images: (a) and (c) images corrupted with noise; (b) and (d) detected edges.

adaptivity, the current approach offers an expanded set of adjustable parameters, in the form of the RBF centers and widths, which allow more accurate modeling of the users' responses. Experiments have shown that the current approach outperforms conventional image matching approaches, and satisfactory results are achieved within a very small number of iterations. In addition, the proposed technique is general and can be directly integrated into any image database where the indexing features are arranged in vector form.

We also propose the adoption of a modular neural network for the purpose of characterizing edge information in the front-end feature extraction module, which is an important preprocessing step prior to the further extraction of texture and shape information. Unlike previous edge detection approaches, where numerical threshold values have to be explicitly supplied, the current approach allows users to directly select the significant edge pixels from the image, which are then used as network training examples for the extraction of common edge prototypes. From the experimental results, it is seen that the network is capable of generalizing the information from a few sparse sketches to detect all the prominent edges in images from both the training and the test set, and no retraining of the network is required for applying the approach to noisy images, thus providing robust identification of the user's preferred features.

References

[1] W.Y. Ma and B.S. Manjunath, Edge flow: a framework of boundary detection and image segmentation, in *Proc. IEEE Conf. Comput. Vision Pattern Recognition,* pp. 744–749, 1997.

[2] D. Zhong and S.F. Chang, Video object model and segmentation for content-based video indexing, in *Proc. IEEE Int. Conf. Circuits Syst.,* pp. 1492–1495, 1997.

[3] K.C. Liang and C.C.J. Kuo, Progressive indexing, retrieval and transmission of wavelet compressed image database, in *Proc. SPIE 3169,* pp. 190–199, 1997.

[4] J. Peng, B. Bhanu, and S. Qing, Probabilistic feature relevance learning for content-based image retrieval, *Comput. Vision Image Understanding,* vol. 75, no. 1/2, pp. 150–164, 1999.

[5] Y. Rui, T.S. Huang, M. Ortega, and S. Mehrotra, Relevance feedback: a power tool for interactive content-based image retrieval, *IEEE Trans. Circuits Syst. Video Technol.,* vol. 8, no. 5, pp. 644–655, 1998.

[6] T. Gevers and A.W.M. Smeulders, PicToSeek: combining color and shape invariant features for image retrieval, *IEEE Trans. Image Proc.,* vol. 9, no. 1, pp. 102–119, 2000.

[7] I.J. Cox, M.L. Miller, T.P. Minka, T.V. Papathomas, and P.N. Yianilos, The Bayesian image retrieval system, picHunter: theory, implementation and psychophysical experiments, *IEEE Trans. Image Proc.,* vol. 9, no. 1, pp. 20–37, 2000.

[8] B.S. Manjunath and W.Y. Ma, Texture features for browsing and retrieval of image data, *IEEE Trans. Pattern Anal. Machine Intelligence,* vol. 18, no. 8, pp. 837–842, 1996.

[9] Y. Rui, T.S. Huang, S. Mehrotra, and M. Ortega, A relevance feedback architecture in content-based multimedia information retrieval systems, in *Proc. IEEE Workshop on Content-Based Access Image Video Libraries,* pp. 82–89, 1997.

[10] Y. Rui, T.S. Huang, and S. Mehrotra, Content-based image retrieval with relevance feedback in MARS, *Proc. IEEE Int. Conf. Image Processing,* pp. 815–818, 1997.

[11] G. Salton and M.J. McGill, *Introduction to Modern Information Retrieval,* New York, McGraw-Hill, 1983.

[12] Y. Rui, M. Ortega, and T. Huang, Information retrieval beyond the text document, *Library Trends,* vol. 48, no. 2, pp. 437–456, 1999.

[13] M. Ortega, Y. Rui, K. Chakrabarti, and A. Warshavsky, Supporting ranked Boolean similarity queries in MARS, *IEEE Trans. Knowledge Data Engineering,* vol. 10, no. 6, pp. 905–925, 1998.

[14] S. Mehrotra, Y. Rui, K. Chakrabarti, M. Ortega, and T.S. Huang, Multimedia analysis and retrieval system, in *Proc. 3rd Int. Workshop Information Retrieval Sys.,* pp. 39–45, 1997.

[15] R.C. Gonzalez and R. Woods, *Digital Image Processing,* Reading, MA, Addison-Wesley, 1992.

[16] J. Canny, A computational approach to edge detection, *IEEE Trans. Pattern Anal. Machine Intelligence,* vol. 8, no. 6, pp. 679–698, 1986.

[17] J.J. Shen and S.S. Castan, An optimal linear operator for step edge detection, *CVGIP: Graphical Models Image Proc.,* vol. 54, no. 2, pp. 112–133, 1992.

[18] J.A. Anderson, *An Introduction to Neural Networks,* Cambridge, MA, MIT Press, 1995.

[19] S. Haykin, *Neural Networks: A Comprehensive Foundation,* New York, MacMillan, 1994.

[20] J. Moody and C.J. Darken, Fast learning in networks of locally-tuned processing units, *Neural Computation,* vol. 1, no. 2, pp. 281–294, 1989.

[21] J.H. Friedman, Flexible metric nearest neighbor classification, Tech. Rep., Dept. of Statistics, Stanford University, 1994.

[22] J.A. Lay and L. Guan, Image retrieval based on energy histograms of the low frequency DCT coefficients, *Proc. IEEE Int. Conf. Acoustics Speech Signal Proc.,* pp. 3009–3012, 1999.

[23] R. Anand, K. Mehrotra, C.K. Mohan, and S. Ranka, Efficient classification for multiclass problems using modular neural networks, *IEEE Trans. Neural Networks,* vol. 6, no. 1, pp. 117–124, 1995.

[24] B.L.M. Happel and J.M.J. Murre, Design and evolution of modular neural network architectures, *Neural Networks,* vol. 7, no. 6–7, pp. 985–1004, 1994.

[25] S.Y. Kung and J.S. Taur, Decision-based neural networks with signal/image classification applications, *IEEE Trans. Neural Networks*, vol. 6, no. 1, pp. 170–181, 1995.

[26] S.Y. Kung, M. Fang, S.P. Liou, M.Y. Chiu, and J.S. Taur, Decision-based neural network for face recognition system, *Proc. Int. Conf. Image Processing,* pp. 430–433, 1995.

[27] S.H. Lin, S.Y. Kung, and L.J. Lin, Face recognition/detection by probabilistic decision-based neural networks, *IEEE Trans. Neural Networks,* vol. 8, no. 1, pp. 114–132, 1997.

[28] L. Wang, S.A. Rizvi, and N.M. Nasrabadi, A modular neural network vector predictor for predictive image coding, *IEEE Trans. Image Proc.,* vol. 7, no. 8, pp. 1198–1217, 1998.

[29] L. Wang, S.Z. Der, and N.M. Nasrabadi, Automatic target recognition using a feature-decomposition and data-decomposition modular neural network, *IEEE Trans. Image Proc.,* vol. 7, no. 8, pp. 1113–1121, 1998.

[30] T. Kohonen, *Self-Organizing Maps,* Berlin, Springer-Verlag, 2nd ed., 1997.

[31] B. Kosko, *Neural Networks and Fuzzy Systems,* Englewood Cliffs, NJ, Prentice-Hall, 1992.

12

Applications of Neural Networks to Biomedical Image Processing

Tülay Adali
University of Maryland

Yue Wang
Catholic University or America

Huai Li
University of Maryland

12.1 Introduction

Fueled by the rapid growth in the development of medical imaging technologies and the increasing availability of computing power, biomedical image processing emerged as one of the most active research areas of recent years. With their rich information content, biomedical images are opening entirely new areas of research and are posing new challenges to researchers. Neural networks, among other approaches, have demonstrated a growing importance in the area and are increasingly used for a variety of biomedical image processing tasks. These include detection and characterization of disease patterns, analysis (quantification and segmentation), compression, modeling, motion estimation, and restoration of images from a variety of imaging modalities such as magnetic resonance (MR), positron emission tomography (PET), ultrasound, radiography, and mammography images. For a recent collection of examples of neural network applications to biomedical signal and image processing, see the papers in references [1] and [9].

This chapter concentrates on two specific application areas that are increasingly important: image analysis (quantification and segmentation) and computer assisted (aided) diagnosis (CAD) system design. Both applications demonstrate the unique ways neural structures and learning algorithms can effectively be used in the biomedical domain.

The image analysis application discussed here demonstrates an example of unsupervised learning with a finite mixture network that is intimately related to the radial basis function network. We show that the image context can be modeled by a localized mixture model and that the final image segmentation can be achieved by a probabilistic constraint relaxation network. We give examples of the application of the framework in analyses of MR and mammographic images.

The second application, CAD design, demonstrates two specific ways neural networks can be used for classification (detection) type tasks in biomedical image processing. In the first application, meaningful features that identify the disease patterns of interest are extracted and input into a neural classifier. The second CAD system introduced herein relies on a convolutional neural network

0-8493-2359-2/01/$0.00+$1.50

(CNN) to extract features of disease patterns internally and, hence, to learn to distinguish them from non-disease patterns. We show application of the first CAD to mass detection in mammograms and the second CAD, based on CNN, is applied to detection of clustered microcalcifications.

12.2 Biomedical Image Analysis

Model-based image analysis aims at capturing the intrinsic character of images with few parameters and is also instrumental in helping to understand the nature of the imaging process. Key issues in image analysis include model selection, parameter estimation, imaging physics, and the relationship of the image to the task (how the image is going to be utilized) [2, 3]. Stochastic model-based image analysis has been the most popular among the model-based image analysis methods as, most often, imaging physics can be modeled effectively with a stochastic model. For example, the suitability of standard finite normal mixture models has been verified for a number of medical imaging modalities [4]–[7]. This section discusses a complete treatment of stochastic model-based image analysis that includes model and model order selection, parameter estimation, and final segmentation. We focus on models that use finite mixtures and show examples in MR and mammographic image analysis.

In image analysis, we can treat pixel and context modeling separately, assuming that each pixel can be decomposed into a pixel image and a context image. Pixel image is defined as the observed gray level associated with the pixel, and finite mixture models have been the most popular pixel image models. In particular, standard finite normal mixtures (SFNMs) have been widely used in statistical image analysis, and efficient algorithms are available for calculating the parameters of the model. Furthermore, by incorporating statistical properties of context images, where context image is defined as the membership of the pixel associated with different regions, a localized SFNM formulation can be used to impose local consistency constraints on context images in terms of a stochastic regularization scheme [8].

The next section describes the finite mixtures model and addresses identification of the model, i.e., estimation of the parameters of the model and the model order selection. Section 12.2.2 discusses approaches to modeling context and address segmentation of the MR image into different tissue components.

12.2.1 Pixel Modeling

Imagine a digital image of $N \equiv N_1 \times N_2$ pixels. Assume that this image contains K regions and that each pixel is decomposed into a pixel image x and a context image l. By ignoring information regarding the spatial ordering of pixels, we can treat context images (i.e., pixel labels) as random variables and describe them using a multinomial distribution with unknown parameters π_k. Since this parameter reflects the distribution of the total number of pixels in each region, π_k can be interpreted as a prior probability of pixel labels determined by the global context information. Thus, the relevant (sufficient) statistics are the pixel image statistics for each component mixture and the number of pixels of each component. The marginal probability measure for any pixel image, i.e., the finite mixtures distribution, can be obtained by writing the joint probability density of x and l and then summing the joint density over all possible outcomes of l, i.e., by computing $p(x_i) = \Sigma_l p(x_i, l)$, resulting in a sum of the following general form:

$$p_{\mathbf{r}}(x_i) = \sum_{k=1}^{K} \pi_k p_k(x_i), \quad i = 1, \ldots, N \tag{12.1}$$

where x_i is the gray level of pixel i. $p_k(x_i)$s are conditional region probability density functions (PDFs) with the weighting factor π_k, satisfying $\pi_k > 0$, and $\Sigma_{k=1}^{K} \pi_k = 1$. The generalized Gaussian

PDF given region k is defined by [10]:

$$p_k(x_i) = \frac{\alpha\beta_k}{2\Gamma(1/\alpha)} \exp\left[-|\beta_k(x_i - \mu_k)|^\alpha\right], \quad \alpha > 0, \quad \beta_k = \frac{1}{\sigma_k}\left[\frac{\Gamma(3/\alpha)}{\Gamma(1/\alpha)}\right]^{1/2} \tag{12.2}$$

where μ_k is the mean, $\Gamma(\cdot)$ is the gamma function, and β_k is a parameter related to the variance σ_k by

$$\beta_k = \frac{1}{\sigma_k}\left[\frac{\Gamma(3/\alpha)}{\Gamma(1/\alpha)}\right]^{1/2}. \tag{12.3}$$

When $\alpha \gg 1$, the distribution tends to a uniform PDF; for $\alpha < 1$, the PDF becomes sharper; for $\alpha = 2.0$, one has the Gaussian (normal) PDF; and for $\alpha = 1.0$, one has the Laplacian PDF. Therefore, the generalized Gaussian model is a suitable model to fit the histogram distribution of those images whose statistical properties are unknown since the kernel shape can be controlled by selecting different α values. The finite Gaussian mixture model for $\alpha = 2$ is also commonly referred to as the standard finite normal mixture model which is the identification we adopt in this chapter. It can be written as

$$p_k(x_i) = \frac{1}{\sqrt{2\pi}\sigma_k} \exp\left(-\frac{(x_i - \mu_k)^2}{2\sigma_k^2}\right) \quad i = 1, 2, \ldots, N \tag{12.4}$$

where μ_k and σ_k^2 are the mean and variance of the kth normal kernel and K is the number of normal components.

The whole image can be closely approximated by an independent and identically distributed random field $\mathbf{X}$. The corresponding joint PDF is

$$P(\mathbf{x}) = \prod_{i=1}^{N} \sum_{k=1}^{K} \pi_k p_k(x_i) \tag{12.5}$$

where $\mathbf{x} = [x_1, x_2, \ldots, x_N]$, and $\mathbf{x} \in \mathbf{X}$. Based on the joint probability measure of pixel images, the likelihood function under finite mixture modeling can be expressed as

$$\mathcal{L}(\mathbf{r}) = \prod_{i=1}^{N} p_{\mathbf{r}}(x_i) \tag{12.6}$$

where $\mathbf{r} : \{K, \alpha, \pi_k, \mu_k, \sigma_k, k = 1, \ldots, K\}$ denotes the model parameter set. Note that $p_{\mathbf{r}}(x_i)$ refers to the joint density defined in Equation (12.1); however, we have added the subscript $\mathbf{r}$ to emphasize that it is a parameterized density.

Maximization of the likelihood yields parameters for the chosen distribution given the observations, i.e., the pixel images. Once the model is chosen, identification addresses the estimation of local region parameters $(\pi_k, \mu_k, \sigma_k, k = 1, \ldots, K)$ and the structural parameters (K, α). In particular, the estimation of the order parameter K is referred to as model order selection.

12.2.1.1 Parameter Estimation

With an appropriate system likelihood function, the objective of model identification is to estimate the model parameters by maximizing the likelihood function. This is equivalent to minimization of relative entropy between the image histogram $p_{\mathbf{x}}(u)$ and the estimated PDF $p_{\mathbf{r}}(u)$, where u is the gray level [11, 12] as relative entropy measures the information theoretic distance between two distributions and is zero only when the two distributions match.

There are a number of approaches to perform the maximum likelihood (ML) estimation of finite mixture distributions [13]. The most popular method is the expectation–maximization (EM) algorithm [14, 15]. EM algorithm first calculates the posterior Bayesian probabilities of the data based on the observations and obtains the current parameter estimates (E-step). It then updates parameter estimates using generalized mean ergodic theorems (M-step). The procedure moves back and forth between these two steps. The successive iterations increase the likelihood of the model parameters being estimated. A neural network interpretation of this procedure is given by Perlovsky and McManus [16].

We can use relative entropy (the Kullback–Leibler distance) [17] for parameter estimation, i.e., we can measure the information theoretic distance between the histogram of the pixel images, denoted by $p_{\mathbf{x}}$, and the estimated distribution $p_{\mathbf{r}}(u)$ which we define as the global relative entropy (GRE):

$$D\left(p_{\mathbf{x}} \| p_{\mathbf{r}}\right) = \sum_{u} p_{\mathbf{x}}(u) \log \frac{p_{\mathbf{x}}(u)}{p_{\mathbf{r}}(u)} . \tag{12.7}$$

It can be shown that, when relative entropy is used as the distance measure, distance minimization is equivalent to the ML estimation of the model parameters [11, 12].

For the case of the FGGM model, the EM algorithm can be applied to the joint estimation of the parameter vector and the structural parameter α as follows [14]:

EM Algorithm

1. For $\alpha = \alpha_{\min}, \ldots, \alpha_{\max}$:
   - $m = 0$, given initialized $\mathbf{r}^{(0)}$.
   - E-step: for $i = 1, \ldots, N,\ k = 1, \ldots, K$, compute the probabilistic membership:

$$z_{ik}^{(m)} = \frac{\pi_k^{(m)} p_k(x_i)}{\sum_{k=1}^{K} \pi_k^{(m)} p_k(x_i)} \tag{12.8}$$

   - M-step: for $k = 1, \ldots, K$, compute the updated parameter estimates:

$$\begin{cases} \pi_k^{(m+1)} = \frac{1}{N} \sum_{i=1}^{N_1 N_2} z_{ik}^{(m)} \\ \mu_k^{(m+1)} = \frac{1}{N\pi_k^{(m+1)}} \sum_{i=1}^{N} z_{ik}^{(m)} x_i \\ \sigma_k^{2(m+1)} = \frac{1}{N\pi_k^{(m+1)}} \sum_{i=1}^{N} z_{ik}^{(m)} \left(x_i - \mu_k^{(m+1)}\right)^2 \end{cases} \tag{12.9}$$

   - When $|GRE^{(m)}(p_{\mathbf{x}} \| p_{\mathbf{r}}) - GRE^{(m+1)}(p_{\mathbf{x}} \| p_{\mathbf{r}})| \leq \epsilon$ is satisfied, go to step 2. Otherwise, $m = m + 1$ and go to E-Step.
2. Compute GRE, and go to step 1.
3. Choose the optimal $\hat{\mathbf{r}}$ which corresponds to the minimum GRE.

However, the EM algorithm generally has the reputation of being slow, since it has a first order convergence in which new information acquired in the expectation step is not used immediately [18]. Recently, a number of online versions of the EM algorithm were proposed for large scale sequential learning [11, 13, 19, 20]. Such a procedure eliminates the need to store all the incoming observations and changes the parameters immediately after each data point, allowing for high data rates. Titterington et al. [13] present a stochastic approximation procedure that is closely related to the probabilistic self-organizing mixtures (PSOM) algorithm we introduce below. Other similar formulations for normal mixture parameter estimation are due to Marroquin and Girosi [19] and Weinstein et al. [20].

For the adaptive estimation of the SFNM model parameters, we can derive an incremental learning algorithm by simple stochastic gradient descent minimization of $D(p_{\mathbf{x}}||p_{\mathbf{r}})$ [5, 11] given in Equation (12.7) with $p_{\mathbf{r}}$ given by Equation (12.4):

$$\mu_k{}^{(t+1)} = \mu_k^{(t)} + a(t)\left(x_{t+1} - \mu_k^{(t)}\right) z_{(t+1)k}^{(t)} \tag{12.10}$$

$$\sigma_k^{2(t+1)} = \sigma_k^{2(t)} + b(t)\left[\left(x_{t+1} - \mu_k^{(t)}\right)^2 - \sigma_k^{2(t)}\right] z_{(t+1)k}^{(t)} \tag{12.11}$$

$$k = 1, \ldots, K$$

where $a(t)$ and $b(t)$ are introduced as learning rates, two sequences converging to zero, and ensuring unbiased estimates after convergence.

Updates for the constrained regularization parameters, π_k in the SFNM model, are obtained using a recursive sample mean calculation based on a generalized mean ergodic theorem [21]:

$$\pi_k^{(t+1)} = \frac{t}{t+1}\pi_k^{(t)} + \frac{1}{t+1} z_{(t+1)k}^{(t)} \,. \tag{12.12}$$

Hence, the updates given by Equations (12.10), (12.11), and (12.12), together with an evaluation of Equation (12.8) using Equation (12.4), provide the incremental procedure for computing the SFNM component parameters. Their practical use requires a strong mixing condition and a decaying annealing procedure (learning rate decay) [21]–[23]. For details of the derivation, see Wang et al. [9, 11]. In finite mixture parameter estimation, the algorithm initialization must also be carried out carefully. Wang et al. [24] introduced an adaptive Lloyd–Max histogram quantization (ALMHQ) algorithm for threshold selection which is also well suited to initialization in an ML estimation. It can be used for initializing the network parameters: μ_k, σ_k^2, and π_k, k, $1, 2, \ldots, K$.

12.2.1.2 Model Order Selection

The determination of the region parameter K directly affects the quality of the resulting model parameter estimation and, in turn, affects the result of segmentation. In a statistical problem formulation such as the one introduced in the previous section, the use of information theoretic criteria for the problem of model determination arises as a natural choice. Two popular approaches are Akaike's information criterion (AIC) [25], and Rissanen's minimum description length (MDL) [26]. Akaike proposes the selection of the model that gives the minimum AIC, which is defined by

$$\mathrm{AIC}\left(K_a\right) = -2\log\left(\mathcal{L}\left(\hat{\mathbf{r}}_{ML}\right)\right) + 2K_a \tag{12.13}$$

where $\hat{\mathbf{r}}_{ML}$ is the maximum likelihood estimate of the model parameter set $\mathbf{r}$, and K_a is the number of free adjustable parameters in the model [4, 25] and is given by $3K - 1$ for the SFNM model. The AIC selects the correct number of the image regions K_0 such that

$$K_0 = \arg\left\{\min_{1\le K\le K_{\mathrm{MAX}}} \mathrm{AIC}\left(K_a\right)\right\} \,. \tag{12.14}$$

Rissanen addresses the problem from a quite different point of view. He reformulates the problem explicitly as an information coding problem in which the best model fit is measured such that high probabilities are assigned to the observed data, while at the same time the model itself is not too complex to be described [26]. The model is selected by minimizing the total description length defined by

$$\mathrm{MDL}\left(K_a\right) = -\log\left(\mathcal{L}\left(\hat{\mathbf{r}}_{ML}\right)\right) + 0.5K_a\log(N) \,. \tag{12.15}$$

Similarly, the correct number of distinctive image regions K_0 can be estimated as

$$K_0 = \arg\left\{ \min_{1 \le K \le K_{\text{MAX}}} \text{MDL}(K_a) \right\} . \tag{12.16}$$

It is also worth noting that Schwartz arrives at the same formulation by using Bayesian arguments [27]. Wax and Kailath [28] provide a good introduction to model order selection for signal processing.

12.2.2 Context Modeling and Segmentation

Once the pixel model is estimated, the segmentation problem is the assignment of labels to each pixel in the image. A straightforward solution is to label pixels into different regions by maximizing the individual likelihood function $p_k(x)$, i.e., by performing ML classification. Usually, this method may not achieve a good performance since it does not use local neighborhood information in the decision. The CBRL algorithm [29] is one approach that can incorporate the local neighborhood information into the labeling procedure and, thus, improve the segmentation performance. The CBRL algorithm to perform/refine pixel labeling based on the localized FGGM model can be defined as follows [7].

Let ∂i be the neighborhood of pixel i with an $m \times m$ template centered at pixel i. An indicator function is used to represent the local neighborhood constraints $R_{ij}(l_i, l_j) = I(l_i, l_j)$, where l_i and l_j are labels of pixels i and j, respectively. Note that pairs of labels are now either compatible or incompatible. Similar to the procedure described in Hummel and Zucker [29], one can compute the frequency of neighbors of pixel i which has the same label values k as at pixel i:

$$\pi_k^{(i)} = p\left(l_i = k | \mathbf{l}_{\partial i}\right) = \frac{1}{m^2 - 1} \sum_{j \in \partial i, j \neq i} I\left(k, l_j\right) \tag{12.17}$$

where $\mathbf{l}_{\partial i}$ denotes the labels of the neighbors of pixel i. Since $\pi_k^{(i)}$ is a conditional probability of a region, the localized FGGM PDF of gray-level x_i at pixel i is given by:

$$p\left(x_i | \mathbf{l}_{\partial i}\right) = \sum_{k=1}^{K} \pi_k^{(i)} p_k\left(x_i\right) \tag{12.18}$$

where $p_k(x_i)$ is given in Equation (12.2). Assuming gray values of the image are conditional independent, the joint PDF of $\mathbf{x}$, given the context labels $\mathbf{l}$, is

$$P(\mathbf{x}|\mathbf{l}) = \prod_{i=1}^{N} \sum_{k=1}^{K} \pi_k^{(i)} p_k\left(x_i\right) \tag{12.19}$$

where $\mathbf{l} = (l_i : i = 1, \ldots, N)$.

It is important to note that the CBRL algorithm can obtain a consistent labeling solution based on the localized FGGM model Equation (12.18). Since $\mathbf{l}$ represents the labeled image, it is consistent if $S_i(l_i) \ge S_i(k)$, for all $k = 1, \ldots, K$ and for $i = 1, \ldots, N$ [29], where

$$S_i(k) = \pi_k^{(i)} p_k\left(x_i\right) . \tag{12.20}$$

Now we can define

$$A(\mathbf{l}) = \sum_{i=1}^{N} \left(\sum_{k} I\left(l_i, k\right) S_i(k) \right) \tag{12.21}$$

as the average measure of local consistency, and

$$LC_i = \sum_k I\,(l_i, k)\, S_i(k), \quad i = 1, \ldots, N \tag{12.22}$$

represents the local consistency based on $\mathbf{l}$. The goal is to find a consistent labeling $\mathbf{l}$ which can maximize Equation (12.21). In the real application, each local consistency measure LC_i can be maximized independently. Hummel and Zucker have shown that when $R_{ij}(l_i, l_j) = R_{ji}(l_j, l_i)$, if $A(\mathbf{l})$ attains a local maximum at $\mathbf{l}$, then $\mathbf{l}$ is a consistent labeling [29].

Based on the localized FGGM model, $l_i^{(0)}$ can be initialized by the ML classifier,

$$l_i^{(0)} = \arg\left\{\max_k \; p_k\,(x_i)\right\}, \quad k = 1, \ldots, K\,. \tag{12.23}$$

Then, the order of pixels is randomly permutated and each label l_i is updated to maximize LC_i, i.e., classify pixel i into kth region if

$$l_i = \arg\left\{\max_k \; \pi_k^{(i)}\, p_k\,(x_i)\right\}, \quad k = 1, \ldots, K \tag{12.24}$$

where $p_k(x_i)$ is given in Equation (12.2), $\pi_k^{(i)}$ is given in Equation (12.17). By considering Equations (12.23) and (12.24), we can give a modified CBRL algorithm as follows [7]:

CBRL Algorithm

1. Given $\mathbf{l}^{(0)}$, $m = 0$.
2. Update pixel labels:
   - Randomly visit each pixel for $i = 1, \ldots, N$.
   - Update its label l_i according to:

$$l_i^{(m)} = \arg\left\{\max_k \pi_k^{(i)(m)}\, p_k\,(x_i)\right\}\,.$$

3. When $\frac{\Sigma(\mathbf{l}^{(m+1)} \oplus \mathbf{l}^{(m)})}{N_1 N_2} \leq 1\%$, stop; otherwise, $m = m + 1$, and repeat step 2.

12.2.3 Application Examples

We present two examples to demonstrate the application of the stochastic model-based image analysis scheme described in Sections 12.2.1 and 12.2.2. Although tissue quantification and image segmentation may be simultaneously performed [30, 32, 33], a more accurate result can be achieved if the two objectives are considered separately [11, 34]. Guided by the two information theoretic criteria, our algorithm proceeds by fitting an SFNM with model order selection to the histogram of pixel images and then constructing a consistent relaxation labeling of the context images. A summary of the major steps in implementation is

1. For each value of K, perform an ML tissue quantification by applying the EM algorithm (Equations (12.8) and (12.9)).
2. Scan the values of $K = K_{\min}, \ldots, K_{\max}$ by using AIC in Equation (12.13) and MDL Equation (12.15) to determine the suitable number of tissue types K_0.
3. Select the result of tissue quantification corresponding to the value of K_0 determined in step 2.

4. Initialize image segmentation using the ML classification method Equation (12.23).
5. Finalize tissue segmentation by CBRL (implementing Equation (12.24)).

For this study, we use data consisting of three adjacent, T1-weighted MR images parallel to the AC-PC line. Since the skull, scalp, and fat in the original brain images do not contribute to the brain tissue, we edited the MR images to exclude nonbrain structures prior to tissue quantification and segmentation, as explained by Wang and colleagues [8, 9]. This also helps us achieve better quantification and segmentation of brain tissues by delineation of other tissue types that are not clinically significant [30, 31, 34]. The extracted brain tissues are shown in Figure 12.1.

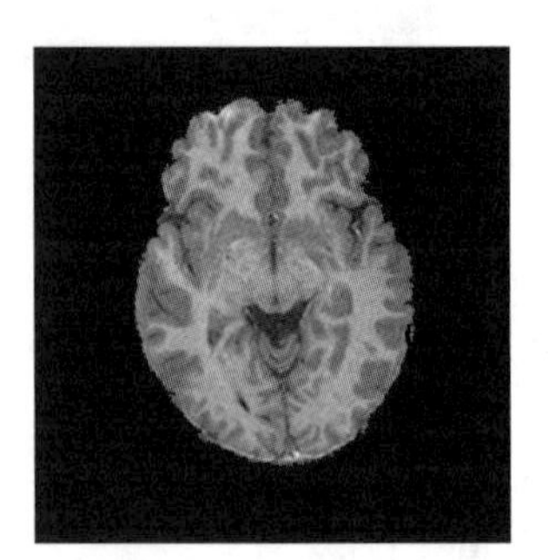
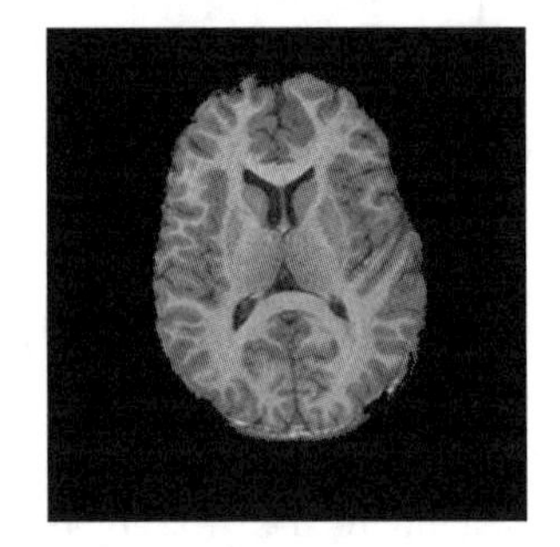
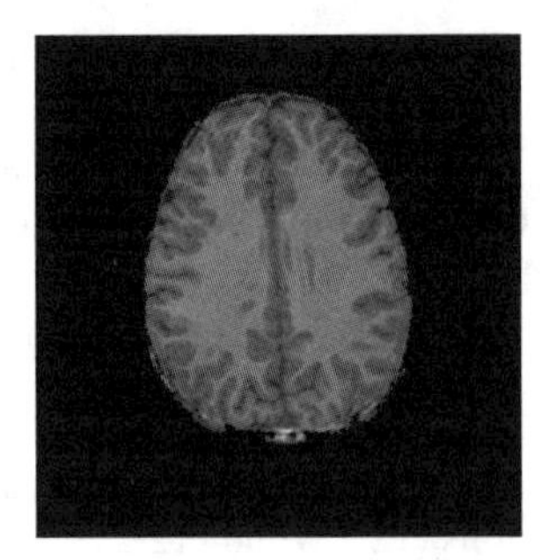

12.1 Three sample MR brain tissues.

Evaluation of different image analysis techniques is a particularly difficult task, and the dependability of evaluations by simple mathematical measures such as squared error performance is questionable. Therefore, most of the time, the quality of the quantified and segmented image usually depends heavily on the subjective and qualitative judgments. Besides the evaluation performed by radiologists, we use the GRE value to reflect the quality of tissue quantification.

The brain is generally composed of three principal tissue types, i.e., white matter (WM), gray matter (GM), cerebrospinal fluid (CSF), and their combinations, called the partial volume effect. We consider the pair-wise combinations as well as the triple mixture tissue, defined as CSF-white-gray (CWG). More importantly, since the MRI scans clearly show the distinctive intensities at local brain areas, the functional areas within a tissue type need to be considered. In particular, the caudate nucleus and putamen are two important local brain functional areas. In our complete image analysis framework, we allow the number of tissue types to vary from slice to slice, i.e., we do consider adaptability to different MR images. We let $K_{\min} = 2$ and $K_{\max} = 9$ and calculate AIC(K) (Equation (12.13)) and MDL(K) (Equation (12.15)) for $K = K_{\min}, \ldots, K_{\max}$. The results with these three criteria all suggest that the three sample brain images chosen contain six, eight, and six tissue types, respectively. According to the model fitting procedure using information theoretic criteria, the minima of these criteria indicate the most appropriate number of tissue types, which is also the number of hidden nodes in the corresponding PSOM (mixture components in SFNM).

When performing the computation of the information theoretic criteria, we use PSOM to iteratively quantify different tissue types for each fixed K. The PSOM algorithm is initialized by the adaptive Lloyd–Max histogram quantization [24]. For slice 2, the results of final tissue quantification with $K_0 = 7, 8, 9$ are shown in Table 12.1 corresponding to $K_0 = 8$, where a GRE value of 0.02–0.04 nats is achieved. These quantified tissue types agree with those of a physician's qualitative analysis results [11].

The CBRL tissue segmentation for slice 2 is performed with $K_0 = 7, 8, 9$, and the algorithm is initialized by ML classification (Equation (12.23)) [13]. CBRL updates are terminated after five to ten iterations since further iterations produce almost identical results. The segmentation results are

TABLE 12.1 Result of Parameter Estimation for Slice 2

Tissue Type	1	2	3	4	5	6	7	8
π	0.0251	0.0373	0.0512	0.071	0.1046	0.1257	0.2098	0.3752
μ	38.848	58.718	74.400	88.500	97.864	105.706	116.642	140.294
σ^2	78.5747	42.282	56.5608	34.362	24.1167	23.8848	49.7323	96.7227

shown in Figure 12.2. It is seen that the boundaries of WM, GM, and CSF are successfully delineated. To see the benefit of using information theoretic criteria in determining the number of tissue types, the decomposed tissue type segments are given in Figure 12.3 with $K_0 = 8$. As can be observed in Figures 12.2 and 12.3, the segmentation with eight tissue types provides a very meaningful result. The regions with different gray levels are satisfactorily segmented; specifically, the major brain tissues are clearly identified. If the number of tissue types were underestimated by one, tissue mixtures located within putamen and caudate areas would be lumped into one component, though the results are still meaningful. When the number of tissue type is overestimated by one, there is no significant difference in the quantification result, but white matter has been divided into two components. For $K_0 = 8$, the segmented regions represent eight types of brain tissues: (a) CSF, (b) CG, (c) CGW, (d) GW, (e) GM, (f) putamen area, (g) caudate area, and (h) WM, as shown in Figure 12.3. These segmented tissue types again agree with the results of radiologists' evaluations [11].

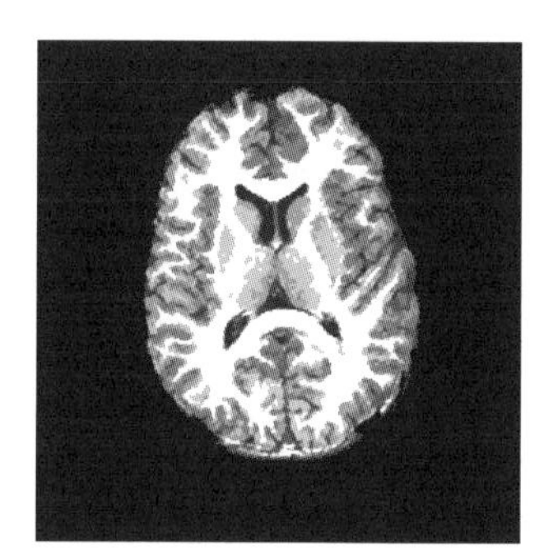
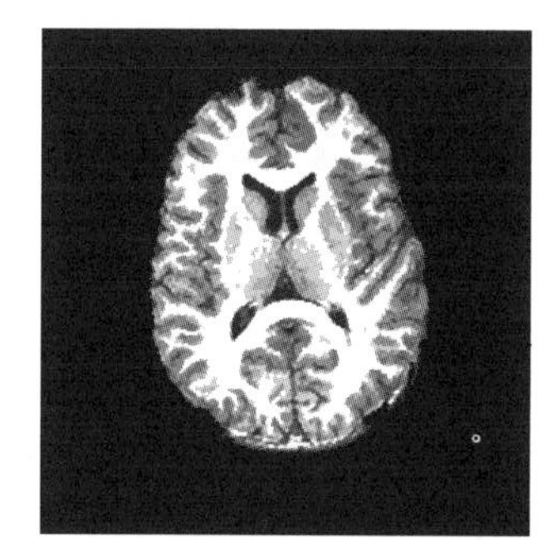
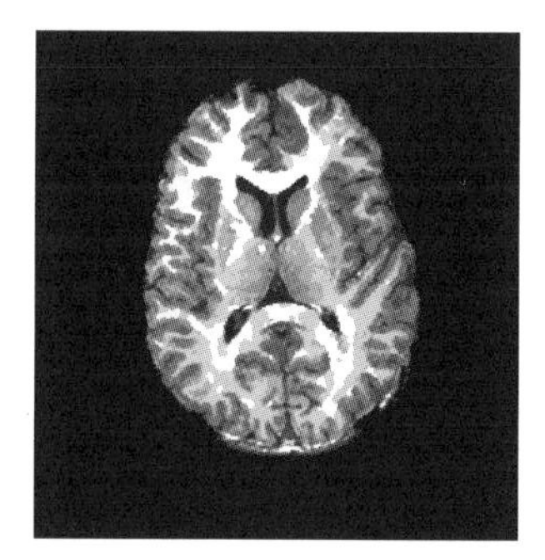

12.2 Results of tissue segmentation for slice 2 with $K_0 = 7, 8, 9$ (from left to right).

Another possible application area for the image analysis framework we introduced is in segmentation and extraction of suspicious mass areas from mammographic images. With an appropriate statistical description of various discriminate characteristics of both true and false candidates from the localized areas, an improved mass detection can be achieved in computer aided diagnosis. Preprocessing is an important step in image analysis for most applications. In this example, one type of morphological operation is derived to enhance disease patterns of suspected masses by cleaning up unrelated background clutters, and then image segmentation is performed to localize the suspected mass areas using a stochastic relaxation labeling scheme [7, 35]. Results are shown in Figure 12.4.

The mammograms for this study were selected from the Mammographic Image Analysis Society (MIAS) database and the Brook Army Medical Center (BAMC) database created by the Department of Radiology at Georgetown University Medical Center. The areas of suspicious masses were identified by an expert radiologist based on visual criteria and biopsy proven results. The BAMC films were digitized with a laser film digitizer (Lumiscan 150) at a pixel size of 100 μm $\times$ 100 μm and 4096 gray levels (12 bits). Before the method was applied, the digital mammograms were smoothed by averaging 4×4 pixels into one pixel. According to radiologists, the size of small masses is 3–15 mm in effective diameter. A 3 mm object in an original mammogram occupies 30 pixels in a digitized image with a 100 μm resolution. After reducing the image size by four times, the object

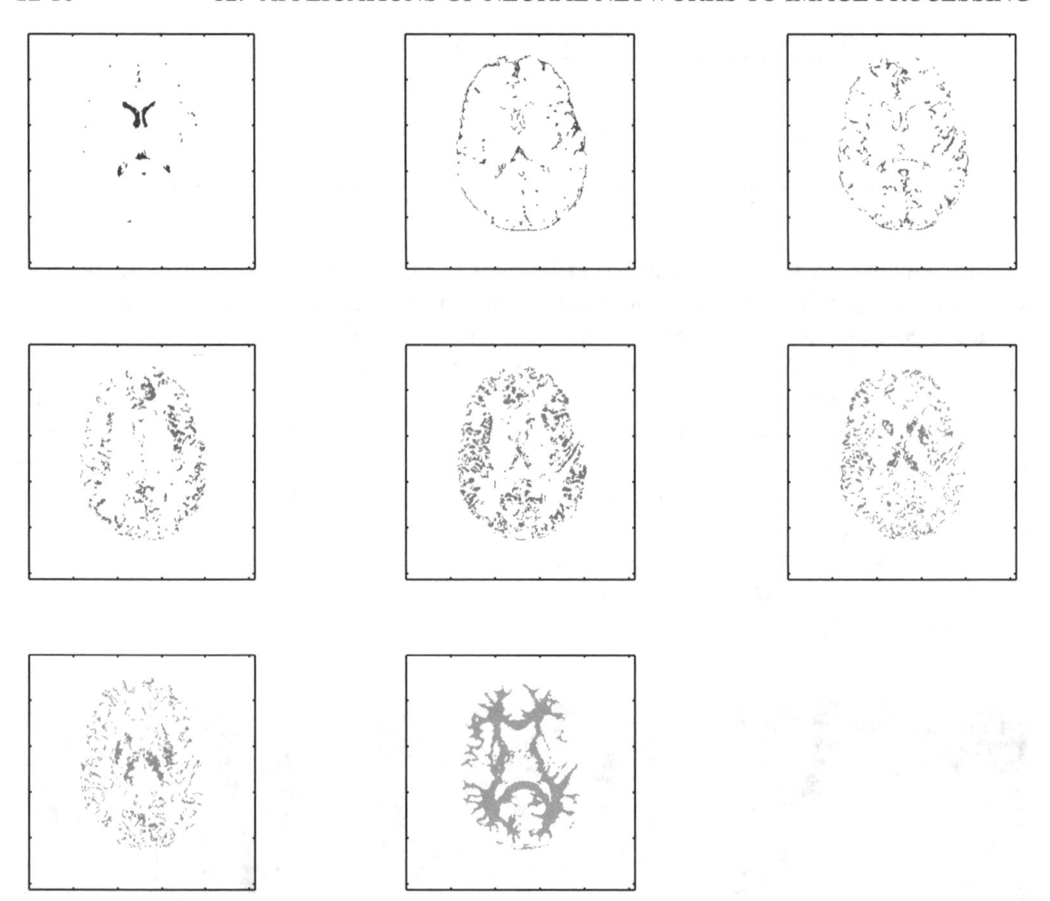

12.3 Results of tissue type decomposition for slice 2. They represent eight types of brain tissues: CSF, CG, CGW, GW, GM, putamen area, caudate area, and WM (left to right, top to bottom).

will occupy the range of about 7 to 8 pixels. The object with the size of 7 pixels is expected to be detectable by any computer algorithm. Therefore, size reduction can be applied for mass detection and can save computation time.

Consider the use of the FGGM model and the two information criteria, AIC and MDL, to determine the mixture number K. Tables 12.2 and 12.3 show the AIC and MDL values with different K and α of the FGGM model based on one sample original mammogram. As can be observed from the tables, even with different values for α, for all cases, AIC and MDL values are minimum when $K = 8$. This indicates that AIC and MDL are relatively insensitive to the change of α. With this observation, we can decouple the relation between K and α and choose the appropriate value of one while fixing the value of the other. Figure 12.5a and b shows two examples of AIC and MDL curves with different K and fixed $\alpha = 3.0$. Figure 12.5a is based on the original, and Figure 12.5b is based on the enhanced mammogram. With the original mammogram, both criteria achieve the minimum when $K = 8$. Figure 12.5b indicates that $K = 4$ is the appropriate choice for the number of meaningful regions for the mammogram enhanced by dual morphological operation, which is reasonable since the numbers of effective regions are expected to decrease after background correction. The results of parameter estimation with $K = 8$ and different values of α are shown in Figure 12.6.

The order of the model is thus fixed at $K = 8$, and the value of α is changed for estimating the FGGM model parameters using the EM algorithm given in Section 12.2.2 with the original mammogram. The GRE value between the histogram and the estimated FGGM distribution is used

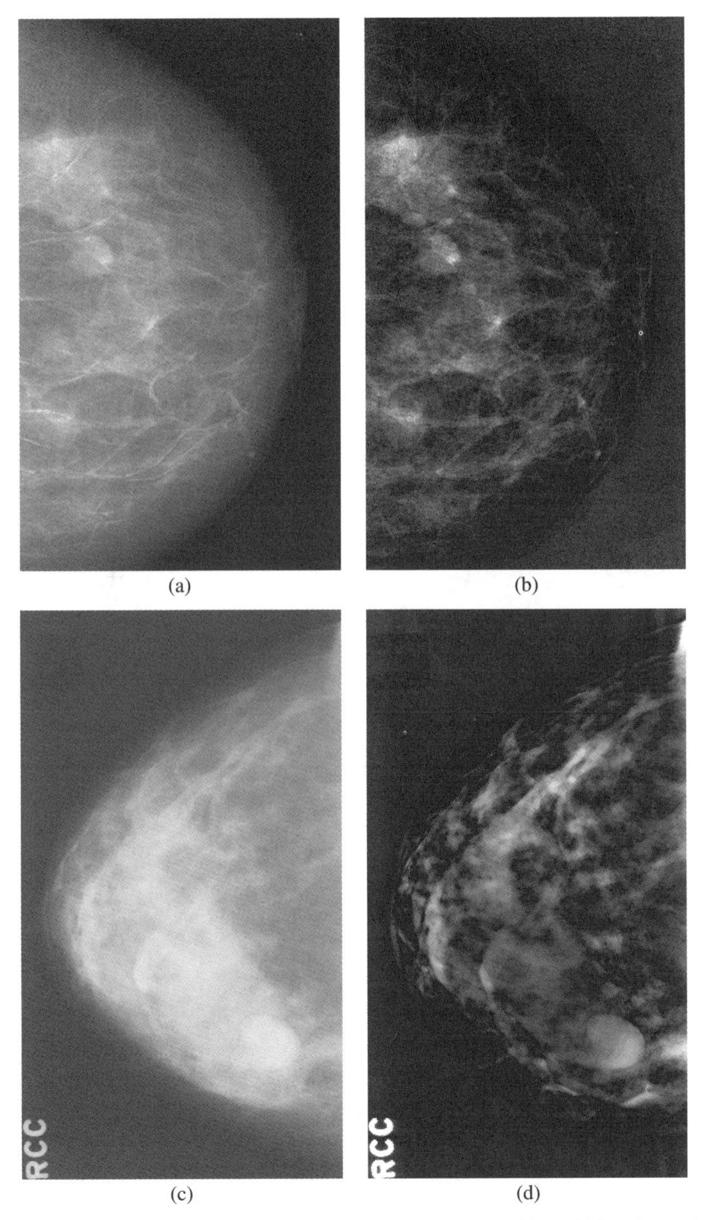

12.4 Examples of mass enhancement: (a) and (c) original mammograms; (b) and (d) enhanced mammograms.

as a measure of the estimation bias, and it is noted that GRE achieves a minimum distance when the FGGM parameter $\alpha = 3.0$, as shown in Figure 12.6. A similar result is obtained when the EM algorithm is applied to the enhanced mammogram with $K = 4$. This indicates that the FGGM model might be better than the SFNM model ($\alpha = 2.0$) in modeling mammographic images when the true statistical properties of mammograms are generally unknown, though the SFNM has been successfully used in a large number of applications, as shown in our previous example. Hence, the choice of the best model to describe the data depends on the nature of the data for the given problem. For details of this experiment, see Li et al. [7].

After determination of all model parameters, every pixel of the image is labeled to one region (from 1 to K) based on the CBRL algorithm. Then, the brightest region, which corresponds to label

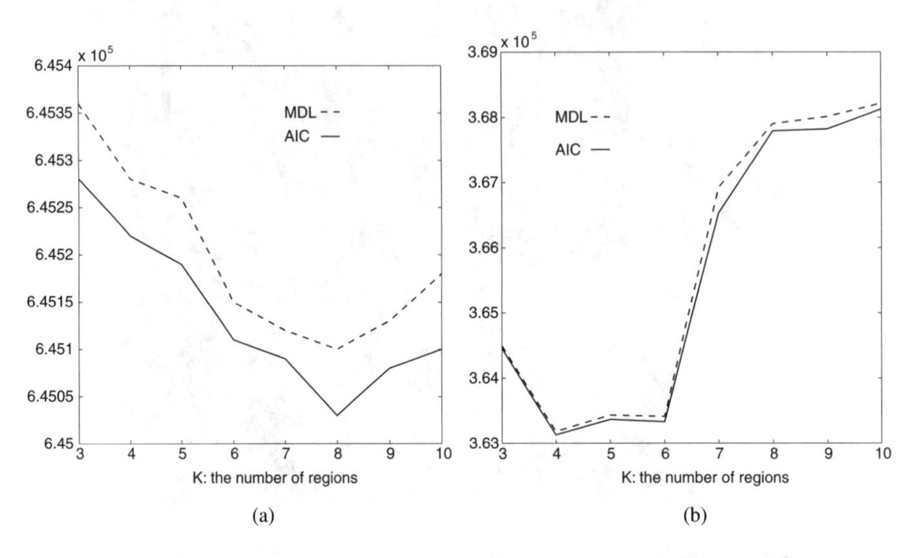

12.5 AIC and MDL curves as functon of the number of regions K: (a) results based on the original mammogram (Optimal $K = 8$); (b) results based on the enhanced mammogram (Optimal $K = 4$).

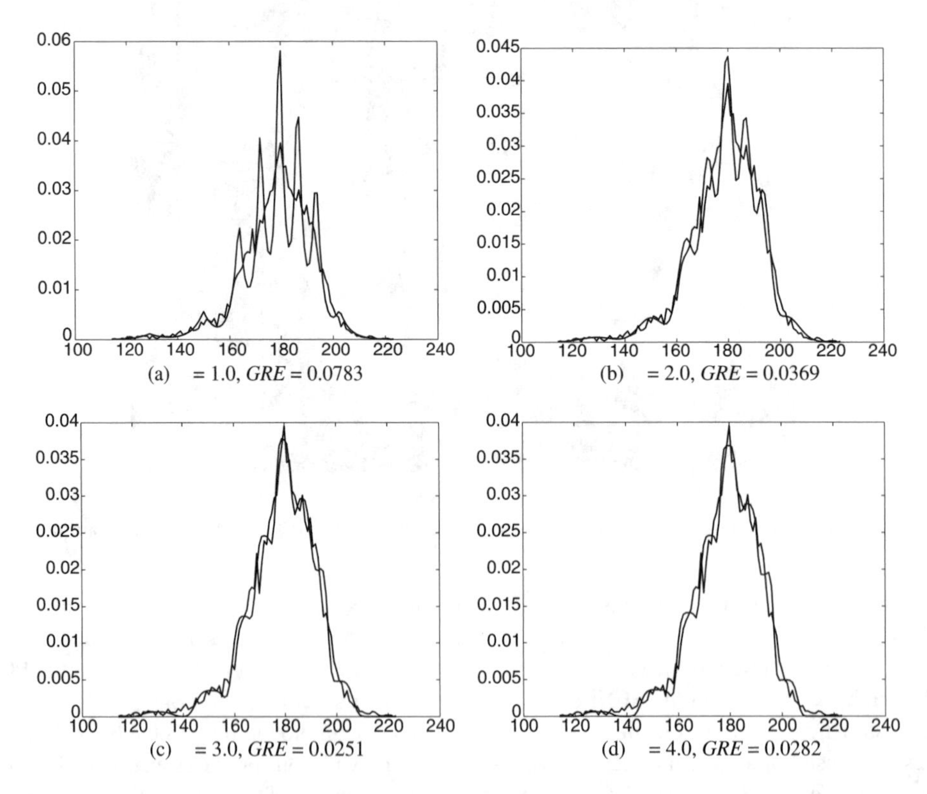

12.6 The comparison of learning curves and histograms of the original mammogram with different α values for $K = 8$ (Optimal $\alpha = 3.0$).

TABLE 12.2 Computed AIC Values for the FGGM Model with Different α

K	$\alpha = 1.0$	$\alpha = 2.0$	$\alpha = 3.0$	$\alpha = 4.0$
2	651250	650570	650600	650630
3	646220	644770	645280	646200
4	645760	644720	645260	646060
5	645760	644700	645120	646040
6	645740	644670	645110	645990
7	645640	644600	645090	645900
8	645550 (min)	644570 (min)	645030 (min)	645850 (min)
9	645580	644590	645080	645880
10	645620	644600	645100	645910

TABLE 12.3 Computed MDL Values for the FGGM Model with Different α

K	$\alpha = 1.0$	$\alpha = 2.0$	$\alpha = 3.0$	$\alpha = 4.0$
2	651270	650590	650630	650660
3	646260	644810	645360	646350
4	645860	644770	645280	646150
5	645850	644770	645280	646100
6	645790	644750	645150	646090
7	645720	644700	645120	645930
8	645680 (min)	644690 (min)	645100 (min)	645900 (min)
9	645710	644710	645140	645930
10	645790	644750	645180	645960

TABLE 12.4 Comparison of Segmentation Error Resulting from Noncontextual and Contextual Methods

Method	Soft Classification	Bayesian Classification	CBRL
GRE Value	0.0067	0.4406	0.1578

K, plus a criterion of closed isolated area, is chosen as the candidate region of suspicious masses, as shown in Figure 12.7. These results are noted to be highly satisfactory when compared to outlines of the lesions [7]. Also, similar to the previous example, GRE values can be used to assess the performance of the final segmentation. Table 12.4 shows our evaluation data from three different segmentation methods when applied to these real images.

12.3 CAD System Design

In order to improve detection and classification in clinical screening and/or diagnosis using radiographic images, many CAD systems have been developed within the last decade. Among others, the development of CAD systems for breast cancer screening and/or diagnosis has received particular attention [36]–[47]. This attention might be attributed to the fact that the role of a CAD system is better defined as complementary to radiologists' clinical duties, i.e., CAD systems can be used for tasks that the radiologists cannot perform well or find difficult to perform. Because of generally larger size and complex appearance of masses, especially the existence of spicules in malignant lesions, as compared to microcalcifications, feature-based approaches are widely adopted in many CAD systems for breast cancer screening [36]–[39], [41, 44]. Kegelmeyer et al. has reported initially promising results for detecting spiculated tumors based on local edge characteristics and Laws texture features [44]. Zwiggelaar et al. developed a statistical model to describe and detect the abnormal pattern of linear structures of spiculated lesions [36]. Karssemeijer and te Brake [37] proposed to identify stellate distortions by using the orientation map of line-like structures, while Petrick et al. showed reduction of false positive detection by combining breast tissue composition information [39]. Zhang et al. used the Hough spectrum to detect spiculated lesions [41].

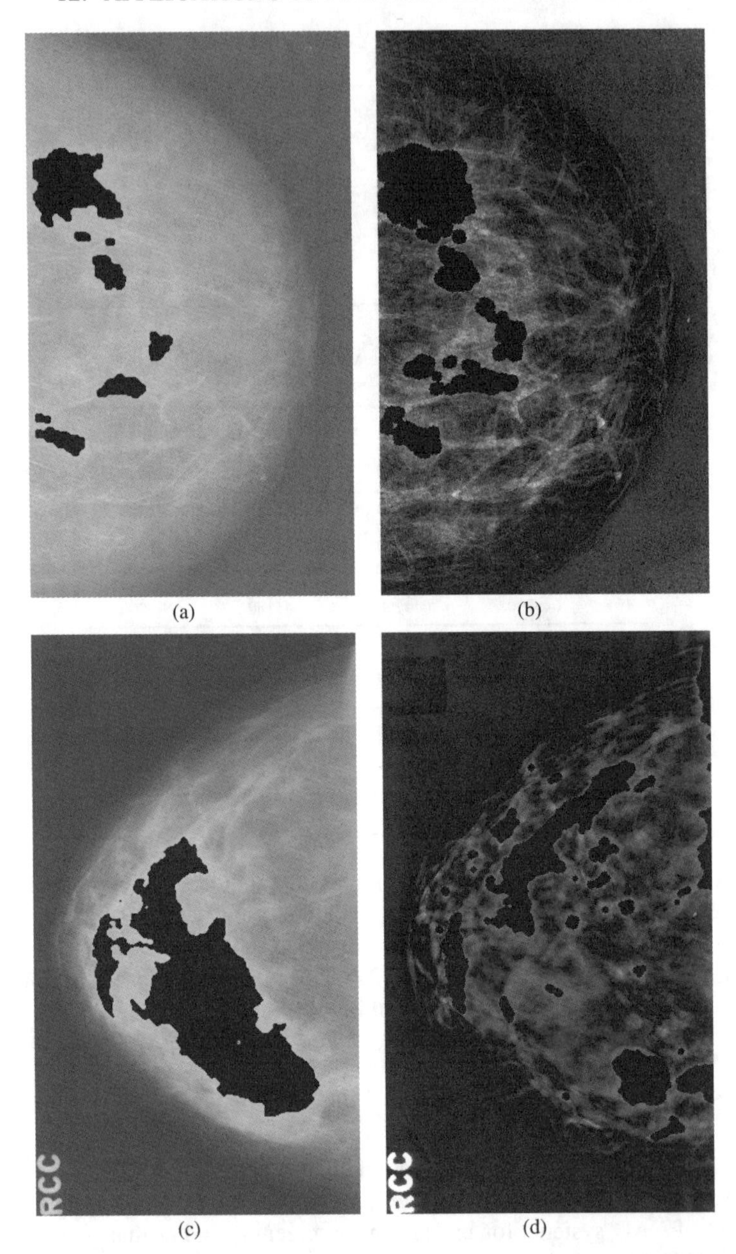

12.7 Segmentation results for suspected masses based on the original mammogram (a) and (c); (b) and (d) results based on the enhanced mammogram, $K = 4, \alpha = 3.0$.

As is the case in most classification type applications, the first and most critical step in CAD design is the construction of the database (choice of cases to include preprocessing of data, extraction and definition of relevant of features, and labeling of data, i.e., identification of classes). The next step involves design of the classifier, which typically is a problem in a high-dimensional space, requiring use of complex classifier structures due to the inherent complexity of the problem. For this reason, modular network structures that aim at partitioning the problem into simpler sets that are then weighted to form the decisions (e.g., as those discussed in Chapter 5) are particularly attractive solutions for the task. Section 12.3.1 introduces such a modular network and discusses its application to a carefully constructed featured knowledge database of suspicious mass sites for breast cancer screening/detection.

Another approach in CAD systems is to choose a network structure that can extract relevant features of disease patterns internally rather than defining explicit features. The second part of this chapter introduces an example of this approach and shows that convolutional neural networks can be effectively used for this task and applied to CAD design for breast mammography.

12.3.1 Feature-Based Modular Networks for CAD

In the following sections we describe the two main steps in the design of a feature-based CAD system: construction of a featured database and the database mapping, i.e., design of the modular neural network for performing the classification task. Even though our concentration in the discussion to follow is on CAD for breast cancer, most of the discussion and methodology is applicable to a variety of CAD design tasks such as electrocardiogram beat classification [42] and detection of malignant melonoma [43].

12.3.1.1 Feature Extraction

Even though feature extraction has been a key step in most pattern analysis tasks, the procedure is often carried out intuitively and heuristically. The general guidelines are

1. Discrimination — features of patterns in different classes should have significantly different values.
2. Reliability — features should have similar values for patterns of the same class.
3. Independence — features should not be strongly correlated to each other.
4. Optimality — some redundant features should be deleted. A small number of features is preferred for reducing the complexity of the classifier. Among a number of approaches for the task, principal component analysis has, by far, been the most widely used approach.

Many useful image features have been suggested by the image processing and pattern analysis communities [3, 48, 49]. These features can be divided into three categories, intensity features, geometric features, and texture features, whose values are calculated from the pixel matrices of the region of interest (ROI). Though these features are mathematically well defined, they may not be complete since they cannot capture all relevant aspects of human perception. Thus, we suggest inclusion of several additional expert-suggested features to reflect the radiologists' experiences. The typical features are summarized in Table 12.5, while Figure 12.8 shows the raw image of the corresponding featured sites.

(a)

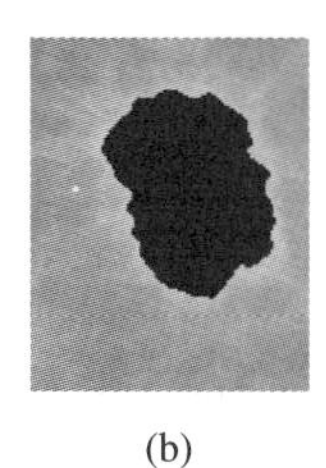
(b)

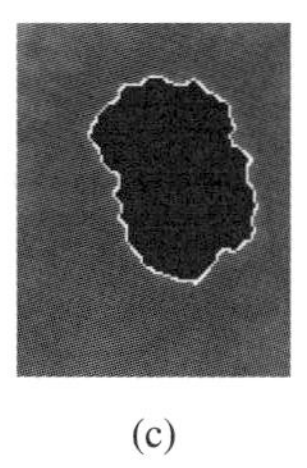
(c)

12.8 One example of mass segmentation and boundary extraction: (a) mass patch; (b) segmentation; and (c) boundary extraction.

TABLE 12.5 Summary of Mathematical Features

Feature Subspace	Features
A. Intensity Features	1. Contrast measure of ROI
	2. Standard derivation inside ROI
	3. Mean gradient of ROI's boundary
B. Geometric Features	1. Area measure
	2. Circularity measure
	3. Deviation of the normalized radial length
	4. Boundary roughness
C. Texture Features	1. Energy measure
	2. Correlation of co-occurrence matrix
	3. Inertia of co-occurrence matrix
	4. Entropy of co-occurrence matrix
	5. Inverse difference moment
	6. Sum average
	7. Sum entropy
	8. Difference entropy
	9. Fractal dimension of ROI surface

The joint histogram of the feature point distribution extracted from true and false mass regions is studied, and the features that can better separate the true and false mass regions are selected for further study. Our experience has suggested that three features, the site area, two measures of compactness (circularity), and difference entropy, led to better discrimination and reliability. They are defined as:
1. Compactness 1:

$$C_1 = \frac{A_1}{A} \tag{12.25}$$

where A is the area of the actual suspected region and A_1 is the area of the overlapping region of A and the effective circle A_c, defined as the circle whose area is equal to A and is centered at the corresponding centroid of A.
2. Compactness 2:

$$C_2 = \frac{P}{4\pi A} \tag{12.26}$$

where P is the boundary perimeter and A is the area of region.
3. Difference Entropy:

$$DH_{d,\theta} = -\sum_{k=0}^{L-1} p_{x-y}(k) \log p_{x-y}(k) \tag{12.27}$$

where

$$p_{x-y}(k) = \sum_{i=0}^{L-1}\sum_{j=0}^{L-1} p_{d,\theta}(i,j), \ |i-j| = k\,. \tag{12.28}$$

Several important observations are worth reiteration:

- The knowledge database that will be used by the CAD system is constructed from the cases selected by both lesion localization and human expert experience. This joint set provides more complete information and, during the interactive decision making, allows the CAD system to provide input when the cases are missed by the localization procedure but presented to the system by the radiologists.
- The knowledge database is defined quantitatively in a high-dimensional feature space. It provides not only the knowledge for training the neural network classifier, but also an objective base for evaluating the quality of feature extraction or a network's learning capability and the online visual explanation possibility.

- The assignment of the cases' class memberships (e.g., mass and non-mass classes) is supervised by the radiologists or pathological reports. A complete knowledge database includes three subsets: raw data of mass-like sites, corresponding feature points, and class membership labels.

12.3.1.2 Database Mapping

The decision making support by a CAD system addresses the problem of mapping a knowledge database given a finite set of data examples. The mapping function can therefore be interpreted as a quantitative representation of the knowledge about the mass lesions contained in the database [50]. Instead of mapping the whole data set using a single complex network, it is more practical to design a set of simple class subnets with local mixture clusters, each of which represents a specific region of the knowledge space. Inspired by the principle of divide-and-conquer in applied statistics, probabilistic modular neural networks (PMNNs) have become increasingly popular in machine learning research [16, 22, 50, 53, 56, 57]. This section presents PMNN applications to the problem of mapping from a feature database for mass detection.

Assume that the data points x_i in a database come from M classes $\{\omega_1, \ldots, \omega_r, \ldots, \omega_M\}$, and each class contains K_r clusters $\{\theta_1, \ldots, \theta_k, \ldots, \theta_{K_r}\}$, where ω_r is the model parameter vector of class r, and θ_k is the kernel parameter vector of cluster k within class r. Further assume that, in our training data set (which should be a representative subset of the whole database), each data point has a one-to-one correspondence to one of the classes, denoted by its class label l_{ir}^*, defining a supervised learning task, but the true memberships of the data to the local clusters are unknown, defining an unsupervised learning task. The class index r introduced here should not be confused with the parameter vector $\mathbf{r}$ introduced in Section 12.2.1.

For the model of local class distribution, since the true cluster membership for each data point is unknown, we can treat cluster labels of the data as random variables, denoted by l_{ik} [58]. By introducing a probability measure of a multinomial distribution with an unknown parameter π_k to reflect the distribution of the number of data points in each cluster, the relevant (sufficient) statistics are the conditional statistics for each cluster and the number of data points in each cluster. The class conditional probability measure for any data point inside the class r, i.e., the standard finite mixture distribution (SFMD), can be obtained by writing down the joint probability density of the x_i and l_{ik} and then summing it over all possible outcomes of l_{ik}, as a sum of the following general form:

$$f\left(u|\omega_r\right) = \sum_{k=1}^{K_r} \pi_k g\left(u|\theta_k\right) \tag{12.29}$$

where $\pi_k = P(\theta_k|\omega_r)$ with a summation equal to one, and $g(u|\theta_k)$ is the kernel function of the local cluster distribution. Note that the formulations given in Equations (12.4) and (12.29) are intimately related. The mixture model in Equation (12.4) is for modeling the pixel image distribution over the whole image and the pixel images are scalar valued quantities, whereas here, in Equation (12.29), we are assuming a mixture distribution within each class and, hence, we specify the class index in the formulation and modeling the feature vector distribution; therefore, u will typically be multidimensional.

Also important to note are the following: (1) all data points in a class are identically distributed from a mixture distribution; (2) the SFMD model uses the probability measure of data memberships to the clusters in the formulation instead of realizing the true cluster label for each data point; and (3) since the calculation of the data histogram $f_{\mathbf{x}_r}$ from a class relies on the same mechanism as in Equation (12.29), its values can be considered as a sampled version of the true class distribution f_r^*.

For the model of global class distributions, let the prior for each class be given by $P(\omega_r)$, then the sufficient statistics for mapping the database, i.e., the conditional finite mixture distribution (CFMD), is the pair $\{P(\omega_r), f(u|\omega_r)\}$. The posterior probability $P(\omega_r|x_i)$ given a particular observation x_i can be obtained by Bayes rule:

$$P(\omega_r|x_i) = \frac{P(\omega_r)f(x_i|\omega_r)}{p(x_i)} \tag{12.30}$$

where $p(x_i) = \Sigma_{r=1}^{M} P(\omega_r)f(x_i|\omega_r)$. Hence, (1) in order to classify the data points into classes, Equation (12.30) is a candidate as a discriminant function; (2) since defining a supervised learning requires information of l_{ir}^*, the Bayesian prior $P(\omega_r)$ is an intrinsically known parameter and can be easily estimated by $P(\omega_r) = \Sigma_{i=1}^{N} l_{ir}^*/N$; and (3) the only uncertainty in the estimation comes from class likelihood function $f(u|\omega_r)$ that should be the key issue in the follow-on learning process. For simplicity, in the following context we will omit class index r in our discussion when only single class distribution model is concerned, and we will use θ to denote the parameter vector of regional parameter set $\{(\pi_k, \theta_k)\}$.

Given the SFMD in Equation (12.29), the model, model order (the number of clusters within a class distribution), and model parameters can be estimated/learned using the same framework introduced in Sections 12.2.1.1 and 12.2.1.2.

12.3.1.3 Data Classification via Supervised Learning

The objective of data classification is to realize the class membership l_{ir} for each data point based on the observation x_i and the class statistics $\{P(\omega_r), f(u|\omega_r)\}$. It is well known that the optimal data classifier is the Bayes classifier since it can achieve the minimum rate of classification error [23]. Measuring the average classification error by the mean squared error E, it is shown that minimizing E by adjusting the parameters of class statistics is equivalent to directly approximating the posterior class probabilities when dealing with the two-class problem [23, 51]. In general, for the multiple class problem, the optimal Bayes classifier assigns input patterns into classes based on their posterior probability: input x_i is classified into class ω_r if

$$P(\omega_r|x_i) > P(\omega_j|x_i) \tag{12.31}$$

for all $j \neq r$, a procedure that minimizes the average error.

Note that the ultimate aim is the design of the network as an estimator of the posterior class probability. Direct estimation of the posterior class probability $P(\omega_r|x_i)$ requires use of a global type approximator, such as the multilayer perceptron network, while the class conditional density $f(x_i|\omega_r)$ is usually estimated using local approximators such as radial basis function networks. Jordan [54] and Ni et al. [55] present a discussion of the major issues involved in the design for either case. In general, global approximators imply more robust performance at the expense of slower convergence, while the local approximators are very effective if they provide a good match to data structure. A good match of the model to the database will also ensure efficiency in the estimation/learning of parameters. Here, we propose use of local models (finite mixtures, i.e., radial basis type models) within a modular structure increasing the flexibility of the model as well as the efficiency in learning the parameters of the overall model. And since the prior class probability $P(\omega_r)$ is known in supervised learning, the posterior class probability $P(\omega_r|x_i)$ is easily obtained by the Bayes relationship Equation (12.30). Also note that when the ultimate goal of learning is data classification, the question may be asked: learning class likelihoods or decision boundaries? Since, in fact, only the decision boundaries are the quantities of interest, the problem can be reformulated as the learning of class boundaries (much more efficient) rather than class likelihoods (generally time consuming). Thus, an efficient supervised algorithm to learn the class conditional likelihood densities, called decision-based learning [56], is adopted here. The decision-based learning algorithm uses the misclassified data to adjust the density functions $f(u|\omega_r)$, which are initially obtained using the unsupervised learning scheme described previously, so that minimum classification error can be achieved. The algorithm is summarized as follows.

Define the rth class discriminant function $\phi_r(x_i, \mathbf{w})$ as $P(\omega_r)f(x_i|\omega_r)$. Assume a set of training patterns $\mathbf{X}=\{x_i; i = 1, 2, \ldots, M\}$. The set $\mathbf{X}$ is further divided into a positive training set $\mathbf{X}^+=\{x_i; x_i \in \omega_r, i = 1, 2, \ldots, N\}$ and a negative training set $\mathbf{X}^-=\{x_i; x_i \notin \omega_r, i = N+1, N+2, \ldots, M\}$. Define an energy function:

$$E = \sum_{i=1}^{M} l(d(i)) \tag{12.32}$$

where

$$d(i) = \begin{cases} T - \phi_r(x_i, \mathbf{w}) & \text{if } x_i \in \mathbf{X}^+ \\ \phi_r(x_i, \mathbf{w}) - T & \text{if } x_i \in \mathbf{X}^- \end{cases} \tag{12.33}$$

where $T = \max_{\forall j \neq r}(\phi_j(x_i, \mathbf{w}))$. The penalty function l can be either a piecewise linear function

$$l(d) = \begin{cases} \zeta d & \text{if } d \geq 0 \\ 0 & \text{if } d < 0 \end{cases} \tag{12.34}$$

where ζ is a positive constant or a sigmoidal function:

$$l(d) = \frac{1}{1 + \exp^{-d/\xi}} . \tag{12.35}$$

Notice that the energy function E is always large or equal to zero, and only misclassified training patterns contribute to the energy function. Therefore, the misclassification is minimized if E is minimized.

The reinforced and anti-reinforced learning rules are used to update the network:

$$\begin{aligned} &\text{Reinforced Learning:} && \mathbf{w}^{(j+1)} = \mathbf{w}^{(j)} + \eta l'(d(t))\nabla\phi(\mathbf{x}(t), \mathbf{w}) \\ &\text{Anti-reinforced Learning:} && \mathbf{w}^{(j+1)} = \mathbf{w}^{(j)} - \eta l'(d(t))\nabla\phi(\mathbf{x}(t), \mathbf{w}) . \end{aligned} \tag{12.36}$$

If the misclassified training pattern is from the positive training set, reinforced learning will be applied. If the training pattern belongs to the negative training set, we anti-reinforce the learning, i.e., pull the kernels away from the problematic regions.

12.3.1.4 Application Example

This section presents the application of the framework introduced in Sections 12.3.1.1–12.3.1.3 to CAD design for breast cancer. We design the classifier to distinguish true masses from false masses based on the features extracted from the suspected regions. The objective is to reduce the number of suspicious regions and to identify the true masses.

We use the same database described in Section 12.2.3 and select 150 mammograms from the 200 study mammograms in our database. Each mammogram selected contains at least one mass case of varying size and location. The areas of suspicious masses are identified following the proposed procedure with biopsy proven results. Fifty mammograms with biopsy proven masses are selected from the 150 mammograms for training. The mammogram set used for testing contained 46 single-view mammograms which were also selected from the 150 mammograms: 23 normal cases and 23 with biopsy proven masses. The same image size reduction discussed in Section 12.2.3 is employed here as well.

After segmentation, the area index feature is first used to eliminate the non-mass regions. In our study, we set $A_1 = 7 \times 7$ pixels and $A_2 = 75 \times 75$ pixels as the thresholds. A_1 corresponds to the smallest size of masses (3 mm), and an object with an area of 75×75 pixels corresponds to 30 mm in the original mammogram. This indicates that the scheme can detect all masses with sizes up to 30 mm. Masses larger than 30 mm are rare cases in the clinical setting. When the segmented region satisfies the condition $A_1 \leq A \leq A_2$, the region is considered to be suspicious for mass. For representative demonstration, we select a three-dimensional feature space consisting of compactness 1, compactness 2, and difference entropy. These three features have been determined as having the better separation (discrimination) between the true and false mass classes. It should be noted that the feature vector can easily extend to higher dimensions. A training feature vector set is constructed from 50 true mass ROIs and 50 false mass ROIs, then used to train two modular probabilistic decision-based neural networks separately. In addition to the decision boundaries recommended by the computer algorithms, a visual explanation interface has also been integrated with three-dimensional to two-dimensional hierarchical projections. Figure 12.9a shows the database map projection with compactness 1 and difference entropy. Figure 12.9b shows the database map

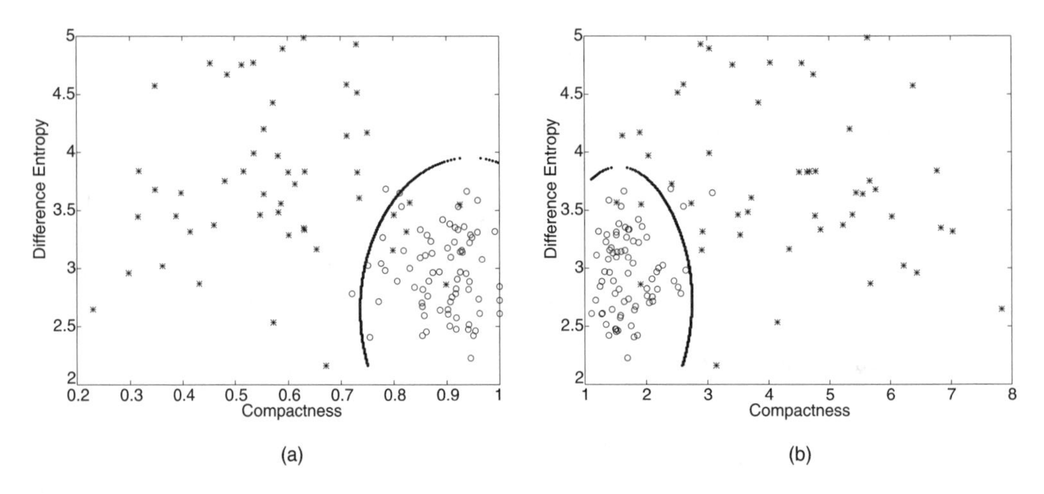

12.9 Classification results: -o- denotes true mass cases; -*- denotes false mass cases. (a) classification using compactness 1; (b) classification using compactness 2.

projection with compactness 2 and difference entropy. Our experience has suggested that the recognition rate with compactness 1 is more reliable than that with compactness 2. In order to have more accurate texture information, the computation of the second-order joint probability matrix $p_{d,\theta}(i, j)$ is based only on the segmented region of the original mammogram. For the shrunk mammograms, we found that the difference entropy had better discrimination with $d = 1$. The difference entropy used in this study was the average of values at $\theta = 0°, 45°, 90°$, and $135°$.

We have conducted a preliminary study to evaluate the performance of the CAD in real case detection, in which 6 to 15 suspected masses per mammogram were detected and classified as requiring further clinical evaluation. We found that the proposed classifier can reduce the number of suspicious masses with a sensitivity of 84% at 1.6 false positive findings per mammogram based on the testing data set containing 46 mammograms (23 of them have biopsy proven masses). Figure 12.10 shows a representative mass detection result on one mammogram with a stellate mass. After the enhancement, ten regions with the brightest intensity were segmented. Using the area criterion, too large and too small regions were eliminated first, and the remaining regions were submitted to the PMNN for further evaluation. The results indicated that the stellate mass lesion was correctly detected.

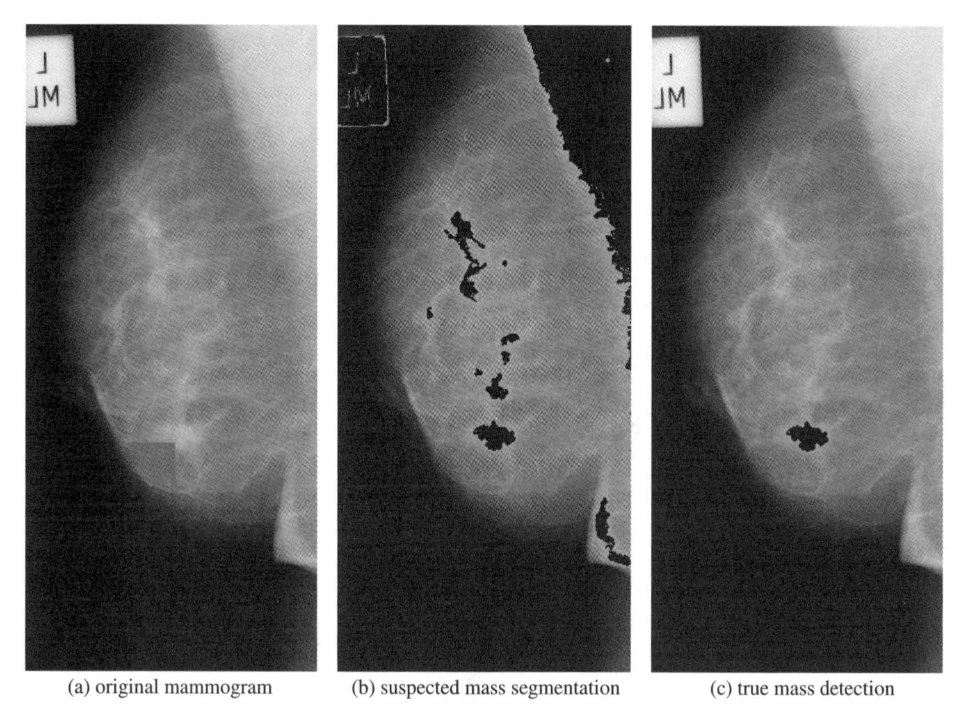

(a) original mammogram (b) suspected mass segmentation (c) true mass detection

12.10 One example of mass detection using the modular neural network classifier.

12.3.2 Convolutional Neural Networks for CAD Design

The CAD introduced in the previous section (Section 12.3.1) first extracts a set of features from the input database and then designs a neural network classifier for the specific detection task using those features. Another option is to use a neural network to automatically extract relevant features from the data set before classification. For this task, the network structure has to be carefully chosen for the given data set and the problem. In what follows, we first describe the convolutional neural networks that can be used to extract relevant features from an image database by carefully selecting the network parameters. We then discuss application of a CNN to detection of clustered microcalcifications.

12.3.2.1 General Architecture of the CNN

The CNN is a simplified version of a "neocognitron," which simulates the network structure and signal propagation in vertebrate animal vision [59, 60].

To explain the structure of a CNN, consider the simple CNN shown in Figure 12.11. A CNN typically consists of an input layer, one or more hidden layers (convolution layers), and an output layer. The input layer of the CNN contains $M \times M$ input nodes that represent $M \times M$ pixels of the ROIs to be recognized. Each convolution layer has local connections with the preceding layer (either the input layer or the previous hidden layer). The nodes in the hidden layer are organized into different groups and the groups between adjacent layers are locally connected by weighting coefficients that are arranged in kernels. For example, as shown in Figure 12.11, the input layer contains $M \times M$ nodes and the kernel size is $K \times K$. The hidden layer is organized in n groups. The number of nodes in each group is $N \times N$ ($N = M - K + 1$ for a $K \times K$ kernel). The total number of links between the input layer and the hidden layer is $n \times K^2 \times N^2$. Learning is constrained such that the kernel weights connecting two groups in the adjacent hidden layers (or between the input and the hidden layers) are shift invariant. As a result, the number of independent links is $n \times K^2$.

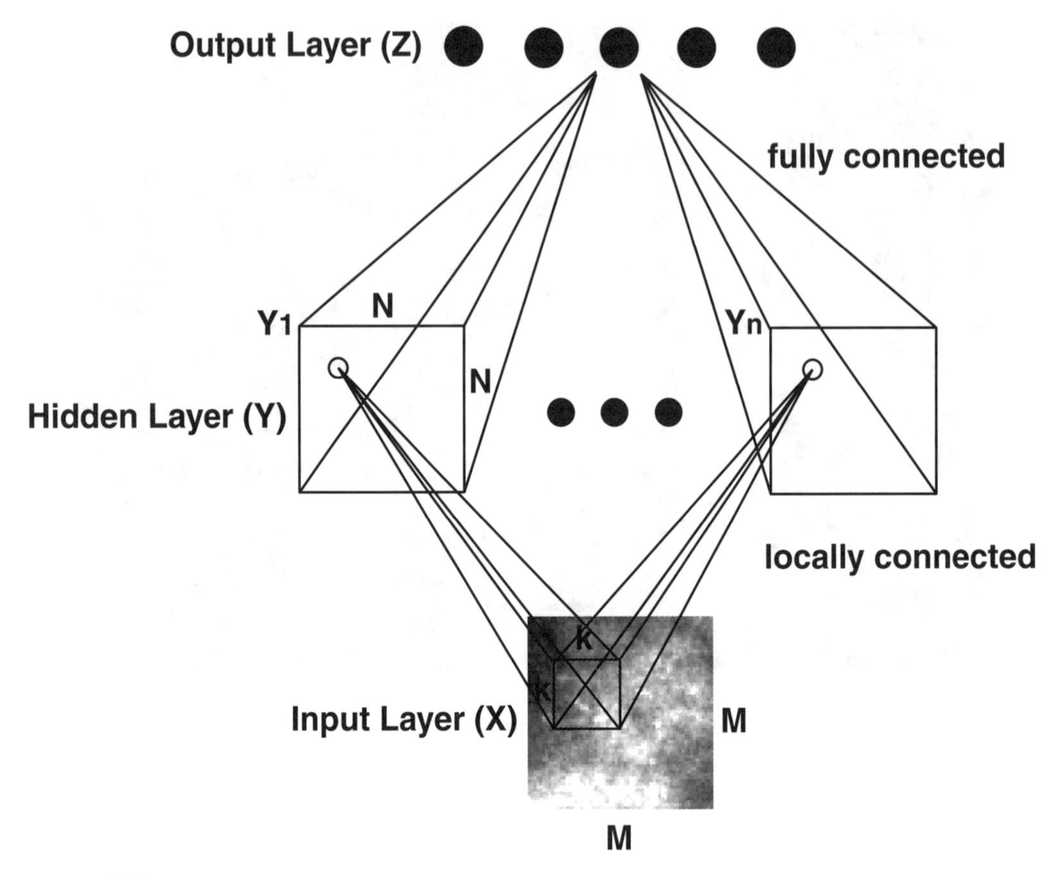

12.11 CNN structure.

The output layer is fully connected to the previous hidden layer. If the output layer contains N_Z nodes, the total number of links are $N_Z \times n \times N^2$.

Similar to the multilayer perceptron network, the signals input into the CNN are convolved with the weight kernels, and the value of the convolution is collected into the corresponding node in the upper layer. The value is further processed by the node through an activation function and produces an output signal. The output signal is forward propagated in a similar manner. It is expected that the CNN first extracts the features in the hidden convolution layers and then classifies these features in the output stage. The convolution kernels are trained to form a set of feature extractors by supervised learning. Each convolution kernel is expected to function as an image analyzer and perform a specific feature-extracting operation on the ROIs. Moreover, the output stage is trained to classify the features at the output layer.

To illustrate the signal propagation and the training process, we consider a one-hidden-layer CNN (Figure 12.11) and define the following:

$X_{i,j}$ = the input signal, $i, j = 1, \ldots, M$

$Y^{n_g}_{i',j'}$ = the output signal in the n_gth group of the hidden layer, $n_g = 1, \ldots, n$, $i', j' = 1, \ldots, N$

Z_o = the output signal at oth node of the output layer, $o = 1, \ldots, N_Z$, N_Z is the total number of output nodes

$v^{n_g}_{lm:(i,j)\to(i',j')}$ = the weighting kernels connecting the node (i', j') of the n_gth group in the hidden layer and the node $(i - l + 1, j - m + 1)$ in the input layer, $l, m = 1, \ldots, K$

$w^{n_g}_{i'j':(i',j')\to(o)}$ = the weighting factors connecting the oth node of the output layer and the node (i', j') of the n_gth group of the hidden layer, $n_g = 1, \ldots, n, i', j' = 1, \ldots, N$.

When the sigmoidal function is used as the activation function, the output signals at the hidden and output layers are given as:

$$Y^{n_g}_{i',j'} = \frac{1}{1 + \exp\{-[\sum_{l=1}^{K} \sum_{m=1}^{K} (v^{n_g}_{lm:(i,j)\to(i',j')} X_{i-l+1,j-m+1}) + a_{i,j}]\}} \tag{12.37}$$

$$Z_o = \frac{1}{1 + \exp\{-[\sum_{n_g=1}^{n} \sum_{i'=1}^{N} \sum_{j'=1}^{N} (w^{n_g}_{i'j':(i',j')\to(o)} Y^{n_g}_{i',j'}) + b_{i',j'}]\}} \tag{12.38}$$

where $a_{i,j}$ and $b_{i',j'}$ are the bias terms. Note that the weighting kernel connecting the input and the hidden layer should be shift invariant,i.e.,

$$v^{n_g}_{lm:(i,j)\to(i',j')} = v^{n_g}_{lm:(i+s,j+s)\to(i'+s,j'+s)} = v^{n_g}_{lm}$$

where s is a shifting factor. For each node, (i', j') corresponds to only one position (i, j) in the input ROIs such that $i' = i - K + 1,\ j' = j - K + 1$.

12.3.2.2 Supervised Training of the CNN

A back-propagation algorithm can be easily derived for training the CNN. We define the cost function to be minimized as

$$E = \frac{1}{2} \sum_{o=1}^{N_Z} [Z_{do} - Z_o]^2 \tag{12.39}$$

where Z_{do} is the desired value of a given training pattern at the oth node of the output layer. The conventional steepest descent delta rule for back-propagation training is applied to update all weighting factors connecting the adjacent layers.

At the hidden layer, weights can be updated as:

$$v^{n_g}_{lm:(i,j)\to(i',j')}(t+1) = v^{n_g}_{lm:(i,j)\to(i',j')}(t) + \alpha \sum_{lm} \left[\beta^{n_g}_{i'j'} X_{i-l+1,j-m+1}\right] \tag{12.40}$$

where α is a gain factor and

$$\beta^{n_g}_{i'j'} = Y^{n_g}_{i',j'} \left[1 - Y^{n_g}_{i',j'}\right] Q^{n_g}_{i',j'} \tag{12.41}$$

and

$$Q^{n_g}_{i',j'} = \sum_{o} \left[w^{n_g}_{i'j':(i',j')\to(o)} \delta_o\right] . \tag{12.42}$$

At the output layer, the weights are updated as

$$w^{n_g}_{i'j':(i',j')\to(o)}(t+1) = w^{n_g}_{i'j':(i',j')\to(o)}(t) + \eta \delta_o Y^{n_g}_{i',j'} \tag{12.43}$$

where η is a gain factor and

$$\delta_o = Z_o [1 - Z_o] [Z_{do} - Z_o] . \tag{12.44}$$

All weights in the CNN are initialized to a small random value, e.g., a random number in the range -0.5 to 0.5. The training process is terminated when the total cost achieves a certain low tolerance.

12.3.2.3 Application Example

Computer automated detection of clustered microcalcifications has been an active area of research. Chan et al. [46, 61] first demonstrated that a difference-image technique can effectively detect microcalcifications on digitized mammograms. Fam et al. [62] and Davies and Dance [63] detected clustered microcalcifications using conventional image processing techniques. In their studies, local thresholding and region growing algorithms were used to segment suspected regions. The segmented objects were then analyzed using size, shape, and gradient measures to detect true clusters of microcalcifications. The detection methods used in these early works included Bayesian classifiers and binary decision trees. Wu et al. [64] used multilayer perceptron networks to detect microcalcifications based on features extracted from the power spectrum of the suspected regions. More recently, Lo et al. [65] proposed a CNN combined with a regional clustering criterion to recognize clustered microcalcifications. This section shows successful application of CNN for CAD design for clustered microcalcification detection using a partial wavelet reconstruction approach to enhance the signal pattern in the ROIs [35].

Evaluation of the CNN classifer we introduced in Sections 12.3.2.1 and 12.3.2.2 is conducted using a database of 91 selected mammograms. Each mamogram is digitized into $2048 \times 2500 \times 12$ bits (for an 8" × 11" area where each image pixel represents a 100 μm square). All mammograms are selected from different patients, and the sizes of all digitized mammograms reduced to $512 \times 625 \times 12$ bits using 4×4 pixel averaging and then processed by the methodology explained earlier in this section. Based on the corresponding biopsy reports, one experienced radiologist evaluates all 91 mammograms and identifies 75 areas containing masses. (Note that the reports record the malignancy of the biopsy specimens. The radiologist only uses them as reference for the identification of masses.) Through the preprocess and the first-step screen based on the circularity test, a total of 125 suspicious areas are extracted from the 91 digitized mammograms.

We randomly select 54 computer-segmented areas where 30 patches are matched with the radiologist's identification and 24 are not. This database is used to train two neural network classifiers: (1) a standard multilayer perceptron (MLP) and (2) a CNN. The structures of both networks are determined through cross-validation using the receiver operating characteristics (ROCs) method.

In the ROC analysis, the distribution of the positive and negative cases can be represented by certain probability distributions. When the two distributions overlap on the decision axis, a cut-off point can be made at an arbitrary decision threshold. The corresponding true-positive fraction (TPF) vs. false-positive fraction (FPF) for each threshold can be drawn on a plane. By indicating several points on the plot, curve fitting can be employed to construct an ROC curve. The area under the curve, which is referred to as Az, can be used as a performance index of the system. In general, the higher the Az value, the better the performance of the system under study. In addition, two other indices, sensitivity (TPF) and specificity (1−FPF), are usually used to evaluate the system performance on the specified point of the ROC curve. In this study, a computer program (LABROC) [66] is employed for the analysis.

We used the database first to determine the best neural network structure. For the CNN, a significantly higher value of Az was obtained when we used a 16×16 pixel region for the input and 5×5 pixels for the convolution kernel size. In addition, the use of two hidden layers resulted in better performance than the use of a single hidden layer. A 3×3 convolution kernel size was used in the second hidden layer. In addition, 12 and 8 groups were used in the first and second hidden layers, respectively. For the MLP, best ROC performance was obtained for a single hidden layer structure with an input layer equal to the total number of pixels in the image, a hidden layer with 125 nodes, and a single output for the binary decision.

For testing the performance of the two networks, we used the remaining 71 computer segmented areas that were not part of the training set. The neural network output values were fed into LABROC, and the results indicated that the areas Az under the ROC curves were 0.781 for the MLP and 0.844

for the CNN. The ROC curves of these two neural networks are shown in Figure 12.12a. We also invited another senior mammographer to conduct an ROC observer study. The mammographer was

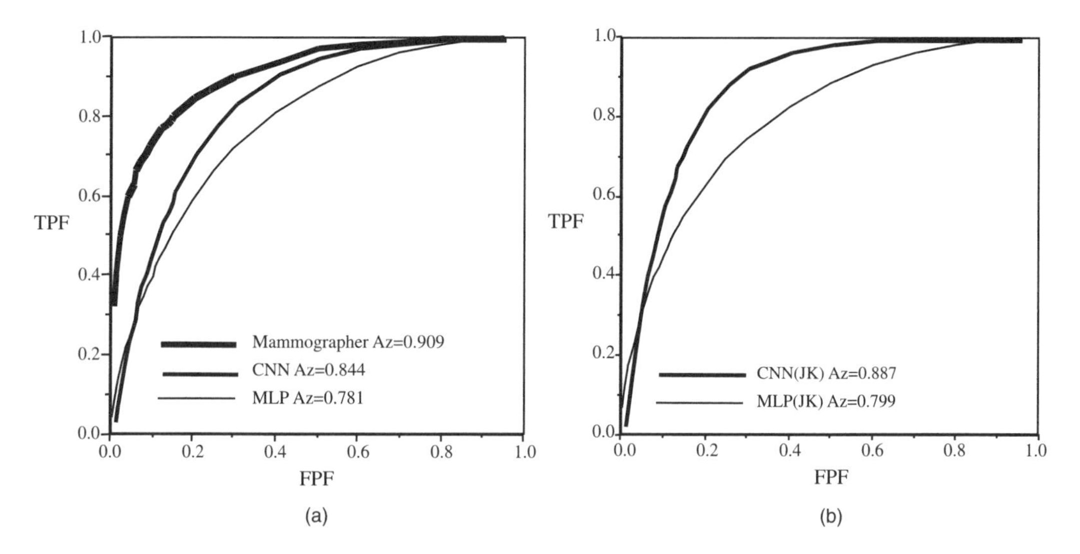

12.12 ROC evaluation results: (a) comparison of ROC curves for the MLP, CNN, and the human observer performance; (b) comparison of ROC curves for the MLP and CNN performance for the leave-one-case-out experiment.

asked to rate each patch using a numerical scale ranging from 0 to 10 regarding its likelihood of being a mass. These 71 numbers were also fed into the LABROC program. The mammographer's performance in Az on this set of test cases was 0.909 and is also shown in Figure 12.12a.

We further conducted a leave-one-out experiment using the same database. In this experiment, we used those patches extracted from 90 of the mammograms for the training and used the patches extracted from the one remaining mammogram as test objects. The procedure was repeated 91 times to allow every suspicious patch from each mammogram to be tested in the experiment. For each individual suspicious area, the computed features were identical to those used in the previous experiment. Again, both neural network classifiers were independently evaluated with the same procedure. The results are shown in Figure 12.12b with Az values of 0.799 for the MLP and 0.887 for the CNN classifier.

References

[1] Applications of Neural Networks in Biomedical Signal Processing special session, *Proceedings of the IEEE International Workshop on Neural Networks for Signal Processing (NNSP),* Amelia Island Plantation, FL, Sept. 1997.

[2] R. Chellappa, Q. Zheng, P. Burlina, C. Shekhar and K. Eom, On the positioning of multi-sensor imagery for exploitation and target recognition, *Proceedings of IEEE,* vol. 85, no. 1, pp. 120–138, Jan. 1997.

[3] A.K. Jain, *Markov Random Fields: Theory and Application,* Boston, Academic Press, 1993.

[4] T. Lei and W. Sewchand, Statistical approach to x-ray CT imaging and its application in image analysis — Part II: a new stochastic model-based image segmentation technique for x-ray CT image, *IEEE Transactions on Medical Imaging,* vol. 11, no. 1, pp. 62–69, Mar. 1992.

[5] Y. Wang and T. Adali, Efficient learning of finite normal mixtures for image quantification, in

Proceedings of the IEEE International Conference in Acoustics, Speech, and Signal Processing, Atlanta, GA, pp. 3422–3425, 1996.

[6] Y. Wang, MR imaging statistics and model-based MR image analysis, Ph.D. dissertation, University of Maryland, Baltimore, May 1995.

[7] H. Li, Y. Wang, K.J.R. Liu, S.C.B Lo, Statistical model supported approach to radiographic mass detection — Part I: improving lesion characterization by morphological filtering and site segmentation, *IEEE Transactions on Medical Imaging,* to appear.

[8] Y. Wang, T. Adali, M.T. Freedman, and S.K. Mun, MR brain image analysis by distribution learning and relaxation labeling, *Proceedings of the 15th Southern Biomedical Engineering Conference,* pp. 133–136, Dayton, OH, Mar. 1996.

[9] Y. Wang, T. Adali, C. Lau, and S.Y. Kung, Quantitative analysis of MR brain image sequences by adaptive self-organizing mixtures, *Journal of VLSI Signal Processing Systems for Signal, Image, and Video Technology,* special issue on neural networks for biomedical image processing, vol. 18, no. 3, pp. 219–239, Apr. 1998.

[10] J. Zhang and J.W. Modestino, A model-fitting approach to cluster validation with application to stochastic model-based image segmentation, *IEEE Transactions on PAMI,* vol. 12, no. 10, pp. 1009–1017, Oct. 1990.

[11] Y. Wang, T. Adali, S.Y. Kung, and Z. Szabo, Quantification and segmentation of brain tissue from MR images: a probabilistic neural network approach, *IEEE Transactions on Image Processing,* special issue on applications of neural networks to image processing, vol. 7, no. 8, pp. 1165–1181, Aug. 1998.

[12] T. Adali, X. Liu, and M.K. Sönmez, Conditional distribution learning with neural networks and its application to channel equalization, *IEEE Transactions on Signal Processing,* vol. 45, no. 4, pp. 1051–1064, Apr. 1997.

[13] D.M. Titterington, A.F.M. Smith, and U.E. Markov, *Statistical Analysis of Finite Mixture Distributions,* New York, John Wiley & Sons, 1985.

[14] A.P. Dempster, N.M. Laird, and D.B. Rubin, Maximum likelihood from incomplete data via the EM algorithm, *Journal of the Royal Statistical Society Series B*, vol. 39, pp. 1–38, 1977.

[15] R.A. Redner and N.M. Walker, Mixture densities, maximum likelihood and the EM algorithm, *SIAM Review,* vol. 26, pp. 195–239, 1984.

[16] L. Perlovsky and M. McManus, Maximum likelihood neural networks for sensor fusion and adaptive classification, *Neural Networks,* vol. 4, pp. 89–102, 1991.

[17] L. Kullback, and R.A. Leibler, On information and sufficiency, *Annals of Mathematics and Statistics,* vol. 22, pp. 79–86, 1951.

[18] L. Xu and M.I. Jordan, On convergence properties of the EM algorithm for Gaussian mixture, Technical Report, MIT Artificial Intelligence Laboratory, Jan. 1995.

[19] J.L. Marroquin and F. Girosi, Some extensions of the k-means algorithm for image segmentation and pattern classification, Technical Report, MIT Artificial Intelligence Laboratory, Jan. 1993.

[20] E. Weinstein, M. Feder, and A.V. Oppenheim, Sequential algorithms for parameter estimation based on the Kullback–Leibler information measure, *IEEE Transactions on Acoustics Speech, and Signal Processing,* vol. 38, no. 9, pp. 1652–1654, 1990.

[21] T.M. Cover and J.A. Thomas, *Elements of Information Theory,* New York, John Wiley & Sons, 1991.

[22] S. Haykin, *Neural Networks: A Comprehensive Foundation,* New York, Macmillan College Publishing Company, 1994.

[23] H.V. Poor, *An Introduction to Signal Detection and Estimation,* New York, Springer-Verlag, 1996.

[24] Y. Wang, T. Adali, and B. Lo, Automatic threshold selection by histogram quantization, *SPIE Journal of Biomedical Optics,* vol. 2, no. 2, pp. 211–217, Apr. 1997.

[25] H. Akaike, A new look at the statistical model identification, *IEEE Transactions on Automatic Control,* vol. 19, no. 6, Dec. 1974.

[26] J. Rissanen, A universal prior for integers and estimation by minimum description length, *The Annals of Statistics,* vol. 11, no. 2, 1983.

[27] G. Schwartz, Estimating the dimension of a model, *The Annals of Statistics,* vol. 6, no. 2, pp. 461–464, 1978.

[28] M. Wax and T. Kailath, Detection of signals by information theoretic criteria, *IEEE Transactions on Acoustics, Speech, and Signal Processing,* vol. 33, no. 2, Apr. 1985.

[29] R.A. Hummel and S.W. Zucker, On the foundations of relaxation labeling processes, *IEEE Transactions on Pattern Analysis and Machine Intelligence,* vol. 5, no. 3, May 1983.

[30] P. Santago and H.D. Gage, Quantification of MR brain images by mixture density and partial volume modeling, *IEEE Transactions on Medical Imaging,* vol. 12, no. 3, pp. 566–574, Sept. 1993.

[31] A.J. Worth and D.N. Kennedy, Segmentation of magnetic resonance brain images using analog constraint satisfaction neural networks, *Information Processing in Medical Imaging,* pp. 225–243, 1993.

[32] L.O. Hall, A.M. Bensaid, L.P. Clarke, R.P. Velthuizen, M.S. Silbiger, and J.C. Bezdek, A comparison of neural network and fuzzy clustering techniques in segmenting magnetic resonance images of the brain, *IEEE Transactions on Neural Networks,* vol. 3, pp. 672–682, 1992.

[33] H.E. Cline, W.E. Lorensen, R. Kikinis, and R. Jolesz, Three-dimensional segmentation of MR images of the head using probability and connectivity, *Journal of Computer Assisted Tomography,* vol. 14, pp. 1037–1045, 1990.

[34] Z. Liang, J.R. MacFall, and D.P. Harrington, Parameter estimation and tissue segmentation from multispectral MR images, *IEEE Transactions on Medical Imaging,* vol. 13, no. 3, pp. 441–449, Sept. 1994.

[35] H. Li, Model-based image processing techniques for breast cancer detection in digital mammography, Ph.D. dissertation, University of Maryland, May 1997.

[36] R. Zwiggelaar, T.C. Parr, J.E. Schumm, I.W. Hutt, C.J. Taylor, S.M. Astley, and C.R.M. Boggis, Model-based detection of spiculated lesions in mammograms, *Medical Image Analysis,* vol. 3, no. 1, pp. 39–62, 1999.

[37] N. Karssemeijer and G.M. te Brake, Detection of stellate distortions in mammograms, *IEEE Transactions on Medical Imaging,* vol. 15, pp. 611–619, 1996.

[38] L. Miller and N. Ramsey, The detection of malignant masses by non-linear multiscale analysis, *Excerpta Medica,* vol. 1119, pp. 335–340, 1996.

[39] N. Petrick, H.P. Chan, B. Sahiner, M.A. Helvie, M.M. Goodsitt, and D.D. Adler, Computer-aided breast mass detection: false positive reduction using breast tissue composition, *Excerpta Medica,* vol. 1119, pp. 373–378, 1996.

[40] W.K. Zouras, M.L. Giger, P. Lu, D.E. Wolverton, C.J. Vyborny, and K. Doi, Investigation of a temporal subtraction scheme for computerized detection of breast masses in mammograms, *Excerpta Medica,* vol. 1119, pp. 411–415, 1996.

[41] M. Zhang, M.L. Giger, C.J. Vyborny, and K. Doi, Mammographic texture analysis for the detection of spiculated lesions, *Excerpta Medica,* vol. 1119, pp. 347–351, 1996.

[42] Y.H. Hu, S. Palreddy, and W.J. Tompkins, Patient-adaptable ECG beat classifier using a mixture of experts approach, *IEEE Transactions on Signal Processing,* vol. 44, no. 9, pp. 891–900, 1997.

[43] M. Hintz-Madsen, L.K. Hansen, J. Larsen, E. Olesen, and K.T. Drzewiecki, Detection of melanoma using neural classifiers, in *Proceedings of the IEEE Workshop on Neural Networks for Signal Processing (NNSP),* Piscataway, NJ, pp. 223–232, 1996.

[44] W.P. Kegelmeyer Jr., J.M. Pruneda, P.D. Bourland, A. Hillis, M.W. Riggs, and M.L. Nipper, Computer-aided mammographic screening for spiculated lesions, *Radiology,* vol. 191, pp. 331–337, 1994.

[45] R.N. Strickland, Tumor detection in non-stationary backgrounds, *IEEE Transactions on Medical Imaging,* vol. 13, no. 3, pp. 491–499, 1994.

[46] H.P. Chan, D. Wei, M.A. Helvie, B. Sahiner, D.D. Alder, M.M. Goodsitt, and N. Petrick, Computer-aided classification of mammographic masses and normal tissue: linear discriminant analysis in texture feature space, *Phys. Med. Biol.,* vol. 40, pp. 857–876, 1995.

[47] M.L. Giger, C.J. Vyborny, and R.A. Schmidt, Computerized characterization of mammographic masses: analysis of spiculation, *Cancer Letters,* vol. 77, pp. 201–211, 1994.

[48] R.M. Haralick, K. Shanmugam, and I. Dinstein, Textural features for image classification, *IEEE Transactions on Systems, Man, and Cybernetics,* vol. SMC-3, no. 6, pp. 610–621, Nov. 1973.

[49] R. Schalkoff, *Pattern Recognition: Statistical, Structural, and Neural Approaches,* New York, John Wiley & Sons, 1992.

[50] Y. Wang, S.-H. Lin, H. Li, and S.-Y. Kung, Data mapping by probabilistic modular network and information theoretic criteria, *IEEE Transactions on Signal Processing,* pp. 3378–3397, Dec. 1998.

[51] H. Gish, A probabilistic approach to the understanding and training of neural network classifiers, in *Proceedings of the IEEE International Conference on Acoustics, Speech, and Signal Processing,* vol. 2, pp. 1361–1364, 1990.

[52] C.E. Priebe, Adaptive mixtures, *Journal of the American Statistical Association,* vol. 89, no. 427, pp. 910–912, 1994.

[53] M.I. Jordan and R.A. Jacobs, Hierarchical mixture of experts and the EM algorithm, *Neural Computation,* vol. 6, pp. 181–214, 1994.

[54] M.I. Jordan, Why the logistic function? A tutorial discussion on probabilities and neural networks, MIT Computational Cognitive Science Technical Report 9503, 1995.

[55] H. Ni, T. Adali, B. Wang, and X. Liu, A general probabilistic formulation for supervised neural classifiers, *Journal of VLSI Signal Processing Systems for Signal, Image, and Video Technology,* Special issue on neural networks for signal processing, vol. 26, nos. 1/2, pp. 141–153, Aug. 2000.

[56] S.Y. Kung, and J.S. Taur, Decision-based neural networks with signal/image classification applications, *IEEE Transactions on Neural Networks,* vol. 1, no. 1, pp. 170–181, Jan. 1995.

[57] S.H. Lin, S.Y. Kung, and L.J. Lin, Face recognition/detection by probabilistic decision-based neural network, *IEEE Transactions on Neural Networks,* Special issue on artificial neural networks and pattern recognition, vol. 8, no. 1, Jan. 1997.

[58] D.M. Titterington, Comments on application of the conditional population-mixture model to image segmentation, *IEEE Transactions on Pattern Analysis and Machine Intelligence,* vol. 6, no. 5, pp. 656–658, Sept. 1984.

[59] K. Fukushima, Neocognitron: a self-organizing neural network model for a mechanism of pattern recognition unaffected by shift in position, *Biological Cybernetics,* vol. 36, pp. 193–202, 1980.

[60] K. Fukushima, Neocognitron: a neural network model for a mechanism of visual pattern recognition, *IEEE Transactions on Systems, Man, and Cybernetics,* vol. 13, no. 5, pp. 826–834, 1983.

[61] H.P. Chan, et al., Improvement in radiologists' detection of clustered microcalcifications on mammograms: the potential of computer-aided diagnosis, in *Investigations on Radiology,* vol. 25, pp. 1102–1110, 1990.

[62] B.W. Fam, S.L. Olson, P.F. Winter, and F.J. Scholz, Algorithm for the detection of fine clustered calcifications on film mammograms, *Radiology,* vol. 169, pp. 333–337, 1988.

[63] D.H. Davies and D.R. Dance, Automatic computer detection of clustered microcalcifications in digital mammograms, *Phys. Med. Biol.,* vol. 35, pp. 1111–1118, 1990.

[64] Y. Wu, K. Doi, M.L. Giger, and M. Nishikawa, Computerized detection of clustered microcalcifications in digital mammograms: application of artificial neural networks, *Med. Phys.,* vol. 19, pp. 555–560, 1992.

[65] S.C. Lo, H.P. Chan, J.S. Lin, H. Li, M.T. Freedman, and S.K. Mun, Artificial convolution neural network for medical image pattern recognition, *Neural Networks,* vol. 8, no. 7/8, pp. 1201–1214, 1995.

[66] C.E. Metz, J.H. Shen, and B.A. Herman, New methods for estimating a binormal ROC curve from continuously distributed test results, in *Proceedings of the Annual Meeting of the American Statistical Association,* Anaheim, CA, 1990.

13

Hierarchical Fuzzy Neural Networks for Pattern Classification[1]

Jinshiuh Taur
National Chung-Hsing University

Sun-Yuan Kung
Princeton University

Shang-Hung Lin
EPSON Palo Alto Laboratories, ERD

13.1 Introduction

Information processing is becoming increasingly important due to the advances of the computing and networking technologies. The systems are required to handle complex, uncertain, and sometimes even contradictory information for a variety of applications. In this chapter, a potential framework of fuzzy neural networks based on hierarchical structures is proposed to provide the ability for robust information processing. Unsupervised and supervised strategies are integrated to train the parameters in the proposed processing framework. Also presented are some promising application examples for biometric authentication, medical image processing, video segmentation, object recognition/detection, and multimedia content-based retrieval.

[1]This research was supported in part by Mitsubishi Electric, ITA, and the R.O.C. National Science Council through Grant NSC 88-2213-E-005-012.

0-8493-2359-2/01/$0.00+$1.50

The parameters in the traditional neural networks usually have no physical meaning, and the initial values are typically selected at random. That is, each individual parameter cannot be directly related to the input or output values. Therefore, it is, in general, impossible to explain or pinpoint the meaning of the network parameters; traditional neural networks can be treated as black boxes whose parameters are obtained by training from example data sets. In contrast, the parameters in fuzzy logic systems can be associated with physical meaning. For example, we can assign a set of parameters to handle the input region with "positive large" values. Consequently, it is easier to design the initial values from the input–output data pairs and to incorporate a human expert's knowledge into fuzzy systems. However, unlike neural networks, the conventional fuzzy systems do not have the ability to adjust themselves to the changing environments.

From the divide-and-conquer point of view, many researchers have proposed modular neural networks [22, 24, 25, 49]. This approach solves a large, complicated task by using smaller and modularized trainable networks (i.e., experts), whose solutions are dynamically integrated into a single coherent network using the trainable gating network. More precisely, the gating network is implemented as a softmax activation function [3, 45]. A local expert's output with a larger (smaller) gating activation will be allocated a greater (lesser) influence on the overall output. In a very similar fashion, fuzzy inference systems (FISs) perform task decomposition based on fuzzy membership functions. The Sugeno-type FIS learning can be viewed as a variation of the modular network (as illustrated in Figure 13.3) where each local expert is expressed as a rule model. It will be shown in this chapter that neural and fuzzy systems share a lot of fundamental characteristics when viewed as modular systems. The fuzzy neural networks (FNNs) are used to denote the modular networks with learning capability. FNNs can enjoy the advantages of both neural networks (e.g., learning and optimization capabilities) and fuzzy systems (e.g., human-like **If-Then** logic rules and ease of incorporating expert knowledge). Based on the concept of modular systems, the hierarchical structure is adopted to design fuzzy neural networks. The hierarchical fuzzy neural networks (HFNNs) are adopted to denote the FNNs designed with this strategy. In this chapter, the building elements of HFNNs are described first. Then, some design examples of this family are presented. Table 13.1 summarizes the acronyms used in this chapter for quick reference.

TABLE 13.1 Acronyms Used in This Chapter

Acronym	Description
DBNN	decision-based neural network
EM	expectation–maximization
FIS	fuzzy inference system
FNN	fuzzy neural network
FPF	false-positive fraction
HFNN	hierarchical fuzzy neural network
LBF	linear basis function
MOE	mixture of experts
MLP	multilayer perceptron
NEFCAR	neuro-fuzzy classifier with adjustable rule importance
NN	neural network
OCON	one-class-one-net
RBF	radial basis function
ROC	receiver operating characteristic
ROI	regions of interest
TPF	true-positive fraction
VQ	vector quantization

Hierarchical fuzzy neural networks (HFNNs) have become a competitive means for many applications from low-level image processing to high-level pattern recognition. In particular, we highlight how HFNNs can play a key role in pattern classification applications. We present examples of texture classification and image/video segmentation with several applications to medical and multimedia processing. The HFNNs can cope well with a variety of cues such as texture, intensity, edge, color, and motion. They are also useful for detection and recognition of high-level features. We shall discuss application examples where HFNNs can successfully facilitate recognition tasks such as detection of bank notes, recognition of human faces, or identification of breast cancer cells.

The chapter is organized as follows. Section 13.2 describes the basic building modules and the hierarchical structures of the fuzzy neural networks. The differences between several modular networks are also discussed. We describe several important HFNN models and their classification applications, according to the hierarchical structures, in Sections 13.3, 13.4, and 13.5. More specifically, the unsupervised clustering expectation–maximization (EM) technique is described in Section 13.3. It can be used to construct a one-level modular network as well as to determine the initial parameters for the individual local modules in a hierarchical network. Therefore, it can be considered as the critical core technology for HFNNs. In Section 13.4, class-level modules and expert-level modules are incorporated to form two-level hierarchical structures. Two multilevel HFNNs are proposed based on the order of the modules adopted in the local networks. The decision-based training strategy is adopted to update the parameters in the network. Finally Section 13.5 presents a hierarchical fuzzy neural classifier (NEFCAR) to show how to improve system performance by integrating neural learning techniques and the fuzzy linguistic structure with both positive and negative rules. The class-level hierarchical structure and fuzzy **If-Then** logic rules are integrated into this classifier.

13.2 Modular Networks and Hierarchical Structures

This section describes the basic building modules and the hierarchical structures of neural networks and fuzzy systems. The similarities and differences between the models are also described. Hierarchical FNNs are constructed based on the commonality of their structural frameworks and functional units.

13.2.1 Modules and Hierarchical Levels

A neural network (NN) can be defined as an architecture comprising massively parallel adaptive processing elements interconnected via structured networks. There are many design options for the cost function, the learning algorithm, the nonlinear function, and the network structure. Ultimately, the design of the artificial neural networks often depends on the chosen applications. The traditional neural networks, exemplified by the multilayer perceptron (MLP), have a connectionist structure. They offer some measure of fault tolerance and distributed representation properties. More importantly, they possess adaptive learning abilities to estimate sampled functions, represent these samples, encode structural knowledge, and infer input–output relationships via association. Its main strength lies in that, given sufficient hidden units, an MLP is a universal approximator; an MLP can approximate any continuous function on a compact subset to any desired accuracy [8]. On the other hand, as depicted in Figure 13.1, the main weakness of the MLP lies in its totally flat structure. A direct consequence of such structural simplicity is often a bulky network, with an excessively large number of hidden units, which, in turn, hampers the convergence of the training process. One effective solution is to incorporate proper hierarchical structure into the networks. The notions of modular networks and functional blocks are essential for hierarchical designs. In particular, the following two types of modules will be relevant to the FNNs for pattern classification:

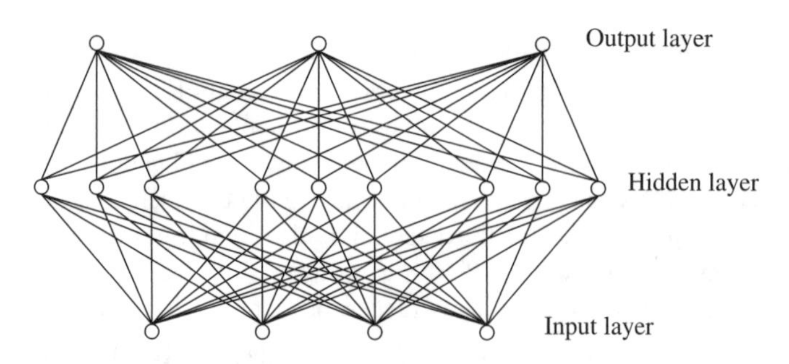

13.1 Multilayer perceptrons. This figure shows an MLP with one hidden layer. The arcs indicate the weights connecting the nodes in different layers.

1. Expert-level (rule-level) modules: the effectiveness of designing a modular fuzzy neural network hinges upon a proper designation of local experts. Each expert serves the function of (1) extracting local features and (2) making local recommendations. For example, one hidden node may be devoted to extracting a certain local feature of particular interest to an expert. The expert level in neural networks is compatible with the rule level in fuzzy systems. (For example, compare Figures 13.2 and 13.3.) The rules in the gating network are used to decide how to combine recommendations from several local experts, with corresponding degrees of confidence.
2. Class-level modules: an important goal of pattern recognition is to determine to which class an input pattern best belongs. Therefore, it is natural to consider class-level modules as the basic partitioning units, where each module specializes in distinguishing its own class from the others. Consequently, the number of hidden nodes (or experts) designated to a particular class is often very small. The class-level modules are adopted by the one-class-one-net (OCON) network. In contrast to expert-level partitioning, this OCON structure facilitates a global (or mutual) supervised training scheme. In global interclass supervised learning, any dispute over a pattern region by (two or more) competing classes may be effectively resolved by resorting to the teacher's guidance. Such a distributed processing structure is also convenient for network upgrading when there is a need to add or remove memberships. Finally, such a distributed structure is also appealing to the design of the RBF networks.

Accordingly, modular networks can be structurally divided into the following categories:

- zero-level (i.e., structurally flat) networks: this is exemplified by the traditional MLP, which has a "single-network" structure, as shown in Figure 13.1.
- one-level modular structures: by adopting the divide-and-conquer principle, the task is first divided into modules and then the individual results are integrated into a final and collective decision. Three typical modular networks are (1) the basic decision-based neural network (DBNN) based on the class-level modules (see Figure 13.4), (2) basic mixture of experts (MOE), which utilizes the expert-level modules (see Figure 13.2), and (3) Sugeno-type fuzzy inference system (see Figure 13.3). See Sections 13.2.2, 13.2.3, and 13.2.4, respectively. In Section 13.3, the one-level FNN based on the EM technique is introduced.
- two-level hierarchical structures: to this end, the divide-and-conquer principle needs to be applied twice: once on the expert-level and again on the class-level. Depending on the order used, this could result in two kinds of hierarchical networks: one has an experts-in-class construct, and another has a classes-in-expert construct. These two hierarchical structures will be elaborated upon in Section 13.4.

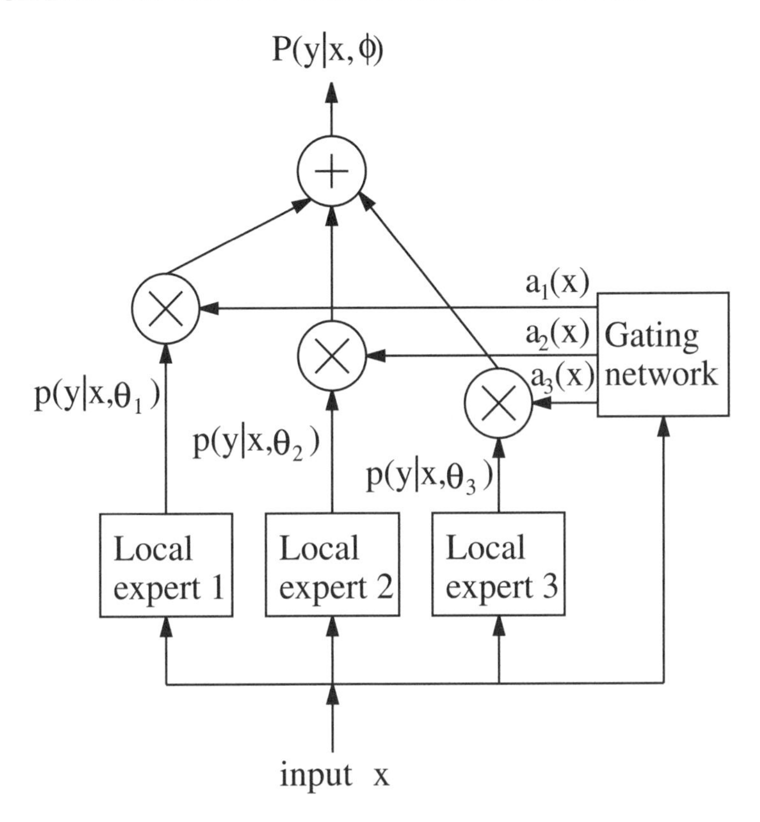

13.2 The baseline MOE architecture. An expert network estimates the pattern's conditional *a posteriori* probability. A baseline MOE comprises two subsystems: local experts and a gating network. The local experts are adaptively trained to extract certain local features particularly relevant to their own local decisions, while the gating network computes the global weights to be applied the local decisions.

One critical decision to the design of the HFNN involves the selection of the basis functions. There are several alternatives for the basis functions of the basic neural units, including:

- The linear basis function (LBF) [54] employs a sigmoid-type threshold function over the linear vector product of the pattern vector and weight vectors. Such a threshold function serves as the basic discriminating unit.
- The radial basis function (RBF) [46, 52] employs an RBF (e.g., a Gaussian kernel) to serve as the activation function. The weighting parameters in the RBF network are the centers, the widths, and the heights of these kernels.

This chapter primarily adopts the RBF-based Gaussian function due to its popularity as well as mathematical succinctness. Nevertheless, the same hierarchical structure and the learning mechanism remain largely applicable to other types of basis or membership functions.

13.2.2 Decision-Based Neural Networks

For most pattern recognition applications, the ultimate goal is to correctly assign an input pattern to the class to which it belongs. Therefore, it is quite natural to consider class-level partitioning as part of a hierarchical design. To introduce a class-level hierarchy into the FNN network structure, the baseline decision-based neural network (DBNN) serves as an illuminating design example [33, 38]. As shown in Figure 13.4, a DBNN has a modular OCON network structure: one subnet is designated

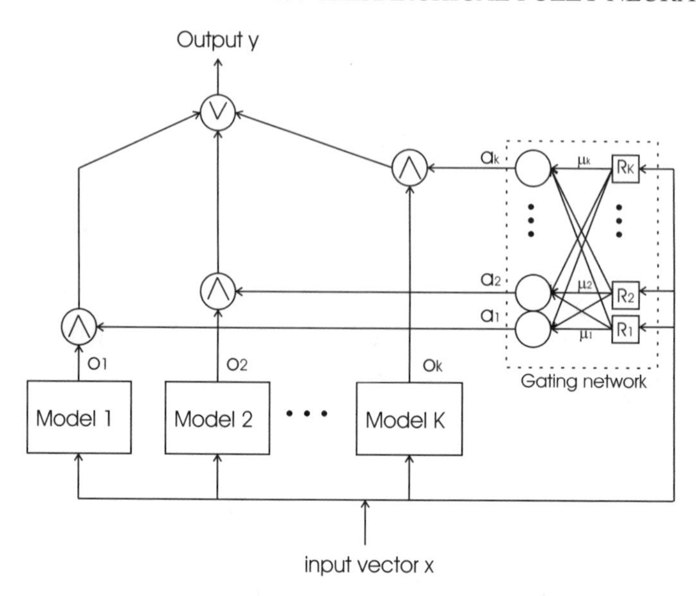

13.3 In a Sugeno-type fuzzy classifier, the vector **x** is input to the models (local experts) and the gating network. The gating network is corresponding to the **If** part of the **If-Then** rule. The R_i node is the rule node which computes the matching degree of the input **x** for Rule i. The nodes after the rule nodes normalize the matching degrees from the rule nodes to produce the weighting factor for the outputs of the local experts. The output y is a function of the outputs from local experts and the weighting factor from the gating network. The $\wedge$ and $\vee$ denote the weighting and the combining operators, respectively. The multiplication and addition are usually adopted to implement these two operations. That is, the output is a linear combination of the outputs from local experts and the weighting factor from the gating network. This corresponds to the defuzzification stage. This figure also represents a basic common framework shared by neural networks and fuzzy inference system. (With permission from S.Y. Kung, J. Taur, and S.H. Lin, Synergistic modeling and applications of hierarchical fuzzy neural networks, *Proceedings of the IEEE,* vol. 87, no. 9, pp. 1550–1574, 1999.)

to represent one object class. For multiclass classification problems, the outputs of the subnets (the discriminant functions) will compete with each other, and the subnet with the largest output values will claim the identity of the input pattern.

The learning scheme of the DBNN consists of two decoupled phases: locally unsupervised and globally supervised learning. The purpose is to simplify a difficult estimation problem by dividing it into several localized subproblems; thereafter, the fine-tuning process would involve minimal resources.

13.2.2.1 Locally Unsupervised Learning via VQ or EM Clustering Method

Several approaches can be used to estimate the number of hidden nodes, or an initial clustering can be determined based on vector quantization (VQ) or EM clustering methods. In the hard-decision DBNN, the VQ-type clustering (e.g., k-mean) algorithm can be applied to obtain initial locations of the centroids. For the probabilistic DBNN, the EM algorithm can be applied to achieve maximum likelihood estimation for each class conditional likelihood density. (Note that once the likelihood densities are available, the posterior probabilities can be easily obtained.)

13.2.2.2 Globally Supervised Learning Rules

Based on VQ or EM clustering, the decision-based learning rule can be applied to further fine tune the decision boundaries. In the second phase of the DBNN learning scheme, the objective

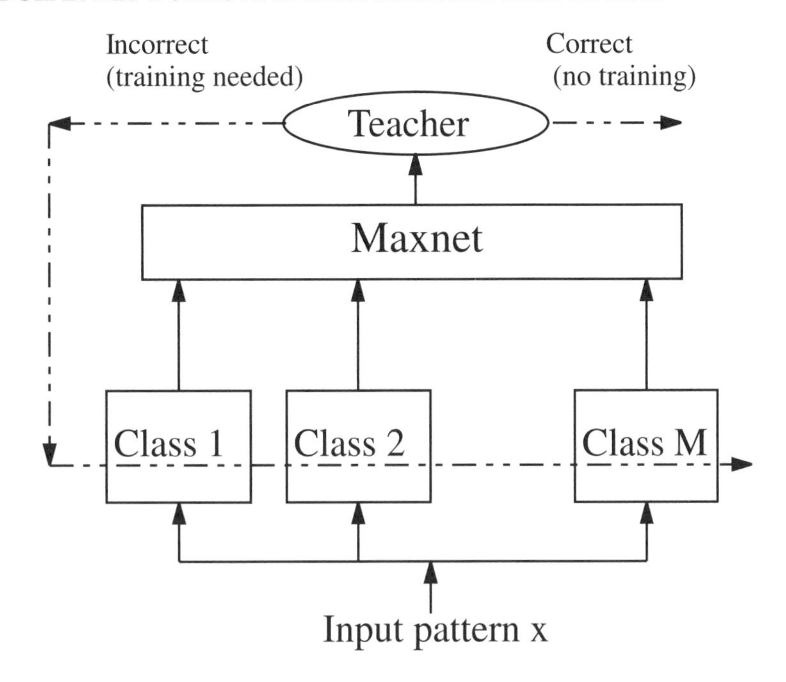

13.4 The baseline configuration of a DBNN. In the DBNN, one subnet is designated to represent one class. The output scores of the subnets compete with each other, and the highest scoring subnet claims the identity of the input pattern. The decision-based learning rule is adopted for fine-tuning the decision boundaries between the classes.

of the learning process changes from maximum likelihood estimation to minimum classification error. Interclass mutual information is used to fine-tune the decision boundaries (i.e., the globally supervised learning). In this phase, DBNN applies a reinforced–anti-reinforced learning rule [33] or a discriminative learning rule [30] to adjust network parameters. Only misclassified patterns are involved in this training phase.

13.2.2.2.1 Reinforced–Anti-Reinforced Learning Rules

Let $\psi(\mathbf{x}, \Theta_i)$ denote the score (discriminant) function of class i. Suppose that the mth training pattern $\mathbf{x}^{(m)}$ is known to belong to class ω_i, and that the leading challenger is denoted $j = \arg\max_{j \neq i} \psi(\mathbf{x}^{(m)}, \Theta_j)$. The learning rule is

$$\begin{array}{ll} \text{Reinforced learning:} & \Theta_i^{(m+1)} = \Theta_i^{(m)} + \eta \nabla \psi\left(\mathbf{x}^{(m)}, \Theta_i\right), \\ \text{Anti-reinforced learning:} & \Theta_j^{(m+1)} = \Theta_j^{(m)} - \eta \nabla \psi\left(\mathbf{x}^{(m)}, \Theta_j\right) \end{array} \tag{13.1}$$

where Θ_i is the weight vector of class i and η is a positive learning rate.

The learning rule is based on a minimal updating principle. The rule tends to avoid or minimize unnecessary side effects due to overtraining. Given one training pattern, there are two scenarios. One is that the pattern is already classified correctly by the current network, in which case there will be no updating attributed to that pattern, and the learning process will proceed with the next training pattern. The second scenario is that the pattern is classified incorrectly to another winning class. In that case, parameters of two classes must be updated. The score of the winning class should be reduced by the anti-reinforced learning rule, while the score of the correct (but not winning) class should be enhanced by the reinforced learning rule.

In the DBNN, the winning class is the one with highest score function. The DBNN learning rule adopts a minimal updating principle so that only the two classes immediately involved in the dispute should be updated. The action towards correcting a mistake is twofold: (1) the reinforced learning rule will be applied to the correct class so as to enhance its score; (2) the anti-reinforced learning rule will be applied to the winning class, which will result in a lower score. After multiple training sweeps, the boundary (or the pattern) should ultimately be placed on the correct side of the pattern (or the boundary).

13.2.3 Mixture of Experts

Among the prominent neural models, the network architecture of the mixture of experts (MOE) [25] has the closest resemblance to fuzzy inference systems. The MOE exhibits an explicit relationship with statistical pattern classification methods. Given a pattern, each expert network estimates the pattern's conditional *a posteriori* probability on the (adaptively tuned or preassigned) feature space. Each local expert network performs multi-way classification over K classes by using either K independent binomial models, each modeling only one class, or one multinomial model for all classes. Moreover, the corresponding output of the gating network represents the associated confidence on each expert. The final system output is the weighted sum of the estimated probabilities from all of the expert networks.

With reference to Figure 13.2, the MOE comprises the following subsystems:

1. local experts: the design of modular neural networks hinges upon the choice of local experts. Usually, a local expert is adaptively trained to extract a certain local feature that is particularly relevant to its local decision. Sometimes, a local expert can be assigned a predetermined feature space. Based on the local feature, a local expert will process a local recommendation.
2. gating network: the gating network serves the function of computing the proper weights to be used for the final weighted decision. A probabilistic rule is used to integrate recommendations from several local experts, taking into account the experts' confidence levels.

The training of the local experts as well as the confidence levels in the gating network of the MOE network is based on the expectation–maximization (EM) algorithm. The objective is to estimate the model parameters so as to attain the highest probability of the training set given the estimated parameters. For a given input $\mathbf{x}$, the posterior probability of generating class $\mathbf{y}$ given $\mathbf{x}$ using K experts can be computed as

$$P(\mathbf{y}|\mathbf{x}, \phi) = \sum_{j=1}^{K} P\left(\mathbf{y}|\mathbf{x}, \Theta_j\right) a_j(\mathbf{x}) \qquad (13.2)$$

where $\mathbf{y}$ is a binary vector and a_j is the probability for weighting the expert outputs. For example, if we consider two classes for a classification problem, then $\mathbf{y}$ is [1 0] or [0 1]. The parameter ϕ is a vector $[\mathbf{V}, \Theta_j]$; $\mathbf{V} = \{\mathbf{V}_j, j = 1 \ldots, K\}$ is the parameter set for the gating network; Θ_j is the parameter set for the jth expert network ($j = 1, \ldots, K$); and $\mathrm{P}(\mathbf{y}|\mathbf{x}, \Theta_j)$ is the output of the jth expert network.

The mixture of experts (MOE) model has been applied to many applications. For application to sunspot time series prediction, a Bayesian framework for inferring the parameters of an MOE model based on ensemble learning by variational free energy minimization proves to be very effective and performs significantly better than single networks [65]. MOE has also been shown to yield very good performance in automated cytology screening applications [23]. For broader application domains, MOE has also been extended to cope with a multi-expert-level tree structure, known as hierarchical mixture of experts [27].

13.2.3.0.2 RBF Neural Networks

In an RBF neural network, each hidden node represents a receptive field with the following normalized Gaussian activation function:

$$a_j(\mathbf{x}) = \frac{\mu_j}{\sum_{k=1}^{K} \mu_k} \tag{13.3}$$

$$\mu_k = \exp\left(-|\mathbf{x} - \mathbf{m}_k|^2 / 2\sigma_k^2\right) \tag{13.4}$$

where $\mathbf{x}$ is the n-dimensional input vector and K is the number of hidden nodes. The parameters $\mathbf{m}_k$ and σ_k^2 denote the mean and variance of the kth Gaussian function. Then, the output $y(\cdot)$ can be computed as the weighted sum of the activation values

$$y(\mathbf{x}) = \sum_{j=1}^{K} o_j a_j(\mathbf{x}) \tag{13.5}$$

where o_j is the height of the jth Gaussian kernel.

It is obvious that if the gating network output a_j in Equation (13.2) is defined as the a_j in Equation (13.3) and the $P(\mathbf{y}|\mathbf{x}, \Theta_j)$ is defined to be a constant o_j, then the RBF neural network becomes an MOE system with a radial basis gating function and constant expert output.

13.2.4 Sugeno's Fuzzy Inference Systems

The fuzzy logic systems, in contrast to connectionist neural networks, offer a structural framework with high-level fuzzy **If-Then** rule thinking and reasoning. The basic idea behind a fuzzy inference system is to incorporate a human's expert experience into the system design. The input–output relationship is described by a collection of fuzzy inference rules (e.g., **If-Then** rules) involving linguistic variables. Fuzzy systems base their decisions on inputs in the form of linguistic variables defined by membership functions which are formulas used to determine the fuzzy set to which a value belongs and the degree of membership in that set. The variables are then matched with the preconditions of linguistics **If-Then** rules (fuzzy logic rules) to calculate the firing strengths of the rules, and the response of each rule is obtained through fuzzy implication. Following the compositional rule of inference, the response of each rule is weighted according to the rule firing strength to generate the appropriate output.

For example, in Sugeno's fuzzy inference system shown in Figure 13.3, the **If-Then** rules in the fuzzy rule base can be expressed as

$$\textbf{If } \mathbf{x} \text{ is } R_j \textbf{ Then } y \text{ is } \text{Model}_j\,.$$

The fuzzification and firing strength are calculated in the rule node. The inference engine deduces its final output from the outputs of the models. For example, such a "defuzzified" output may be calculated as a weighted sum of individual outputs since each model produces crisp output. The weighted average is adopted as the inference procedure. Lin and Lee [37] call this procedure fuzzy reasoning (of the third type).

A multiple-input–single-output (MISO) fuzzy system can take the following fuzzy rules:

$$\begin{cases} \text{Rule 1:} & \textbf{If } x_1 \text{ is } S_1^1 \textbf{ And } x_2 \text{ is } S_2^1 \textbf{ And } \cdots \textbf{ And } x_n \text{ is } S_n^1 \textbf{ Then } y \text{ is } O^1 \\ \text{Rule 2:} & \textbf{If } x_1 \text{ is } S_1^2 \textbf{ And } x_2 \text{ is } S_2^2 \textbf{ And } \cdots \textbf{ And } x_n \text{ is } S_n^2 \textbf{ Then } y \text{ is } O^2 \\ & \vdots \\ \text{Rule } K\text{:} & \textbf{If } x_1 \text{ is } S_1^K \textbf{ And } x_2 \text{ is } S_2^K \textbf{ And } \cdots \textbf{ And } x_n \text{ is } S_n^K \textbf{ Then } y \text{ is } O^K \end{cases} \tag{13.6}$$

where S_l^j and O^j are one of the input and output fuzzy sets, respectively. Computationally, the "**If**" part can be implemented as a fuzzy (or soft) weighting factor, while a fuzzy "**And**" can be replaced by arithmetic multiplication.

Now assume that the membership functions μ_{lj} of the fuzzy sets S_l^j are Gaussian-like functions with mean m_{lj} and variance σ_{lj}^2:

$$\mu_{lj}(x_l) = \exp\left(-\left(x_l - m_{lj}\right)^2 / 2\sigma_{lj}^2\right) . \tag{13.7}$$

The output fuzzy set O^j is assumed to be a fuzzy singleton at o_j from the jth model. With the weighting determined by the **If** part, the defuzzified output is calculated by taking weighted contributions from different model outputs. Just like Equation (13.5) in an RBF neural network, the output y in a centroid defuzzification scheme can be computed as:

$$y = \sum_{j=1}^{K} o_j a_j(\mathbf{x}) \tag{13.8}$$

where

$$a_j = \frac{\mu_j}{\sum_{k=1}^{K} \mu_k} \quad \text{and} \quad \mu_k = \Pi_{l=1}^{n} \mu_{lk}(x_l) . \tag{13.9}$$

13.2.5 Comparison between Modular Networks

This section discusses the similarities and differences of the FIS and MOE networks, which are based on the expert (rule)-level modules. The relationship of network property and the training strategy between an MOE network and the baseline DBNN, which is constructed using class-level modules, is also discussed. Stretching the similarity further, the intersection of fuzzy systems and neural networks actually defines a large family of learning networks. Therefore, a family of fuzzy neural networks is proposed based on the proper combination of class and expert level modules hierarchically.

13.2.5.1 FIS and MOE Networks

It has recently become popular for a fuzzy system to utilize Gaussian membership functions and a centroid defuzzification scheme. This is due, in part, to its capabilities of approximating any real continuous function on a compact set to an arbitrary accuracy, provided sufficient fuzzy logic rules are available [31, 61]. In the neural net literature, it has also been established that neural networks with the normalized radial basis functions (RBFs) as the hidden nodes are universal approximators [52]. Therefore, neural networks and fuzzy systems are similar in terms of their approximating capability. Moreover, by comparing Equations (13.3) and (13.5) with Equations (13.9) and (13.8), it is clear that the aforementioned RBF MOE neural network and fuzzy inference system are essentially equivalent if the σ_{ij}'s in Equation (13.7) are identical for all j, or the σ_k's in Equation (13.3) are independent for each input dimension. Having the same mathematical formulation, they naturally share very similar system architectures. Illuminating evidence is realized by comparing Figure 13.2 and Figure 13.3, representing the MOE modular neural network and Sugeno's fuzzy inference system, respectively.

Therefore, the Sugeno-type FIS and the MOE networks are basically equivalent as long as the gating network of the MOE generates the fuzzy membership values according to the membership functions and the **And** operation in the fuzzy **If-Then** rules. However, there are some subtle differences between the MOE and the Sugeno-type FIS, as listed in the following:

- For the FIS, there usually exist shared parameters for the rule nodes due to the partition of the input space. Thus, the rule nodes can be easily interpreted as linguistic rules. In contrast, the parameters in the MOE network are usually independent.
- The output for each rule of Sugeno-type FIS is usually a (zeroth-order or first-order) polynomial function of the input, while the output for the expert in MOE is usually a nonlinear function.
- If the gating network adopts elliptic basis functions with a general covariance matrix, it becomes difficult to design an equivalent FIS using the rule in Equation (13.6).

13.2.5.2 MOE and DBNN

The MOE and DBNN models share many similarities. For example, both modular structures are based on the divide-and-conquer principle, and both employ the EM algorithm in the training phase. Nevertheless, there are some substantial differences:

- Network properties: each expert network in the MOE estimates the conditional posterior probabilities for all the pattern classes. The output of a local expert is ready to make the classification based on its own local information and expert's perspective. This characteristic suggests that the interclass communication/decision exists on the local network level under an MOE model. In contrast, each neuron in a DBNN estimates the class conditional likelihood density. The interclass communication/decision does not occur until the final subnet output is formed. This enables the absence of interclass communication across the (class) modules of the DBNN. (This, in a sense, achieves a truly distributive processing.)
- Training strategies: the training strategies of these two models are vastly different. During the MOE training, all the training patterns have the power to update every expert. The influence from the training patterns on each expert is regulated by the gating network (which itself is under training) so that, as the training proceeds, the training patterns will have higher influence on the nearby experts and lower influence on those far away. In contrast, unlike the MOE, the DBNN makes use of both unsupervised (EM-type) and supervised (decision-based) learning rules. The DBNN uses only the misclassified training patterns for its globally supervised learning. Moreover, unlike the MOE, which updates all the classes, the DBNN updates only the "winner" class and the class to which the misclassified pattern actually belongs. Its training strategy is to abide by a "minimal updating principle."

13.2.5.3 Hierarchical Fuzzy Neural Networks

The FNNs draw inspiration from innovations within both the neural network and fuzzy logic communities. Such FNNs strive to preserve the structure of the fuzzy systems and, at the same time, maximally exploit unsupervised and supervised learning rules in neural networks. One should be able to learn rules in a hybrid fashion and calibrate them for better total-system performance.

The learning process for an FNN involves mapping sample data to the FNN's network parameters via both unsupervised learning and supervised learning. Unsupervised learning can be used to obtain the initial fuzzy rule base from the sample data while supervised learning is effective in fine-tuning the decision boundaries of the classifier. Both the MOE and DBNN employ the expectation–maximization (EM) algorithm whose derivation will be discussed in Section 13.3.1.

In terms of the structural design, an effective implementation of FNNs hinges upon a combination of locally distributed and hierarchical networks. Local and distributed processing is critical to the robustness of the FNNs. A hierarchical design, on the other hand, often results in a more efficient network structure. Proper incorporation of expert-level modules and class-level modules into a hierarchical FNN can prove advantageous in computation and performance. A hierarchical FNN comprises a variety of fuzzy processing modules, for which EM serves as a basic tool. In addition, the decision-based learning rule proves to be effective in implementing a global (i.e., interclass) supervised training scheme. Recently, there have been many important applications involving fusion of information from completely different sources. The hierarchical FNN structure can be easily extended to cope with multi-channel information processing. Hierarchical fuzzy neural networks with an embedded fusion agent offer an effective approach to channel fusion. The class-level hierarchy of DBNN and the rule-level hierarchy in the FIS may be properly combined to yield fuzzy neural networks useful for specific applications. The structural designs and the associated learning algorithms will be elaborated in the following sections.

13.3 One-Level Modular Structure

For the one-level modular structure, the EM algorithm can be adopted to estimate the probability density and then a Bayesian classification approach can be adopted. For HFNNs, the EM algorithm is a convenient tool to achieve maximum likelihood estimation for each class conditional likelihood density.

13.3.1 Expectation–Maximization (EM) Fuzzy Classifier

Unsupervised learning or clustering rules can be perceived as a result of natural evolution from the traditional statistical clustering and parameter estimation techniques. These often serve as a promising preprocessing step of a pattern recognition system to enhance the performance. Unsupervised learning algorithms may be applied to determine the initial weights for individual local experts. The initial clusters can be trained by vector quantization (VQ) or k-mean clustering techniques [13]. k-mean and VQ are often used interchangeably: they classify input patterns based on the nearest-neighbor rule. k-mean [13] can be treated as a special method for implementing vector quantization (VQ) [20]. The task is to cluster a given data set $\mathbf{X} = \{\mathbf{x}_i | i = 1, \ldots, N\}$ into K groups, each represented by its centroid denoted by $\hat{\mathbf{X}} = \{\mathbf{x}'_j | j = 1, \ldots, K\}$. The nearest-neighbor rule assigns a pattern $\mathbf{x}$ to the class associated with its nearest centroid, e.g., $\mathbf{x}'_i$. k-mean and VQ have simple learning rules and the classification scheme is straightforward. Mathematically, it aims at minimizing the following cost function:

$$E(h; \mathbf{X}) = \sum_{i,j} h_j(\mathbf{x}_i)|\mathbf{x}_i - \mathbf{x}'_j|^2 \tag{13.10}$$

where $h_j(\mathbf{x}_i) = 1$ for the members only, otherwise $h_j(\mathbf{x}_i) = 0$. (For example, $h_j(\mathbf{x}_i) = 1$ could indicate that $\mathbf{x}_i$ is closest to $\mathbf{x}'_j$ among all K centroids in $\hat{\mathbf{X}}$.) The k-mean algorithm [43] provides a simple mechanism for minimizing the sum of squared error with K clusters.

The iterations in the VQ clustering adopt a "hard-decision" rule, i.e., $h_j(\mathbf{x}_i)$ is either one or zero. In this sense, VQ is only a special case of a more general clustering algorithm, i.e., expectation–maximization (EM). The EM algorithm is a well established iterative method for maximum likelihood estimation (MLE) [11] and for clustering mixtures of Gaussian distributions. It serves as a useful tool for estimating distribution parameters and thus results in data clustering. Most importantly, EM introduces a notion of "entropy" (or uncertainty) to induce a fuzzy classification, making it very amenable to the notions of fuzzy **If-Then** rule and fuzzy membership in fuzzy neural models.

13.3.1.1 EM for Fuzzy Neural Networks

The EM algorithm can be perceived as a "soft" version of VQ, thus offering an efficient fuzzy clustering tool for the unsupervised learning phase in training FNNs. In addition, the EM algorithm offers several attractive attributes:

- EM naturally accommodates model-based clustering formulation with one model corresponding to one rule used in the FNN (see Figure 13.3).
- The EM allows the final decision to incorporate prior information. This could be instrumental to multiple-expert or multiple-channel information fusion.

The most common clustering is via either a radial basis function (RBF) or a more general elliptic basis function. In the latter case, the component density $p(\mathbf{x}_i|\Theta_j)$ is a Gaussian distribution, with the model parameter of the jth cluster $\Theta_j = \{\mu_j, \Sigma_j, \pi_j\}$ consisting of the mean vector, the full-rank covariance matrix, and the prior probability.

13.3.1.1.1 EM Algorithm

The problem is to find an optimal estimation of a mixture of Gaussian likelihood functions $\prod_i p(\mathbf{x}_i)$ with respect to $\Theta = \{\Theta_j, j = 1, \ldots, K\}$, given a set of data $\mathbf{X} = \{\mathbf{x}_i | i = 1, \ldots, N\}$ as independent identically distributed samples:

$$p(\mathbf{x}_i) = \sum_{j=1}^{K} \pi_j p(\mathbf{x}_i|\Theta_j) \qquad \sum_{j=1}^{K} \pi_j = 1 \tag{13.11}$$

where Θ_j represents the jth cluster, and π_j denotes its prior probability.

The optimal estimation is obtained by minimizing an energy function E defined from the negative logarithm of $p(\mathbf{x}_i)$:

$$E = -\sum_{i=1}^{N} \log p(\mathbf{x}_i) = -\sum_{i=1}^{N} \frac{\sum_{j=1}^{K} \pi_j p(\mathbf{x}_i|\Theta_j)}{p(\mathbf{x}_i)} \log p(\mathbf{x}_i) \,. \tag{13.12}$$

Define $h_j(\mathbf{x}_i) \equiv \frac{\pi_j p(\mathbf{x}_i|\Theta_j)}{p(\mathbf{x}_i)}$.

Equation (13.12) becomes

$$\begin{aligned} E &= -\sum_{i=1}^{N}\sum_{j=1}^{K} h_j(\mathbf{x}_i) \log p(\mathbf{x}_i) \\ &= \sum_{i=1}^{N}\sum_{j=1}^{K} h_j(\mathbf{x}_i) \left(-\log p(\mathbf{x}_i) + \log\left[\pi_j p(\mathbf{x}_i|\Theta_j)\right] - \log\left[\pi_j p(\mathbf{x}_i|\Theta_j)\right]\right) \\ &= \sum_{i=1}^{N}\sum_{j=1}^{K} h_j(\mathbf{x}_i) \left(\log h_j(\mathbf{x}_i) - \log\left[\pi_j p(\mathbf{x}_i|\Theta_j)\right]\right) \\ &= \sum_{i,j} h_j(\mathbf{x}_i) \log h_j(\mathbf{x}_i) - \sum_{i,j} h_j(\mathbf{x}_i) \log \pi_j - \sum_{i,j} h_j(\mathbf{x}_i) \log p(\mathbf{x}_i|\Theta_j) \,. \end{aligned} \tag{13.13}$$

Note that, $h_j(\mathbf{x}_i)$ equals the probability of $\mathbf{x}_i$ belonging to jth cluster given a prior model ($h_j(\mathbf{x}_i) = Pr(\mathbf{x}_i \in \Theta_j | \mathbf{x}_i, \Theta)$). It can be considered as a "fuzzy" membership function.

The EM problem can be expressed as one which minimizes E with respect to both (1) the model parameters $\Theta = \{\Theta_j, \forall j\}$ and (2) the membership function $\{h_j(\mathbf{x}_i), \forall i, j\}$. The interplay of these two variables can hopefully induce a bootstrapping effect facilitating the convergence process. This is further elaborated below:

- In the E step, while fixing the model parameter $\Theta = \{\Theta_j, \forall j\}$, we find the best cluster probability h_j to optimize E (with constraint $\Sigma_{j=1}^{K} h_j(\mathbf{x}_i) = 1$):

$$h_j(\mathbf{x}_i) \propto \pi_j e^{-s_j(\mathbf{x}_i, \mu_j, \Sigma_j)/\sigma_T} . \tag{13.14}$$

- In the M step, we search for the best model parameter $\Theta = \{\Theta_j, \forall j\}$ which optimizes E, while fixing the cluster probability $h_j(\mathbf{x}_i), \forall i$.

The EM algorithm discussed above is directly applicable to the hierarchical FNNs as discussed in the subsequent section. Note that, in a particular iteration, the parameters to minimize the weighted-squared-error $s_j(\mathbf{x}_i, \mu_j, \Sigma_j)$ can be obtained analytically, which is the special advantage of using RBF-type likelihood functions. On the other hand, if a linear model (e.g., LBF) is chosen to parameterize the likelihood and/or the gating functions, we need an iterative method to achieve the optimal solutions in the iteration. In other words, the EM algorithm becomes a double-loop optimization. For example, Jordan and Jacobs [28] applied a Fisher scoring method called iteratively reweighted least squares (IRLS) to train the LBF MOE network.

13.3.1.1.2 EM vs. k-mean

By rearranging Equation (13.13), we obtain the following energy function [21, 67]:

$$E = \sum_{i,j} h_j(\mathbf{x}_i) s_j(\mathbf{x}_i, \mu_j, \Sigma_j) - \sigma_T \sum_{i,j} h_j(\mathbf{x}_i) \log \pi_j + \sigma_T \sum_{i,j} h_j(\mathbf{x}_i) \log h_j(\mathbf{x}_i) . \tag{13.15}$$

There are three terms in the energy function E:

- The first term is the external energy, where $s_j(\mathbf{x}_i, \mu_j, \Sigma_j)$ denotes a weighted squared error:

$$s_j(\mathbf{x}_i, \mu_j, \Sigma_j) = (\mathbf{x}_i - \mu_j) \Sigma_j^{-1} (\mathbf{x}_i - \mu_j)^T .$$

- The second term represents the internal energy. For each sample $\mathbf{x}_i$, the internal energy term grasps the influence (prior probability) of its neighboring clusters.
- The third term can be interpreted as the (negative) entropy term, which helps induce the membership's fuzziness.

By examining Equation (13.14), we can see that k-mean clustering is a special case of the EM scheme. When Σ_j is an identity matrix and σ_T approaches 0, Equation (13.15) would be reduced into Equation (13.10), which leads to a hard-decision clustering (i.e., with cluster probabilities $h_j(\mathbf{x}_i)$ equal to either 1 or 0). This demonstrates that σ_T plays the same role as the temperature parameter in the simulated annealing method. Note that the probability density function has the form $p(\mathbf{x}_i|\Theta_j) \propto e^{-s_j(\mathbf{x}_i, \mu_j, \Sigma_j)/\sigma_T}$, so the higher the temperature, the greater the entropy. It is a common practice to use some sort of annealing temperature schedule, i.e., starting with a higher σ_T and then gradually decreasing σ_T to a lower value as iterations progress in order to force a more certain classification.

13.3.2 Applications of EM Fuzzy Classifiers

13.3.2.1 Motion-Based Video Segmentation

Robust scene segmentation is a prerequisite for object-based video processing and high-performance video compression. Various approaches to this complex task have been proposed, including classification of motion flow, color/texture segmentation, and dominant-motion extraction. Lin and colleagues [41, 42], applied the EM method to object-oriented motion segmentation, which divides a video scene into different motion regions. The procedure is briefly described below.

Initially, motion clustering is performed upon a selected set of motion feature blocks tracked by a true motion tracker. The feature blocks are represented by the principal components (PCs) of their position and velocity. The motion parameters for each of the clustered feature blocks may be estimated and used as the initial condition for the final segmentation process. The final segmentation and the corresponding motion parameters are iteratively updated by a model-based EM algorithm. The model-based EM is based on minimization of the following energy function (where b denotes the image blocks):

$$E(\mathbf{A}, h) = \sum_{b,j} h_j(b) s_j\left(b, A_j\right) - \sigma_T^2 \sum_{b,j} h_j(b) \log \pi_j(b) + \sigma_T^2 \sum_{b,j} h_j(b) \log h_j(b) \,. \tag{13.16}$$

The first term represents the external (error) energy function, so that each cluster (e.g., jth cluster) would be best fit to a given motion (e.g., affine) model denoted by A_j. The second term represents an internal energy function, which enforces the region smoothness by allowing neighboring blocks of a target block to exercise proportional influence on the classification of that target block. This serves the purpose of forcing the classification to take into account the intensity/texture continuity (i.e., image cues), thus resulting in a smoother segmentation. The third term stands for the entropy function, which encourages a softer classification.

Figure 13.5 shows an example of video scene segmentation containing two moving books shot from a moving camera. Figure 13.5a shows the distribution of the feature blocks in the PC-coordinate.

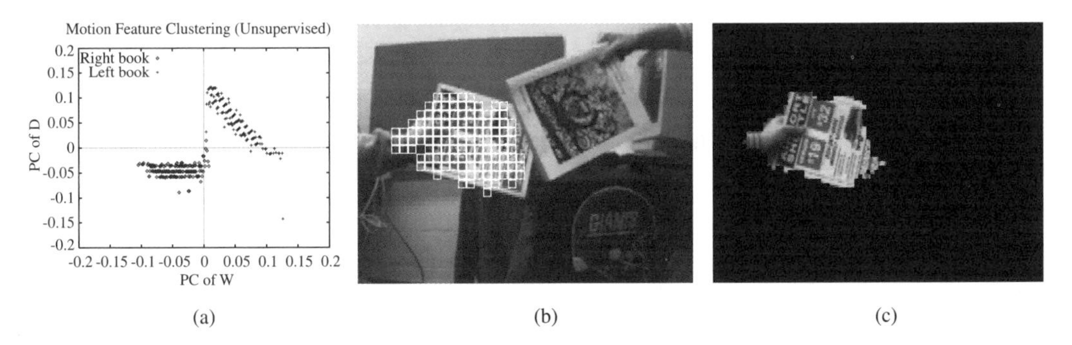

13.5 Motion-based video segmentation result of sequence with two books with moving camera. (a) Distribution in terms of the principal-components (PCs) of the feature blocks obtained by a true motion tracker. Vertical axis: PC of motion (D); horizontal axis: PC of position (W); (b) feature blocks of the left book clustered by EM; and (c) final segmentation (of the left book) by a multi-cue model-based EM. (With permission from S.Y. Kung, J. Taur, and S.H. Lin, Synergistic modeling and applications of hierarchical fuzzy neural networks, *Proceedings of the IEEE*, vol. 87, no. 9, pp. 1550–1574, 1999.)

The unsupervised EM clustering scheme is then adopted to cluster the feature blocks. Figure 13.5b shows the feature blocks classified into the left book. Figure 13.5c demonstrates that the object region of the left book as extracted by the EM-based segmentation.

13.3.2.2 Texture Classification via Intraclass EM Clustering

The texture information can be the gray level of a pixel or the texture features of the neighborhood around a pixel. The objective of texture classification is to determine the boundary of a region where the image has the same textural characteristics. Both the unsupervised and supervised approaches are useful for the texture classification application. If there is no representative training image available in the application, then unsupervised techniques are the only options available.

The EM algorithm described in Section 13.3.1 has been adopted as an effective means for texture classification, which can be used as a core unsupervised clustering technique. Satisfactory performances of the unsupervised EM algorithm for segmenting satellite images and medical images have been reported [9, 44, 53]. Nevertheless, the supervised technique can usually deliver much better segmentation results. An example based on intraclass EM clustering will be described here. As a comparison, another example using interclass supervised learning will be discussed in the subsequent section.

It is assumed that the probability distributions of texture information of different regions in a textured image can be represented by statistical models. The EM algorithm can be adopted to estimate the probability density, and a Bayesian classification approach can be adopted to segment the images. The neighborhood (spatial) information can be considered in the probability distribution model or used in a post-processing stage to produce a smooth segmentation. Popat and Picard [50] applied the EM technique to image segmentation. The training images from a (known) texture class are used to obtain a representative statistical model. The classification is accomplished by centering a neighborhood at each pixel location and choosing for that pixel the class whose conditional probability (given a texture model) is the highest. The preliminary result usually has a "noisy" appearance. One way to smooth the boundary is to make good use of the spatial homogeneity. More precisely, for a pixel to be assigned to a specific class, its neighborhoods must also have reasonably high conditional likelihood (given the same texture model). According to the experimental report [50], the total error rate is below 5% for segmenting a four-square-region image comprising four Brodatz textures. It was also observed that the overall error rate could be greatly reduced (to 1%) by first applying low-pass filtering to perform spatial averaging [9, 44, 53].

13.4 Two-Level Hierarchical Networks

13.4.1 Hierarchical FNNs for Fuzzy Decision

As mentioned in the previous sections, the MOE and DBNN networks adopt the expert-level and class-level partitioning strategies, respectively. A hierarchical FNN configuration should allow the incorporation of both the expert-level and class-level modules. As elaborated below, the selection of the inner blocks vs. the outer blocks will lead to very distinctive hierarchical structures.

13.4.1.1 Experts-in-Class Hierarchical Structures

Figure 13.6 depicts such a structure. The inner blocks comprise expert-level modules, while the outer blocks are on the class level. A typical example of this type of network is the hierarchical DBNN [40], which describes the class discriminant function as a mixture of multiple probabilistic distributions. That is, the discriminant function of the class ω_c in the hierarchical DBNN is a class conditional likelihood density $p(\mathbf{x}_i|\omega_c)$:

$$p(\mathbf{x}_i|\omega_c) = \sum_{k=1}^{K} P\left(E_k|\omega_c\right) p\left(\mathbf{x}_i|\omega_c, E_k\right) \tag{13.17}$$

where $p(\mathbf{x}_i|\omega_c, E_k)$ is the discriminant function of subnet c in expert k, and $p(\mathbf{x}_i|\omega_c)$ is the combined discriminant function for class ω_c. The expert confidence $P(E_k|\omega_c)$ can be learned by the EM algorithm described below. Define $\alpha_k = P(E_k|\omega_c)$ and set the initial value of $\alpha_k = 1/K, \forall k = 1, \ldots, K$. At the iteration step m,

$$h_k^{(m)}(\mathbf{x}_i) = \frac{\alpha_k^{(m)} p(\mathbf{x}_i|\omega_c, E_k)}{\sum_l \alpha_l^{(m)} p(\mathbf{x}_i|\omega_c, E_l)}, \qquad \alpha_k^{(m+1)} = \frac{1}{N}\sum_{i=1}^{N} h_k^{(m)}(\mathbf{x}_i) \; . \tag{13.18}$$

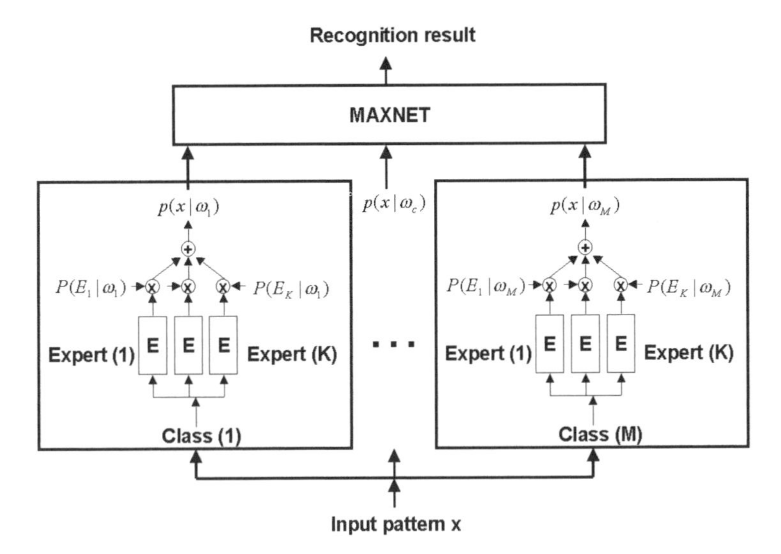

13.6 Experts-in-class hierarchical design: for the applications where there are several experts or information sources, experts-in-class hierarchical scheme can be applied for classification. (The gating networks are omitted in the drawing.) Like the baseline DBNN model, the minimal updating principle can be adopted to train the parameters in the network. $P(E_j|\omega_c)$ serves as the confidence indicator for the jth expert in class c. It is a trainable parameter, and its value is fixed during retrieving time. (With permission from S.Y. Kung, J. Taur, and S.H. Lin, Synergistic modeling and applications of hierarchical fuzzy neural networks, *Proceedings of the IEEE,* vol. 87, no. 9, pp. 1550–1574, 1999.)

Each expert processes only the local features from its corresponding class. The outputs from different experts are linearly combined. The weighting parameters, $P(E_k|\omega_c)$, represent the confidence of expert E_k producing the correct answer for the object class ω_c. Once they are trained in the learning phase, their values remain fixed during the retrieving (or identification) phase. By definition, $\Sigma_{k=1}^{K} P(E_k|\omega_c) = 1$, where K is the number of experts in the subnet ω_c. So it has the property of a probability function. Note that, in conjunction with the expert-level (or rule-level) hierarchy, each hidden node within one class subnet may be used to model a certain local expert (or rule) with a varying degree of confidence, which reflects its ability to interpret a given input vector. The locally unsupervised and globally supervised scheme described in Section 13.2.2 can be adopted to train the OCON network, (see Figure 13.4).

13.4.1.2 Classes-in-Expert Hierarchical Structures

Figure 13.7 depicts such a structure. The inner blocks comprise class modules while the outer blocks are the expert modules. Each expert has its own hierarchical DBNN classifier. The outputs of the hierarchical DBNNs are transformed to the posterior probabilities by softmax functions. In this fusion scheme, the expert weighting $P(E_j|\mathbf{x})$ is a function of input pattern $\mathbf{x}$. Therefore, the importance of individual experts may vary with different input patterns observed.

This network adopts the posterior probabilities of electing a class given $\mathbf{x}_i$ (i.e., $P(\omega_c|\mathbf{x}_i, E_k)$) — instead of the likelihood of observing $\mathbf{x}_i$ given a class (i.e., $p(\mathbf{x}_i|\omega_c, E_k)$) — to model the discriminant function of each cluster. For this version of hierarchical FNN, a new confidence $P(E_k|\mathbf{x}_i)$ is assigned, which stands for the confidence on expert k when the input pattern is $\mathbf{x}_i$. Accordingly, the probability model is modified to become

$$P(\omega_c|\mathbf{x}_i) = \sum_{k=1}^{K} P(E_k|\mathbf{x}_i)\, P(\omega_c|\mathbf{x}_i, E_k) \tag{13.19}$$

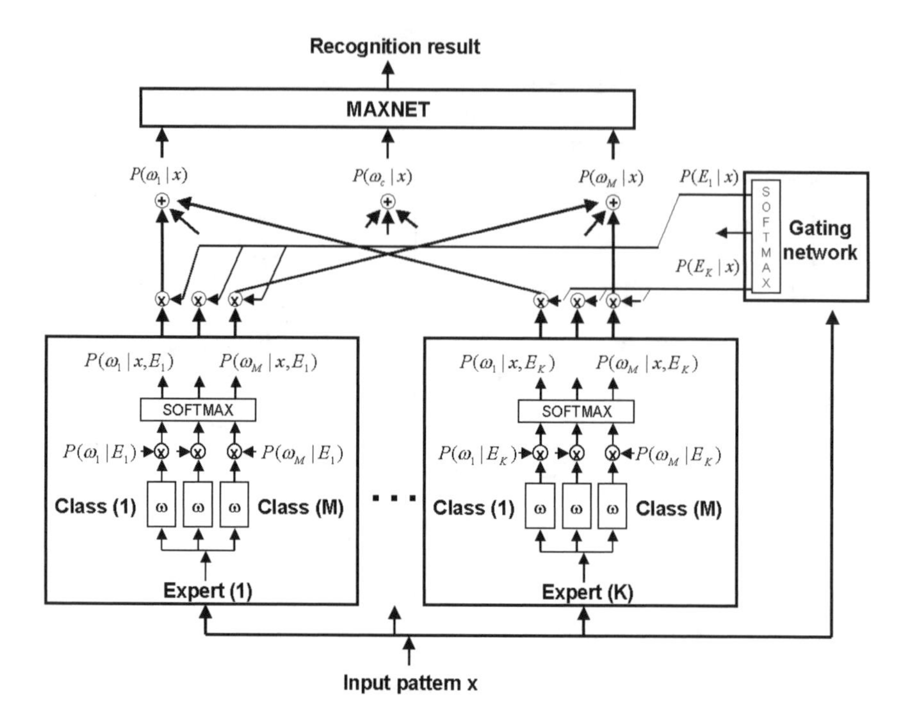

13.7 Classes-in-expert hierarchical design: in this scheme, the expert weighting parameters ($P(E_j|\mathbf{x})$) are functions of the input pattern **x**. The prior probability $P(\omega_i|E_j)$ could either be preassigned or estimated in a similar fashion as other prior probabilities such as $P(\Theta_k|\omega_i, E_j)$ (see Equation 13.18). This network can be viewed as a hybrid model of MOE and DBNNs, where local expert networks serve as local classifiers. When applying such a hierarchical FNN to channel fusion, each channel module can be regarded as a local expert with predetermined feature space. (With permission from S.Y. Kung, J. Taur, and S.H. Lin, Synergistic modeling and applications of hierarchical fuzzy neural networks, *Proceedings of the IEEE*, vol. 87, no. 9, pp. 1550–1574, 1999.)

where

$$P\left(\omega_c|\mathbf{x}_i, E_k\right) = \frac{P\left(\omega_c|E_k\right) p\left(\mathbf{x}_i|\omega_c, E_k\right)}{p\left(\mathbf{x}_i|E_k\right)}, \qquad p\left(\mathbf{x}_i|E_k\right) = \sum_c P\left(\omega_c|E_k\right) p\left(\mathbf{x}_i|\omega_c, E_k\right) \tag{13.20}$$

and the confidence $P(E_k|\mathbf{x}_i)$ can be obtained by the following equation:

$$P\left(E_k|\mathbf{x}_i\right) = \frac{P\left(E_k\right) p\left(\mathbf{x}_i|E_k\right)}{\sum_l P\left(E_l\right) p\left(\mathbf{x}_i|E_l\right)}. \tag{13.21}$$

Equation (13.20) is one type of softmax function. Its weighting parameter $P(\omega_c|E_k)$, just like $P(E_k|\omega_c)$ in Equation (13.17), is made to satisfy the property of a probability function (i.e., $\Sigma_c P(\omega_c|E_k) = 1$). Consequently, $P(\omega_c|E_k)$ can be recursively estimated by EM iterations in Equation (13.18). The term $P(E_k)$ may be interpreted as the confidence-level on expert k, which can be learned by the EM iterations, very similar to Equation (13.18). The confidence level $P(E_k)$ provides the key factor affecting the fusion weight $P(E_k|\mathbf{x}_i)$, which is the output of the softmax gating network. It can also be shown that $P(E_k)$ can be learned by Equation (13.18) with slight modification. We note that, unlike the experts-in-class approach, the fusion weights need to be computed for each testing pattern during the retrieving phase.

13.4.1.2.1 Channel Fusion

The problem of combining the classification power of several classifiers is of great importance to various applications. In many remote sensing, pattern recognition, and multimedia applications, it is not uncommon that different channels or sensors are provided to facilitate the recognition of an object. In addition, for many applications with very high-dimensional feature data, it provides some computational relief to divide feature vectors into several lower-dimensional vectors before integrating them for final decision (i.e., divide-and-conquer).

Several categories of fusion layers have been studied by Abidi and Gonzalez [2]. In the present context, the classes-in-expert hierarchical FNN can be naturally extended to cover the sensor fusion network. To this end, the definition of experts needs to be properly expanded. Now, the local experts include not only (1) the adaptive-trained type, but also (2) the predetermined type. For the former, the feature space (often a certain local region) represented by an expert is adaptively trained in *a posteriori* fashion. The model parameters depend very much on the initial condition the local expert is assigned. As for the predetermined experts, each local expert has a fixed model parameter, as it is designated to extract certain previously known feature space (e.g., high- or low-frequency components). By regarding each sensor as a predetermined local expert, the classes-in-expert hierarchical FNN can be made amenable to sensor fusion applications.

More especifically, the sensor-fusion FNN consists of several classifier channels, each of which receives input vector from its own sensor. Its structure (although not shown) resembles that of the classes-in-expert FNN. The fusion of different channels can be implemented as a (properly gated) linear combination of outputs, with the gating parameters reflecting the confidence measures of the sensor channels. This scheme can make a good use of the Bayesian estimation formulation and also facilitate adoption of EM training of the channel confidence parameters.

13.4.2 Applications of Hierarchical FNNs

13.4.2.1 Texture Classification via Global (Interclass) Supervision

In the above section, the EM classifier does not make a full use of the interclass supervised training, which directly tackles any mutual dispute which might exist between two competing classes. Substantial improvement can be expected by fully utilizing global interclass supervision. This ideia prompted Taur and Tao [56] to propose an experts-in-class hierarchical texture classifier, based on the decision-based (reinforced and anti-reinforced) learning rule. Twelve Brodatz texture images were tested in the experiments, and the hierarchical classifier achieved an extremely low classification error rate (as low as 0.2%). Such a superior performance is partially due to the adoption of global supervision. It is also partially due to the adoption of a novel texture feature, called fuzzy texture spectrum. The fuzzy texture spectrum, based on the relative differences of the gray levels between pixels, appears to be fairly insensitive to noise and changing of the background brightness in texture images.

13.4.2.2 Face Recognition and Content-Based Indexing for Video Browsing

Face recognition is a user-friendly, nonintrusive, and convenient approach to biometric identification. Many neural networks have been proposed for face recognition [4, 7, 19, 35, 40, 60]. Among various recognition approaches, fuzzy decision-based neural networks have shown very good success in this field [40]. By combining facial information with other biometric features such as speech, feature fusion not only enhances accuracy but also provides some fault tolerance, i.e., it can tolerate a temporary corruption of one of the bimodal channels. Such neural networks have also been successfully applied to detecting human faces and locating eyes [38, 39].

In many video applications, browsing through a large amount of video material to find the relevant clips is an extremely important task. The video database indexed by human faces, exemplified by

Figure 13.8, provides users the facility to efficiently acquire video clips about the person of interest. For example, a film-study student may conveniently extract the clips of his/her favorite actor from movie archives to study his/her performance, and a TV news reporter may quickly find, from a news database, the clips containing images of some politician in order to edit headline news.

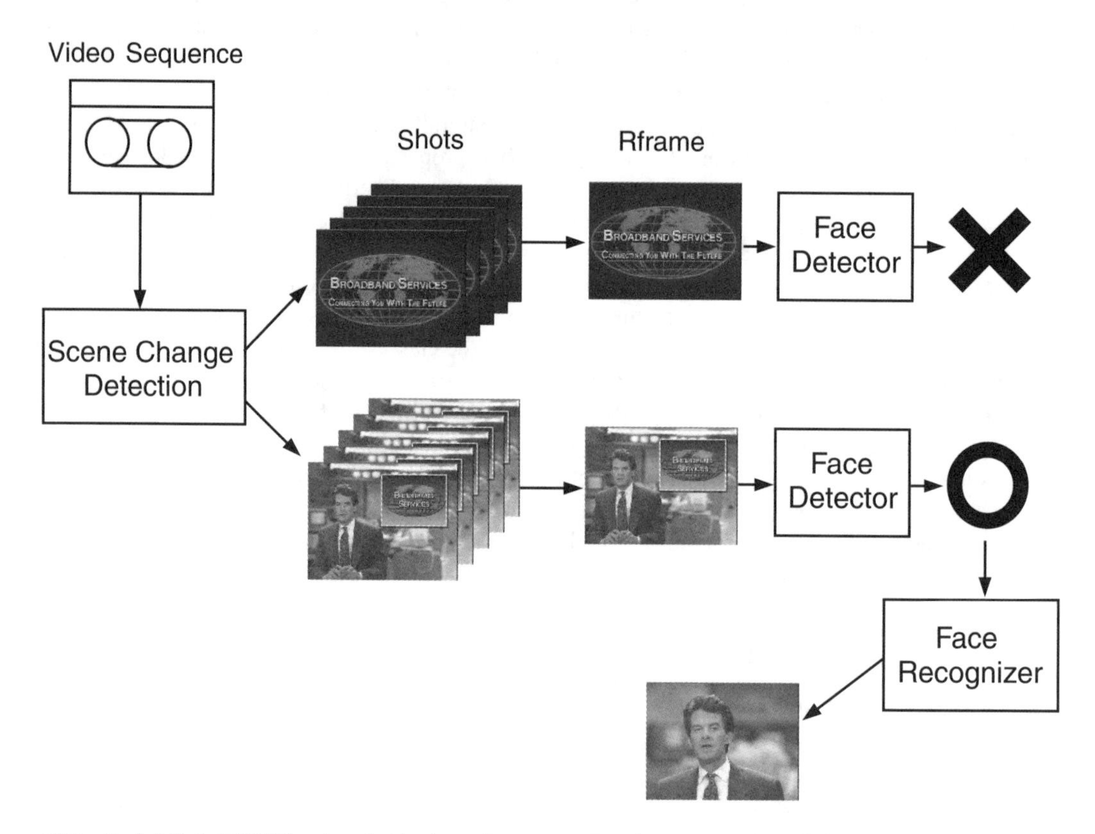

13.8 Probabilistic DBNN face-based video browsing system. Face detector examines all the representative frames to see if they contain human faces, and, if so, the face detector passes the frame to the face recognizer to identify whose face it is. (With permission from S.Y. Kung, J. Taur, and S.H. Lin, Synergistic modeling and applications of hierarchical fuzzy neural networks, *Proceedings of the IEEE,* vol. 87, no. 9, pp. 1550–1574, 1999.)

Fuzzy neural processing presents a promising approach to fast access of audio-visual objects, manipulating them, and presenting them in a highly flexible way. Extracting proper information content inherent in video clips leads to efficient search schemes for content-based retrieval. A video indexing and browsing scheme based on human faces was proposed by Lin and colleagues [39, 40]. The scheme adopts the (experts-in-class) hierarchical FNN for face detection and recognition techniques. The scheme contains three steps. The first step of this face-based video browser is to segment the video sequence by applying a scene change detection algorithm. Scene change detection gives indication of when a new shot starts and ends. Each segment (shot) created by scene change detection can be considered a story unit of this sequence. From every video shot, its representative frame and feed it into a probabilistic DBNN face detector [40]. Those representative frames to which the detector gives high face detection confidence scores are annotated and serve as the indices for browsing.

This scheme can also be helpful for constructing hierarchies of video shots for the purpose of video browsing. One such algorithm [66], for example, proposes using global color and luminance information as similarity measures to cluster video shots in an attempt to build video shot hierarchies. Their similarity metrics enable very fast processing of videos. However, in their demonstration, some shots featuring the same anchorman fail to be grouped together due to insufficient image content understanding. For this type of application, we believe that the existence of similar objects, and human objects in particular, should provide a good similarity measure. As reported in the literature [5, 6], this scheme successfully classifies these shots to the same group.

13.4.2.3 Currency Recognition

Currency recognition is becoming a mandatory module in many color printers and scanners. It detects the presence of specific originals such as currencies, bank notes, or securities and prevents such pictures from being scanned or printed. Though currency recognition is a standard two-dimensional image recognition task, its major challenge is to recognize a wide variety of currencies with all kinds of variations under a very limited computation resource, such as the microprocessor in a \$99 color scanner.

Fuzzy neural networks have been successfully applied to anti-forgery and currency discrimination. A hierarchical experts-in-class DBNN recognizer has been designed to utilize both the local texture features and the global structural information of the registered currency patterns. It is reported that currencies from more than 8 countries on a 50 DPI 8.5" $\times$ 11" scanned page can be detected within 3 seconds on a 132 MHz processor, with a misrecognition rate of less than 0.1% (i.e., no currency pattern out of 1000 tests fails to be detected) and the false detection rate is less than 0.001% (i.e., no noncurrency pattern out of 100,000 tests is falsely detected). Results are shown in Figure 13.9.

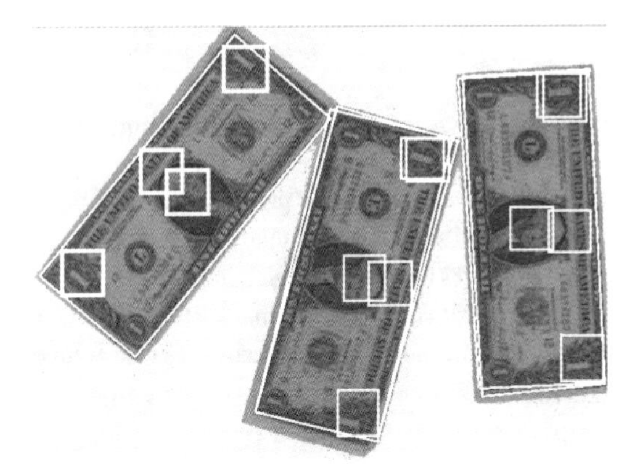

13.9 Money patterns detected by a hierarchical DBNN recognizer. The small boxes indicate the locations of the detected local currency texture features, and the large boxes show the locations of the money patterns. (With permission from S.Y. Kung, J. Taur, and S.H. Lin, Synergistic modeling and applications of hierarchical fuzzy neural networks, *Proceedings of the IEEE,* vol. 87, no. 9, pp. 1550–1574, 1999.)

13.4.2.4 Medical Applications of Experts-in-Class FNNs

13.4.2.4.1 Medical Image Quantification

The problem of image quantification is very different from image segmentation. Compared to image segmentation, which categorizes each image pixel to one of the many image classes (i.e., hard classification), image quantification assigns to pixels the probabilistic (fuzzy) memberships from multiple image classes (i.e., quantitative mapping functions). These memberships carry particular significance beyond the actual segmentation. One example is the determination of the activity involving the transmission of nerve impulses in the selected regions of interest (ROI) in the brain [34]. To assist doctors in analyzing the high activity regions in the positron emission tomography (PET) image of the brain, Wang et al. [63, 64] assigned the image pixels fuzzy membership values from different brain tissue classes. The memberships are created by examining the higher-resolution magnetic resonance (MR) image which is registered to the PET image beforehand.

The fuzzy class memberships are realized by the class conditional likelihood functions in the experts-in-class network. A model fitting scheme is used to estimate the number and kernel of local clusters using information theoretic criteria. The class distribution functions are then obtained by learning generalized Gaussian mixtures where a fuzzy classification of the data is performed. Further classification of the data is treated as a hard Bayesian detection problem, where the decision boundaries between the classes are fine-tuned by the decision-based learning scheme. Successful implementation of this framework has been demonstrated [62, 63].

13.4.2.4.2 Computer Aided Diagnosis

The aforementioned experts-in-class networks can be applied to the computer aided diagnosis for breast cancer detection. The objective is to detect masses (suspicious cancer regions) in digital mammography. Some typical mass cluster appearances on mammograms are displayed in Figure 13.10. In clinic sites, masses are evaluated based on the location, density, size, shape, margins, and the presence of associated calcifications. Note that the knowledge database involving computer assisted diagnosis has long been recognized as fairly complex. In fact, the complexity has little to do with "dimensionality" of the feature space. Therefore, the hierarchical DBNN proves to be a very effective tool for classification. For more details, see Li et al. [36]. A two-class hierarchical DBNN is trained to distinguish the "true masses" from the "false masses" based on the features extracted from the suspected regions:

- A total of 150 mammograms were selected from the mammographic database. Each mammogram contained at least one mass case of varying size and location. Among them, 50 of the mammograms contained the biopsy proven masses (true masses). Note that one mammogram consisted of two breast images taken from different viewing directions. In other words, 300 images were selected.
- The training set was constructed from 50 true mass ROIs and 50 false mass ROIs. Note that there was more than one mass ROI in one mammogram image.
- The test set contained 46 randomly selected single-view mammograms: 23 normal cases and 23 containing biopsy proven masses.
- The feature vector contained two features: compactness and difference entropy. According to our investigation, these two features have the better separation (discrimination) between the true and false mass classes.

Figure 13.10b shows the classification of two classes with our method. In our evaluation study, 6 to 15 suspected masses per mammogram were detected and recommended to physicians for further evaluation. The receiver operating characteristic (ROC) method is used to evaluate the detection performance. When the two distributions overlap on the decision axis, a cut-off point can be made at an arbitrary decision threshold. The corresponding true-positive fraction (TPF) vs. false-positive fraction (FPF) for each threshold can be drawn on a plane, where sensitivity (TPF) and specificity (one minus FPF) are used to evaluate the system performance on the specified point of the ROC curve. The best operating point of the proposed classifier is at a sensitivity of 84%, with a specificity of 82%. At this point, the classifier reaches the performance of 1.6 false positive findings per mammogram, which outperforms the conventional rate at 2.0 [62].

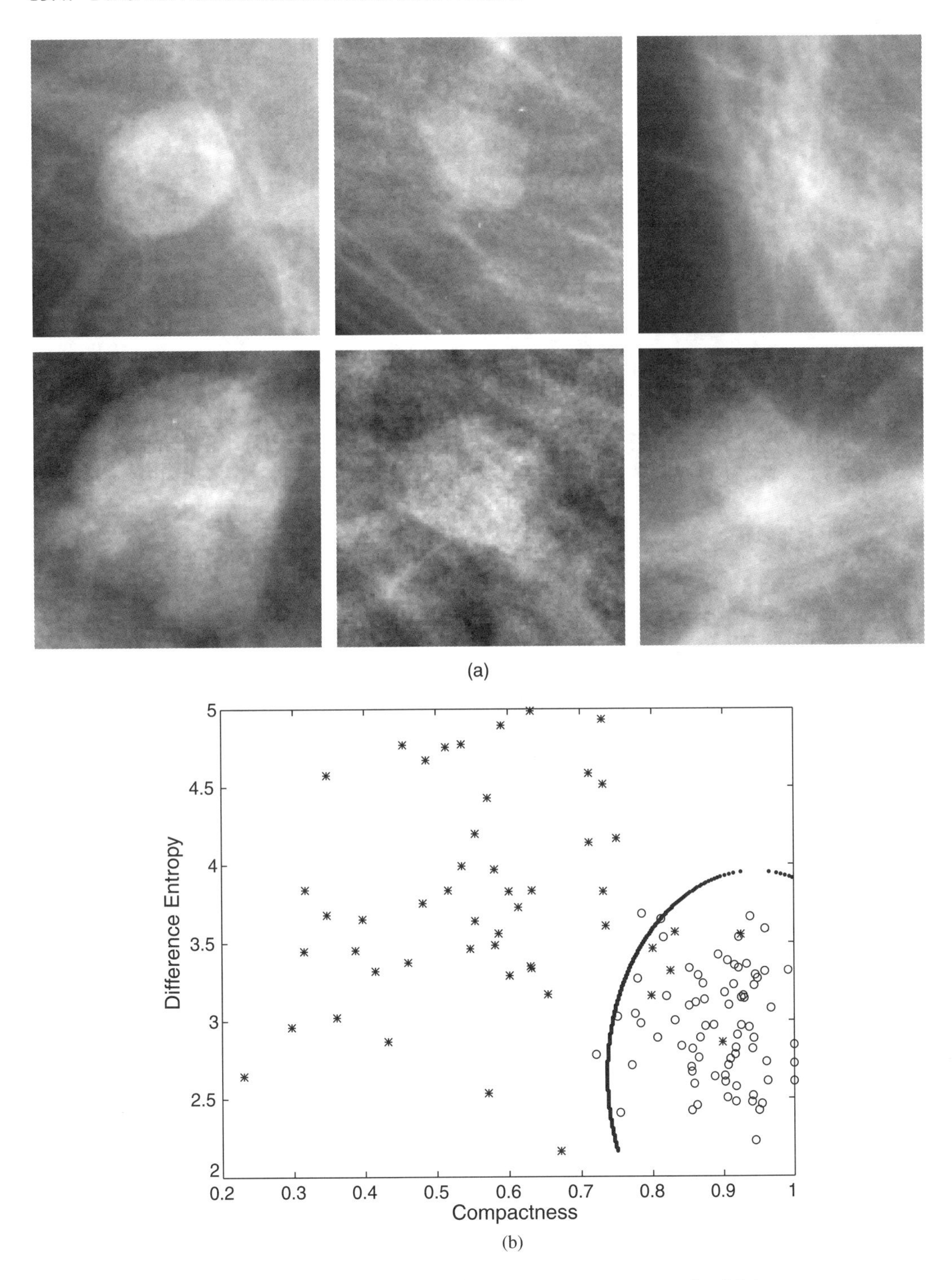

13.10 (a) The typical mass appearances in mammograms; (b) the classification results: "o" denotes true mass cases, "*" denotes false mass cases. Compactness and difference entropy are the features used for classification. Originally, a total of 17 features selected by medical experts were studied in our DBNN clustering. The two-dimensional plot shows the two most representative features which possess the greatest distinguishability. (With permission from S.Y. Kung, J. Taur, and S.H. Lin, Synergistic modeling and applications of hierarchical fuzzy neural networks, *Proceedings of the IEEE,* vol. 87, no. 9, pp. 1550–1574, 1999.)

13.4.2.5 Three-Dimensional Object Recognition via Classes-in-Expert FNN

The classes-in-expert hierarchical fusion network has demonstrated classification improvements on three-dimensional vehicle recognition problems [38]. This is illustrated in Figure 13.11. The experiment used six car models from different view angles to create the training and testing

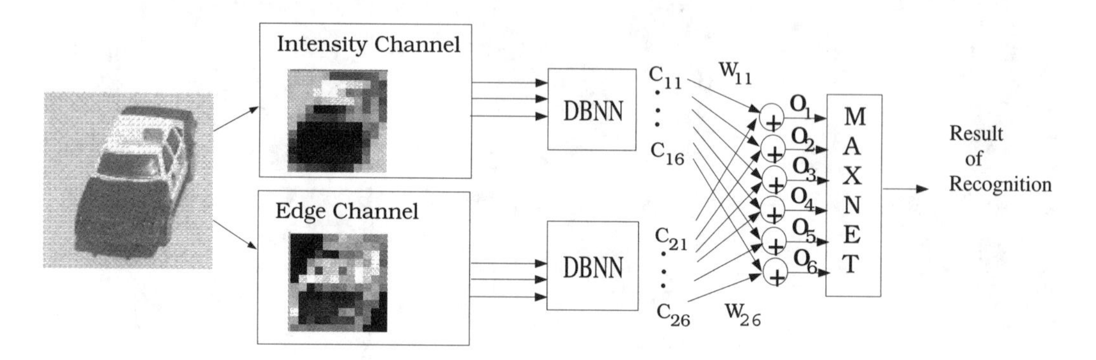

13.11 A classes-in-expert system for car recognition. Given an original image, two experts are adopted to classify various car models using features from different frequency domains. One expert uses the low-frequency information, and the other uses the high-frequency information. The classification results from the two experts are combined by the classes-in-expert fusion scheme. (With permission from S.Y. Kung, J. Taur, and S.H. Lin, Synergistic modeling and applications of hierarchical fuzzy neural networks, *Proceedings of the IEEE,* vol. 87, no. 9, pp. 1550–1574, 1999.)

database. Around 30 images (each with size 256 × 256 pixels) were taken for each car model from various viewing directions. There were a total of 172 examples in the data set. Two classifier channels were built from two different feature extraction methods: one used intensity information, and the other used edge information. Upon fusion of two channels (with 94 and 85% recognition rate each), the recognition rate reached 100%. The fusion model was compared with a single network classifier. The input vectors of these two networks were formed by cascading the intensity vector with the edge vector. Therefore, the input vector dimension becomes $144 \times 2 = 288$. The network is the RBF-type DBNN. The experimental result shows a performance of around 96% recognition rate, which is far inferior to (the perfect rate of) the fusion network.

13.5 Hybrid Hierarchical Network

The HFNNs draw inspiration from innovations within both the neural network and fuzzy logic communities. Such HFNNs strive to preserve the structure of the fuzzy systems and, at the same time, maximally exploit unsupervised and supervised learning rules in neural networks. One should be able to learn rules in a hybrid fashion and calibrate them for better total-system performance. One hybrid design example will be elaborated in the following.

13.5.1 Neuro-Fuzzy Classifiers with Adjustable Rule Importance

The class-level hierarchical structure used in the DBNN and the interpretation of fuzzy **If-Then** logic rules can be combined to establish the connections between the hidden nodes and the output nodes. One good example is the neuro-fuzzy classifier called NEFCAR, which is built upon the OCON structure [57]. Based on the interpretation of fuzzy **If-Then** rules, the connections between the hidden nodes and the output nodes in the OCON structure are established. Both positive and negative rules are utilized, and they are given varying and adjustable rule importances. Simulation studies point to the result that the classification rate can be improved by adding the cross connections. This demonstrates that the system performance may be improved by properly combining neural learning techniques and the fuzzy linguistic structure.

When the neuro-fuzzy network is designed by using the input–output data pairs $(\mathbf{x}^i, f^i)$ from experiments, a rule "If $\mathbf{x}$ is $\mathbf{x}^i$, then f is f^i," can be constructed from each data pair for simplicity. However, when the number of samples is large, the computational cost will make this simple approach inadmissible. In this situation, a clustering algorithm can be applied to find the "representative" centroids of the data and then assign importance factors to the corresponding rules to reflect the numbers of samples covered by the centroids. From this idea, we propose the neuro-fuzzy classifier NEFCAR [57, 58].

13.5.1.1 Architecture of NEFCAR

Let us assume that the input pattern, the number of input patterns, the dimension of the input pattern, the number of class, and the number of rules in class j, are denoted as $\mathbf{x}$, N_x, N, M, and D_j, respectively. The fuzzy rules of NEFCAR for an N-dimensional input pattern $\mathbf{x} = \{x_1, \ldots, x_N\}$ are of the form:

$$\begin{cases} \text{Positive Rule:} & \text{If } x_1 \text{ is } \mu_1 \text{ and } \cdots \text{ and } x_N \text{ is } \mu_N \\ & \quad \text{then } \mathbf{x} \text{ is in class } i \\ \text{Negative Rule:} & \text{If } x_1 \text{ is } \mu_1 \text{ and } \cdots \text{ and } x_N \text{ is } \mu_N \\ & \quad \text{then } \mathbf{x} \text{ is } \textit{not} \text{ in class } k \end{cases} \tag{13.22}$$

where μ_ls are the fuzzy sets with Gaussian-like membership functions. The consequent of the positive rule, "$\mathbf{x}$ is in class i," is represented as a classifier output variable $f_i = 1$. On the other hand, the consequent of the negative rules is represented as an output $f_k = -1$. The schematic diagram of the architecture of the classifier is shown in Figure 13.12. If a rule node is from class j and the output of class j is under consideration, then this rule is regarded as a positive rule. On the other

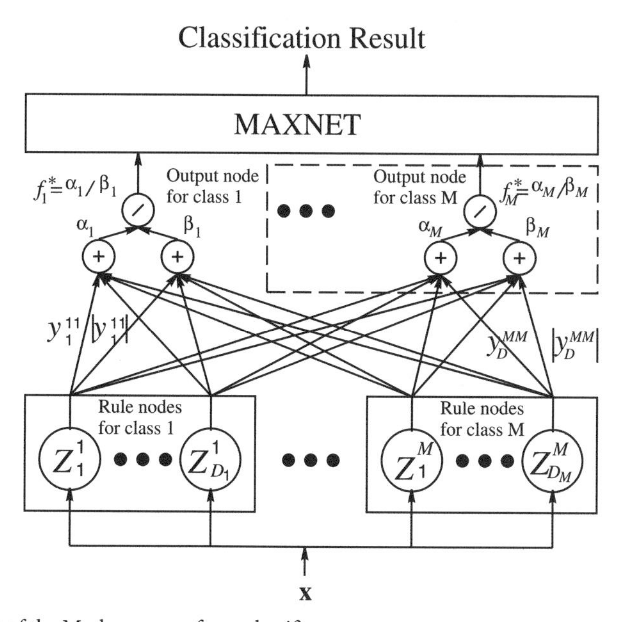

13.12 Block diagram of the M-class neuro-fuzzy classifier.

hand, if the output of class $i(\neq j)$ is under consideration, this rule is designed to behave as a negative rule. Therefore, for a rule node in class j, we effectively have one positive rule and $(M-1)$ negative rules as follows:

$$\begin{cases} \text{Positive Rule:} & \text{If } x_1 \text{ is } \mu_1 \text{ and } \cdots \text{ and } x_N \text{ is } \mu_N \,, \\ & \quad \text{then } f_j = 1 \,. \\ \text{Negative Rule:} & \text{If } x_1 \text{ is } \mu_1 \text{ and } \cdots \text{ and } x_N \text{ is } \mu_N \,, \\ & \quad \text{then } f_1 = -1 \,. \\ & \vdots \\ \text{Negative Rule:} & \text{If } x_1 \text{ is } \mu_1 \text{ and } \cdots \text{ and } x_N \text{ is } \mu_N \,, \\ & \quad \text{then } f_{j-1} = -1 \,. \\ \text{Negative Rule:} & \text{If } x_1 \text{ is } \mu_1 \text{ and } \cdots \text{ and } x_N \text{ is } \mu_N \,, \\ & \quad \text{then } f_{j+1} = -1 \,. \\ & \vdots \\ \text{Negative Rule:} & \text{If } x_1 \text{ is } \mu_1 \text{ and } \cdots \text{ and } x_N \text{ is } \mu_N \,, \\ & \quad \text{then } f_M = -1 \,. \end{cases} \tag{13.23}$$

The importance of the dth rule node in class j to the output of class i is represented by a weighting factor y_d^{ij}. The importance factor is interpreted as duplicating the same rule y_d^{ij} times in the defuzzification procedure for output i. When y_d^{ij} gets larger, the corresponding rule becomes more important to output f_i^*.

Assume that the mean and the variance of the lth (Gaussian-like) membership function of the dth rule for the jth class are denoted as m_{dl}^j and σ_{dl}^j, respectively. Moreover, the height defuzzification approach [12] is adopted to compute the output of each class, and the multiplication is adopted for the "and" operation in the rule in Equation (13.23). Then, the output of class i can be computed using the following formula:

$$f_i^* = \alpha_i / \beta_i \tag{13.24}$$

where

$$\alpha_i = \sum_{d=1}^{D_i} (+1) y_d^{ii} Z_d^i + \sum_{j=1, j\neq i}^{M} \sum_{d=1}^{D_j} (-1) y_d^{ij} Z_d^j \tag{13.25}$$

$$= \sum_{d=1}^{D_i} y_d^{ii} Z_d^i - \sum_{j=1, j\neq i}^{M} \sum_{d=1}^{D_j} y_d^{ij} Z_d^j \tag{13.26}$$

$$\beta_i = \sum_{j=1}^{M} \sum_{d=1}^{D_j} y_d^{ij} Z_d^j \tag{13.27}$$

and

$$Z_d^j = \exp\left(- \sum_{l=1}^{N} \frac{(x_l - m_{dl}^j)^2}{(\sigma_{dl}^j)^2} \right) \tag{13.28}$$

which is the matching degree of the "if" part of the dth rule node in class j. We can further absorb the (+1) and (-1) into y_d^{ij} and obtain

$$\alpha_i = \sum_{j=1}^{M} \sum_{d=1}^{D_j} y_d^{ij} Z_d^j \quad (13.29)$$

$$\beta_i = \sum_{j=1}^{M} \sum_{d=1}^{D_j} |y_d^{ij}| Z_d^j . \quad (13.30)$$

Therefore, we can consider (y_d^{ij})s as weighting parameters in the network shown in Figure 13.12. From the above equations, it is obvious that

$$-1 \leq f_i^* \leq 1 \text{ , for } i = 1, \ldots, M .$$

The classification procedure is described as follows. The pattern $\mathbf{x}$ is input to each rule node which computes the matching degree (Z_d^j) of the "if" part of the rule. Then the output of each class (f_i^*) is computed according to the weighting of each rule. The class, c, which has the largest output is identified. That is,

$$c = \arg\left(\max_i f_i^*\right) . \quad (13.31)$$

The pattern is classified into class c if the confidence measure is large enough. Similarly, if we are dealing with a two-class application, the shaded region and the weights connected to it, which are shown in Figure 13.12, can be removed. In this situation, the sample is classified into class 1 if $f_1^* > 0$. Otherwise, it is classified into class 2.

13.5.1.2 Training Strategy

The locally unsupervised and globally supervised technique is adopted. That is, for the parameters in the network of a given class, we utilize an unsupervised k-mean clustering method to obtain the initial values using the patterns in the same class. Also training patterns from all classes are used to update the classifier after the initialization using the gradient descent approach. In decision-based training, the teacher only indicates to which class the current pattern should belong. There are no target values for the training patterns. Only the misclassified patterns are used to train the system through the reinforced and anti-reinforced rules. On the other hand, in the approximation-based approach, the squared errors between output values and the teacher values for all the training data are taken into consideration. For training NEFCARs, we adopt a strategy which combines the approximation-based and decision-based training strategies.

NEFCARs can provide the confidence measure of each classification easily. If the pattern is from class i, we can define the confidence measure as

$$C_m^i = \left(\sum_{d=1}^{D_i} y_d^{ii} Z_d^i\right) / y_{\max} \quad (13.32)$$

where $y_{\max}$ is defined as

$$y_{\max} = \max_{d,i,j} y_d^{ij} . \quad (13.33)$$

The C_m^i measures the normalized sum of matching degrees of the rule antecedent of the rules from class i.

In the training phase, confidence measure can be used to avoid outliers. If C_m^i is smaller than a threshold T_c for a training sample, then this sample is ignored in this iteration to avoid the training on outlier and possible numerical difficulties. Let C_{ma} denote the average of the confidence measure, that is,

$$C_{ma} = \frac{1}{N_x} \sum_{i=1}^{M} \sum_{x \in \text{ Class } i} C_m^i$$

where N_x denotes the total number of patterns. The C_{ma} is calculated for each epoch of training. When C_{ma} becomes small in the training process, it indicates that the rules in each class cannot model the data very well on average. Although the error rate can be small for the training set, the generalization performance cannot be guaranteed to be small. This situation sometimes results from overtraining.

In the retrieving phase, if the output i has the largest output value, the test pattern **x** will be classified into class i with confidence measure C_m^i. If C_m^i is smaller than a certain threshold, the pattern will be left undecided.

13.5.1.3 Updating Formula

Let the teacher vector for a pattern from class k be denoted as $T_k = \{t_1, t_2, \ldots, t_M\}$ and have the value

$$\begin{cases} t_i = -1, & i \neq k \\ t_i = +1, & i = k \, . \end{cases} \tag{13.34}$$

The goal of training is to minimize the mean squared difference between the output f_i^* and the teacher value t_i for the patterns with error that is above a noise tolerance level $(1-n_t)$. Since Gaussian-like functions are adopted as the membership functions, the error back-propagation algorithm can be easily implemented to calculate the gradients for all the parameters in the neuro-fuzzy classifier. The gradient from the ith output node can be computed as

$$\begin{cases} g_{ij} = 0, & abs(e_i) < 1 - n_t \\ g_{ij} = \frac{\partial e_i^2}{\partial w_j}, & abs(e_i) \geq 1 - n_t \end{cases} \tag{13.35}$$

where w_j represents one of the parameters in the set $\{y_d^{ij}, m_{dl}^j, \sigma_{dl}^j\}$.

Assume that the current training pattern is from class k. Furthermore, let i and j denote the class indexes of the output node and the rule node, respectively. Then the parameter can be adjusted by the updating rule:

$$w_j^{p+1} = w_j^p - \sum_{i=1}^{M} g_{ij} \, \gamma(i, j, k) \tag{13.36}$$

where p is the iteration index and γ is a weighting factor, which will be explained below.

For the architecture in Figure 13.12, we have three types of training gradient information for a pattern from class k according to which output node is under consideration and to which class the rule belongs:

$$
\begin{array}{lll}
\text{1. reinforced learning:} & & \\
\quad g_{ij},\ j = k & \gamma = \eta_1 & \\
\text{2. anti-reinforced learning:} & & \\
\quad g_{ij},\ i = k,\ \text{and}\ j \neq k, & \gamma = \eta_2 & \\
\quad g_{ij},\ i \neq k,\ j \neq k,\ \text{and}\ i = j, & \gamma = \eta_2 & \\
\text{3. cross-reinforced learning:} & & \\
\quad g_{ij},\ i \neq k,\ j \neq k,\ \text{and}\ i \neq j, & \gamma = \eta_3 &
\end{array}
\tag{13.37}
$$

In the first situation, the updating will try to increase the absolute value of the outputs of the rule nodes and the absolute values of the importance weighting factors for the rules from the same class as training pattern class k to decrease the error. We call it "reinforced learning." In the second case, the updating will try to decrease the absolute value of the outputs of the rule nodes and the absolute values of the importance weighting factors for the rules from classes other than k. This type of training is called anti-reinforced learning. In the last case, the training will try to increase the outputs of the rule nodes and the absolute values of the importance weighting factors and is called "cross-reinforced learning." Usually, reinforced learning will increase the confidence measure defined in Equation (13.32), while anti-reinforced learning and cross-reinforced learning will decrease the confidence measure.

Although the cross-reinforced learning can also help the network reduce the training error, it may result in degrading the generalization performance. In Equation (13.37), different types of training are assigned different weighting γ to avoid degrading the generalization capability. Let the weighting factors for the first, second, and third type be denoted as η_1, η_2, and η_3, respectively. Therefore, in our design,

$$\eta_3 \leq \eta_2 \leq \eta_1$$

and η_3 is sometimes set to zero.

13.5.2 Applications of NEFCAR Hierarchical Classifier

Biometric identification techniques can be applied to many practical applications in the area of automation and information security. Moreover, computer technology has advanced rapidly in recent years. It will make biometric identification a safe and useful approach [19, 35, 40, 59, 60]. Among these biometric identification methods, face recognition is a very convenient and effective approach. Based on NEFCARs, this section presents an online face detection and recognition system which consists of four major subsystems: (1) region of interest (ROI) detection, (2) face detection, (3) face localization, and (4) face recognition. The flow chart of the algorithm is depicted in Figure 13.13.

13.5.2.1 ROI Detection

In order to save the computation time for face detection using the NEFCAR, we would like to find the regions of interest in which there exists a human face with high confidence. Moreover, some complex background can be filtered out, which simplifies the design of other subsystems. The information from motion and the skin color are used to obtain the ROIs. We first identify the rectangular regions that contain large areas of skin color. Then, motion information is used to further reduce the number of ROIs.

13.5.2.1.1 Skin Color

To alleviate the influence from the illumination, we project the points in the normalized RGB space onto the plane determined by the points with coordinates (0,0,1), (0,1,0), and (1,0,0) along the

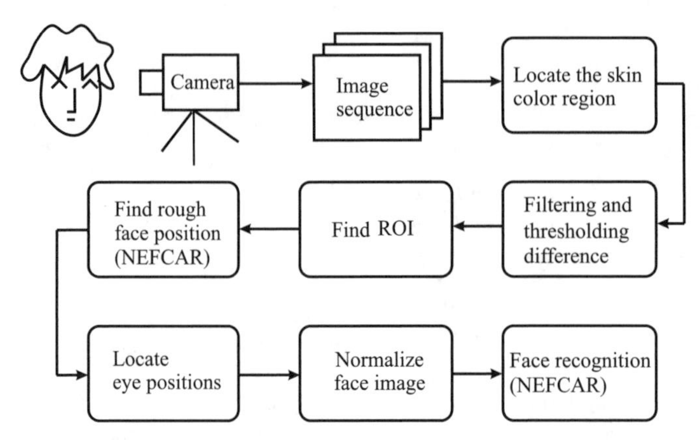

13.13 Flow chart of the face localization system.

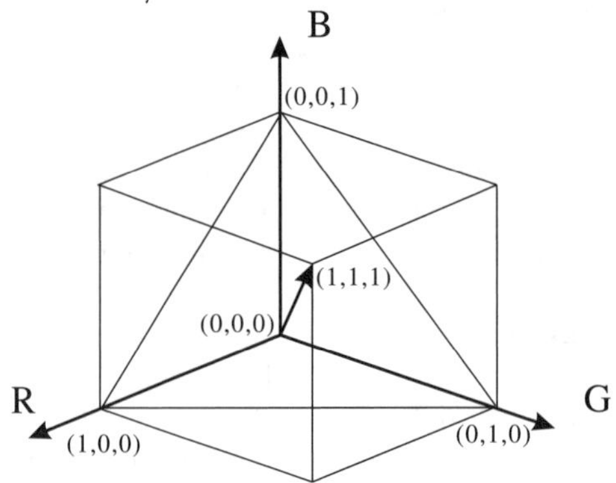

13.14 This figure shows that the points in the cube of the normalized RGB space can be projected to the plane defined by (0,0,1), (0,1,0), and (1,0,0) along the [1 1 1] direction. (With permission from J. Taur and C.W. Tao, A new neuro-fuzzy classifier with application to online face detection and recognition, *Journal of VLSI Signal Processing Systems,* vol. 26, no. 3, 2000.)

[1 1 1] direction (see Figure 13.14). On this plane, we can define a new two-dimensional coordinate system. On this new coordinate system, a Gaussian mixture defined as

$$p(\mathbf{x}) = \sum_{j=1}^{M} p_n\left(\mathbf{x}|\omega_j\right) P\left(\omega_j\right) \tag{13.38}$$

is used to model the distribution of the skin color, where $P(\omega_j)$ is the prior probability of the jth Gaussian component, and $p_n(\mathbf{x}|\omega_j)$ is the Gaussian distribution with mean vector μ_j and covariance matrix Σ_j of the jth component. The EM algorithm is adopted to obtain the parameters in the Gaussian mixture model [10]. If $p(\mathbf{x})$ for a pixel is larger than a threshold, it is considered a pixel belonging to skin region. Figure 13.15a shows the regions obtained by the skin color information.

13.5.2.1.2 Motion Information

The images are first transformed into gray-scale images. The difference image is calculated from two consecutive images to find the regions with moving objects. If the difference is larger than a threshold, the value of the pixel is set to one; otherwise it is set to zero. The result is shown in Figure 13.15b. For each ROI obtained previously, we can calculate the ratio of the area of pixels with a value of one to the area of the ROI. If the ratio is too small, the ROI will be considered as a still object of skin color and will be ignored. This process can remove some still background regions that are classified as skin regions.

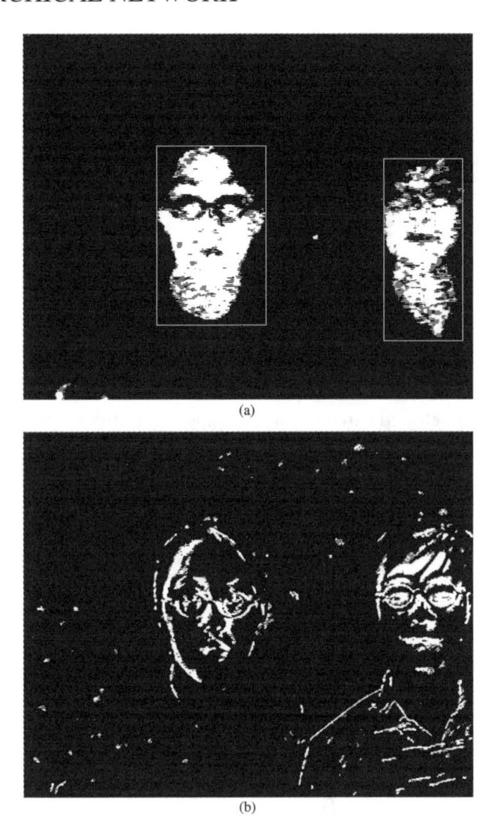

13.15 In image (a), the pixels classified to be skin pixels are shown in white. In image (b), the white pixel indicates that the difference between the gray levels of two consecutive images is large. The final ROIs are indicated by the boxes in image (a). (With permission from J. Taur and C.W. Tao, A new neuro-fuzzy classifier with application to online face detection and recognition, *Journal of VLSI Signal Processing Systems,* vol. 26, no. 3, 2000.)

13.5.2.2 Face Detection

A two-class NEFCAR is adopted to detect the face. If the face is detected in a connected region in an ROI, the final position is computed as the weighted position at the original resolution using the confidence measure at the detected positions. We assume that there exists at most one face in each ROI. Therefore, if more than one connected region is detected, the region with the largest sum of the confidence measure is selected.

13.5.2.2.1 Image Database

To save the storage space and the processing time, we first work on the still images, which are taken using a digital camera. These images can be considered the ROIs obtained from the color and motion information. In the training and test procedure, images from 75 people with three different view angles (frontal 45° to the right, 0°, 45° to the left) are used (see Figure 13.16 for typical images). The sizes of faces vary from about 160 × 115 to 200 × 150 pixels.

13.5.2.2.2 Feature Vector

To alleviate the harmful influences from hair style, ornaments, or facial expressions, we adopt a normalized T-shape image block, which covers the eyes and nose, as the feature vector (see the right image in Figure 13.16 and the image in Figure 13.18). The feature area is averaged and down-sampled by a factor of eight. This process can further reduce the influence from some variations, for example, eye glasses. Then the mean of the feature vector is removed and the variance is normalized to one. For the training patterns, we manually select the center positions of the eyes (p_1 and p_2)

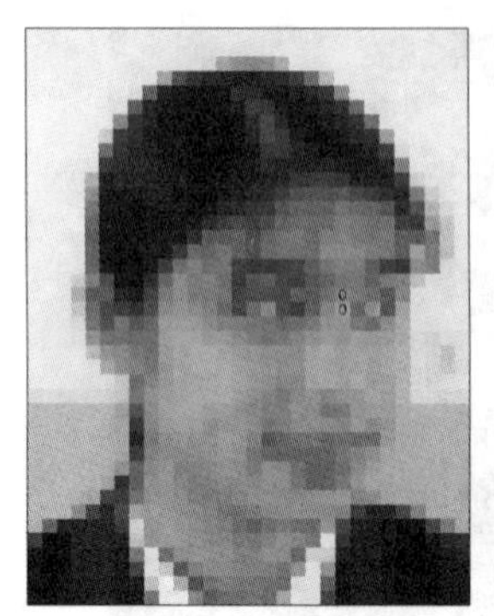
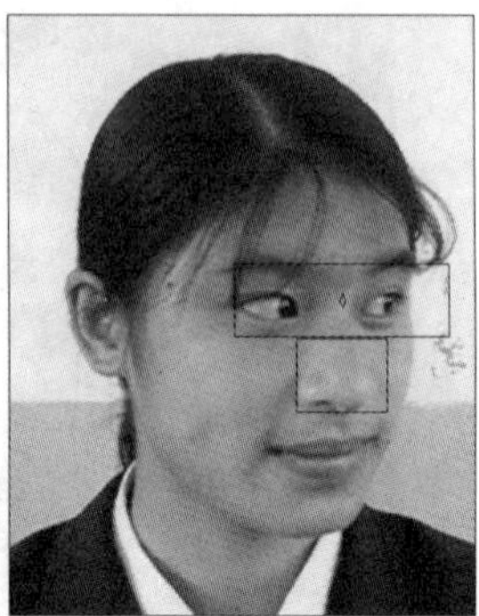

13.16 This figure shows a typical detected situation for the database of still images. The left image shows the down-sampled images and the detected face positions (marked with circles). The right image shows the images at the original resolution. The feature region (within boxes) and the final detected position (marked with ◇) are shown. (With permission from S.Y. Kung, J. Taur, and S.H. Lin, Synergistic modeling and applications of hierarchical fuzzy neural networks, *Proceedings of the IEEE,* vol. 87, no. 9, pp. 1550–1574, 1999.)

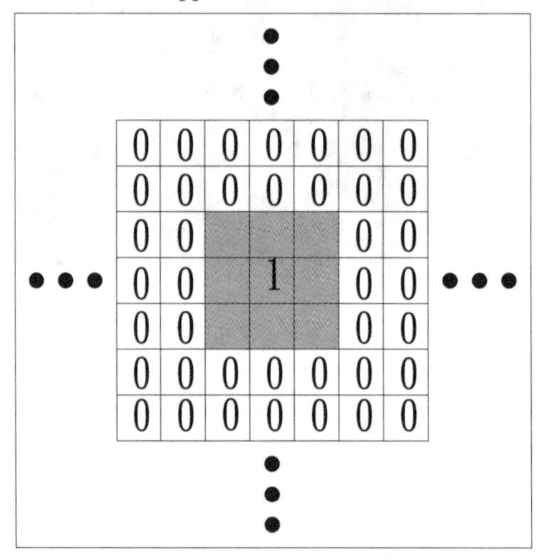

13.17 This figure shows the positions of positive and negative training patterns. "1" and "0" are used to denote the positions of the positive and negative patterns, respectively. The mask m_g is indicated as the gray 3×3 region.

by using the mouse. The position for a positive sample in the image is then obtained by averaging the center positions ($(p_1 + p_2)/2$). That is, a positive sample will be generated from the pixels in the T-shape image block at $(p_1 + p_2)/2$. The pixels in the image outside a mask m_g centered at the positive sample are considered the positions of negative patterns. The size of the mask m_g is 3×3 in the down-sampled images (see Figure 13.17). The number of training patterns thus obtained is more than 60,000. The same feature vector is used for face detection and recognition.

13.5.2.2.3 Results of Face Detection

If the classification rate is computed for the decision at each pixel, the overall error rate will be extremely low. However, since the goal is to locate the face, it would be more meaningful to use the final detection error as the performance measure. When evaluating the performance of the classifier, if the face is detected within the mask m_g centered at the desired position, the detection is considered to be correct. Otherwise, a false detection occurs. If the confidence measure is too low for the detection, it is left undecided (rejected). The training accuracy (images with 45° to the right and 0°) is 100% correct. The test accuracy on the third set of images (45° to the left) is 93.33%

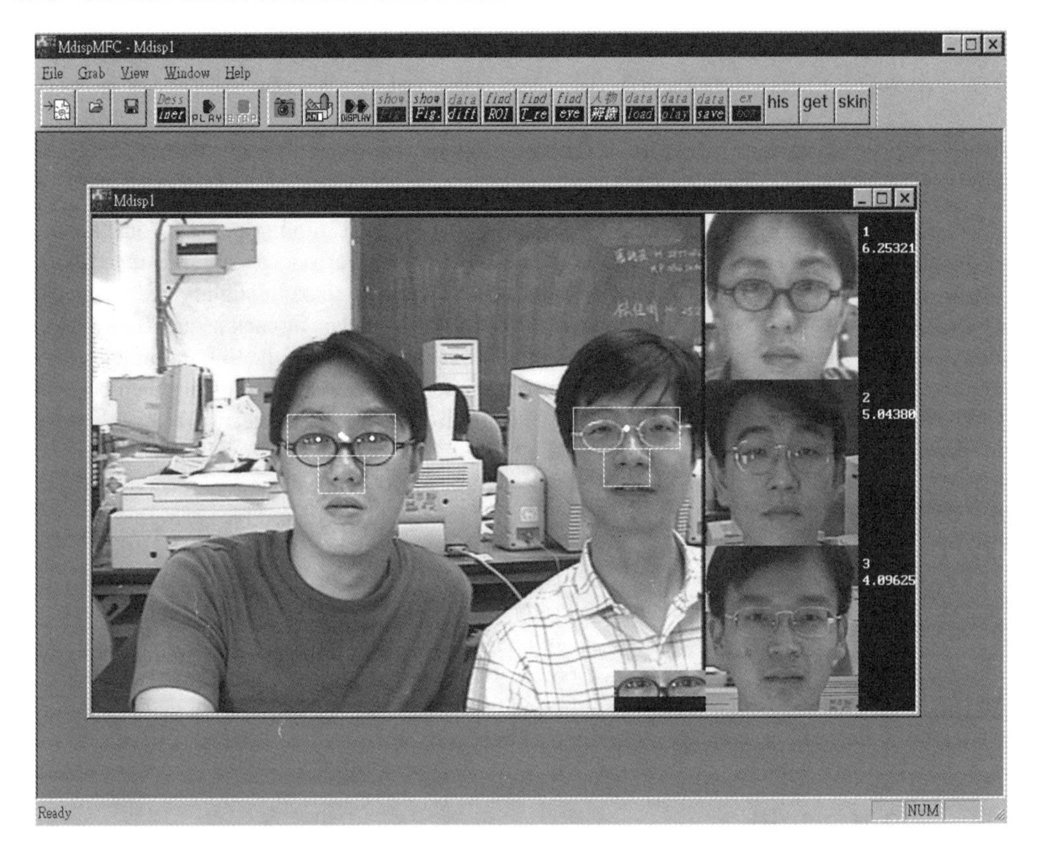

13.18 This figure shows a typical result of the online face detection situation. The T-shape feature region is shown with boxes. Detected positions are marked with white dots. The eye positions are shown as white dots and the refined face position is also shown. The system lists top three candidates in decreasing order of confidence values (shown on the right-hand side). (With permission from J. Taur and C.W. Tao, A new neuro-fuzzy classifier with application to online face detection and recognition, *Journal of VLSI Signal Processing Systems,* vol. 26, no. 3, 2000.)

correct, 5.33% undetected, and 1.33% with wrong positions. The typical detected still face is shown in Figure 13.16.

The trained two-class NEFCAR is applied to the online face detection. A typical result is shown in Figure 13.18. The accuracy of the face position can be further improved by an eye-localization procedure, which is explained next.

13.5.2.3 Face Localization and Recognition

After we find the rough position of the face at lower resolution in the face detection subsystem, we can use two eye-shape masks to find the accurate eye positions at the original resolution. The center point of the eye positions is used as the face position. The face image is rotated to the upright position according to the eye positions, and the size is also normalized so that the distance of the eye positions is 55 pixels. A nonaliasing spatial transform algorithm [16] is used to normalize the detected image. Then the corresponding face feature can be extracted. As shown in Figure 13.18, two faces are detected. We assume that the face closest to the center of the camera will be considered the object to be recognized in an access control application.

A multi-class NEFCAR is trained to classify the located face into one of the people in the database. In order to tolerate the possible inaccuracy from the eye localization, each training image is rotated by (-2, 2) degrees, resized by a factor of (0.95, 1.05), and shifted (up, down, left, right) by two pixels.

Therefore, 45 feature vectors are extracted from each face image. The graphic user interface of the system and the result of performing the recognition task are shown in Figure 13.18.

13.5.2.4 Experiment Results of the Online System

The database for the training and testing of the online face detection and recognition system consists of 25 people. When recording the image sequence, the sampling period of images is set to 0.1 seconds, and ten images are saved for each sequence. For one person, we recorded two sequences, in which the person was asked to nod his/her head or shake it slightly, respectively. A total of 500 images were collected. The first, third, and fifth images of each sequence are used to train a multi-class NEFCAR for face recognition. The face positions in the training images for the face recognition subsystem are selected using the mouse. The feature vectors are then computed from the T-shape regions at these positions. The NEFCAR used for face detection is exactly the one described in Section 13.5.2.2, which is trained using only the database with still images. Note that the people in the database with still images and the people in the online database are totally different. For the 500 images, the error rates of face detection, face localization, and face recognition are 1% (5/500), 0.606% (3/495), and 1.219% (6/492), respectively. (Among the six misclassified images, four images rank second and one image ranks third.) Therefore, the total error rate for the whole system is 2.8%. However, if the whole image sequence is considered the unit of recognition (i.e., we take the majority of classification results in ten images), the error rate becomes 0%. If each image is processed separately, the system takes 1.667 seconds on average to classify a person, including 0.969 seconds, 0.365 seconds, 0.178 seconds, and 0.155 seconds to find the ROI, detect and locate the face, normalize the face, and classify the face, respectively.

13.6 Conclusion

This chapter proposed a family of hierarchical fuzzy neural networks which incorporate an adaptive and modular design of neural networks into the basic fuzzy logic systems. Several important models critical to the development of the hierarchical FNN family were studied. In addition, for robust processing, hierarchical structures involving both expert (rule) modules and class modules are incorporated into the FNNs. Unsupervised (e.g., EM) learning and interclass supervised learning (e.g., decision-based learning) are integrated into the hierarchical FNNs. Theoretically, the hierarchical FNN family adopts a probabilistic soft-decision training strategy and a hierarchical structure which reflects (expressive) knowledge of experts. Practically, the proposed FNN family represents a robust information processing system for classification and data fusion. It can yield performance advantages and can be useful to a broad spectrum of application domains. As demonstrated in the chapter, several exemplifying classification applications have been built upon such a hierarchical model including biometric authentication, medical image processing, video segmentation, object recognition/detection, and multimedia content-based retrieval.

References

[1] S. Abe and R. Thawonmas, A fuzzy classifier with ellipsoidal regions, *IEEE Transactions on Fuzzy System,* vol. 5, no. 3, 358–368, 1997.

[2] M.A. Abidi and R.C. Gonzalez, *Data Fusion in Robotics and Machine Intelligence,* Academic Press, Boston, 1992.

[3] J.S. Bridle, Probabilistic interpretation of feedforward classification network outputs, with relationships to statistical pattern recognition, in F. Fogelman and J. Herault, Editors, *Neuro-Computing: Algorithms, Architectures, and Applications,* Springer-Verlag, London, 1991, pp. 227–236.

[4] R. Brunelli and T. Poggio, Face recognition: features versus templates, *IEEE Transactions on Pattern Analysis and Machine Intelligence,* vol. 15, pp. 1042–1052, 1993.

[5] Y. Chan, S.H. Lin, and S.Y. Kung, Video indexing and retrieval, in B. Sheu and M. Ismail, Editors, *Multimedia Technology for Applications,* IEEE Press, New York, pp. 253–281, 1998.

[6] Y. Chan, S.H. Lin, Y.P. Tan, and S.Y. Kung, Video shot classification using human faces, *Proceedings of the IEEE International Conference on Image Processing,* pp. 843–846, Lausanne, Switzerland, 1996.

[7] I.J. Cox, J. Ghosn, and P. Yianilos, Feature-based face recognition using mixture distance, Tech. Rep. 95-09, Research Institute, 1995.

[8] G. Cybenko, Approximation by of a sigmoidal function, *Mathematics of Control, Signals and Systems,* vol. 2, pp. 303–314, 1998.

[9] Y. Delignon, A. Marzouki, and W. Pieczynski, Estimation of generalized mixtures and its application in image segmentation, *IEEE Transactions on Image Processing,* vol. 6, no. 10, pp. 1364–1375, 1997.

[10] M.M. Dempster, N.M. Laird, and D.B. Rubin, Maximum likelihood from incomplete data via the EM algorithm, *Journal of the Royal Statistical Society,* Series B, vol. 39, pp. 1–38, 1997.

[11] A. Dempster, N. Laird, and D. Rubin, Maximum likelihood from incomplete data via the EM algorithm, *Journal of Royal Statistical Society,* B39, pp. 1–38, 1976.

[12] D. Driankov, H. Hellendoorn, and M. Reinfrank, *An Introduction to Fuzzy Control,* Springer-Verlag, New York, 1993.

[13] R.O. Duda, P.E. Hart, and D.G. Stork, *Pattern Classification,* Gath Wiley Interscience, New York, 2001.

[14] S.H. Lai and M. Fang, Robust and automatic adjustment of display window width and center for MR images, *Proceedings of SPIE Symposium on Medical Imaging: Image Perception,* vol. 3340, pp. 105–116, San Diego, CA, Feb. 1998.

[15] S.H. Lai and M. Fang, A neural network based system for optimal medical image visualization with fast online adaptation capabilities, *Proceedings of the 32nd Annual Conference on Information Sciences and Systems,* pp. 715–720, Princeton, NJ, March 1998.

[16] K.M. Fant, A nonaliasing, real-time spatial transform technique, *IEEE Computer Graphics and Applications,* vol. 6, pp. 71–80, January 1986.

[17] R. Fisher, The use of multiple measurements in taxonomic problems, *Annual Eugenics,* vol. 7 (part II), pp. 179–188, 1936.

[18] K. Funahashi, On the approximate realization of continuous mappings by neural networks, *Neural Networks,* vol. 2, pp. 183–192, 1989.

[19] F. Goudail, E. Lange, T. Iwamoto, K. Kyuma, and N. Otsu, Face recognition system using local autocorrelations and multiscale integration, *IEEE Transactions on Pattern Analysis and Machine Intelligence,* vol. 18, no. 10, 1996.

[20] R.M. Gray, Vector quantization, *IEEE ASSP Magazine,* vol. 1, pp. 4–29, 1984.

[21] R.J. Hathaway, Another interpretation of the EM algorithm for mixture distributions, *Statistics and Probability Letters,* vol. 4, pp. 53–56, 1986.

[22] S. Haykin, *Neural Networks: A Comprehensive Foundation,* Macmillan College Publishing Company, New York, 1994.

[23] J.N. Hwang and E. Lin, Mixture of discriminative learning experts of constant sensitivity for automated cytology screening, *1997 IEEE Workshop on Neural Networks for Signal Processing,* pp. 152–161, Amelia Island, FL, September 1997.

[24] R.A. Jacobs, M.I. Jordan, and A.G. Barto, Task decomposition through competition in a modular connectionist architecture: the what and where vision tasks, *Cognitive Science,* vol. 15, pp. 219–250, 1991.

[25] R.A. Jacobs, M.I. Jordan, S.J. Nowlan, and G.E. Hinton, Adaptive mixtures of local experts, *Neural Computation,* vol. 3, pp. 79–87, 1991.

[26] J.S.R. Jang, C.T. Sun, and E. Mizutani, *Neuro-Fuzzy and Soft Computing,* Prentice-Hall, Englewood Cliffs, NJ, 1997.

[27] M.I. Jordan and R.A. Jacobs, Hierarchies of adaptive experts, in *Advances in Neural Information Systems,* vol. 4, Morgan Kaufmann, San Mateo, CA, 1992, pp. 985–992.

[28] M.I. Jordan and R.A. Jacobs, Hierarchical mixtures of experts and the EM algorithm, *Neural Computation,* vol. 6, pp. 181–214, 1994.

[29] B.H. Juang, S.Y. Kung, and C.A. Kamm, Editors, *Proceedings of the IEEE Workshops on Neural Networks for Signal Processing,* Volumes I to VII, IEEE Press, New York, 1991–1997.

[30] B.H. Juang and S. Katagiri, Discriminative learning for minimum error classification, *IEEE Transactions on Signal Processing,* vol. 40, no. 12, pp. 3043–3054, 1992.

[31] B. Kosko, Fuzzy systems are universal approximators, *Proceedings of the IEEE International Conference on Fuzzy Systems,* pp. 1153–1162, San Diego, March 1992.

[32] S.Y. Kung, *Digital Neural Networks,* Prentice-Hall, Englewood Cliffs, NJ, 1993.

[33] S.Y. Kung and J.S. Taur, Decision-based neural networks with signal/image classification applications, *IEEE Transactions on Neural Networks,* vol. 6, no. 1, pp. 170–181, 1995.

[34] C. Lau, T. Adali, and Y. Wang, Co-registration of PET/MR brain images by multi-feature correlation matching, in *Procedings of the 15th Southern Biomedical Engineering Conference,* Dayton, OH, March 1996, pp. 301–304.

[35] S. Lawrence, C.L. Giles, A.C. Tsoi, and A.D. Back, Face recognition: a convolutional neural network approach, *IEEE Transactions on Neural Networks,* vol. 8, no. 1, pp. 98–113, 1997.

[36] H. Li, Y. Wang, K.J.R. Liu, S.H.B. Lo, and M.T. Freedman, Statistical model supported approach to radiographic mass detection, Part I: improving lesion characterization by morphological filtering and site segmentation, and Part II: decision making through minimax entropy modeling and modular neural networks, *IEEE Transactions on Medical Imaging,* 1999.

[37] C.T. Lin and C.S. Lee, *Neural Fuzzy Systems: A Neuro-Fuzzy Synergism to Intelligent Systems,* Prentice-Hall, Englewood Cliffs, NJ, 1996.

[38] S.H. Lin, Biometric identification for network security and access control, Ph.D. dissertation, Department of Electrical Engineering, Princeton University, Princeton, NJ, 1996.

[39] S.H. Lin, Y. Chan, and S.Y. Kung, A probabilistic decision-based neural network for location deformable objects and its applications to surveillance system and video browsing, in *IEEE International Conference on Acoustics, Speech and Signal Processing,* pp. 3554–3557, Atlanta, GA, 1996.

[40] S.H. Lin, S.Y. Kung, and L.J. Lin, Face recognition/detection by probabilistic decision-based neural networks, *IEEE Transactions on Neural Networks,* special issue on artificial neural network and pattern recognition, vol. 8, no. 1, pp. 114–132, 1997.

[41] Y. Lin, Object oriented scene segmentation from visual motion Ph.D. dissertation, Department of Electrical Engineering, Princeton University, 1998.

[42] Y. Lin, Y.K. Chen, and S.Y. Kung, A principal component clustering approach to object-oriented motion segmentation and estimation, *Journal of VLSI Signal Processing Systems,* vol. 17, pp. 163–188, 1997.

[43] M. MacQueen, Some methods for classification and analysis of multivariate observation, In L.M. LeCun and J. Neyman, Editors, *Proceedings of the 5th Berkeley Symposium on Mathematical Statistics and Probabilities,* vol. 1, University of California Press, Berkeley, 1967, pp. 281–297.

[44] P. Masson and W. Pieczynski, SEM algorithm and unsupervised statistical segmentation of satellite images, *IEEE Transactions on Remote Sensing,* vol. 31, no. 3, pp. 618–633, 1993.

[45] P. McCullagh and J.A. Nelder, *Generalized Linear Models,* 2nd edition, Chapman & Hall, London, UK, 1989.

[46] J. Moody and C. Darken, Fast learning in networks of locally-tuned processing units, *Neural Computing,* vol. 1, pp. 281–294, 1989.

[47] D. Nauck, U. Nauck, and R. Kruse, Generating classification rules with the neuro-fuzzy system NEFCLASS, *Proceedings of the Biennial Conference of the North American Fuzzy Information Processing Society,* Berkeley, CA, 1996.

[48] D. Nauck and F. Klawonn, Neuro-fuzzy classification initialized by fuzzy clustering, *Proceedings of the Fourth European Congress on Intelligent Techniques and Soft Computing,* Aachen, 1996.

[49] S.J. Nowlan, and G.E. Hinton, Evaluation of adaptive mixtures of competing experts, in *Advances in Neural Information Processing Systems,* vol. 3, Morgan Kaufmann, San Mateo, CA, 1991, pp. 774–780.

[50] K. Popat and R.W. Picard, Cluster-based probability model and its applications to image and texture processing, *IEEE Transactions on Image Processing,* vol. 6, pp. 268–284, 1997.

[51] Y. Wang, A. Reibman, F. Juang, T. Chen, and S.Y. Kung, Editors, *Proceedings of the IEEE Workshops on Multimedia Signal Processing,* IEEE Press, Princeton, NJ, 1997.

[52] T. Poggio and F. Girosi, Networks for approximation and learning, *Proceedings of the IEEE,* vol. 78, pp. 1481–1497, 1990.

[53] J.C. Rajapakse, J.N. Giedd, and J.L. Rapoport, Statistical approach to segmentation of single-channel cerebral MR images, *IEEE Transactions on Medical Imaging,* vol. 16, no. 2, p. 176–185, 1997.

[54] D.E. Rumelhart and J.L. McClelland and the PDP Research Group, *Parallel Distributed Processing (PDP): Exploration in the Microstructure of Cognition,* vol. I, MIT Press, Cambridge, MA, 1986.

[55] J.S. Taur and S.Y. Kung, Fuzzy decision neural networks and applications to data fusion, *Proceedings of the IEEE Workshops on Neural Networks for Signal Processing,* vol. III, pp. 171–180, Linthicum Heights, MD, Sept. 1993.

[56] J.S. Taur and C.W. Tao, Texture classification using a fuzzy texture spectrum and neural network, *Journal of Electronic Imaging,* vol. 7, no. 1, pp. 29–35, 1998.

[57] J.S. Taur and C.W. Tao, Face detection using neuro-fuzzy classifiers, in *Proceedings of the International Symposium on Multimedia Information Processing,* Taiwan, December 1998, pp. 309–314.

[58] J.S. Taur and C.W. Tao, An online face detection and recognition system using neuro-fuzzy classifier, in *Proceedings of the International Symposium on Multimedia Information Processing,* December 1999, pp. 297–302.

[59] J.S. Taur and C.W. Tao, A new neuro-fuzzy classifier with application to online face detection and recognition. Accepted for publication in the *Journal of VLSI Signal Processing Systems.*

[60] D. Valentin, H. Abdi, A.J. O'Tool, and G.W. Cottrell, Connectionist models of face processing: a survey, *Pattern Recognition,* vol. 27, pp. 1209–1230, 1994.

[61] L.X. Wang, *Adaptive Fuzzy Systems and Control: Design and Stability Analysis,* Prentice-Hall, Englewood Cliffs, NJ, 1995.

[62] Y. Wang, S.H. Lin, H. Li, S.Y. Kung, Data mapping by probabilistic modular networks and information theoretic criteria, *IEEE Transactions on Signal Processing,* vol. 46, no. 12, pp. 3378–3397, 1998.

[63] Y. Wang, T. Adali, S.Y. Kung, and Z. Szabo, Quantification and segmentation of brain tissue from MR images: a probabilistic neural network approach, *IEEE Transactions on Image Processing,* special issue on applications of neural networks to image processing, vol. 7, no. 8, pp. 1165–1181, 1998.

[64] Y. Wang, T. Adali, C. Lau, and S.Y. Kung, Quantitative analysis of MR brain image sequences by adaptive self-organizing mixtures, *Journal of VLSI Signal Processing Systems,* special issue on neural networks for biomedical image processing, vol. 18, no. 3, pp. 219–2490, 1998.

[65] S.R. Waterhouse, D. MacKay, and A.J. Robinson, Bayesian methods for mixtures of experts, *Advances in Neural Information Processing,* vol. 8, pp. 351–357, Nov. 1995.

[66] M.M. Yeung, B.L. Yeo, W. Wolf, and B. Liu, Video browsing using clustering and scene transitions on compressed sequences, in *Proceedings, SPIE, Multimedia Computing and Networking,* vol. 2417, pp. 399–413, Feb. 1995.

[67] A.L. Yuille, P. Stolorz, and J. Utans, Statistical physics, mixtures of distributions, and the EM algorithm, *Neural Computation,* vol. 6, pp. 334–340, 1994.

Index

A

B

E

F

G

H

I

N

O

S

T

U

V

W

Z